Atlas of Procedures in Neonatology

Fifth Edition

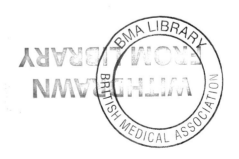

Atlas of Procedures in Neonatology

Fifth Edition

Senior Editor

Mhairi G. MacDonald, MBChB, DCH, FAAP, FRCPE, FRCPCH

Professor of Pediatrics
George Washington University
School of Medicine and Health Sciences
Washington, DC

Co-Editor

Jayashree Ramasethu, MBBS, DCH, MD, FAAP

Associate Professor of Clinical Pediatrics
Georgetown University Medical Center
Program Director, Neonatal Perinatal Medicine Fellowship Program
Division of Neonatal Perinatal Medicine
MedStar Georgetown University Hospital
Washington, DC

Associate Editor

Khodayar Rais-Bahrami, MD, FAAP

Professor of Pediatrics
George Washington University
School of Medicine and Health Sciences
Program Director, Neonatal-Perinatal Fellowship Program
Division of Neonatal-Perinatal Medicine
Children's National Medical Center
Washington, DC

With 59 Contributors

Illustrators
Judy Guenther
Virginia Schnoonover
Jennifer Smith

 Wolters Kluwer | Lippincott Williams & Wilkins
Health

Philadelphia · Baltimore · New York · London
Buenos Aires · Hong Kong · Sydney · Tokyo

Acquisitions Editor: Rebecca Gaertner
Product Manager: Nicole Walz
Vendor Manager: Bridgett Dougherty
Senior Manufacturing Manager: Benjamin Rivera
Marketing Manager: Kimberly Schonberger
Design Coordinator: Terry Mallon
Production Service: Aptara, Inc.

Printed in China

Library of Congress Cataloging-in-Publication Data

Atlas of procedures in neonatology / senior editor, Mhairi G. MacDonald;
co-editors, Jayashree Ramasethu, Khodayar Rais-Bahrami. – 5th ed.
  p. ; cm.
  Procedures in neonatology
  Includes bibliographical references and index.
  ISBN 978-1-4511-4410-9 (hardback : alk. paper)
  I. MacDonald, Mhairi G. II. Ramasethu, Jayashree. III. Rais-Bahrami,
Khodayar. IV. Title: Procedures in neonatology.
  [DNLM: 1. Infant, Newborn, Diseases–therapy–Atlases. 2. Infant,
Newborn, Diseases–therapy–Outlines. 3. Intensive Care,
Neonatal–Atlases. 4. Intensive Care, Neonatal–Outlines.
  5. Neonatology–methods–Atlases. 6. Neonatology–methods–Outlines.
WS 17]
  618.92′0028–dc23
                                              2012016637

Care has been taken to confirm the accuracy of the information presented and to describe generally accepted practices. However, the authors, editors, and publisher are not responsible for errors or omissions or for any consequences from application of the information in this book and make no warranty, expressed or implied, with respect to the currency, completeness, or accuracy of the contents of the publication. Application of the information in a particular situation remains the professional responsibility of the practitioner.

The authors, editors, and publisher have exerted every effort to ensure that drug selection and dosage set forth in this text are in accordance with current recommendations and practice at the time of publication. However, in view of ongoing research, changes in government regulations, and the constant flow of information relating to drug therapy and drug reactions, the reader is urged to check the package insert for each drug for any change in indications and dosage and for added warnings and precautions. This is particularly important when the recommended agent is a new or infrequently employed drug.

Some drugs and medical devices presented in the publication have Food and Drug Administration (FDA) clearance for limited use in restricted research settings. It is the responsibility of the health care provider to ascertain the FDA status of each drug or device planned for use in their clinical practice.

To purchase additional copies of this book, call our customer service department at (800) 638-3030 or fax orders to (301) 223-2320. International customers should call (301) 223-2300.

Visit Lippincott Williams & Wilkins on the Internet: at LWW.com. Lippincott Williams & Wilkins customer service representatives are available from 8:30 am to 6 pm, EST.

10 9 8 7 6 5 4 3 2 1

"This book is dedicated to multidisciplinary health care teams worldwide, and their trainees, who strive every day to provide exemplary evidence-based intensive care to sick neonates."

Contributors

M. Kabir Abubakar, MD, FAAP
Associate Professor of Clinical Pediatrics
Director, Neonatal ECMO Program
Division of Neonatal–Perinatal Medicine
MedStar Georgetown University Hospital
Washington, DC

Hany Aly, MD
Professor
Departments of Pediatrics and Obstetrics & Gynecology
The George Washington University School of Medicine and the
    Health Sciences
Director
Division of Newborn Services
The George Washington University Hospital
Washington, DC

Jacob V. Aranda, MD, PhD
Professor and Vice Chair for Research
Division Director
Department of General Pediatrics
Division of Neonatal–Perinatal Medicine
The Children's Hospital at SUNY Downstate Medical Center
Brooklyn, New York

Monisha Bahri, MD, MBBS, FAAP
Attending Physician
Department of Neonatology/Pediatrics
Washington Hospital Center
Washington, DC

Aimee M. Barton, MD, FAAP
Assistant Professor
Division of Neonatal–Perinatal Medicine
MedStar Georgetown University Hospital
Washington, DC

Alan Benheim, MD, FACC, FAAP
Pediatric Cardiology Associates, P.C.
Fairfax, Virginia
Clinical Assistant Professor
Department of Pediatrics-Pediatric Cardiology
University of Virginia School of Health Sciences
Charlottesville, Virginia

Vadim Bronshtein, MD
Department of Neonatal–Perinatal Medicine
Children's Hospital at Downstate
SUNY Downstate Medical Center NEO
Brooklyn, New York

A. Alfred Chahine, MD, FACS, FAAP
Chief of Pediatric Surgery
MedStar Georgetown University Hospital
Attending Pediatric Surgeon
Children's National Medical Center
Associate Professor of Surgery and Pediatrics
The George Washington University School of Medicine and the
    Health Sciences
Washington, DC

Ela Chakkarapani, MBBS, MRCPCH
Senior Registrar and Research Fellow
Department of Neonatology
University of Bristol
St. Michael's Hospital
Bristol, United Kingdom

Kimberly M. Chan, MD
Department of Internal Medicine
Axminster Medical Group
Los Angeles, California

Robert D. Christensen, MD
Director, Neonatology Research
Intermountain Healthcare
Salt Lake City, Utah

Yu-Chen Jennie Chung, MD
Neonatal–Perinatal Medicine Fellow
Division of Neonatal–Perinatal Medicine
Georgetown University Hospital
Washington, DC

Linda C. D'Angelo, RN, BSN, CWOCN
Wound, Ostomy and Continence Nurse
Shady Grove Adventist Hospital
Rockville, Maryland

Manju Dawkins, MD
Attending Physician
Department of Dermatology
Bronx Lebanon Hospital Center
Bronx, New York

William F. Deegan, III, MD
The Retina Group of Washington
Chevy Chase, Maryland, and Alexandria and Fairfax,
    Virginia

Jennifer A. Dunbar, MD
Ophthalmology/Pediatric Ophthalmology
Loma Linda University Medical Center
San Bernardino, California

Ross M. Fasano, MD
Director, Chronic Transfusion Program
Division of Hematology, Transfusion Medicine
Children's National Medical Center
Assistant Professor of Pediatrics
The George Washington University School of Medicine and the
    Health Sciences
Washington, DC

LCDR Rebecca J. Fay, MD
Attending Neonatologist
Department of Pediatrics, Division of Neonatology
Naval Medical Center Portsmouth
Portsmouth, Virginia
Assistant Professor of Pediatrics
Uniformed Services University of Health Sciences
Bethesda, Maryland

Laura A. Folk, RNC-NIC, BSN, MEd
Staff Nurse
Neonatal Intensive Care Unit
MedStar Georgetown University Hospital
Washington, DC

Rebecca M. Ginzburg, JD
Associate General Counsel of Boston University
Lecturer in Law
Boston University School of Law
Boston, Massachusetts

Dorothy Goodman, BSN, RN, CWOCN
Wound Ostomy Continence Nurse
MedStar Georgetown University Hospital
Washington, DC

Allison M. Greenleaf, RN, MSN, CPNP
Pediatric Nurse Practitioner
Department of Pediatrics
Division of Neonatal–Perinatal Medicine
MedStar Georgetown University Hospital
Washington, DC

Ashish O. Gupta, MD
Neonatal–Perinatal Medicine Fellow
Division of Neonatal–Perinatal Medicine
MedStar Georgetown University Hospital
Washington, DC

Gary Hartman, MD
Clinical Professor of Surgery
Chief, Division of Pediatric Surgery
Stanford University School of Medicine
Stanford, California
Associate Vice President of Medical Affairs
Lucile Packard Children's Hospital
Palo Alto, California

Hosai Hesham, MD
Department of Otolaryngology
Georgetown University Hospital
Washington, DC

Chahira Kozma, MD
Professor of Pediatrics
Chief, Division of Genetics
MedStar Georgetown University Hospital
Washington, DC

Margaret Mary Kuczkowski, MSN, CPNP
Neonatal Intensive Care Unit
MedStar Georgetown University Hospital
Washington, DC

Victoria Tutag Lehr, BSPharm, PharmD
Associate Professor
Department of Pharmacy Practice
EACPHS Wayne State University
Clinical Pharmacy Specialist Pain Management
Children's Hospital of Michigan
Detroit, Michigan

Mirjana Lulic-Botica, BSc, RPh, BCPS
Neonatal Clinical Pharmacy Specialist
Hutzel Women's Hospital
Detroit Medical Center
Detroit, Michigan

Secelela Malecela, MD
Assistant Professor of Pediatrics
Division of Neonatal–Perinatal Medicine
MedStar Georgetown University Hospital
Washington, DC

Kathleen A. Marinelli, MD, IBCLC, FABM, FAAP
Associate Professor of Pediatrics
University of Connecticut School of Medicine
Farmington, Connecticut
Attending Neonatologist and Lactation Specialist
Connecticut Children's Medical Center
Hartford, Connecticut

An N. Massaro, MD
Assistant Professor of Pediatrics
The George Washington University School of Medicine and the
    Health Sciences
Co-Director of Research, Division of Neonatology
Children's National Medical Center
Washington, DC

Gregory J. Milmoe, MD
Associate Professor of Otolaryngology-Head & Neck Surgery
Georgetown University School of Medicine
Washington, DC

M. A. Mohamed, MD, MPH
Associate Professor of Pediatrics and Global Health
The George Washington University School of Medicine and
    Health Sciences
Washington, DC

Susan H. Morgan, MEd, CCC-A
Director of Audiology
Department of Otolaryngology Head & Neck Surgery
MedStar Georgetown University Hospital
Washington, DC

Sepideh Nassabeh-Montazami, MD, FAAP
Assistant Professor of Pediatrics
Division of Neonatal Perinatal Medicine
MedStar Georgetown University Hospital
Washington, DC

Nickie Niforatos, MD
Fellow, Fetal and Transitional Medicine
Department of Neonatology
Children's National Medical Center
Washington, DC

John North, MD
Perinatal Medicine & Neonatal Medicine and Pediatrics
Fairfax Neonatal Associates
Falls Church, Virginia

Wendy M. Paul, MD
Assistant Professor, Department of Pathology
George Washington University School of Medicine and the
    Health Sciences
Director, Point of Care Testing and Satellite Testing
Associate Director, Transfusion Medicine
Children's National Medical Center
Washington, DC

Majid Rasoulpour, MD
Professor Emeritus
Department of Pediatrics
University of Connecticut School of Medicine
Farmington, Connecticut
Pediatric Nephrologist
Connecticut Children's Medical Center
Hartford, Connecticut

Mary E. Revenis, MD
Assistant Professor of Pediatrics
Children's National Medical Center
George Washington University School of Medicine and the
    Health Sciences
Washington, DC

Lisa M. Rimsza, MD
Professor and Associate Chair of Research
Department of Pathology
University of Arizona
Tucson, Arizona

Dora C. Rioja-Mazza, MD, FAAP
Attending Neonatologist
Department of Pediatrics
Division of Neonatology
Reston Hospital Center
Reston, Virginia

Priyanshi Ritwik, BDS, MS
Associate Professor
Postgraduate Program Director
Department of Pediatric Dentistry
LSU School of Dentistry
Director, Special Children's Dental Clinic
Children's Hospital, New Orleans
New Orleans, Louisiana

Anne S. Roberts, MD
Surgery Resident
MedStar Georgetown University Hospital
Washington, DC

Jeanne M. Rorke, RNC, NNP, MSN
Neonatal Nurse Specialist
Neonatal Intensive Care Unit
MedStar Georgetown University Hospital
Washington, DC

Mariam M. Said, MD
Assistant Professor of Pediatrics
Department of Pediatrics
The George Washington University School of Medicine and
    Health Sciences
Attending Neonatologist
Department of Neonatology
Children's National Medical Center
Washington, DC

Thomas Sato, MD
Professor of Surgery
Division of Pediatric Surgery
Children's Hospital of Wisconsin
Medical College of Wisconsin
Milwaukee, Wisconsin

Melissa Scala, MD
Neonatal–Perinatal Medicine Fellow
Division of Neonatal Perinatal Medicine
MedStar Georgetown University Hospital
Washington, DC

Suna Seo, MD
Neonatal–Perinatal Medicine Fellow
Division of Neonatal–Perinatal Medicine
MedStar Georgetown University Hospital
Washington, DC

Billie Lou Short, MD
Professor of Pediatrics
The George Washington University School of Medicine and the
    Health Sciences
Chief, Division of Neonatology
Children's National Medical Center
Washington, DC

Lamia Soghier, MD, FAAP
Assistant Professor of Pediatrics
The George Washington University School of Medicine and the
    Health Sciences
Attending Physician
Division of Neonatology
Department of Pediatrics
Children's National Medical Center
Washington, DC

Martha C. Sola-Visner, MD
Assistant Professor of Pediatrics
Children's Hospital Boston
Harvard Medical School
Boston, Massachusetts

Ganesh Srinivasan, MD, DM, FAAP
Assistant Professor Pediatrics and Child Health (Neonatology)
Director, Neonatal–Perinatal Fellowship Program
University of Manitoba
Researcher
Manitoba Institute of Child Health
Winnipeg, Manitoba, Canada

Keith Thatch, MD
Pediatric Surgery Intensivist
Clinical Lecturer
University of Michigan Health System
Ann Arbor, Michigan

Marianne Thoresen, MD, PhD
Professor of Neonatal Neuroscience
School of Clinical Sciences
University of Bristol
Bristol, United Kingdom
Professor of Physiology
Institute of Basic Medical Sciences
University of Oslo
Oslo, Norway

Gloria B. Valencia, MD
Division Chief NICU Director
Department of Pediatrics
Neonatology and Perinatal Medicine
SUNY Downstate Medical Center
Brooklyn, New York

S. Lee Woods, MD, PhD
Medical Director
Center for Maternal and Child Health
Maryland State Department of Health and Mental Hygiene
Baltimore, Maryland

Preface

"Neonatology is a taxing field: strenuous, demanding, confusing, heartbreaking, rewarding, stimulating, scientific, personal, philosophical, cooperative, logical, illogical, and always changing." From the preface to the first edition of the *Atlas of Procedures in Neonatology, 1983.*

The preface to the first edition of the *Atlas of Procedures in Neonatology* was written approximately 8 years after the first sub-board examination in Neonatal-Perinatal Medicine was held in the United States. In the preface, emphasis was placed upon the rapid development of new technology and the decreasing size (<1.5 k) and maturity (<32 weeks' gestation) of the patients in the neonatal intensive care unit.

Thirty years later, patient size (≈400 g) and maturity (≈22 to 23 weeks' gestation) are at a nadir, having reached the current limits of newborn viability. Thus, over the years, our patients have become increasingly fragile and challenged to withstand the stress of living with extremely immature organs plus the additional stress and trauma associated with the very therapy required to keep them alive. New therapies and technologies continue to develop (e.g., Brain and Whole Body Cooling, new Chapter 45), "old" therapies have been re-established for use in very premature infants (e.g., Bubble Nasal Continuous Positive Airway Pressure, new Chapter 35).

Since the landmark report of the Institute of Medicine, "To Err is Human," was published in 1999, the paradigm of medical care has been focused on patient safety, and nowhere is it more important than in the neonatal intensive care unit. Errors in this vulnerable patient population can have devastating, damaging, and serious immediate and long-term consequences. Teamwork and the use of evidence-based guidelines have had a significant impact on some complications of intensive care, such as catheter-related bloodstream infections, which were previously thought to be inevitable. However, we noted as we prepared this edition, some previously unreported complications of long-established procedures, and numerous isolated case reports of "unusual complications," making them not uncommon at all. Such reports serve to emphasize that the neonatologist must remain vigilant, and not only continuously monitor the impact of the technologic and other advances specific to their own field, but also the impact of advances in the other specialties that contribute to neonatal intensive care.

In this edition, we have replaced the procedures DVD with a Website. Contents include fully searchable text, an image bank, and videos. To the video collection, we have added lumbar puncture, radial artery puncture, intraosseous infusion, bubble CPAP, and pericardiocentesis, continuing the tradition established with the fourth edition to include both commonly performed procedures and vital emergency procedures that trainees may have infrequent opportunity to perform.

In the 1980s, procedures performed on neonates were practiced on animals and homemade simulators. In 2012, simulators include sophisticated, interactive model humans, capable of testing not only practical skills but also the reasoning process involved in making good therapeutic decisions (see Educational Principles of Simulation-Based Procedural Training, new Chapter 1). No simulation equipment can currently replicate the fragility of the extremely preterm infant, but this will undoubtedly change over the next few years. We recognize that, in order to decrease risk and improve patient safety, the crucial element in simulated training is not so much the expensive and technologically advanced model as the opportunity to practice critical skills repeatedly in a safe environment, with precise measurements of performance and constructive feedback.

The above quote from the first edition of the *Atlas of Procedures in Neonatology* remains as pertinent today, for the fifth edition, as it was 30 years ago.

Mhairi G. MacDonald, MBChB,
DCH, FAAP, FRCPE, FRCPCH

Jayashree Ramasethu, MBBS, DCH, MD, FAAP

Khodayar Rais-Bahrami, MD, FAAP

The rapid advances in neonatology in the last 15 years have brought with them a welter of special procedures. The tiny, premature, and the critically ill term neonate is attached to a tangle of intravenous lines, tubes, and monitoring leads. As a result, more and more procedures are done at the bedside in the intensive-care nursery, rather than in a procedure room or operating room. With these technical advances has come the opportunity for more vigorous physiologic support and monitoring. With them also has come a whole new gamut of side-effects and complications. The old dictum to leave the fragile premature undisturbed is largely ignored. It is therefore the responsibility of those who care for sick newborns to understand the complications as well as the benefits of new procedures and to make systematic observations of their impact on both morbidity and mortality. Unfortunately, the literature on outcome and complications of procedures is widely scattered and difficult to access. Manuals that give directions for neonatal procedures are generally deficient in illustrations giving anatomic detail and are often cursory.

We are offering *Atlas of Procedures in Neonatology* to meet some of these needs. A step-by-step, practical approach is taken, with telegraphic prose and outline form. Drawings and photographs are used to illustrate anatomic landmarks and details of the procedures. In several instances, more than one alternative procedure is presented. Discussion of controversial points is included, and copious literature citations are provided to lead the interested reader to source material. A uniform order of presentation has been adhered to wherever appropriate. Thus, most chapters include indications, contraindications, precautions, equipment, technique, and complications, in that order.

The scope of procedures covered includes nearly all those that can be performed at the bedside in an intensive-care nursery. Some are within the traditional province of the neonatologist or even the pediatric house officer. Others, such as gastrostomy and tracheostomy, require skills of a qualified surgeon. Responsibility for procedures such as placement of chest tubes and performance of vascular cutdowns will vary from nursery to nursery. However, some details of surgical technique are supplied for even the most invasive procedures to promote their understanding by those who are responsible for sick neonates. We hope this will help neonatologists to be more knowledgeable partners in caring for babies and will not be interpreted as a license to perform procedures by those who are not adequately qualified.

The book is organized into major parts (e.g., "Vascular Access," "Tube Placement," "Respiratory Care"), each of which contains several chapters. Most chapters are relatively self-contained and can be referred to when approaching a particular task. However, Part I, "Preparation and Support," is basic to all procedures. Occasional cross referencing has been used to avoid repetitions of the same text material. References appear at the end of each part.

Many persons have contributed to the preparation of this atlas, and we are grateful to them all. Some are listed under Acknowledgments, and others have contributed anonymously out of their generosity and good will. Special thanks is due to Bill Burgower, who first thought of making such an atlas and who has been gracious in his support throughout this project.

If this atlas proves useful to some who care for sick newborns, our efforts will have been well repaid. Neonatology is a taxing field: strenuous, demanding, confusing, heartbreaking, rewarding, stimulating, scientific, personal, philosophical, cooperative, logical, illogical, and always changing. The procedures described in this atlas will eventually be replaced by others, hopefully more effective and less noxious. In the meantime, perhaps the care of some babies will be assisted.

Mary Ann Fletcher, MD

Mhairi G. MacDonald, MBChB,
FRCP(E), DCH

Gordon B. Avery, MD, PhD

Contents

Section VI   Respiratory Care

Section VII   Tube Replacement

Section VIII   Transfusions

Section IX   Miscellaneous Procedures

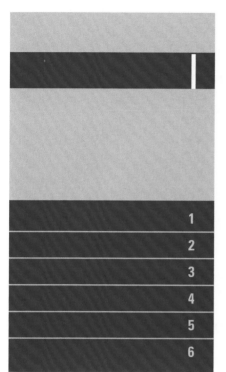

Preparation and Support

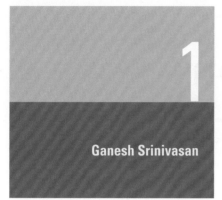

1

Educational Principles of Simulation-Based Procedural Training

Ganesh Srinivasan

The Need

The traditional see one, do one, teach one, *and hope not to harm one* apprentice model of graduated responsibility in the care of real patients and for acquisition of clinical, procedural, and leadership skills has been termed "education by random opportunity." The rationalization of work hours during residency and fellowship training, the increasing breadth of technical skills required in neonatology, and the limited opportunity to acquire competence in the context of safety and time provide us with both a challenge and an opportunity to revisit traditional training and embrace innovative learning strategies. The educational strategies best suited to address acquisition of procedural skills include supervised clinical experiences, simulated experiences, and audiovisual review. Simulation enables repeated procedural exposure in a safe environment without compromising patient safety, that is, see a lot, simulate and train a lot, teach and assist a lot, *and harm none* (1–10). Although animal and other models have been used to teach and practice procedures used in neonates for the past 4 decades (Fig. 1.1A–E and Table 1.1) (11), the role of simulation-based training has made a paradigm shift in the past 15 years to an educational experience that helps address the need for integrated acquisition of technical skills, behavioral skills (including ability to work as part of a team), and cognitive skills—factors where deficits identified and not corrected may lead to adverse outcomes. For example, the Neonatal Resuscitation Program™ has embraced simulation-based resuscitation training methodology to teach and evaluate competence in neonatal resuscitation (12). This chapter serves as a general overview of the current underlying educational principles of simulation-based training in neonatology (13–18).

Definition

Modern-day simulation is an immersive instructional strategy that is used to replace or amplify real experiences with guided experiences that evoke or replicate substantial aspects of the real world in a fully interactive manner.

The Theory of Simulation-Based Learning

Bloom's Taxonomy

According to Bloom's taxonomy of learning (Fig. 1.2), knowledge and comprehension are the simplest levels of learning. Simulation, when used with the goal of improving practice, can allow the learner to move from knowledge or comprehension to application, analysis, and synthesis, which are better indicators of competence.

Adult Learners

1. Are self-directed and self-regulated in their learning
2. Are predominantly intrinsically motivated to learn
3. Have previous knowledge and experience that are an increasing resource for learning
4. Through this previous experience, they form mental models that guide their behavior
5. Use analogical reasoning in learning and practice

The process of having an experience (concrete experience), reflecting on the experience (reflective observation), developing mental models (abstract conceptualization), and testing that mental model (active experimentation) is based on Kolb's experiential learning cycle (Fig. 1.3).

Kolb's Experiential Learning Cycle

1. **Concrete experience (feeling):** Simulations provide concrete experiences that stress the learner, causing a significant change of body state to foster meaningful reflection of learner identified knowledge gaps.
2. **Reflective observation (watching):** Debriefing provides the opportunity for learners to reflect on the simulation and their performance. The learner observes before making a judgement and seeks optimal comprehension by viewing the experience from different

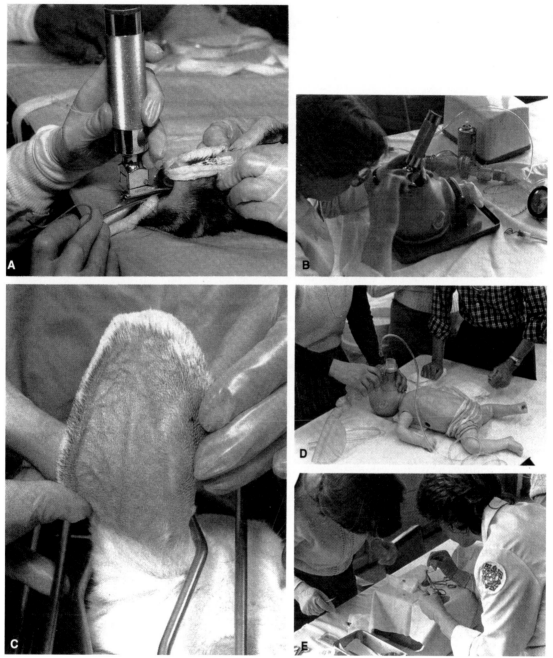

FIG. 1.1. Teaching models (**A**) A ferret is used to demonstrate endotracheal intubation. (**B**) An infant intubation model (Resusci Intubation Model, Laerdal Medical, Armonk, NY) is used to practice endotracheal intubation. A viewing port in the back of the head allows demonstration of anatomic relationships. (**C**) A rabbit's ear has been shaved to demonstrate vessels for intravenous placement. (**D**) A resuscitation model (Resusci Baby, Laerdal Medical) is used to practice bag and mask ventilation. (**E**) An umbilical cord is used to practice catheter insertion. The cord is placed in an infant feeding bottle, filled with normal saline, and supported inside a cardboard box. The end of the cord projects through a cut nipple. (From *Neonatology: Pathophysiology and Management of the Newborn, 4th ed.* Philadelphia: JB Lippincott;1994, p. 37.)

perspectives. The educators can facilitate the process by providing an objective view of the learner's performance.

3. **Abstract conceptualization (thinking):** Is the logical analysis of ideas and acting on intellectual understanding of a situation by the learner, and helps pro-

vide the educator with the opportunity to clarify the same. This results in a new mental model and understanding.

4. **Active experimentation (doing):** This new mental model and understanding, developed by the learner, requires immediate testing by active experimentation,

TABLE 1.1   Teaching Models Used to Teach Procedures

Manikin (Small Dolls with Soft Vinyl Skin)
To teach tracheotomy care:
  Create a hole in the doll's neck with a sharp instrument—a corkscrew works well.
  Insert a size 1 or size 0 tracheotomy tube.
  Tie the ties, and use as a model to teach proper suctioning and skin care techniques.
To teach umbilical catheter managements:
  Puncture the doll's anterior abdomen using a 16-gauge Medicut needle.
  Insert needle through the doll's front and back, then remove.
  Thread an umbilical catheter through from front to back.
  Insert blunt needles onto catheter at both ends. An IV bag containing water tinted with red food coloring can be attached to the posterior end of the catheter
    to simulate blood.
To teach technique for drawing samples for blood gases:
  Insert a three-way stopcock into the umbilical catheter anteriorly and attach IV bag and tubing.
This system also can be used to teach arterial and venous blood pressure monitoring by transducer.
  To simulate arterial pressure, wrap a blood pressure cuff around the partially filled IV bag and inflate to 60–70 torr.
  For a venous line, inflate to 5–10 torr.

Resusci Head[a]
The model head used for endotracheal intubation can be modified to teach orogastric and nasogastric feeding by attaching a reservoir to the esophageal opening.

Rabbits
To teach placement of chest tube:
  Anesthetize a rabbit weighing approximately 2 kg using xylazine, 8.8 mg/kg IM. Wait 10 min, then administer ketamine HCI, 50 mg/kg IM.
  Place the rabbit on its back and shave or clip the chest hair as closely as possible. Use a commercial depilatory to remove remaining hair.
  Restrain the rabbit's fore- and hindpaws securely.
  Surgically drape the rabbit.
  Place electrodes on the chest wall for attachment to a cardiorespiratory monitor. Changes in ECG tracing due to the pneumothorax can then be
    demonstrated.
  Insert chest tube.

Weanling Kittens
To teach endotracheal intubation:
  Use kittens weighing 1–1.5 kg.
  Withhold food 8 h before intubation; however, allow water intake.
  Give ketamine HCI 20 mg/kg IM.
  Wait 10 min for full effect of ketamine HCI.
Examine larynx after every four or five attempts at intubation. If the laryngeal area is traumatized, allow 7–10 d for recovery.

Ferrets
To teach endotracheal intubation
  Withhold food 8 h before intubation; however, allow water intake.
  Give ketamine HCI, 5 mg/kg IM, and acepromazine maleate, 0.55 mg/kg IM, and allow to take effect.
  Maintain anesthesia with 40% of original dose IM as needed. If necessary, control sneezing with 0.5 mg/kg IM of diphenhydramine.
  Apply bland ophthalmic ointment to eyes to prevent desication.
Examine larynx for signs of trauma, as for kittens, and allow recovery between training sessions. Evidence of trauma was noted in 100% of ferrets after 10 intubations.

Placenta and Cord
To teach insertion of IV infusion lines and umbilical vessel catheters:[b]
  Preserve placenta and cord by freezing in *individual* containers.
  Allow 3–4 h for thawing before use.
  Use vessels on the fetal surface of the placenta to demonstrate insertion of peripheral IV needles and cannulae. Blood drawing also can be demonstrated.
  Cut a 15-cm length of cord to demonstrate the anatomy of the umbilical stump and the technique for arterial and venous catheterization. The cord may be
    placed in an infant's feeding bottle that contains saline. One end of the cord then protrudes through a suitably cut nipple and can be pulled out of the bot-
    tle for each attempt at the procedure.

[a]Laerdal Medical, Armonk, NY.
[b]Use of this model is not recommended unless HIV and hepatitis B virus status of source is known.
From: Avery GB, *Neonatology: Pathophysiology and Management of the Newborn*, 4th ed. Philadelphia: JB Lippincott; 1994.

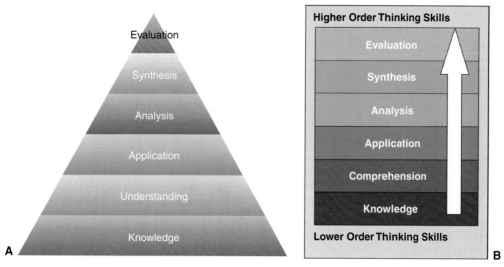

FIG. 1.2. **A:** From Doug Devitre. http://retechtraining.wordpress.com/2008/07/16/how-adults-learn-to-use-technology-effectively/(with permission). **B:** From Andrew Churches http://edorigami.wikispaces.com/Bloom%27s+-+Introduction (with permission)

in order to imprint new knowledge and effect long-term changes in practice.

Depending on the situation or environment, the learner may enter the learning style at any point and will best learn the new task if they practice all four modes in Kolb's cycle.

For example, *learning to place a radial arterial line:*

Reflective observation: Thinking about placing a radial line and watching another person place a line

Abstract conceptualization: Understanding the theory, indications and contraindications, hand

washing and safety, and having a clear grasp of the concept

Concrete experience: Receiving practical tips and techniques from an expert

Active experience: Getting the opportunity and attempting to place a line under supervision

Procedural Skill Learning

Procedural skill learning occurs in three phases

Cognitive phase: In the cognitive phase, the learner must learn why the procedure might be necessary, recognize

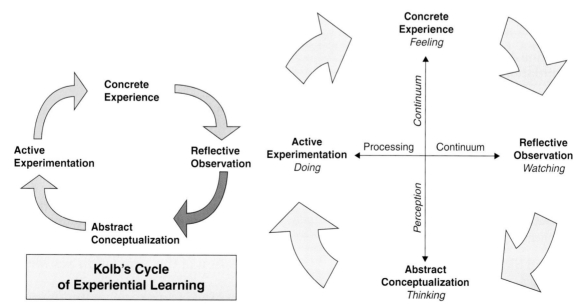

FIG. 1.3. **Kolb's experiential cycle** forms the basis for adult simulation-based education. (Image by Karin Kirk from http://serc.carleton.edu/introgeo/enviroprojects/what.html with permission [Left] and Clark DR [Right] from ref 17, with permission.)

the indications and the contraindications for the procedure, and gain a general understanding of what is involved in the procedure. The learner's attention is focused by providing orientation and instructions for performance and establishing specific goals for "prepractice" activities. Modeling during prepractice, through demonstration or video, is effective for teaching movement strategies, spatial information, and sequential and spatial skills for dynamic tasks, including surgical skills.

Development phase: The goal in the development phase is to achieve mastery of the skill by repeated purposeful practice and feedback. Mastery learning and deliberate practice involves the learner performing the skill until it is performed without error, taking as much time as necessary to ensure that the skill is performed correctly. The approach using distributed practice (i.e., several short sessions of practice rather than one long session) has also been shown to be effective in procedural skill acquisition and retention.

Automated phase: The automated phase involves perfecting the skill by improving the ability to distinguish essential from nonessential stimuli and continuing to practice the skill after competency is achieved. This results in a decreasing need for thought processing as the skill develops.

Simulation-Based Training

Simulation-based training is pertinent to and can be incorporated into all aspects of procedural skills training.

The key components of simulation-based training include:

A. Identifying and Elucidating the Learning Objectives Specifically Amenable to Simulation

Clarity of planned learning objectives is integral to planning a useful simulation

B. Prepractice Activities in Preparation for Simulation

1. Didactic training sessions
2. Prereading material
3. Audiovisual aids such as training videos

C. Choosing the Optimal Simulator (Tables 1.1–1.4)

1. High-fidelity simulators
2. Low-fidelity simulators
3. Procedural trainers
4. Miscellaneous special training simulators

D. A Defined Simulation Environment

1. At a clinical learning and simulation facility
2. At the hospital or patient care facility
3. Adjacent to site where patient care is to be provided, and just before performing the procedure on the patient ("just-in-place and just-in-time training")

4. Telesimulation using appropriate audiovisual telecommunication equipment for outreach training

E. Prescenario Briefing

1. Ensure confidentiality and respectfulness.
2. Acquaint participants with the capabilities of the simulator.
3. Clarify simulator strengths and weaknesses.
4. Enter into the "fiction contract": The learner agrees to suspend judgement of realism for any given simulation, in exchange for the promise of learning new knowledge and skills. (This helps to keep the focus on the learning objectives.)
5. Discuss the root of the scenarios.

F. Running the Appropriately Realistic, Challenging, and Well-designed Scenario

1. Rehearse in advance
2. Thoughtful use of actor confederates and props to simulate realism
3. Choose the appropriate start, optimal duration, and finish
4. Achieve an optimal alert and activated state in the participants

G. Recording and Identifying the Knowledge and Performance Gaps of the Participants During the Scenario

1. Focused observation and recording
2. Use of checklists
3. Use of video

H. Postscenario Debriefing

Postscenario debriefing is the heart of the simulation:

1. Debriefing may focus on actions or both frames (internal images of reality) and actions and help trainees make sense of, learn from, and apply simulation experience to change frames of thought and resulting actions. The goal is to provide objective evaluative feedback.
2. The good judgement approach to debriefing, as advocated by the Institute of Medical Simulation at Harvard, consists of four phases
   a. **Preview phase:** Helps focus the debriefing content
   b. **Reactions phase:** Clears the air and sets the stage for discussion of feelings and facts
   c. **Understanding phase:** Promotes understanding of learner's performance, and explores the basis for learner's actions, using advocacy and enquiry
   d. **Summary phase:** Distills lessons learned for future use; what worked well, what should be changed

I. Evaluation of the Simulation Session

Acknowledgements to:

Dr. Mhairi Macdonald
Dr. Jenny Rudolph

TABLE 1.2	Commercially Available Low-Fidelity Manikin-Based Task Training Simulators: Are Focused on Single Skills and Permit Learners to Practice in Isolation

Name	Manufacturer	Approx. Cost	Description	Simulator
Baby Ivy	Laerdal	$520	Simulated infant head with internally molded scalp veins designed for practicing neonatal peripheral venous access. Life-size neonate head with internally molded scalp veins Peripheral IV line insertion and removal for fluid and medication administration after patient stabilization Infusible veins allow realistic flash to confirm proper placement Maintenance and securing of line Mounted on a hard-side case	
Baby Stap	Laerdal	$460	Reproduction of a neonatal infant positioned for the practice of lumbar puncture techniques. Lateral decubitus position Upright position Realistic interchangeable spine with spinal cord may be palpated for location of correct puncture site Fluid may be infused	
Baby Umbi	Laerdal	$460	Female newborn infant reproduction designed for the practice of umbilical catheterization. Retractable umbilical cord for actual catheterization Two arteries and vein molded into umbilical cord facilitate: Low umbilical artery catheter High umbilical artery catheter Umbilical vein catheter Securing and dressing procedures may be practiced	
Baby Arti	Laerdal	$435	Lifelike reproduction of an infant arm with bony structures allows students to master the technique of neonatal radial artery puncture. Percutaneous puncture site in radial artery Mechanical radial artery pulse generator provides realistic arterial pressure Simulated blood may be infused for blood backflow in syringe Replaceable skin and artery ensures longevity of model Mounted on a base	

(continued)

TABLE 1.2	Commercially Available Low-Fidelity Manikin-Based Task Training Simulators: Are Focused on Single Skills and Permit Learners to Practice in Isolation (*Continued*)

Name	Manufacturer	Approx. Cost	Description	Simulator
Laerdal Intraosseous Trainer	Laerdal	$440	The Laerdal Intraosseous Trainer is designed for training in infant intraosseous infusion techniques. • Intraosseous needle insertion • Aspiration of simulated bone marrow • Replaceable pads are prefilled with simulated bone marrow	
Infant IV Leg	Laerdal	$200	The Infant IV Leg is designed for training extremity venipuncture procedures and IV fluid administration in the superficial veins of the foot. • Venous access in the medial and malleolus sites • Venipuncture possible in medial and lateral malleolus sites • Heel stick simulation • Fluid may be infused for realistic flashback	
Laerdal® Infant Airway Management Trainer	Laerdal	$500–650	Realistic anatomy of the tongue, oropharynx, epiglottis, larynx, vocal cords, and trachea Practicing of oral and nasal intubation Practicing use of laryngeal mask airway Correct tube placement can be checked by practical inflation test Bag-valve-mask ventilation can be practiced Sellick maneuver can be performed Stomach inflation Realistic tissue simulation	

(continued)

TABLE 1.3	Medium-Fidelity Manikin-Based Simulators: Provide a More Realistic Representation But Lack Sufficient Cues for the Learner to Be Fully Immersed in the Situation

Name	Manufacturer/ URL	Approx. Cost	Capabilities	Simulator
Nita Newborn	Laerdal (http://www. laerdal.com/us/doc/376/ Nita-Newborn)	$622	The Nita Newborn is a model of a 4-lb, 16" newborn female with realistic landmarks and articulation for vascular access procedures Nose and mouth openings allow placement[a] of nasal cannulae, endotracheal tubes, nasotracheal tubes and feeding tubes Standard venipuncture in various sites facilitating blood withdrawal, fluid infusion and heparinization Median, basilic and axillary sites in both arms Saphenous and popliteal veins in right leg External jugular and temporal veins Central catheter insertion, securing, dressing and maintenance PICC line insertion, securing, dressing and maintenance Umbilical catheterization	
Newborn Anne	Laerdal (http://www. laerdal.com/us/doc/222/ Newborn-Anne#)	$1,900	Newborn Anne accurately represents a full-term (40 weeks), 50th percentile newborn female, measuring 21" and weighing 7 lbs. The airway is designed to allow for training in all aspects of newborn airway management, including the use of positive-pressure airway devices, and the placement of ET tubes and LMAs. The torso includes functionality to relieve a tension pneumothorax via needle decompression. The patent umbilicus has a manually generated pulse and can be assessed, cut, and catheterized for IV access. Newborn Anne features IO access in both legs.	

TABLE 1.3	Medium-Fidelity Manikin-Based Simulators: Provide a More Realistic Representation But Lack Sufficient Cues for the Learner to Be Fully Immersed in the Situation (*Continued*)

Name	Manufacturer/ URL	Approx. Cost	Capabilities	Simulator
Neonatal Resuscitation Baby	Laerdal (http://www.laerdal.com/us/doc/1077/Neonatal-Resuscitation-Baby)	$929	Anatomically accurate head and airway with landmarks, trachea, esophagus, stomach, and simulated lungs Oropharyngeal and nasopharyngeal airway insertion with right mainstem intubation and suctioning Realistic chest rise and fall with BVM ventilation Realistic practice of chest compressions Umbilical cord with two arteries and one vein facilitating high and low UAC and umbilical vein catheterization Use of shoulder roll permitted NG/OG tube insertion, care, medication administration, and removal possible Gastric lavage and gavage capable	
Newborn Simulators	Laerdal (http://www.laerdal.com/us/doc/223/Newborn-Simulators)	$41	Newborn simulator with realistic articulation Neonatal monitoring • Head and chest circumference, head to heel length, weight and abdominal girth • Application and setup of thoracic impedance monitor, pulse oximeter sensor and transcutaneous PO$_2$ monitor and electrode application Neonatal treatments such as eye prophylaxis (Crede's Treatment), thermoregulation and phototherapy Parent explanation for bathing, holding, feeding, dressing and setup of home apnea monitor Includes hospital wristband and diaper.	

Nursing Baby

Laerdal (http://www.laerdal.com/us/doc/225/Nursing-Baby)

$1,800–$3,000

Normal, bulging, and depressed fontanelles for assessment and diagnosis
Head with anatomical landmarks, trachea, and esophagus, along with simulated lungs and stomach allow the practice of many procedures, including NG, OG, tracheal care, and suctioning
Bilateral deltoid and bilateral thigh IM injections are possible
Articulating IV arm and IV leg allow for practice of IV cannulation, medication administration, site care, and maintenance
Medication and fluid administration through IO infusion allowed via tibia access with landmarks at the tibial tuberosity and medial malleolus
Gastrostomy tube opening for care and feeding
Presents normal and abnormal heart, breath, and bowel sounds for auscultation
Interchangeable genitalia allows for urinary catheterization with fluid return, rectal temperature simulation, and administration of suppositories

S100 Susie® and Simon® Newborn Advanced Care Simulator

Gaumard (http://www.gaumard.com/the-susie-and-simon-newborn-advanced-care-simulator/)

$420–$1,200

Soft and flexible face skin
Self-molded hair
Realistic eyes
NG exercises to demonstrate tube feeding and gastric suction
Simulated ear canal
Soft arms and legs rotate within the torso body for lifelike feel and position
Soft hands, feet, fingers, and toes
Heel stick and finger prick technique
Soft upper body skin over torso for "babylike" feel
Bathing and bandaging activity
IM injection in upper thigh
Interchangeable male organ
Urethral passage and bladder
Male and female catheterization
Removable internal tanks
Enema administration

(continued)

TABLE 1.3 Medium-Fidelity Manikin-Based Simulators: Provide a More Realistic Representation But Lack Sufficient Cues for the Learner to Be Fully Immersed in the Situation (*Continued*)

Name	Manufacturer/ URL	Approx. Cost	Capabilities	Simulator
S107 Multipurpose Patient Care and CPR Infant	http://www.gaumard.com/ multipurpose-patient-care-and-cpr-infant-s107/	$845	All features of the S100 Newborn, as well as: External stoma sites with internal tanks Oral, nasal, and digital intubation Place OP/NP tubes Right/left mainstem bronchi Place nasal and oral gastric tubes Suctioning BVM with realistic chest rise Chest compression Umbilical catheterization IO infusion IV arm with variable, palpable pulses	
V800 Nita Newborn™	Gaumard (http://www. gaumard.com/nita-newborn-v800l)	$800	An anatomically correct 4-lb, 16″ female newborn for dressing care, securing and maintenance of vascular access devices in infants, including standard venipuncture, central venous catheter, umbilical catheter, and PICC. Right and left arms with accessible median basilic and axillary veins Right leg with saphenous and popliteal veins Neck and head area with frontal, postauricular, temporal and external jugular veins Simulated, translucent skin allows visualization of underlying veins Veins are self-sealing Nasal and oral openings for placement of nasal cannulae, nasogastric tubes and feeding tubes, permitting practice of suctioning, securing, dressing, and cleansing	

(continued)

S320 PEDI® Airway Trainer Newborn

Gaumard (http://www.gaumard.com/pedi-airway-trainer-newborn-s320/)

$520 to $650

- Complete upper torso with realistic chest cavity containing heart, lungs, and stomach
- Fully articulating head, neck, and jaw permitting head-tilt/chin lift, jaw thrust and neck extension into the sniffing position
- Anatomically accurate mouth, tongue, airway, and esophagus designed to illustrate the profound differences between intubating an infant, a child or an adult
- Nasal passage permits placement of NP tube
- Soft neck with cricoid cartilage permits classic Sellick maneuver needed to provide a better view of the vocal cords and/or minimize gastric reflux
- Realistic trachea, bronchi, and lungs permit observable unilateral or bilateral lung expansion under positive-pressure ventilation
- Narrow, floppy, slightly curved epiglottis
- Anteriorly positioned vocal cords
- Realistic 3.8-mm airway, narrowing below the vocal cords

S320.100/101 PEDI® Blue Neonatal Simulator with SmartSkin™ Technology

Gaumard (http://www.gaumard.com/pedi-blue-neonate-simulator-with-newborn-hal-body-s320-101/)

$2,000–$5,000

- Full size articulating neonate
- Realistic airway with tongue, vocal cords, trachea, and esophagus for airway management exercises
- Heart, lungs, ribs, stomach, and liver
- Oral or nasal intubation plus suctioning
- Cricoid prominence permits the Sellick maneuver
- Bilateral lung expansion with realistic chest rise
- Practice intubation using a Miller 1 blade and uncuffed 2.5 ET tube
- View peripheral and central cyanosis as well as healthy skin tone
- Practice umbilical catheterization and simulate pulsatile element with use of handheld squeeze bulb
- Simulate neonatal CPR with either two-thumb "encircling" technique or two finger alternate compression method
- Practice delicate IO access with optional IO leg
- Practice injection and IV techniques with optional training arm

TABLE 1.3   Medium-Fidelity Manikin-Based Simulators: Provide a More Realistic Representation But Lack Sufficient Cues for the Learner to Be Fully Immersed in the Situation (*Continued*)

Name	Manufacturer/ URL	Approx. Cost	Capabilities	Simulator
S108 PREMIE™ Blue Simulator with SmartSkin™ Technology	Gaumard (http://www.gaumard.com/premie-blue-simulator-with-smartskin-technology-s108/)	$2,100	28-week articulating PREMIE Realistic airway with tongue, vocal cords, trachea, and esophagus for airway management exercises Heart, lungs, airway, and ribs Simulate "heel stick" maneuver for capillary blood sample BVM or CPR exercises Intubation plus suctioning Bilateral lung expansion with realistic chest rise View peripheral and central cyanosis as well as healthy skin tone Use monitor to select rates of improvement and deterioration Watch skin color change in response to the efforts of your student Pulse umbilicus using squeeze bulb Practice placement of umbilical lines Simulate CPR with either two-thumb "encircling" technique or two finger alternate compression method Practice delicate IO access Practice injection and IV techniques	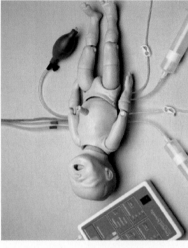

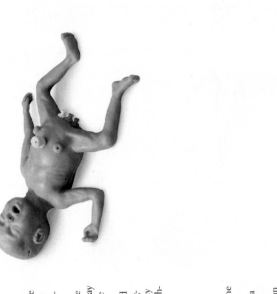

**Life/form®
Micro-Preemie
Simulator**

Nasco (http://www.enasco.
com/product/
LF01212U)

$250

25-week gestation

- Breathing: Pulse bulb to manually simulate breathing rate volume.
- Ventilation: Molded-in lung produces a visible chest rise when ventilated by mouth; trachea and pharynx are not anatomically correct but will accept a functioning endotracheal tube.
- GI: One nostril will accept a functioning NG tube (tube passes through the body and liquids will either drain away from the body or into the diaper); optional stoma can be plugged into a permanent site on the abdomen.
- Umbilicus: Soft, lifelike umbilicus has a patent vein and two arteries; umbilical stump functions like a cork, plugging into a small cavity molded into the abdomen (cavity can be used as a reservoir for blood drawn through a catheter or to receive fluids and the drain exits from the diaper area); a separate umbilicus represents an optional omphalocele.
- IV access: Several typical sites have embedded tubing that can accept an IV catheter; one is functional, allowing the administration of fluids, which will drain from the diaper area.
- Chest tube: A permanent site in the baby's side accepts a nonfunctioning chest tube.
- Neural tube defect: An optional structure representing an open neural tube defect can be inserted into the back.
- Various monitors, sensors, electrodes, etc., can be attached to the manikin wherever needed.

*a*Nita Newborn does not have intubation capabilities.
BVM, bag-valve-mask; CPR, cardiopulmonary resuscitation; ET, endotracheal; IO, intraosseous; LMA, laryngeal mask airway; NG, nasogastric; NP, nasopharyngeal; OC, orogastric; OP, oropharyngeal; PICC, peripherally inserted central catheter; UAC, umbilical artery catheter.

TABLE 1.4	Commercially Available High-fidelity Manikin-Based Simulators: Provide Adequate Cues to Allow for Full Immersion, Respond to Treatment Interventions, and Provide Feedback				
Name	**Manufacturer**	**Price**	**Picture**		**URL**
S3010 Newborn HAL® Mobile Team Trainer	Gaumard	$20,000–$40,000			http://www.gaumard.com/newborn-hal-s3010/
S3009 Premie HAL®	Gaumard	$20,000–$40,000			http://www.gaumard.com/s3009-premie-hal/
SimNewB™	Laerdal	$20,000–$40,000			http://www.laerdal.com/us/doc/88/SimNewB
SimBaby™	Laerdal	$30,000–$45,000			http://www.laerdal.com/SimBaby

TABLE 1.4	Commercially Available High-fidelity Manikin-Based Simulators: Provide Adequate Cues to Allow for Full Immersion, Respond to Treatment Interventions, and Provide Feedback (*Continued*)				
Name	**Manufacturer**	**Price**	**Picture**		**URL**
BabySIM	METI	$30,000–$45,000			http://www.meti.com/products_ps_baby.htm
PDA Baby	Simulaids	$10,500			http://www.simulaids.com/401.htm

References

1. Anderson JM. Educational perspectives. *NeoReviews.* 2005;6:e411.
2. Anderson JM, Warren JB. Using simulation to enhance the acquisition and retention of clinical skills in neonatology. *Semin Perinatol.* 2011;35:59.
3. Arafeh JM. Simulation-based training: the future of competency? *J Perinat Neonatal Nurs.* 2011;25:171.
4. Ballard HO, Shook LA, Locono J, et al. Novel animal model for teaching chest tube placement. *J Ky Med Assoc.* 2009;107:219.
5. Cates LA. Simulation training: a multidisciplinary approach. *Adv Neonatal Care.* 2011;11:95.
6. Cates LA, Wilson D. Acquisition and maintenance of competencies through simulation for neonatal nurse practitioners: beyond the basics. *Adv Neonatal Care.* 2011;11:321.
7. Gaba DM. The future vision of simulation in health care. *Qual Saf Health Care.* 2004;13(Suppl 1):i2.
8. Halamek LP. Teaching versus learning and the role of simulation-based training in pediatrics. *J Pediatr.* 2007;151:329.
9. Halamek LP. The simulated delivery-room environment as the future modality for acquiring and maintaining skills in fetal and neonatal resuscitation. *Semin Fetal Neonatal Med.* 2008;13:448.
10. Halamek LP, Kaegi DM, Gaba DM, et al. Time for a new paradigm in pediatric medical education: teaching neonatal resuscitation in a simulated delivery room environment. *Pediatrics.* 2000;106:E45.
11. MacDonald MG, Johnson B. Perinatal outreach education. In: Avery GB, Fletcher MA, Macdonald MG, eds. *Neonatology: Pathophysiology and Management of the Newborn,* 4th ed. Philadelphia, PA: JB Lippincott Co.; 1994:32.
12. Kattwinkel J, Perlman JM, Aziz K, et al. Neonatal resuscitation: 2010 American Heart Association Guidelines for Cardiopulmonary Resuscitation and Emergency Cardiovascular Care. *Pediatrics.* 2010;126:e1400.
13. Murphy AA, Halamek LP. Educational perspectives. *NeoReviews.* 2005;6:e489.
14. Rudolph JW, Simon R, Dufresne RL, et al. There's no such thing as "nonjudgmental" debriefing: a theory and method for debriefing with good judgment. *Simul Healthc.* 2006;1:49.
15. Ericsson KA. Deliberate practice and the acquisition and maintenance of expert performance in medicine and related domains. *Acad Med.* 2004;79(10 Supp):S70.
16. Institute of Medicine. *To Err is Human: Building a Safer Health System.* Washington, DC: National Academies Press; 2000.
17. Clark DR. (2012). Kolb's Learning Styles and Experiential Learning Model. Updated July 13, 2011. http://nwlink.com/~donclark/hrd/styles/kolb.html. Accessed April 23, 2012.
18. Rodgers DL. High-fidelity patient simulation: a descriptive white paper report. http://sim-strategies.com/downloads/Simulation%20White%20Paper2.pdf. Accessed April 23, 2012.
19. Institute for Medical Simulation Comprehensive Instructor Workshop and Graduate Course material Copyright, all pages, Center for Medical Simulation, 2004–2011. Also personal communication JW Rudolph.

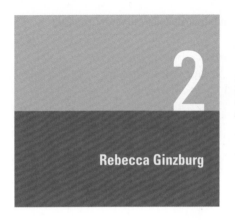

2 Informed Consent for Procedures

Rebecca Ginzburg

The primacy of a patient's personal autonomy is the foundation of most modern professional guidelines and case law concerning informed consent. Because every individual has the right to determine what happens to his or her own body, the individual must ultimately make decisions about which medical procedures he or she will undergo. For that individual's decision to be meaningful, it must be made with full information about the procedure.

In the context of neonates, the notion of personal autonomy is more attenuated, but the requirements of informed consent are no less stringent. The law of every state in the United States requires the parent or legal guardian's consent before a minor receives medical treatment (with certain exceptions, such as in emergencies and treatment of "mature" or "emancipated" minors, e.g., a pregnant minor) (1–3). The presumption, then, is that parents or legal guardians will make treatment decisions based on the information provided by the treating physician. If the information disclosed is inadequate, inaccurate, or unclear, the parent or guardian is not placed in an optimal position to make a treatment decision.

Legal Consequences of Failure to Provide Adequate Disclosure

Failure to provide adequate informed consent may give rise to claims of negligence, assault, and inadequate informed consent (4–7).

Negligence: To establish negligence, a plaintiff (usually a patient or patient's next of kin or guardian) must show that the health care provider(s) had a duty to the patient, that the provider breached that duty, that the patient suffered an injury, and that the breach caused the injury. A health care provider has duties to his or her patients. In the neonatal intensive care unit (NICU), these duties arise because the patient's well-being has been entrusted to the NICU health care team, directed by a physician, based on the team's superior medical knowledge and, either explicitly or implicitly, the team's ability to provide the requested treatment. A priority physician duty is to explain disease process, prognosis, and the range of possible treatments with their individual risks and benefits. Although a treating physician may

delegate the responsibility for obtaining informed consent, he or she needs to keep in mind that when the treating physician fails to ensure that parents or guardians are provided with all the information that they require to make a decision, in a language and manner that the parents or guardians fully understand, the treating physician fails to fulfill his or her duty to the patient. If injury results that was not covered in the informed consent process, the treating physician may be liable for this injury, as may other members of the health care team who were involved in the performance of the procedure (8,9).

A plaintiff may (alternatively or additionally) make a medical malpractice claim for failure to provide adequate disclosure. Medical malpractice is a type of negligence, so the elements required for a prima facie case are the same. The plaintiff must show that the health care provider owed the patient a duty, that the provider breached this duty, that the patient suffered an injury, and that the breach caused the injury. The duty to the patient is, again, based on the provider–patient relationship. To show that a provider breached this duty, the standard of care must be established; when the alleged breach was a failure to obtain informed consent, the standard may depend on the disclosure that a "reasonable" physician would make or that a "reasonable" patient would find material (these standards are discussed in more detail below).

A medical malpractice suit may succeed when a patient (or the patient's parent or guardian) did not receive adequate disclosure and the patient was injured during the procedure, even if the physician performed the procedure competently. If further disclosure would have resulted in a decision that the patient would not undergo the procedure, there has been malpractice because the health care team failed to disclose all material facts. The treating physician would then be liable for all injuries resulting from the procedure (10).

Battery: Battery is unwanted physical contact. In some states, a physician or other health care provider may face a medical battery claim if he or she treats a patient without first getting informed consent or gets consent that does not adequately cover all aspects of the treatment (4). Except in an emergency no procedure other than the one(s) to which the parent or guardian has agreed may be performed. This includes a modification to a procedure that is beyond the scope of the consent (11). It is immaterial whether the provider's intention was to help the patient, whether the procedure was successful, or whether the health care provider was otherwise negligent (12,13). Although damages may be more difficult to prove when the alleged battery was a successful procedure, courts may assess punitive damages (which may not be covered by malpractice insurance) and licensing boards may levy their own penalties (4).

Inadequate Informed Consent: Some state laws also provide for a separate cause of action for failure to secure informed consent (14–16). To prove such a claim, the plaintiff must generally show that the physician or designee failed to inform the patient, parent, or guardian of a material fact relating to the proposed treatment; that consent to the treatment was given without awareness of the material fact; that a reasonably prudent patient, parent, or guardian, in a similar circumstance, would have refused to consent to the treatment if informed of such material fact; and that injuries resulted from the treatment. Like a medical malpractice claim, a failure to secure informed consent claim may succeed even if the procedure was performed without negligence or there is insufficient evidence to support a battery claim (4,17).

Specific and General Informed Consent

There are two kinds of informed consent: general and specific. A patient, parent, or guardian may give a general informed consent (sometimes called a "blanket consent") when the patient is admitted to the hospital and will require ongoing clinical intervention by a number of health care providers. The patient, parents, or guardians may be kept informed of the specifics of procedures during the hospital stay, but they may not be informed of every intervention. A general informed consent will cover routine medical care that a patient may receive while in the hospital, such as drawing blood or administering a nonexperimental medication. The hospital administration will define what constitutes routine care, depending on community and professional standards. The procedures considered routine may also vary depending on the hospital unit to which a patient is admitted.

In the NICU, specific informed consent is required when a procedure falls outside of routine intensive care provided to most patients in the unit. Examples of nonroutine procedures might be surgery for a congenital or acquired defect, renal dialysis, and extracorporeal membrane oxygenation. In such nonroutine cases, parents or guardians must receive sufficient information specific to the procedure to permit them to make a fully informed decision.

It is important to document both general and specific informed consent. In the case of general informed consent, the patient, parent, or guardian is likely to be asked to sign a written consent; these consents should be retained with the patient's records. For specific informed consents, a written or oral disclosure (in many cases, both) is required. In the case of oral disclosure, the individual obtaining consent should summarize in the patient chart, in reasonable detail, the information provided. If consent is obtained by telephone, a witness should listen to the telephone conversation and co-sign the summary in the patient chart.

What is Adequate Disclosure?

Disclosures about proposed procedures should be presented in terms and in a language that the patient, parents, or guardians can fully understand. At minimum, the treating physician should ensure that the following are explained:

1. the procedure;
2. the long- and short-term risks and benefits of the procedure;
3. the alternatives, including doing nothing; and
4. the long- and short-term risks and benefits of the alternatives and doing nothing.

Disclosures should include information about the frequency and severity of the adverse potential consequences and the likelihood, duration, and degree of anticipated benefits from the treatment(s). There is a potential to overload the consentee with information; the patient, parent, or guardian does not need to hear every possible risk, especially if the problem is extremely unlikely to occur. However, the provider should consider the disclosure carefully when there is a low risk of a problem materializing but the consequences are death or severe morbidity.

U.S. state courts have generally endorsed one of two approaches to determine whether a disclosure is sufficient: the physician-centered approach and the patient-centered approach. The physician-centered approach measures the disclosure against the accepted practice among other physicians; it asks what a reasonable physician would disclose. At trial, the court would expect testimony of medical experts to establish the standard disclosure for a given procedure (4,18).

The patient-centered approach considers what information a reasonable patient (or patient's parents or legal guardians) would regard as significant to deciding whether to go forward with the procedure (19,20). At trial, a medical expert's testimony might be valuable to explain the kinds of risks attendant to a procedure; however, expert testimony would not be necessary to show whether a particular fact was material to making the decision whether to proceed (21).

Neither approach is without its problems. The physician-centered approach is problematic because the standard disclosure may not actually include sufficient information. In addition, a disclosure sufficient for one patient, parent, or guardian may not be sufficient for another; by failing to take into account the patient's unique circumstances, the physician may fail to protect the patient's autonomy (21). The patient-centered approach, on the other hand, will at times require considerable time and effort, often in circumstances where time may be limited. In addition, though the patient-centered approach is meant to be based on what the parties knew before the procedure and applied objectively, in practice it can be difficult to apply so rigidly.

For these reasons, courts considering informed consent issues often end up with an approach that looks more like a hybrid of the physician-based and patient-based approaches: A physician should consider what other physicians in the field would disclose in the circumstances; what this patient, parent, or guardian would want to know about the options; and his or her competence with both medical terms and with the language in use (21). There is a lot to keep in mind—including the need to consider federal or state law, hospital rules, and professional association guidelines, along with the particular circumstances of the patient and/or family. If difficult issues arise, the physician should consider consulting with hospital legal counsel before proceeding.

Adequate Informed Consent in the Context of Neonates

As discussed, the doctrine of informed consent is based, in part, on the idea that respect for a patient's personal autonomy is primary. When the patient is a neonate and, therefore, cannot express autonomy, informed consent is more complicated than when the patient is a competent adult. By necessity, obtaining informed consent from a neonatal patient is really a matter of obtaining "informed permission" from the patient's parent or guardian (22). When seeking this permission, the physician must exercise judgment with respect to whether the parent or guardian is competent to make the necessary decisions and, ultimately, whether the parent or guardian's decisions are in the best interest of the patient. At the same time, the treating physician must be careful not to simply substitute his or her judgment for that of the parents' or guardians'.

Coercion, Manipulation, and Persuasion

Consent that is not freely given is not consent. For that reason, the health care provider must be careful that his or her interactions with a neonate's parents or guardians are free from coercion, whether by implicit or explicit threats or inducements (22). For example, the provider should not give the impression that the quality of the neonate's treatment will suffer if the parents or guardians do not consent to a procedure, and the provider should not make any additional support (monetary or otherwise) for the neonate contingent on consent. Obviously, manipulating the parents or guardians by deliberately providing incomplete or untrue information is unacceptable. Given that there is an information imbalance between the parties, it is especially important that the information the parents or guardians receive is accurate. However, there is no requirement that the

physician be impartial and hide his or her opinion, as long as this opinion is based on medical evidence and professional experience, rather than religious or personal bias. It is appropriate for the physician to make a case for a particular intervention, and the parents or guardians will expect recommendations.

Competency of Parents or Guardians and the State

Consent is valid only if the consenting party is legally competent to give consent. The health care provider may begin with the assumption that the neonate's parents or guardians are competent, capable of understanding and balancing the medical information provided, and capable of making and communicating a decision. However, if there are indications that the parents or guardians are not competent, the treating physician should not act on their proffered consent or refusal and should consult hospital legal counsel before proceeding. Some examples of circumstances in which one may question competency to consent include parents or guardians who abuse drugs or alcohol, who show signs of untreated mental illness, or who are minors.

The parents or guardians should not be disqualified from making medical decisions simply because they speak a foreign language. In addition, even when parents or guardians are able to make themselves understood, their understanding of the prevailing language may not be optimal. Thus, all efforts should be made to provide the information in the primary language of the parents or guardians, including locating a qualified medical interpreter or interpreting service (23).

Absent Parents or Guardians

Under common law, when an adult patient requires emergency life-saving treatment, a physician may assume the patient's informed consent for that treatment. Similarly, in an emergency, a physician may assume informed consent if an infant's parent or guardian is absent (or otherwise unable to make the necessary decision) (1).

An infant's parents or guardians may delegate the right to make medical decisions for the infant to another person. To do so, the parents or guardians must have the right to make decisions in the first place and must be legally and medically competent to decide to delegate their rights. In addition, the proxy taking over the decision making must be legally and medically competent to make the medical decisions. If the parents or guardians are absent and have made no delegation, state law may determine the proxy (usually there is a hierarchy of family members but an unrelated proxy, *guardian ad litem*, may be appointed). In any event, the physician should be sure that he or she inquires about, and documents in the patient chart, the source and extent of the proxy's authority (4).

When one parent is absent, the parents' marital status and the custody arrangement for the infant may be important. If the parents are married, consent of only one of the parents will be adequate in most states. However, if the parents are not married or there has been a legal separation or divorce, obtaining proper consent may be more complicated. Whether one parent or the other (or both) have the legal right to make medical decisions will depend on state law, as well as judicial orders or settlement agreements, if they exist. With help from hospital legal counsel, if necessary, the physician should determine whether the parent present can legally provide consent for the infant.

Best Interests of the Patient

When a competent adult patient refuses a procedure that would save his life, the treating physician must respect the patient's choice. With neonatal patients, this is more complicated. A physician has a duty to the infant patient to provide medical care appropriate to the patient's needs, which is a duty separate from the physician's responsibilities to the patient's parents or guardians. The physician's duty to the patient persists even if the patient's parent or guardian refuses to consent to a needed procedure or requests a nonmedically indicated procedure. Both the physician and the parent or guardian are required to act in the "best interest of the child" and, generally, the parent or guardian's medical decision is presumed to be in the best interest of the child (22). The physician is not entirely powerless to overcome that presumption, however.

When a physician considers a parent or guardian's medical decision to justify intervention (or the physician otherwise questions the competency of the parent or guardian), the hospital may decide to notify the appropriate government agency overseeing child welfare or to petition a court directly, depending on state law. The state may appoint a *guardian ad litem* or take custody of the infant temporarily to determine what would be in the infant's best interests. These "intrusion[s] into and interference[s] with familial relationships between a parent and child can rise to the level of a substantive due process violation" (24). Parents have brought suits claiming as much in cases where the state (in the form of a state-run hospital, state agency, or court) took away the parents' right to make medical decisions for their children. However, for a parent's claim that the state's action violated the parent's substantive due process rights, a court must find that the state's actions "shock ...the conscience" (25). This is a very fact-dependent determination; when serious, irreparable consequences may result if a procedure is not performed, the court is likely to find that there has been no substantive due process violation.

The other side of the due process coin is procedural due process: Were the state's procedures to deprive an individual of his rights in a particular circumstance constitutionally adequate? "The family is not beyond regu-

lation in the public interest, however, nor are rights of parenthood beyond limitation" (24,26). Even in the context of refusing medical treatment on medical grounds, courts have held that a parent's "right to practice religion and make parental decisions does not include the liberty to expose a child to ill health or death" (24,26). Though parents and guardians have primary responsibility for a child's health care decisions, the state also has an interest in protecting those who cannot protect themselves (*parens patriae*) and in the "health, safety, welfare of the children within its borders" (13,24,25). So long as the state only deprives a parent of the right to make medical decisions for his or her child in service of those legitimate state interests, a court is likely to find that there has been no violation of the parent's procedural due process rights. This is true even where the parent has not had notice or an opportunity to be heard prior to the state's action; if the delay while giving notice or holding a hearing may further harm the child, the state may act without notice or a hearing (24).

The risk in such a system is that physicians, with the weight of the state behind them, will take the right to make medical decisions away from parents and guardians, even when the parents and guardians have made an informed decision not to consent. Because the state's decisions are necessarily informed by the treating physician, the balance of power in these situations is decidedly tilted toward the physician. However, the state's interest and, therefore, its power to override the parent or guardian's decisions "diminishes as the severity of a [child's] affliction and the likelihood of death increase" (27,28). There must be proof that the procedure in question is the best way to serve the child's welfare; it cannot only be that the procedure would prolong the child's life for some minimal amount of time. The legal presumption is that the parents or guardians make health care decisions, and that is so even when the choice may be to stop treatment of a very ill child. The physician should be careful not to disregard a parent or guardian's considered decisions, though the physician may disagree strongly (22). Although a physician may not simply refuse to continue care of (abandon) a patient, neither is the physician obliged to provide patient care which he or she considers unethical or not in the patient's best interest. In this circumstance, the treating physician, with the full knowledge and participation of the parents or guardians, may refer the case for consideration by an ethics committee and/or to another physician who is willing to follow the treatment plan requested by the parents or guardians.

References

1. American Academy of Pediatrics, Committee on Pediatric Emergency Medicine. Consent for emergency medical services for children and adolescents. *Pediatrics.* 2003;111(3):703.
2. *Bartal v. Brower*, 993 P.2d 629 (Kan. 1999).

3. *Belcher v. Charleston Area Med. Ctr.*, 422 S.E.2d 827 (W. Va. 1992).
4. American Academy of Pediatrics. Clinical report—consent by proxy for nonurgent pediatric care. *Pediatrics*. 2010;126:1022.
5. *Bourgeois v. McDonald*, 622 So. 2d 684, 688 (La. Ct. App. 1993).
6. *K.A.C. v. Benson*, 527 N.W.2d 553 (Minn. 1995).
7. *Canterbury v. Spence*, 464 F.2d 772 (D.C. Cir. 1972), *cert. denied*, 409 U.S. 1064 (1972).
8. *Berkey v. Anderson*, 82 Cal. Rptr. 67 (Cal. 1969).
9. *Dow v. Permanente Med. Group*, 90 Cal. Rptr 747 (Cal. 1970).
10. *Backlund v. Univ. of Wash.*, 975 P.2d 950 (Wash. 1999).
11. *Miller v. HCA, Inc.*, 118 S.W.3d 758 (Tex. 2003).
12. *Newmark v. Williams*, 588 A.2d 1108 (Del. 1991).
13. Svoboda JS, Van Howe RS, Dwyer JG. Informed consent for neonatal circumcision: an ethical and legal conundrum. *J Contemp Health Law Policy*. 2000;17:84.
14. Wash. Rev. Code § 7.70.050 (2011).
15. Alaska Stat. §09.55.556 (Michie 1976).
16. N.Y. Pub. Health Law §Sec. 2805-d (McKinney 2007).
17. *McQuitty v. Spangler*, 976 A.2d 1020 (Md. 2009).
18. Solomon D. Informed consent for routine infant circumcision: a proposal. NY *Law Sch Law Rev.* 2007/08;52:215.
19. *Arato v. Avedon*, 858 P.2d 598 (Cal. 1993).
20. *MacDonald v. U.S.*, 767 F. Supp. 1295, 1310 (M.D. Pa. 1991).
21. *Canterbury v. Spence*, 464 F.2d 772,791–92 (D.C. Cir. 1972).
22. American Academy of Pediatrics, Committee on Bioethics. Informed consent, parental permission, and assent in pediatric practice [reaffirmed October 2006]. *Pediatrics*. 1995;95(2):314.
23. Department of Health and Human Services, Office for Civil Rights. Guidance to Federal Financial Assistance Recipients Regarding Title VI Prohibition Against National Origin Discrimination Affecting Limited English Proficient Persons. Available at: http://www.hhs.gov/ocr/civilrights/resources/specialtopics/lep/policyguidancedocument.html. Accessed August 3, 2011.
24. *Novak v. Cobb County-Kennestone Hosp. Auth.*, 849 F. Supp. 1559(N.D. Ga. 1994).
25. *Bendiburg v. Dempsey*, 707 F.Supp. 1318, 1324 (N.D. Ga 1989).
26. *Prince v. Mass.*, 321 U.S. 158 (1944).
27. *M.N. v. Southern Baptist Hosp. of Florida, Inc.*, 648 So. 2d 769, 771 (Fla. App. 1 Dist. 1994).
28. *Superintendent of Belchertown State Sch. v. Saikewicz*, 370 N.E.2d 417 (Mass. 1977).

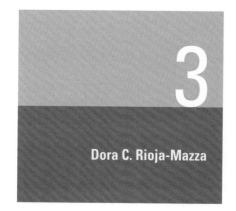

3 Maintenance of Thermal Homeostasis

Dora C. Rioja-Mazza

A. Definitions

1. *Homeostasis:* Fundamental mechanism whereby living things regulate their internal environment within tolerable limits, thus keeping a dynamic equilibrium and maintaining a stable, constant condition. From the Greek *homeo* (same, like) and *stasis* (stable state) (1).
2. *Normal body temperature:* The core body temperature is maintained by the term infant within the range of 36.5°C to 37.5°C, and the skin temperature, from 0.5°C to 1°C lower (2).
3. *Neutral thermal environment:* The range of ambient temperature required for the infant (for each gestational age and weight) to keep a normal body temperature and a minimal basal metabolic rate (2–4).
4. *Thermoregulation:* Mechanisms by which the infant tries to balance heat production and heat loss to accommodate the thermal environment (5–7).
5. *Cold stress:* The infant senses heat loss as a stress and responds with increased heat production and peripheral vasoconstriction, with centralization of circulation, in an effort to maintain the core temperature (8).
6. *Hypothermia:* Heat losses exceed heat production, dropping the infant's temperature below the normal range of 36.5°C to 37.5°C (97.7°F to 99.5°F) (9).
   a. *Mild hypothermia (cold stress):* 36°C to 36.4°C (96.8°F to 97.5°F)
   b. *Moderate hypothermia:* 32°C to 35.9°C (89.6°F to 96.6°F)
   c. *Severe hypothermia:* Below 32°C (89.6°F)
7. *Hyperthermia:* An increase in the infant's temperature to above 37.5°C (99.5°F), due to a warm environment. Hyperthermia is less common than hypothermia but is equally dangerous. Clinically, it may be difficult to distinguish hyperthermia from fever (infectious origin); therefore, always consider both causes in any increase in temperature (9).

B. Background

1. Effects of hypothermia:
   a. Hypothermia may have severe consequences in newborn infants and may even lead to arrhythmias and death (10,11).
   b. *Peripheral vasoconstriction:* Acrocyanosis, paleness, and coldness to touch
   c. Respiratory distress, apnea, and bradycardia (12,13)
   d. Depletion of caloric reserves and hypoglycemia, causing a shift to anaerobic metabolism and lactic acid production (14,15)
   e. Increased oxygen consumption and metabolic demands result in metabolic acidosis—a strong pulmonary vasoconstrictor inducing hypoxemia and central cyanosis (16–18).
   f. *Mobilization of norepinephrine, TSH, T_4 and free fatty acids:* Norepinephrine release promotes pulmonary hypertension and pulmonary ventilation–perfusion mismatch (19).
   g. Decreased cardiac output, increased systemic vascular resistance, and decreased intestinal and cerebral blood flow (11)
   h. Decreased number, activation, and aggregation of platelets (11)
   i. Impaired neutrophil release and function (11)
   j. Risk of kernicterus at low levels of serum bilirubin (20)
   k. Poor weight gain with chronic hypothermia (21)
   l. Controlled hypothermia may have a neuroprotective effect in term and near-term infants with moderate to severe hypoxic ischemic encephalopathy (22,23).
2. Effects of hyperthermia or overheating (9)
   a. *Peripheral vasodilatation:* The skin is hot, the extremities are red, and the face is flushed. Diaphoresis present in full-term infants. Skin temperature is higher than core temperature.
   b. Apnea, tachypnea
   c. Tachycardia and hypotension
   d. The infant assumes a spread-eagle posture.
   e. *Hyperactivity and irritability:* The infant becomes restless and cries, then feeds poorly, with lethargy and hypotonia.
   f. If hyperthermia is severe, shock, seizures, and coma may occur.
   g. If the increase in temperature is due to hypermetabolism (infection), paleness, vasoconstriction, cool extremities, and a core temperature higher than skin temperature may be noted.

3. Factors affecting heat loss
   a. Infant
      (1) Large surface area relative to body mass
      (2) Relatively large head with highly vascular fontanelle
      (3) Skin maturation/thickness, epidermal barrier functionally mature at 32 to 34 weeks. Transepidermal water loss may be 10 to 15 times greater in preterm infants of 25 weeks' gestation (2).
      (4) Decreased stores of subcutaneous fat and brown adipose tissue in more premature infants (7)
      (5) Inability to signal discomfort or trigger heat production (shivering) (7)
   b. Environment (3,4)
      (1) Physical contact with cold or warm objects (conduction)
      (2) Radiant heat loss or gain from proximity to hot or cold objects (radiation)
      (3) Wet or exposed body surfaces (evaporation)
      (4) Air currents in nursery or in incubator fan (convection)
      (5) Excessive or insufficient coverings or clothing
   c. Other factors
      (1) *Metabolic demands of disease:* Asphyxia, respiratory distress, sepsis (11)
      (2) Pharmacologic agents (e.g., vasodilating drugs, maternal analgesics, and unwarmed IV infusions, including blood products) (11)
      (3) Medical stability of infant prior to procedure
      (4) Thermogenic response matures with increase in postconception age (4)

C. Indications

1. Maintenance of thermal homeostasis is necessary at all times, but particular attention should be paid when the neonate is undergoing diagnostic or therapeutic procedures.
2. Avoids increase in insensible water loss (IWL) and improves caloric utilization

D. Equipment, Techniques, and Complications

1. Prevention of heat loss in the delivery room
   a. Warm environment (Table 3.1), room temperature >25°C; place infant on a radiant warmer, dry the skin with a prewarmed towel, and then remove any wet towels immediately (9,14,24).
   b. Use occlusive plastic blankets/bags (2,10,25) (Fig. 3.1).
      (1) Polyethylene bags (20 cm × 50 cm) prevent evaporative heat loss in infants <29 weeks' gestation. Their diathermancy allows transmission of radiant heat to the infant. Immediately after delivery, open the bag under the radiant warmer; wrap the wet infant's body from the shoulders down, and dry only the head. Place hat on head. Remove the wrap after the infant has been stable in the neonatal intensive care unit (NICU), in a humidified environment, for 1 hour.
      (2) *Environment:* Maintains temperature and reduces IWL by 25% (24,25)
      (3) *Access:* Allows neonatal resuscitation (secure airway, intubation, and chest compressions), but vascular access is limited
      (4) *Asepsis:* Limited by access
      (5) *Precautions:* Record core temperature every 5 to 10 minutes until infant is stable.
      (6) *Complications:* Hyperthermia, skin maceration, risk of infection
   c. Hats (2,10,26)
      (1) Stockinette caps are not effective in reducing heat loss in term infants in the delivery room; there is insufficient evidence in preterm infants.
      (2) Woolen hats may reduce or prevent heat loss in term infants in the delivery room.
2. Prevention of heat loss in the NICU
   a. Rigid plastic heat shields (heat shielding)
      (1) *Environment:* Reduces IWL by 25% (27)
      (2) *Access:* Very limited
      (3) *Asepsis:* Limited by access
      (4) *Precautions:* Avoid direct skin contact.
      (5) *Complications:* Hyperthermia, skin maceration, risk of infection
   b. Heat lamp: As an extra heat source (28)
      (1) *Environment:* Increased IWL
      (2) *Access:* Limited by other equipment used (open incubator, bassinette walls)
      (3) *Asepsis:* May be affected by limited access
      (4) *Precautions:* Record temperature every 5 to 10 minutes or use a continuous monitor. To avoid

TABLE 3.1	Room Temperatures and Humidity by Gestational Age and Birthweight		
Gestational Age (wks)	**Birthweight (g)**	**Delivery/Stabilization Room**	**Humidity**
≤26	≤750	26–27°C (78–80°F)	50%
27–28	750–1,000		
29–32	1,001–1,500	≥22°C (≥72°F)	
33–36	1,501–2,500		None
37–42	≥2,501	≥21°C (≥70°F)	

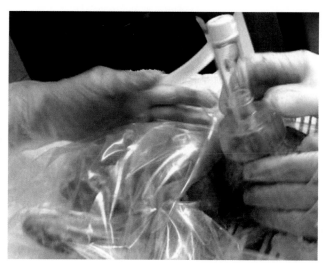

FIG. 3.1. Extremely low-birthweight preterm newborn wrapped in occlusive polyethylene sheet during resuscitation.

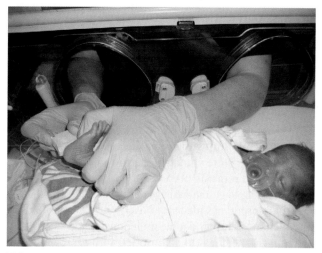

FIG. 3.2. All aspects of homeostasis are maintained during a procedure by use of incubator portholes, swaddling, comfortable position, and sucrose/analgesia pacifier.

burns, do not place oily substances on infant's skin. Avoid heating incubator thermometer; apply manual temperature control (33°C to 35°C) when using an open incubator. Keep infant approximately 60 to 90 cm from lamp bulb, and cover infant's eyes and genitals to protect from the light.

    (5) *Complications:* Cooling or overheating of isolette due to failure to detach the thermistor from infant; dehydration

  c. *Warming mattress:* Extra heat source, for transport or radiology procedures (e.g., MRI). Effective in preventing and treating hypothermia in very-low-birthweight infants (<1,500 g) in the delivery room (2,10,24)

    (1) *Environment:* Heating through conduction; reduces heat requirements and IWL

      (a) Heated water-filled mattress (keep at 37°C)

      (b) Exothermic crystallization of sodium acetate mattress (Transwarmer Infant Transport Mattress, Prism Technologies, San Antonio, Texas) with a postactivation temperature of 39°C ± 1°C

    (2) *Access:* Limited only by other equipment used

    (3) *Asepsis:* Limited only by other equipment used

    (4) *Precautions:* Record temperature every 10 to 20 minutes or use an infant servocontrol (ISC) continuous monitor.

    (5) *Complications:* Hypothermia, hyperthermia, burns

3. Mechanical devices to maintain temperature

  a. *Thermal resistor (thermistor):* A probe placed on the anterior abdominal wall or interscapular area. Use a servocontrol incubator/radiant warmer to keep infant's temperature between 36°C and 36.5°C (4,28)

  b. *Convection-warmed incubator:* (Fig. 3.2)

    (1) *Environment:* Creates a microclimate for each infant. ISC triggered by skin or air temperature; temperature can also be set manually. Double plastic walls, insulated mattress, and forced-heated/humidified air minimize IWL and maintain temperature.

    (2) *Access:* Impeded by portholes, especially when working with assistants. Improved with new incubators/warmers to allow better access (e.g., Giraffe OmniBed neonatal care station [GE Medical Systems, Waukesha, Wisconsin])

    (3) *Asepsis:* Impossible to maintain wide sterile field and infant position

    (4) *Precautions:* Take infant's temperature before and after procedure. Use ISC and ensure that thermistor remains in place. Add an extra heat source (heat lamp) for unstable infants or stressful procedures. Clinical deterioration may require lifting the protective shield.

    (5) *Complications:* Hyperthermia, hypothermia, unexpected break of aseptic field

  c. *Radiant warmed bed:* For unstable infants (28)

    (1) *Environment:* Increases IWL by 50% in small preterm infants.

    (2) *Access:* Unimpeded access to infants receiving intensive care

    (3) *Asepsis:* Ability to maintain infant position and wide sterile field; also allows assistants to participate

    (4) *Precautions:* Keep infant 80 to 90 cm from radiant heat. For premature infants, heat shielding must be added. Increase fluid infusions. Record temperature every 5 to 10 minutes or use a continuous monitor. To avoid burns, do not place oily substances on infant's skin.

    (5) *Complications:* Hyperthermia and dehydration

E. Special Circumstances/Considerations

1. Regulate room temperature to one optimal for infant (28°C to 30°C) (9).
2. Prewarm all heating units, including radiant warmers and incubators.
3. Remember that very-low-birthweight preterm infants and infants during the immediate newborn adaptation period are more vulnerable to hypothermia and IWL. This risk remains present for the first 2 to 4 weeks according to gestational age at birth.
4. For transport outside of the NICU, use a heated, battery-operated transport double-walled incubator.
5. Plug incubator into wall outlet during procedure to allow battery to charge.
6. Be aware that anesthesia may inhibit the infant's thermoregulatory capabilities.
7. Warm all anesthetic and respiratory gases to body temperature, and humidify.
8. *Gastroschisis/omphalocele:* These abdominal wall defects increase the risk of heat loss, fluid imbalance, and visceral damage. The infant may be placed in a "bowel bag" from the torso down, or the entire abdomen may be wrapped in clean, clear plastic wrap. Avoid visceral ischemia by keeping intestines directly above the abdominal wall defect or keep the infant in right lateral decubitus position (29).
9. *Neural tube defects:* Keep the infant in the prone position, cover the lesion with sterile gauze (soaked in warmed sterile saline), and then wrap the trunk circumferentially with a dry gauze. Finally, cover the dry gauze with plastic wrap to minimize insensible water losses and prevent hypothermia (30).

References

1. *Stedman's Medical Dictionary.* 27th ed. Baltimore: Lippincott Williams & Wilkins; 2000.
2. Bissinger RL, Annibale DJ. Thermoregulation in very-low-birthweight infants during the golden hour. *Adv Neonatal Care.* 2010;10:230.
3. LeBlanc M. Relative efficacy of an incubator and an open warmer in producing thermoneutrality for the small premature infant. *Pediatrics.* 1982;69:439.
4. Knobel R, Holditch-Davis D. Thermoregulation and heat loss prevention after birth and during neonatal intensive-care unit stabilization of extremely low-birthweight infants. *J Obstet Gynecol Neonatal Nurs.* 2007;36:280.
5. Silverman WA, Sinclair JC. Temperature regulation in the newborn infant. *N Engl J Med.* 1966;274:146.
6. Brück K. Temperature regulation in newborn infant. *Biol Neonate.* 1961;3:65.
7. Ellis J. Neonatal hypothermia. *J Neonatal Nurs.* 2005;11:76.
8. Lyon AJ, Pikaar ME, Badger P, et al. Temperature control in very low birthweight infants during first five days of life. *Arch Dis Child Fetal Neonatal Ed.* 1997;76(1):F47.
9. Department of Reproductive Health and Research (RHR), World Health Organization. *Thermal Protection of the Newborn: A Practical Guide.* Geneva, Switzerland: World Health Organization; 1997.
10. McCall EM, Alderdice F, Halliday HL, et al. Interventions to prevent hypothermia at birth in preterm and/or low birthweight babies. *Cochrane Database Syst Rev.* 2010;(1):CD004210.
11. Zanelli S, Buck M, Fairchild K. Physiologic and pharmacologic considerations for hypothermia therapy in neonates. *J Perinatol.* 2011;31:377.
12. Thoresen M, Whitelaw A. Cardiovascular changes during mild therapeutic hypothermia and rewarming in infants with hypoxic-ischemic encephalopathy. *Pediatrics.* 2000;106:92.
13. Gebauer CM, Knuepfer M, Robel-Tillig E, et al. Hemodynamics among neonates with hypoxic-ischemic encephalopathy during whole-body hypothermia and passive rewarming. *Pediatrics.* 2006; 117:843.
14. Kattwinkel J, Perlman JM, Aziz K, et al; The International Liaison Committee on Resuscitation (ILCOR), American Heart Association. Neonatal resuscitation: 2010 American Heart Association Guidelines for cardiopulmonary resuscitation and emergency cardiovascular care. *Pediatrics.* 2010;126:e1400.
15. Doctor BA, O'Riordan MA, Kirchner HL, et al. Perinatal correlates and neonatal outcomes of small for gestational age infants born at term gestation. *Am J Obstet Gynecol.* 2001;185:652.
16. Hassan IA-A, Wickramasinghe YA, Spencer SA. Effect of limb cooling on peripheral and global oxygen consumption in neonates. *Arch Dis Child Fetal Neonatal Ed.* 2003;88:F139.
17. Marks KH, Lee CA, Bolan CD Jr, et al. Oxygen consumption and temperature control of premature infants in a double-wall incubator. *Pediatrics.* 1981;68(1):93.
18. Hey EN. The relation between environmental temperature and oxygen consumption in new-born baby. *J Physiol.* 1969;200: 589.
19. Soll RF. Heat loss prevention in neonates. *J Perinatol.* 2008; 28:S57.
20. Ritter DA, Kenny JD, Norton HJ, et al. A prospective study of free bilirubin and other risk factors in the development of kernicterus in premature infants. *Pediatrics.* 1982;69:260.
21. Glass L, Silverman WA, Sinclair JC. Effects of the thermal environment on cold resistance and growth of small infants after the first week of life. *Pediatrics.* 1968;41:1033.
22. Shankaran S, Laptook AR, Ehrenkranz RA, et al; for the National Institute of Child Health and Human Development Neonatal Research Network. Whole-body hypothermia for neonates with hypoxic-ischemic encephalopathy. *N Engl J Med.* 2005;353: 1574.
23. Higgins RD, Raju TN, Perlman J, et al. Hypothermia and perinatal asphyxia: executive summary of the National Institute of Child Health and Human Development workshop. *J Pediatr.* 2006;148: 170.
24. Bhatt DR, White R, Martin G, et al. Transitional hypothermia in preterm newborns. *J Perinatol.* 2007;27:S45.
25. Vohra S, Roberts RS, Zhang B, et al. Heat loss prevention (HeLP) in the delivery room: a randomized controlled trial of polyethylene occlusive skin wrapping in very preterm infants. *J Pediatr.* 2004; 145:750.
26. Lang N, Bromiker R, Arad I. The effect of wool vs cotton head covering and length of stay with the mother following delivery on infant temperature. *Int J Nurs Stud.* 2004;41:843.
27. Symonds ME, Lomax MA. Maternal and environmental influences on thermoregulation in the neonate. *Proc Nutr Soc.* 1992; 51:165.
28. Korones SB. An encapsulated history of thermoregulation in the neonate. *Neoreviews.* 2004;5:e78.
29. Sheldon RE. The bowel bag: a sterile, transportable method for warming infants with skin defects. *Pediatrics.* 1974;53(2): 267.
30. Das UG, Leuthner SR. Preparing the neonate for transport. *Pediatr Clin North Am.* 2004;51:581.

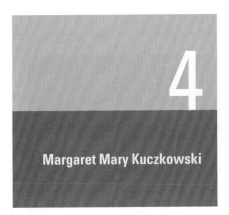

4 Methods of Restraint

Margaret Mary Kuczkowski

Physical restraints are required for proper positioning for certain procedures. Infants may also need to be restrained to prevent accidental injury or interference with treatment (i.e., removal of feeding tubes, catheters). Select the least restrictive but most appropriate restraint for the individual patient.

A. Definitions

1. *Physical restraint*: "Any device, garment, material, or object that restricts a person's freedom of movement or access to one's body" (1)

B. Indications

1. Required for procedures that require proper positioning to maintain asepsis and facilitate access to patient (IV placement, lumbar punctures, etc) (1)
2. To reduce the risk of interference with treatment (removal of feeding tubes, IV access, mechanical ventilation, etc.) (2)
3. To prevent movement artifact for radiographic studies, and MRI (3)
4. To prevent accidental injury

C. Contraindications

Restraints Should not Be Utilized

1. When close observation of the patient could protect against potential injury or potential interference with treatment (1,2)
2. When a change in treatment or medication regimen could protect against potential injury or interference with treatment (1,2)
3. When modification of the patient's environment (decreased stimuli, appropriate developmental positioning, reduced noise) could protect against potential injury or interference with treatment (1,2)
4. When use of a restraint could compromise patient care, procedures, or emergency access (1)

D. Techniques

Restraints for Procedures/Positioning

Whole Body Restraints

1. Mummy Restraint
   a. *Purpose*: Safe temporary method for restraining infants for treatment or examination; allows unimpeded access to head and scalp; individual extremities can be released for access for examination or treatment (1,2)
   b. Equipment
      (1) Clean blanket or small sheet
      (2) Safety pins or other device for securing final blanket fold
   c. Procedure (1)
      (1) Open blanket or sheet.
      (2) Fold one corner toward the center.
      (3) Place infant on blanket, with shoulders at fold and feet toward opposite corner (Fig. 4.1A).
      (4) With infant's right arm flexed and midline, tuck right side of blanket across trunk and under left side of body (Fig. 4.1B).
      (5) Fold lower corner up toward head and tuck under left shoulder (Fig. 4.1C).
      (6) With infant's left arm flexed and midline, tuck left side of blanket across trunk and under right side of body. Be sure to secure arms under blanket (Fig. 4.1D).
2. Commercial restraints for special procedures
   a. A "papoose board" is a flat padded board with canvas straps and Velcro closures and is often used for circumcisions in neonates.
   b. Specially designed sterile wraps to restrain newborn infants for umbilical venous catheterization or for lumbar punctures (Fig. 4.2A–C)
   c. Vacuum immobilization bags (MedVac Infant Immobilizer Bag, CFI Medical Solutions, Fenton, Michigan) are useful for performing MRI and CT scans in newborn infants and usually eliminate the need for sedation (3).

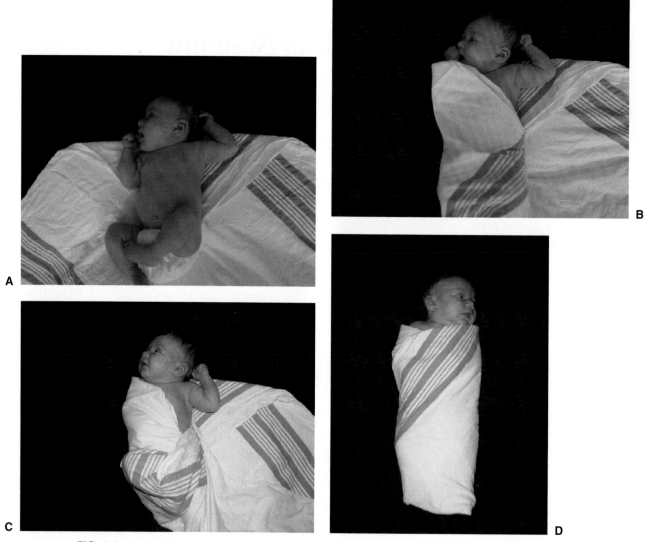

FIG. 4.1.   **A:** Mummy restraint: Steps (1)–(3). **B:** Mummy restraint: Step (4). **C:** Mummy restraint: Step (5). **D:** Mummy restraint: Step (6).

Extremity Restraints

1. Extremity restraint (wrist or ankle) (Fig. 4.3)
    a. *Purpose:* Immobilization of one or more extremities; protects infant from interfering with or removing treatment regimens (IV access, feeding tube, endotracheal tube, etc.)
    b. Equipment
        (1) Commercially available restraint (sheepskin and/or foam padding) for larger infants
        OR
        (1) Roll of gauze or gauze pads
        (2) Adhesive tape
        (3) Safety pins or other securing device
    c. Procedure
        (1) Open gauze and fold in half lengthwise to reinforce material.

        (2) Wrap wrist or ankle with gauze at least three times to create secure restraint. *Caution:* Do not wrap gauze too tight; this might interfere with distal circulation.
        (3) Use adhesive tape to ensure that gauze does not unravel.
        (4) Secure restraint to mattress, blanket, or light sandbag with safety pin.
2. Mitten Restraint
    a. *Purpose:* Thumbless device to restrain or cover hand; eliminate infant's ability to grasp and possibly dislodge necessary treatment regimens (IV access, feeding tube, endotracheal tube, etc.), prevent infant from scratching self or removing dressings, interfering with maintenance of skin integrity
    b. Equipment
        (1) Commercial mittens

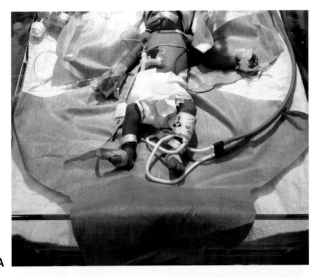

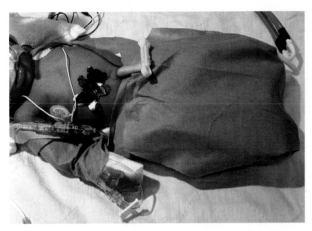

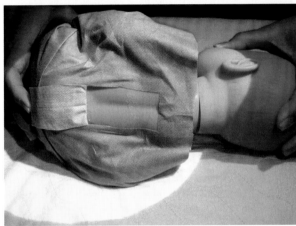

FIG. 4.2. **A, B:** Neowrapi: Wrap to immobilize arms and legs before placement of umbilical catheters (Patent pending; picture provided courtesy of M. Peesay, MD and C. Papageorgopoulos, BSN, RN). **C:** Lumbar Wrapi: wrap to immobilize baby prior to lumbar puncture (Patent pending; picture provided courtesy of M. Peesay, MD and C. Papageorgopoulos, BSN, RN).

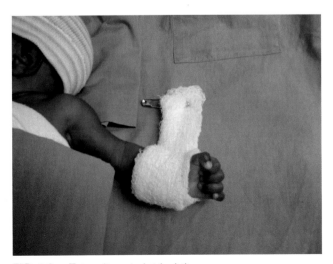

FIG. 4.3. Extremity restraint (wrist).

OR
- (1) Stockinette material (cut to fit individual infant)
- (2) Adhesive tape
- (3) Safety pins or other securing device (optional)

c. Procedure
- (1) Place infant's hand inside stockinette.
- (2) Secure stockinette by applying tape to stockinette material and fastening around infant's wrist. *Caution:* Do not wrap tape too tight; this might interfere with distal circulation.
- (3) Tie end of stockinette in order to isolate fingers inside the stockinette material.
- (4) Secure restraint to mattress, blanket, or light sandbag with safety pin (optional).

3. Elbow restraint (freedom splint) (Fig. 4.4)
   a. *Purpose:* Reduces ability of infant to flex elbow
   b. Equipment

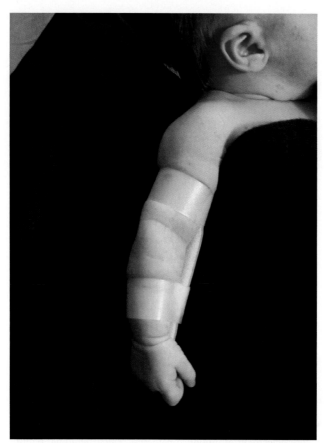

FIG. 4.4.   Elbow restraint.

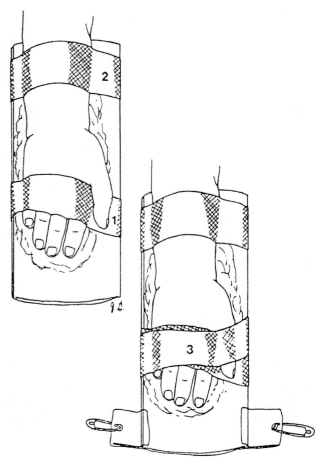

FIG. 4.5.   Restraint for vascular access—wrist and forearm. Tape is applied in order, 1 through 3, as shown.

    (1) Commercially available restraints (sheepskin and/or foam padding) for larger infants

OR

    (1) Foam-padded armboard
    (2) Adhesive tape
    (3) Additional padding material (i.e., cotton balls, gauze pads)

  c. *Procedure:*
    (1) Cut four pieces of tape (appropriate size; tape should not completely encircle extremity).
    (2) Extend upper extremity.
    (3) Place armboard under elbow to eliminate the ability to flex joint.
    (4) Tape extremity securely to armboard. Tape should be applied above and below elbow joint.
    (5) Pad bony prominences with cotton as needed.

Restraints for Vascular Access

Restraints can be used to secure IV access and prevent accidental dislodgement.

 1. Equipment
  a. Restraint device (i.e., armboard). Armboards vary in size; a larger infant may require an armboard that is 1 to 2 cm wider than the hand/foot and extends from the proximal joint to the distal joint. However, to maintain functional position and natural curvature of the hand at rest for long-term restraint, the armboard can be shorter in length to allow for curvature of fingers around the end of the board.
  b. *Adhesive tape:* Transparent tape is recommended for visualization of IV site especially during continuous infusion.
  c. Additional padding material (i.e., cotton balls, gauze pads)

 2. Procedure
  a. Ensure that the infant's extremity is in a developmentally appropriate position.
  b. Assess skin integrity where restraint is to be applied.
  c. Apply restraint board using transparent tape. Do not allow tape to encircle extremity. Three pieces of tape should sufficiently restrain the extremity and allow for visualization of the tips of fingers (Fig. 4.5) or toes (Fig. 4.6 A&B). The sequence of tape allows for functional positioning of thumb and ankle.
  d. Pad bony prominences and maintain natural curvature of extremities (especially the hand and fingers).

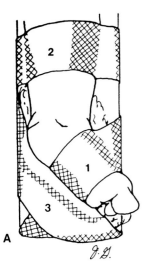

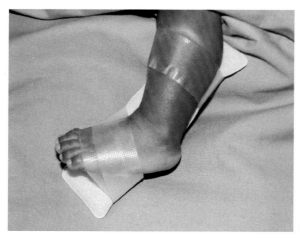

FIG. 4.6. A: Restraint for vascular access—foot and ankle. Tape is applied in order 1 through 3, as shown. B: Foot and ankle restraint for vascular access on premature infant.

E. Precautions

1. Restraints should be a last resort after other reasonable alternatives have failed, including close observation, treatment and/or medication change, modification of environment, etc. Document use of alternative methods (1).

2. For restraints during procedures, proper techniques for analgesia, sedation, and distraction (pacifier, touch, sound, etc.) may be necessary in addition to the restraint (2).

3. Developmentally supportive restraints may still be preferable to excessive use of sedative drugs (3).

4. Family education regarding the need, procedure, and time frame for the use of the restraint is required. Provide an opportunity for collaboration with the family. If possible, remove the restraints when the family is visiting (1).

5. Weigh equipment required for restraints (i.e., armboards) prior to use. If possible, maintain a list of the weights of common restraint materials in use when weighing infants for monitoring daily growth.

6. Evaluate the patient and proper use, placement, and position of restraint according to patient need, hospital policy, and regulatory agency requirement. Regulatory agencies such as the Joint Commission, the U.S. Food and Drug Administration (FDA), and the Centers for Medicare and Medicaid Services (CMS) publish standards of medical care regarding the safe use and legal requirements for restraint implementation and maintenance (1,4,5).

7. Ensure that the infant is in a proper and functional position that promotes flexion and midline positioning of upper and lower extremities.
   a. *Rationale:* Prevention of contractures and support of self-calming techniques of neonates (prone, side-lying) (Figs. 4.7 and 4.8) (4).

8. Pad bony prominences and maintain natural curvature of extremities (especially the hand and fingers)

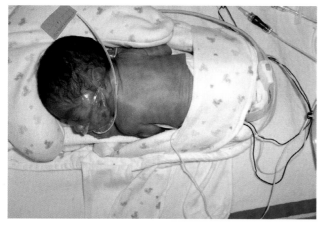

FIG. 4.7. Prone positioning during procedures and at rest provides for improved breathing and sleep, lower expenditure of energy, and more stable physiologic functioning. Care must be taken to create positioning support of the trunk and hips.

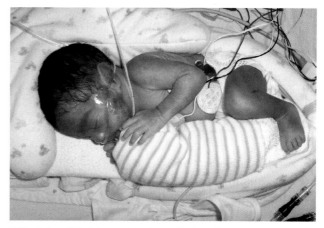

FIG. 4.8. Side-lying positioning is the best alternative to prone for procedures and sleeping. This position allows for more midline positioning of the upper and lower extremities. Nesting support increases postural stability and decreases arching of the back.

a. *Rationale:* Prevents contractures and neurovascular injury; preserves skin integrity; reduces friction and pressure to skin from restraint material (1)

9. When utilizing tape for securing an extremity to a board, use transparent tape when possible to allow for careful and complete assessment of the underlying skin. Do not apply tape too securely, as it may impede circulation. Tips of all digits should remain visible for assessment.

10. Restraints on the upper or lower extremities need to be assessed at least hourly (and/or according to hospital policy and regulatory agency requirement (the Joint Commission, CMS) for
    a. Skin Integrity, including excoriation, erythema, and edema
    b. Pulses
    c. Temperature
    d. Color
    e. Capillary Refill
    f. Range of Motion (ROM) (1)

11. Check for possible constriction by inserting a finger between infant's skin and the secured restraint (2).
    a. *Rationale:* Constriction from a tight restraint can cause neurovascular injury and impede circulation.

12. Specific assessments related to oxygenation, musculoskeletal system, and cardiorespiratory conditions need to be performed in relation to the restraint device and its usage (1).

13. Observe any treatment equipment for proper positioning and patency, especially in close proximity to the restraint device (kinked IV access, dislodgement of catheters, etc.) (1).

14. Attach restraint to a fixed location on bed (if necessary), maintaining the opportunity for quick release and regular vascular checks (safety pin, secure tucking, etc.). Do not attach restraint to equipment that can be moved (crib side rails, incubator doors), as injury may occur. Quick release allows for mobility and access in an emergency (1,2).

15. Document restraint use and, if required, obtain physician order (see hospital policy and/or regulatory agency requirement (the Joint Commission, CMS) (1,2).

16. Remove restraint at the earliest time possible.

F. Complications

1. Failure of restraint resulting in self-injury and/or interference with treatment
2. Neurovascular impairment (1)
3. Impairment of skin integrity (i.e., pressure ulcer formation, necrosis) (1)

4. Contractures or positional deformity/paralysis from prolonged immobility (1)
5. Limb injury (fracture or dislocation) from movement of infant without release of secured restraint or from securing restraint to movable object (e.g., crib side rails, isolette doors) (1)
6. Impairment or compromise of medical state, including oxygenation, musculoskeletal system, and cardiorespiratory conditions (1)
7. Increased agitation or irritability (1)
8. Extravasation injury leading to impairment of skin integrity, tissue necrosis, infection, and/or nerve and tendon damage (6)

G. Special Considerations

1. A temporary alternative to restraint usage during procedures is *therapeutic holding.* This is defined as the "use of a secure, comfortable, temporary holding position that provides close physical contact with the parent or caregiver for 30 minutes or less" (2). Staff must properly prepare the parent or caregiver and provide proper supervision throughout the procedure.

2. The American Academy of Pediatrics has outlined recommendations addressing infant sleep positioning to reduce the risk of sudden infant death syndrome. In terms of positioning the infant, they should be placed in a "supine position (wholly on their back)" (7). Therefore, when returning the patient to a sleep and/or recovery position following a procedure, health care professionals should endorse and model this behavior for parents and caregivers whenever possible.

References

1. Perry AG, Potter PA. *Clinical Nursing Skills and Techniques.* 7th ed. St. Louis: Mosby/Elsevier; 2010.
2. Hockenberry MJ, Wilson D. *Wong's Nursing Care of Infants and Children.* 9th ed. St. Louis: Elsevier Mosby; 2011.
3. Mathur AM, Neil JJ, McKinstry RC, et al. Transport, monitoring, and successful brain MR imaging in unsedated neonates. *Pediatr Radiol.* 2008;38:260.
4. Vergara ER, Bigsby R. *Developmental & Therapeutic Interventions in the NICU.* Baltimore: Paul H. Brookes; 2004.
5. The Joint Commission. *Comprehensive Accreditation Manual for Hospitals.* Chicago: The Joint Commission; 2012.
6. Ramasethu J. Prevention and management of extravasation injuries in neonates. *NeoReviews.* 2004;5(11):c491.
7. American Academy of Pediatrics. Policy Statement: The changing concept of sudden infant death syndrome: diagnostic coding shifts, controversies regarding the sleeping environment, and new variables to consider in reducing risk. *Pediatrics.* 2005;116(50): c1245.

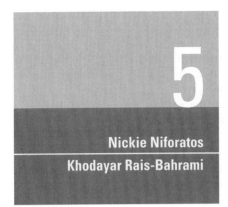

5

Nickie Niforatos
Khodayar Rais-Bahrami

Aseptic Preparation

A. Definitions

1. Antiseptic
   a. Bactericidal or bacteriostatic substance that can be safely applied to skin
   b. Not reliable as a sporicidal
   c. Reduces but does not eliminate bacterial counts on the skin
      (1) Has an immediate effect
      (2) Has variable residual activity by binding to the stratum corneum of the skin
2. Disinfectant
   a. Chemical germicidal substance
   b. Not reliable as a sporicidal
   c. Too harsh to be used on skin
3. Resident flora
   a. Organisms, usually of low virulence, which survive and multiply on skin and can be cultured repeatedly (e.g., *Staphylococcus epidermidis*)
   b. Cannot be completely eradicated without destroying the skin
   c. Regenerate rapidly on skin when surgical gloves are worn
4. Transient flora
   a. Organisms, occasionally pathogenic, but do not survive and multiply on skin (e.g., gram-negative organisms such as *Escherichia coli*)
   b. Can be transmitted to patients from the hands of health care workers
   c. Do not usually remain on the skin for more than 24 hours
   d. Can be eradicated completely by hand washing with antiseptic solutions

B. Background

Bloodstream bacterial infection is an extremely common complication of prematurity. The majority of etiologic pathogens are nosocomial, most often transmitted by health care personnel. Use of aseptic technique is critical in reducing the number of bloodstream infections as well as in decreasing the number of contaminated blood cultures, which in turn leads to a decrease in the unnecessary use of antibiotics and the potential for antibiotic resistance. Protocols and procedures for aseptic technique in neonatal intensive care units (NICUs) are constantly being re-evaluated and updated, and hand hygiene guidelines are routinely published by the U.S. Centers for Disease Control (CDC) (1,2). Hospital managers continuously develop and update strict policies and regulations (3) as well as quality improvement projects aimed to promote adherence to aseptic technique and hand hygiene (4).

C. Indications

1. Preparation of patient's skin and the hands of personnel prior to performing a procedure
   a. To remove transient flora
   b. To decrease and temporarily suppress most resident skin flora
2. Decontamination of hands after a procedure

D. Contraindications

1. Iodine solutions for preparation of skin in premature and low-birthweight infants (may cause skin and thyroid problems in high concentrations) (5)
2. Halogenated bisphenols (e.g., hexachlorophene) for preparation of skin in premature and low-birthweight infants (see E7), or used on burned or denuded skin of all infants
3. Hypersensitivity to halogenated bisphenols
4. Hypersensitivity to chlorhexidine
5. Chlorhexidine for preparation of external auditory meatus

E. Precautions

1. Universal (6,7)
   a. *Definition:* A method of infection control in which all human blood and certain human body fluids are treated as if known to be contaminated with HIV, hepatitis B virus, and other blood-borne pathogens.
   b. *Indications:* Reasonably anticipated risk of skin, eye, mucous membrane, or parenteral contact with

blood or other potentially infectious materials, including semen, vaginal secretions, cerebrospinal fluid, synovial fluid, pleural fluid, pericardial fluid, peritoneal fluid, amniotic fluid, saliva, and any body fluid that is visibly contaminated with blood.

c. Major components
   (1) Use gloves when touching blood, body fluids, mucous membranes, or nonintact skin and when handling items or surfaces soiled with blood or body fluids.

(2) Use a mask and eye protection during procedures that might generate splashing or droplets in the air.
(3) Use a gown or a plastic apron when splashing of blood or body fluid is likely.
(4) Wash hands carefully if they become contaminated with blood or body fluids.
(5) Take extraordinary care when handling needles and other sharp objects, and dispose of them in puncture-resistant containers.

TABLE 5.1 A Comparison of Commonly Used Antiseptics (8,9)

Considerations	Alcohol (70%–90%)	Iodine (1%)	Iodophor	Chlorhexidine	Hexachlorophene (3%)	Chloroxylenol (PCMX) (0.5%–3.5%)
1. Indications	Hand washing Skin preparation minor procedures Preparation of external auditory canal	Surgical hand washing Skin preparation	Surgical hand washing Skin preparation	Hand washing (4%) Skin preparation (0.5% in 70% alcohol)	Hand washing Use limited to term infants during epidemics of MRSA	Hand washing (active agent in antimicrobial soaps) Skin and wound disinfection
2. Effective concentration						
a. Nontoxic	Yes	Hypothyroidism	Hypothyroidism	Yes Local ototoxicity	CNS vacuolation	Yes
b. Nonsensitizing	Yes	No	Yes	Yes	Yes	Low
c. Nonirritating	Burns in preterm neonates	No	Yes	Yes	Yes	Yes
3. Mode of action	Protein denaturation	Oxidation	Oxidation	Cell wall disruption	Cell wall disruption	Cell wall disruption and enzyme inactivation
4. Bactericidal	Yes	Yes	Yes	Yes	No	Yes
5. May be used with detergent	No	No	Yes	Yes	Yes	Neutralized by nonionic surfactants
6. Persistent local action	No	Yes	Yes	Yes	Yes with repeated use	Yes
7. Effective against						
a. Gram-positive bacteria	Yes	Yes	Yes	Yes	Yes	Good (Strep > Staph)
b. Gram-negative bacteria	Yes	Yes	Yes	Yes	No	Fair
c. Spores	No	No	No	No	No	No
d. Tubercle bacillus	Yes	Yes	No	No	No	Fair
e. Viruses	Lipophilic only	Yes	Yes	Yes	Yes	Fair
f. Fungi	Yes	Yes	Yes	Yes	Yes	Fair
8. Use associated with resistance	No	No	No	Contamination	Yes	Ineffective against *Pseudomonas*
9. Rapid action	Yes	Yes	No (4–5 min)	Yes	No	Intermediate
10. Easily inactivated by extraneous organic matter	Maybe (inactivated by nonbacterial protein)	Yes	No (good for crevice and fat penetration)	No	Yes	Minimal

MRSA, methicillin resistant staphylococcus aureus; CNS, central nervous system; EDTA, ethylenediaminetetra-acetic acid; Strep, *Streptococcus* species; Staph, *Staphylococcus* species.

(6) Exclude from patient care all personnel with exudative lesions or weeping dermatitis until these conditions have resolved.

2. Recognize that no antiseptic is totally effective or without risk (Table 5.1).

3. Always allow antiseptics and disinfectants to dry before starting procedure.
   a. A drying time of at least 30 seconds is required for optimal effect (10).
   b. Contamination of instruments with antiseptic is undesirable and may invalidate specimens taken for culture.
   c. If hand disinfectants are not allowed to dry, alcohol-based disinfectant vapors can accumulate inside incubators (11).

4. Avoid removal of iodophor preparations prior to procedure. Removal negates the residual slow-release effect.

5. After the procedure, remove iodophor from all but immediate area of procedure to prevent absorption through skin (5,12,13).

6. Never allow antiseptic to pool under infant. Skin damage may result (14).

7. Use hexachlorophene for skin preparation in newborns only as recommended by the American Academy of Pediatrics (15).
   a. Use only in term infants during outbreak of *Staphylococcus aureus* infection if other infection-control measures have been unsuccessful.
   b. Wash off solution completely, and never use for routine bathing of infants.

8. Reapply alcohol prior to each attempt at procedure or with any delay, as efficacy is short-lived and flora will regenerate quickly.

9. Keep all antiseptics away from eyes.

10. Store antiseptics in closed containers. Reusable dispensers should be thoroughly cleaned, dried, and refilled frequently. Disposable containers are available.

11. Gloving cannot be used as an alternative to hand washing.
    a. The warm, wet skin surface under gloves offers an ideal environment for bacterial multiplication.
    b. Gloves are not completely impermeable to microorganisms.
    c. Latex and vinyl gloves offer comparable permeability, but vinyl gloves leak more readily.

F. Special Circumstances

1. In clinical situations where traditional hand-washing facilities are unavailable, such as during patient transport, alcohol-based hand rinses, foams, or wipes may be used for hand cleaning. When an alcohol solution is used, make three to five applications of 3 to 5 mL each and rub hands well until completely dry. Gloves should be used as otherwise indicated. This technique is not adequate when hands are soiled with organic matter.

2. In medical emergencies, aseptic technique should be used as allowed by the situation, with at least antiseptic skin preparation of the patient, use of gloves, and a sterile field as large as possible under the circumstances.

3. Personnel suffering from allergies to antimicrobial soaps may wash thoroughly for 3 to 5 minutes with plain soap or 70% isopropanol with glycerin prior to gloving (8).

4. Personnel suffering from skin cracking due to frequent use of antiseptic soaps may use moisturizing skin products or barrier creams after hand washing. Products with a bacteriostatic ingredient, such as gels containing 60% ethanol, and emollients are safe and effective in reducing skin problems (8). Containers with a flip top, rather than a screw cap, are recommended. Routine hand decontamination can be done with soap and water or alcohol-based hand rubs (8).

5. Non—latex-containing gloves should be available for staff with latex allergy and to avoid allergic reactions in the patient, particularly in susceptible patients such as those with myelomeningocele (16).

G. Technique (See Procedures Website for Video)

A 3- to 5-minute "scrub" (vigorous washing up to the elbows) is necessary when entering the nursery. Subsequently, a 15- to 30-second hand washing is indicated prior to and after each patient contact.

1. Preparation for a minor procedure
   a. Definition of a minor procedure
      (1) Short duration (5 to 10 minutes); noncomplex
      (2) Does not involve an area, such as the central nervous system (CNS), which is especially vulnerable to infection
      (3) Does not require skin incision
      (4) Includes blood drawing, placement of percutaneous peripheral venous line, bladder tap, punch-skin biopsy
   b. Preparation of personnel
      (1) Wear cap/beard cover if hair is likely to contaminate the field.
      (2) Remove all jewelry from hands and arms.
      (3) Wash hands, wrist, forearms, and elbows, using a small amount of antiseptic preparation (e.g., iodophor or chlorhexidine). Iodophor preparations appear to be equally effective when applied with disposable sponges or brushes. Vigorous scrubbing with a brush leads to skin breakdown and possible contamination and is contraindicated. Be sure to include between the fingers and the lateral surface of the fifth finger.
      (4) Clean nails with stick.
      (5) Wash/scrub hands and forearms to elbow with antiseptic for an additional 2 to 3 minutes.

(6) Rinse hands and forearms with running water, keeping them elevated above elbows.

(7) Use towel to shut off water if knee- or foot-operated faucets are not available.

(8) Dry hands with a clean towel prior to drying forearms.

(9) Wear gloves.

c. Preparation of patient skin

(1) If necessary, cut hair in area of procedure with small scissors, taking care not to nick skin. Avoid shaving, as it may compromise skin and increases the risk of infection.

(2) Apply antiseptic.

(a) Alcohol may be used. Preparation with iodophor may be optimal, but color tends to obscure underlying vessels.

(b) Apply three times in circles progressing away from procedure site.

(c) Apply with some friction.

(d) Allow to dry. Do not wipe off antiseptic.

(e) Never touch skin after application of antiseptic and before initiation of the procedure.

(f) If using alcohol, reapply it prior to every attempt at procedure.

2. Preparation for a major procedure

a. Definition of major procedure

(1) Invasive or involving skin incision

(2) Includes central line placement, cutdown, chest tube, lumbar puncture

(3) Duration longer than 5 to 10 minutes

b. Masks, drapes, and gowns. Clothing is an important barrier to microorganisms shed into the air from the skin and mucous membranes. Surgical masks and gowns must be registered by the FDA to demonstrate safety and efficacy (17).

(1) Put on cap and mask.

(2) Clean nails and "scrub" as for minor procedure, but continue for 4 to 5 minutes.

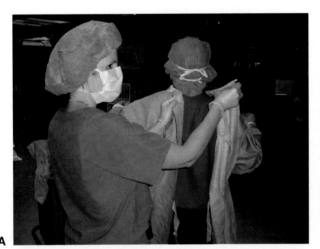
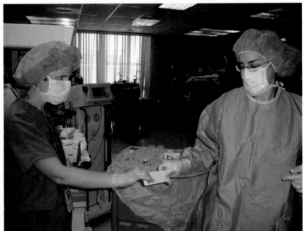
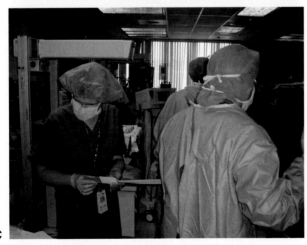
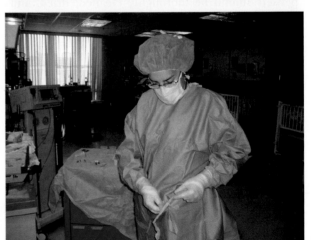

FIG. 5.1.   Correct technique for putting on a sterile gown. Operator is assisted into gown. **A:** The assistant pulls the gown up and back over the operator's shoulders by grasping the inside surface and ties the neck ties at the back of the operator's neck. **B:** Operator hands tip (protected with a removable cardboard tab) of sterile tie to assistant. **C, D:** Operator carries the tie around to the front where the operator takes tie (without the cardboard tab) and ties the gown.

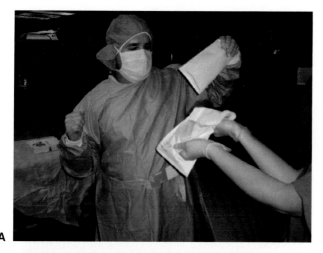

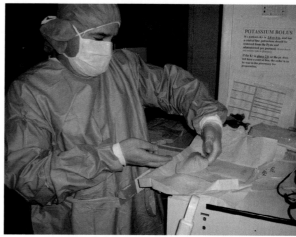

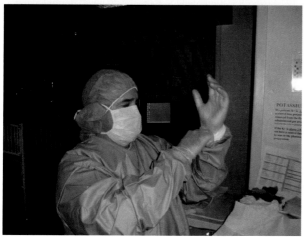

FIG. 5.2. Correct technique for putting on sterile gloves. **A:** Assistant has opened outer pack, allowing removal of uncontaminated inner pack by operator. **B:** Correct method for lifting second glove with gloved hand to avoid contact with skin as second glove is pulled up over sleeve ends. **C:** Pulling first glove up over sleeve ends. The inside surface of the glove is never touched by the gloved hand.

(3) Rinse forearms and hands, keeping them elevated above elbows.

(4) Dry hands and then forearms with *two sterile towels*. Keep wrists and hands elevated until drying is complete.

(5) Put on *sterile gown* with the aid of an assistant (Fig. 5.1).

(6) Put on *sterile gloves*, without contaminating external surface with ungloved hand (Fig. 5.2).

  (a) Have assistant open packet without contaminating contents.

  (b) Pull gloves well over sleeve ends.

c. Preparation of patient skin

(1) Prior to procedure, have assistant:

  (a) Wash area, if soiled, with soap and water.

  (b) If necessary, remove hair using small scissors, taking care not to nick skin. Do not shave the area.

(2) Apply antiseptic with three separate sponges. Start at center of circle, and work centrifugally to at least 5 cm outside immediate area of procedure. Alcohol (70%) should not be used. An

iodophor preparation is commonly used in nurseries in the United States.

(3) Allow antiseptic to dry. Do not wipe off antiseptic prior to procedure.

H. Complications

1. Dry skin caused by repeated use
2. Hexachlorophene
   a. Transcutaneous absorption with CNS vacuolation (8)
   b. Possible teratogenicity when used for hand washing by a pregnant staff member (18)
3. Iodine
   a. Burns
   b. Allergic contact dermatitis has been reported (19).
   c. Skin absorption/hypothyroidism (5,12,13)
      (1) A high incidence of transient neonatal hypothyroidism has been observed in premature infants in Europe after routine skin cleansing with iodine. The same high incidence has not been noted in North America. This difference in incidence may be due to the prior iodine status of the neonate.

4. Iodophor (5,12,13)
   a. Burns possible when allowed to pool under infant
   b. Absorption through skin reported in burn patients and neonates
   c. Alteration of thyroid function
5. Chlorhexidine
   a. Similarity in name and preparation has led to some confusion between chlorhexidine and hexachlorophene. These compounds are different in structure and properties (Table 5.1).
   b. Sensorineural deafness when instilled into middle ear; ocular toxicity with direct exposure to eye (20)
   c. Burns possible when allowed to pool under infant
   d. Absorption through skin and from umbilical stump (21). No associated pathology was documented.
   e. Contamination with gram-negative organisms has been reported, in particular *Pseudomonas* and *Proteus* species (22).
   f. There is no evidence that the detergent or alcohol preparations are susceptible to contamination.
6. Alcohol
   a. Burns in premature infants (23)
   b. Exposure to high concentrations of alcohol vapors in incubators (11)
7. Latex
   a. Allergy in operators
   b. Allergy in infants with neural tube defects (16)

References

1. Centers for Disease Control and Prevention. Guidelines for environmental infection control in health-care facilities. *MMWR Recomm Rep.* 2003;52(10):1.
2. Centers for Disease Control and Prevention [Internet]. 2011 Guidelines for the prevention of intravascular catheter-related infections. http://www.cdc.gov/hicpac/BSI/BSI-guidelines-2011.html. Accessed April 24, 2012.
3. Kilbride HW, Powers R, Wirtschafter DD, et al. Evaluation and development of potentially better practices to prevent neonatal nosocomial bacteremia. *Pediatrics.* 2003;111:504.
4. Pittet D. Improving adherence to hand hygiene practice: a multidisciplinary approach. *Emerg Infect Dis.* 2001;7:234.
5. Linder N, Davidovitch N, Reichman B, et al. Topical iodine-containing antiseptics and subclinical hypothyroidism in preterm infants. *J Pediatr.* 1997;131(3):434.
6. Siegel JD, Rhinehart E, Jackson M, et al; the Healthcare Infection Control Practices Advisory Committee 2007 Guideline for isolation precautions: preventing transmission of infectious agents in healthcare aettings. http://www.cdc.gov/hicpac/2007IP/2007isolationPrecautions.html. Accessed April 24, 2012.
7. Centers for Disease Control and Prevention. Recommendations for preventing transmission of human immunodeficiency virus and hepatitis B virus to patients during exposure-prone invasive procedures. *MMWR Recomm Rep.* 1991;40(8):1.
8. Boyce JM, Pittet D. Guideline for Hand Hygiene in Health-Care Settings: recommendations of the Healthcare Infection Control Practices Advisory Committee and the HICPAC/SHEA/APIC/IDSA Hand Hygiene Task Force. *Infect Control Hosp Epidemiol.* 2002;23(S12):S3.
9. Garland JS, Alex CP, Uhing MR, et al. Pilot trial to compare tolerance of chlorhexidine gluconate to povidone-iodine antisepsis for central venous catheter placement in neonates. *J Perinatol.* 2009;29(12):808. Epub 2009 Oct 8.
10. Intravenous Nurses Society. Intravenous nursing standards of practice. *J Intraven Nurs.* 1998;21:51.
11. Paccaud C, Vernez M, Berode N, et al. Hand-disinfectant alcoholic vapors in incubators. *J Neonatal Perinatal Med.* 2011;4(1):15.
12. Brown RS, Bloomfield S, Bednarek FJ, et al. Routine skin cleansing with povidone–iodine is not a common cause of transient neonatal hypothyroidism in North America: a prospective controlled study. *Thyroid.* 1997;7:395.
13. Kovacikova L, Kunovsky P, Lakomy M, et al. Thyroid function and ioduria in infants after cardiac surgery: comparison of patients with primary and delayed sternal closure. *Pediatr Crit Care Med.* 2005;6(2):154.
14. Wilkinson AR, Baum JD, Keeling JW. Letter to the editor: superficial skin necrosis in babies prepared for umbilical arterial catheterization. *Arch Dis Child.* 1981;56:237.
15. American Academy of Pediatrics, American College of Obstetricians and Gynecologists. *Guidelines for Perinatal Care.* 5th ed. Elk Grove Village, IL: American Academy of Pediatrics; Washington, DC: American College of Obstetricians and Gynecologists; 2002.
16. Majed M, Negat F, Khashab ME, et al. Risk factors for latex sensitization in young children with myelomeningocele. *J Neurosurg Pediatr.* 2009;4(30):285.
17. Sehulster L, Chinn RYW. Guidelines for Environmental Infection Control in Health-Care Facilities. Recommendations of CDC and the Healthcare Infection Control Practices Advisory Committee (HICPAC). *MMWR Recomm Rep.* 2003;52(RR10:1.
18. Check W. New study shows hexachlorophene is teratogenic in humans. *JAMA.* 1978;240:513.
19. Lee SK, Zhai H, Maibach HI. Allergic contact dermatitis from iodine preparations: a conundrum. *Contact Dermatitis.* 2005;52:184.
20. Brickwell PG. Sensorineural deafness following myringoplasty operations. *J Laryngol Otol.* 1971;85:957.
21. Agett PJ, Cooper LV, Ellis SH, et al. Percutaneous absorption of chlorhexidine in neonatal cord care. *Arch Dis Child.* 1981;56:878.
22. Wishart MM, Riley TV. Infection with *Pseudomonas maltophilia.* Hospital outbreak due to contaminated disinfectant. *Med J Aust.* 1976;2:710.
23. Upadhyayula S, Kambalapalli M, Harrison CJ. Safety of anti-infective agents for skin preparation in premature infants. *Arch Dis Child.* 2007;92:646.

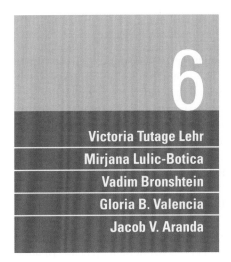

6

Analgesia and Sedation in the Newborn

Victoria Tutage Lehr

Mirjana Lulic-Botica

Vadim Bronshtein

Gloria B. Valencia

Jacob V. Aranda

A. Introduction

The American Academy of Pediatrics (AAP) Prevention and Management of Pain and Stress in the Neonate statement emphasizes the need for humane treatment of pain in infants (1). Historically, barriers to adequate pain management in neonates have been related to the question of pain perception in the newborn (2,3). This question is no longer debated and, in the past 25 years, great strides have been made in the assessment and management of pain in newborns (4). Procedural analgesia for neonates is well established (1,5–8). However, pain management and sedation practices continue to vary among practitioners (4,9–12). There is an overall paucity of pharmacokinetic (PK) and pharmacodynamic (PD) data for many analgesics and sedatives secondary to the varying infant gestational ages and weights. Studies in critically ill neonates are complicated by co-morbid conditions, genetic polymorphisms, complex drug regimens, and ethical issues (12–16). Neonatal pain management requires careful selection and dosing of medications, appropriate assessment and monitoring, and the ability to promptly recognize and manage adverse effects. Improvements in neonatal pain management have been driven by advances in the knowledge of developmental neurobiology, developmental pharmacokinetics and pharmacodynamics of analgesics; and the development of age-appropriate tools for pain assessment and of current best evidence in clinical practice for this vulnerable population (17–20).

This chapter offers general guidelines for the management of analgesia and sedation in newborn infants undergoing procedures that are frequently performed in neonates who require care in the neonatal intensive care unit (1,5–8,11). Selection of the optimal sedative for the management of stress in ventilated infants is less clear and is beyond the scope of this chapter (21,22).

B. Definitions

1. *Analgesia:* A condition in which nociceptive stimuli are perceived but not interpreted as pain; usually accompanied by sedation without loss of consciousness (23).

2. *Conscious sedation:* A medically controlled state of depressed consciousness that allows protective reflexes to be maintained, retains the ability to maintain a patent airway independently and continuously, and permits appropriate responses by the patient (1).

3. *Deep sedation:* A medically controlled state of depressed consciousness or unconsciousness from which the patient is not easily aroused. It may be accompanied by a partial or complete loss of protective reflexes and includes the inability to maintain a patent airway independently and respond purposefully to stimulation (1)

4. *Tolerance:* The ability to resist the action of a drug or the requirement for increasing doses of a drug, with time, to achieve a desired effect (23,24)

5. *Withdrawal:* The development of a substance-specific syndrome that follows the cessation of, or reduction in, intake of a psychoactive substance previously used or administered regularly (23)

6. *Neonatal abstinence syndrome:* Onset of withdrawal symptoms in neonates upon cessation of an agent associated with physical dependence (23,24)

C. General Indications

1. Any condition or procedure known to be painful (1,11,17) (see E)

2. Physiologic indications consistent with perception of pain (8,18–20)
   a. Tachycardia
   b. Tachypnea
   c. Elevated blood pressure (with secondary increase in intracranial pressure)
   d. Decreased arterial oxygen saturation
   e. Hyperglycemia secondary to hormonal and metabolic stress responses

3. Behavioral indications consistent with perception of pain (8,18–20)
   a. Simple motor responses (i.e., withdrawal of an extremity from a noxious stimulus)

b. Facial expressions (i.e., grimace)
c. Altered cry (primary method of communicating painful stimuli in infancy)
d. Agitation

D. Specific Indications

1. Analgesia
   In general, the potency of analgesic treatment selected should be related directly to the anticipated or assessed level of pain (1,7).
   a. Mild pain
      (1) Nonpharmacologic approaches (see H)
      (2) Local and/or topical anesthesia
      (3) Nonopioid analgesics (e.g., acetaminophen)
   b. Moderate and severe pain
      (1) IV opioid analgesics (see E)
      (2) Local and/or topical anesthesia
      (3) Benzodiazepines (see E)
2. Sedation
   Sedatives may be co-administered with analgesics to enhance the anticipated benefits. Because of the escalated risks associated with deep sedation, conscious sedation should be the usual clinical endpoint.
   a. Benzodiazepines (see E)
   b. Chloral hydrate (see E)
   c. Nonpharmacologic approaches (see H)

E. Precautions

1. Be aware, when assessing patients, that
   a. The clinical assessment of pain in the newborn is imprecise. The Neonatal Pain Agitation and Sedation Scale (N-PASS) was recently developed to assess ongoing pain, agitation and sedation levels in term and premature neonates (19). Neonatal pain scales vary in content, utility, reliability, and ease of use and include physiologic, behavioral, and contextural parameters (18–20,25) (see Appendix A.1).
   b. Physiologic and behavioral indicators of pain are nonspecific and may be related to many other factors.
      Ideally, a neonatal pain scale would be fast and easy to use; have reliability and validity for term, preterm, ventilated, and sedated neonates; be able to discriminate between other states (e.g., hunger); and account for confounding factors (e.g., medications, sepsis, cardiac disease) that may reduce the specificity of behavioral and physiologic responses. In reality, however, these scales show varying degrees of sensitivity and specificity (which markedly effects interpretation), a wide interrater variability of pain scores that can reduce the sensitivity, and behavioral responses of the preterm or neurologically impaired neonate (which can reduce the specificity of the pain assessment) (20).

c. Intubated neonates receiving muscle relaxants may have altered physiologic indicators and completely ablated behavioral indicators.
d. A high index of suspicion is required to identify newborn infants in pain (1,8,18).

2. Be aware, when medicating patients, that:
   a. There are numerous potential complications associated with analgesic and sedative agents (Appendix A.2) (26–28). Commonly used sedatives and analgesics for the pediatric patient are listed in Appendix A.2.
   b. Large inter- and intraindividual variations in response have been documented (26–30). In addition, data have been steadily accumulating on the PK/PD of sedatives and analgesics in the newborn (31–34). Neonates, especially premature neonates, have immature hepatic microsomal enzyme systems which mature over 3 to 6 months (15). Many drugs, including morphine, are metabolized by these systems; therefore, these neonates will have significant increases in half-life (>50%) compared with adults and older children for these agents (29,30). The glomerular filtration rate (GFR) is decreased during the first week of life, affecting the elimination of active metabolites of opioids (e.g., morphine) (29,30). Preterm infants will primarily produce the M3G metabolite of morphine, which has antianalgesic properties and a longer half-life compared with morphine (30). Neonates have a large percentage of body mass as water and a decreased plasma concentration of albumin and alpha-glycoprotein (12,15). These variables influence the PK/PD of sedatives, analgesics and concomitant medications, which may interact with these agents (34).
   c. Medications must always be titrated slowly (1,6–8,26).
   d. Co-administration of opioids, benzodiazepines, and other sedatives may result in greatly exaggerated respiratory depressant effects, including apnea (26). This combination requires a decrease in dosage of each medication.
3. Resuscitation equipment and medications should be immediately available. Be prepared to support ventilation and perform tracheal intubation if needed; respiratory depression is a common side effect of a number of analgesic and sedative agents (21).
4. Be aware that
   a. Newborn infants who have developed tolerance to a sedative or analgesic agent, by either direct or in utero exposure, may exhibit symptoms of the neonatal abstinence syndrome upon abrupt cessation of the drug or administration of the appropriate reversal agent (e.g., naloxone or flumazenil) (24,35). For example, naloxone administered to opioid-dependent neonates may precipitate acute, severe withdrawal symptoms (24).

b. Chronic analgesic therapy with agents known to induce tolerance, such as opioids, should be weaned gradually, with close monitoring for evidence of withdrawal symptoms. Administration of semisynthetic opioids, such as fentanyl, produces tolerance more rapidly in infants and young children compared with the natural opioids (35). Tolerance may be produced within 3 to 5 days with fentanyl, compared with 1 to 2 weeks for morphine (21,35). Fentanyl is frequently used in neonates undergoing very painful procedures because of its rapid onset of analgesia, hemodynamic stability, and ability to prevent pain-induced increase in pulmonary vascular resistance (21,35).

5. When using analgesics for a painful procedure
   a. Consider both the duration and the intensity of anticipated pain when selecting medications and methods. For example, short procedures with mild to moderate discomfort, such as lumbar puncture, may be best managed with topical and local anesthetics (1,5–8).
   b. Minimize the number of painful episodes. Multiple procedures performed at the same time may avoid the need for repeated administration of analgesics.
   c. Ensure that oxygen, suction, airway, resuscitation equipment, and reversal agents are readily available.
   d. Follow nothing-by-mouth guidelines for surgery.
   e. Have a nurse or other professional not involved in the procedure constantly monitor respirations, pulse oximetry, heart rate, and level of consciousness.

6. Chloral hydrate, is no longer regarded as a first-line, safe sedative for infants or young children (36–38). This agent should be used with caution in neonates (particularly premature neonates) secondary to the risk of hyperbilirubinemia and accumulation of toxic metabolites. For these reasons, a single dose only is recommended if other agents are not appropriate or available.

F. Advantages and Disadvantages of Commonly Used Agents in the Pediatric Patient

See Appendix A.2

G. Complications

See Appendix A.2

H. Nonpharmacologic Approaches

1. Swaddling and skin-to-skin contact during heel-stick procedures has been shown to reduce behavioral pain responses (1,6).
2. Nonnutritive sucking has been demonstrated to significantly reduce crying in response to painful stimuli (1,6).

3. Sucrose (1,6,8,39)
   a. Infants who drank 2 mL of a 12% sucrose solution prior to blood collection via heel stick cried 50% less than control infants during the same procedure.
   b. Infants who received sucrose on a pacifier prior to and during circumcision cried significantly less than control infants.
   c. 2 mL of 12% to 50% sucrose administered orally 2 minutes prior to the procedure is an effective neonatal analgesic with few adverse effects. However, there is one report of lower neurodevelopmental scores in preterm infants (n = 103; <31 weeks' gestational age) associated with repeated doses of sucrose for analgesia (39). The safe maximum dose of sucrose is unknown.

I. Contraindications

1. There are no absolute contraindications to using analgesia and/or sedation when deemed clinically appropriate.
2. Be aware of the potential side effects associated with the specific agent selected and take the proper precautions.

References

1. Lemons JA, Blackmon LR, Kanto WP, et al. American Academy of Pediatrics: Prevention and Management of Pain in the Neonate: An Update. http://aappolicy.aappublications.org/cgi/content/full/pediatrics;118/5/2231. Accessed August 7, 2011.
2. Anand KJS. Clinical importance of pain and stress in preterm neonates. *Biol Neonate.* 1998;73:1.
3. Anand KJS, Hickey PR. Pain and its effects in the human neonate and fetus. *N Engl J Med.* 1987;317:1321.
4. Simons SH, van Dijk M, Anand KS, et al. Do we still hurt newborn babies? A prospective study of procedural pain and analgesia in neonates. *Arch Pediatr Adolesc Med.* 2003;157:1058.
5. Tutag Lehr V, Taddio A. Practical approach to topical anesthetics in the neonate. *Semin Perinatol.* 2007;31:323.
6. Anand KJS, Johnston CC, Oberlander TF, et al. Analgesia and local anesthesia during invasive procedures in the neonate. *Clin Ther.* 2005;27:884.
7. Vitali SH, Camerota AJ, Arnold JH. Anaesthesia and analgesia in the newborn. In: Macdonald MG, Mullett MD, Sechia MMK, eds. *Neonatology: Pathophysiology and Management of the Newborn.* 6th ed. Philadelphia: Lippincott Williams & Wilkins; 2005:1557.
8. Mathew PJ, Mathew JL. Assessment and management of pain in infants. *Postgrad Med J.* 2003;79:438.
9. Porter FL, Wolf CM, Gold J, et al. Pain and pain management in newborn infants: a survey of physicians and nurses. *Pediatrics.* 1997;100:626.
10. McLaughlin CK, Hull JG, Edwards WH, et al. Neonatal pain: a comprehensive survey of attitudes and practices. *J Pain Symptom Manage.* 1993;8:7.
11. Barker DP, Rutter N. Exposure to invasive procedures in neonatal intensive care unit admission. *Arch Dis Child Fetal Neonatal Ed.* 1995;72:47.
12. Leeder JS. Developmental and pediatric pharmacogenomics. *Pharmacogenomics.* 2003;4:331.
13. Warrier I, Du W, Natarajan G, et al. Patterns of drug utilization in a neonatal intensive care unit. *J Clin Pharmacol.* 2006;46:449.
14. Anand KJS, Aranda JV, Berde CB, et al. Analgesia for Neonates: study design and ethical issues. *Clin Ther.* 2005;27:814.
15. Kearns GL, Abdel-Rahman SM, Alander SW, et al. Developmental pharmacology. *N Engl J Med.* 2003;349:1157.

16. Bjorkman S. Prediction of drug disposition in infants and children by means of physiologically based pharmacokinetic (PBPK) modeling: theophylline and midazolam as model drugs. *Br J Clin Pharmacol.* 2005;59:691.

17. Johnson CC, Collinge JM, Henderson SJ, et al. A cross-sectional survey of pain and pharmacological analgesia in Canadian neonatal intensive care units. *Clin J Pain.* 1997;13:308.

18. Stevens BJ, Pillai RR, Oberlander TE, et al. Assessment of pain in neonates and infants. In: Anand KJS, Stevens BJ, McGrath PJ, eds. *Pain in Neonates and Infants.* 3rd ed. Edinburgh: Elsevier; 2007:67.

19. Hummel P, Puchalski M, Creech SD, et al. Clinical reliability and validity of the N-PASS: neonatal pain, agitation and sedation scale with prolonged pain. *J Perinatol.* 2008;28:55.

20. Johnston CC, Stevens BJ, Yang F, et al. Differential response to pain by very premature infants. *Pain.* 1995;61:471.

21. Aranda JV, Carlo W, Hummel P, et al. Analgesia and sedation during mechanical ventilation in neonates. *Clin Ther.* 2005; 27:877.

22. Anand KJ, Barton BA, McIntosh N, et al. Analgesia and sedation in preterm neonates who require ventilatory support: results of the NOPAIN trial. Neonatal Outcome and Prolonged Analgesia In Neonates. *Arch Pediatr Adolesc Med.* 1999;153:331.

23. American Psychiatric Association. *Diagnostic and Statistical Manual of Mental Disorders.* 4th ed. text rev. Washington, DC: American Psychiatric Press; 2000.

24. Franck L, Vilardi J. Assessment and management of opioid withdrawal in ill neonates. *Neonatal Netw.* 1995;14:39.

25. McRae ME, Rourke DA, Imperial-Perez FA, et al. Development of a research-based standard for assessment, intervention, and evaluation of pain after neonatal and pediatric cardiac surgery. *Pediatr Nurs.* 1997;23:263.

26. Cote CJ, Karl HW, Notterman DA, et al. Adverse sedation events in pediatrics: analysis of medications used for sedation. *Pediatrics.* 2000;106:633.

27. Cote CJ, Notterman DA, Karl HW, et al. Adverse sedation events in pediatrics: a critical incident analysis of contributing factors. *Pediatrics.* 2000;105:805.

28. Morriss FG, Abramowitz PW, Nelson PS, et al. Risk of adverse drug events in neonates treated with opioids and the effect of a bar-code-assisted medication administration system. *Am J Health Syst Pharm.* 2011;68:57.

29. Barrett DA, Barker DP, Rutter N, et al. Morphine, morphine-6-glucuronide, morphine-3-glucuronide pharmacokinetics in new born infants receiving diamorphine infusions. *Br J Clin Pharmacol.* 1996;41:531.

30. Bhat R, Abu-Harb M, Chari G, et al. Morphine metabolism in acutely ill preterm newborn infants. *J Pediatr.* 1992;120:795.

31. Bjorkman S. Prediction of drug disposition in infants and children by means of physiologically based pharmacokinetic (PBPK) modeling: theophylline and midazolam as model drugs. *Br J Clin Pharmacol.* 2005;59:691.

32. Shah PS, Shah VS. Propofol for procedural sedation/anaesthesia in neonates. *Cochrane Database Syst Rev.* 2011;(3): CD007248.

33. Chana SK, Anand KJS. Can we use methadone for analgesia in preterm infants? *Arch Dis Child Fetal Neonatal Ed.* 2001;85:F79 doi:10.1136/fn.85.2.F79.

34. Jacqz-Aigrain E, Burtin P. Clinical pharmacokinetics of sedatives in neonates. *Clin Pharmacokinet.* 1997;36:449.

35. Frank LS, Vilardi J, Durand D, et al. Opioid withdrawal in neonates after continuous infusions of morphine or fentanyl during extracorporeal membrane oxygenation (ECMO). *Am J Crit Care.* 1998;7:364.

36. Lambert GH, Muraskas J, Anderson CL, et al. Direct hyperbilirubinemia associated with chloral hydrate administration in the newborn. *Pediatrics.* 1990;86:277.

37. Reimche LD, Sankaran K, Hindmarsh KW, et al. Chloral hydrate sedation in neonates and infants—clinical and pharmacologic considerations. *Dev Pharmacol Ther.* 1989;12:57.

38. Mayers DJ, Hindmarsh KW, Sankaran K, et al. Chloral hydrate disposition following single-dose administration to critically ill neonates and children. *Dev Pharmacol Ther.* 1991;16:71.

39. Johnston CC, Filinon F, Snider L, et al. Routine sucrose analgesia during the first week of life in neonates younger than 31 weeks postconceptual age. *Pediatrics.* 2002;110:523.

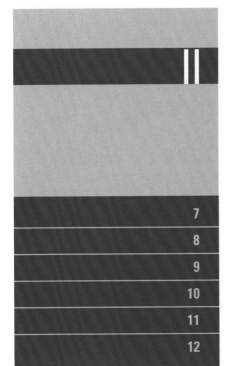

Physiologic Monitoring

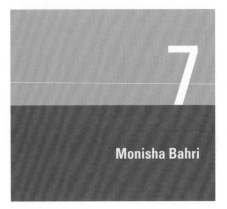

7

Temperature Monitoring

Monisha Bahri

Temperature measurement is an important part of normal newborn care. Accurate measurement is important to detect deviations from normal and also for optimal incubator and radiant warmer function.

The purpose of monitoring temperature is to maintain the infant in a thermoneutral environment zone. This is defined as the narrow range of environmental temperature in which the infant maintains a normal body temperature without increasing metabolic rate and hence oxygen consumption.

Temperature monitoring may be done intermittently or continuously. The site of measurement may be core (rectum, esophagus, or tympanic) or surface (skin, axilla). Although rectal temperature measurement remains the standard, the axillary route is preferred, especially for preterm neonates. The various methods are discussed further in this chapter.

Intermittent Temperature Monitoring

A. Equipment

1. Mercury-in-glass thermometer
   a. Benchmark standard
   b. Determination time >3 minutes.
   c. Risk of breakage/mercury poisoning from vaporized mercury (1).
   d. The American Academy of Pediatrics (AAP) recommends that mercury thermometers be removed from medical offices, medical facilities, and homes (1).
   e. No longer used in neonatal units
2. Electronic digital thermometers (Fig. 7.1)
   a. Most widely used
   b. Thermometer is a small hand-held device.
   c. Temperature sensor may be a thermistor or thermocouple.
   d. Temperature is sensed by the probe; the signal is then processed electronically and displayed digitally. There is an audible signal at the end of the determination time window.
   e. Determination time is <45 seconds.
   f. Resolution is 0.1°C.
   g. Probe-type electronic thermometers are designed to be used with disposable probe covers.

3. Infrared electronic thermometry
   a. Sensitive infrared sensor detects infrared energy radiation from the site of measurement (e.g., tympanic membrane for aural thermometers or skin sites over temporal artery, forehead, and axilla).
   b. The sensor converts the infrared signal to an electrical signal.
   c. Electrical signal is then processed and displayed digitally as temperature.
   d. Determination time is <2 seconds.
   e. Designed to be used with disposable sensor head covers.
   f. Cost-effective (2)

B. Limitations

1. Temperature measurements can vary from axillary sites depending on the environment (e.g., radiant warmer, open crib, or incubator) (3).
2. Axillary temperatures are usually significantly lower that rectal temperatures in newborns (mean ± SD, $0.27 \pm 0.20°C, p < 0.05$) (4)
3. Although speed and ease of operation with infrared thermometry may offer advantages over traditional clinical methods of temperature measurement, studies have failed to show an adequate correlation between infrared ear thermometer readings and rectal or axillary measurements in newborns (5,6). Infrared thermometry is not the preferred method in situations where precision in body temperature measurement is needed.

C. Precautions

1. Probe-type electronic thermometers
   a. Always use disposable probe cover.
   b. Do not force probe, as perforation can occur (e.g., in rectal measurement).
2. Infrared thermometers
   a. Always use disposable sensor head covers.
   b. Do not force sensor head into the ear canal.
   c. Do not use in infants with middle ear disease.
   d. Do not use in very low-birthweight infants because of inappropriate speculum size. Sensor head may

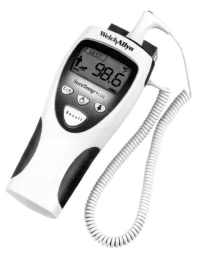

FIG. 7.1. Electronic thermometers: Probe thermometer. (Courtesy of Welch Allyn, New York, USA.)

not be small enough for low-birthweight infants weighing <1,000 g.
  e. Erroneous readings may result from
    (1) Not having the probe lined up with the tympanic membrane
    (2) The presence of heavy cerumen
    (3) The presence of serous otitis media (7)

D. Technique

1. Probe-type electronic thermometers
   a. Apply disposable probe cover to the probe.
   b. For core temperature, insert probe into the rectum (2 to 3 cm).
   c. For noninvasive approximation of core temperature, place the probe in the axilla (Fig. 7.2) (8–10).
   d. Hold the probe in place and wait for an audible beep before removing the probe.

  e. Read temperature and return the probe to its compartment to deactivate the unit.
2. Infrared thermometers
   a. Apply disposable cover to the sensor head.
   b. Gently insert tapered end into the ear canal.
   c. While holding the unit steady, depress the trigger.
   d. Remove from the ear canal and read temperature.
   e. Remove used disposable cover.

E. Complications

1. Inaccurate reading (11–14)
2. Tissue trauma
   a. Rectal or colonic perforation (11,15,16)
   b. Pneumoperitoneum (17)
   c. Peritonitis
3. Risk of trauma to the tympanic membrane
4. Thermometer housing unit can transmit infection; disinfect after each use.

Continuous Temperature Monitoring

A. Purpose

1. Provides reliable continuous monitoring of neonatal body temperature
2. Provides trend of temperature over time
3. Provides automated environmental control (Fig. 7.3)
4. Probes used for continuous core temperature monitoring may be used for servocontrol of cooling blankets in whole-body cooling protocols (Chapter 45).

B. Background

1. Sites used may be *surface* (e.g., skin over the abdomen) or *core* (e.g., rectum, esophagus).

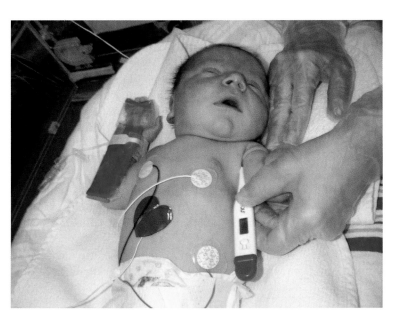

FIG. 7.2. Axillary temperature being taken with an electronic probe thermometer. The probe is held perpendicular to the patient, and the arm is held securely against the side of the chest.

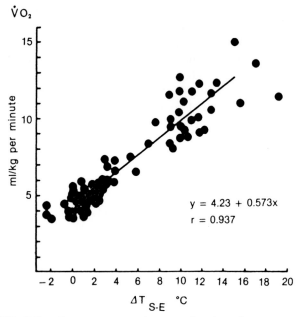

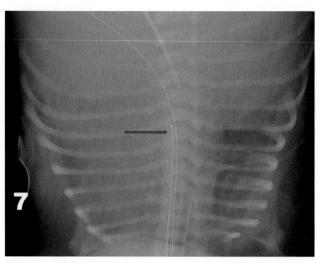

FIG. 7.4. Chest x-ray showing esophageal temperature probe, used for servocontrolling of cooling blanket in whole-body cooling protocol.

FIG. 7.3. Oxygen consumption as a function of temperature gradient between skin and environment. (From Adamsons K Jr, Gandy GM, James LS. The influence of thermal factors upon oxygen consumption of the newborn human infant. *J Pediatr.* 1965;66:495, with permission.)

2. Thermistor probes (most widely used)
   a. The thermistor is a resistive device, having a high negative temperature coefficient of resistance, so that its resistance decreases proportionately as the temperature increases.
   b. As the resistance of the thermistor changes, the electrical current flowing through the probe changes proportionally.
   c. The level of current detected by the electronic monitor is converted to thermal units.
3. Thermocouple probes
   a. The thermocouple probe is a very small bead made up of the junction of two dissimilar metals.
   b. The bead generates a very small voltage proportional to temperature.
   c. The voltage generated by the bead is measured by the monitor and converted to thermal units.
   d. The thermocouple and the thermistor are not interchangeable.
   e. Battery-powered interface devices are available that allow the use of thermocouple probes with thermistor-compatible monitors
   f. Thermocouple probes are less expensive than thermistors.

C. Indications

1. Continuous temperature monitoring and servocontrol for whole-body cooling (Fig. 7.4)

2. Automatic control of heater output of radiant warmer or incubator

D. Contraindications

1. Rectal route in tiny infants

E. Equipment Specifications: Hardware and Consumables

1. Continuous temperature monitoring may be a component of the bedside monitor, free-standing, or incorporated into a radiant warmer or incubator.
2. Capabilities of the neonatal temperature monitor should include:
   a. Resolution to 0.1°C
   b. Temperature display in both Fahrenheit and Centigrade
3. Most free-standing temperature monitors are battery-powered.
4. The monitors employ a thermistor or thermocouple.
5. Monitors using thermistors are identified as Yellow Springs Instrument Co.(YSI) 400- or YSI 700-compatible.
   a. YSI 400-compatible probes are single-element devices.
   b. YSI 700-compatible probes are dual-element devices.
   c. YSI 400 and YSI 700 probes are physically identical and are available in the same configurations but are electrically different and will not work interchangeably.
6. Monitors using thermocouple probes are identified as such, and the probe connection is different from the thermistor type.

TABLE 7.1	Site for Temperature Monitoring	
Site	**Range (°C)**	**Application**
Surface		
1. Abdomen over liver	36–36.5	Servocontrol
2. Axillary	36.5–37	Noninvasive approximation of core temperature
Core		
1. Sublingual	36.5–37.5	Quick reflection of body change
2. Esophageal	36.5–37.5	Reliable reflection of changes
	33.5	Target temperature in whole-body cooling protocols
3. Rectal	36.5–37.5	Slow reflection of changes
	34–35	Target temperature in head cooling protocols associated with mild systemic hypothermia

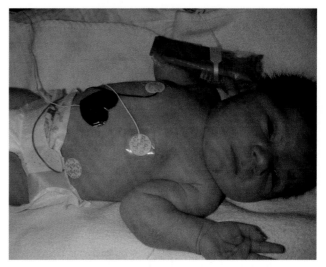

FIG. 7.5. Skin probe properly placed on infant (note that probe has protective foil cover and lies flat on the skin surface).

7. Probes for both thermistors and thermocouples are available in different configurations for different sites. For example:
   a. Surface skin probe
   b. Tympanic membrane thermocouple probe

F. Precautions

1. Do not apply skin probes to broken or bruised skin.
2. Do not apply skin probes over clear plastic dressings.
3. Do not use fingernails to remove skin surface probes.
4. Do not force core probes during insertion.
5. Do not reuse disposable probes.
6. Shield skin probe with reflective pad if used with radiant warmer or heat lamp.
7. When using servocontrol mechanisms for environmental control, take intermittent temperatures at other sites to monitor effectiveness (18,19).

G. Technique

1. Skin surface probe (Table 7.1)
   a. Prepare the skin using an alcohol pad to ensure good adhesion to the skin.
   b. Cover probe with a reflective cover pad (foil-covered foam adhesive pad, incorporated in the disposable probe) (Fig. 7.5). Probe must be covered with an aluminum foil disk to reflect back the added heat from devices such as radiant warmers, phototherapy lights, infrared warming lights, and any other external radiant heat-generating sources (20).
   c. Apply probe over the liver in the supine infant.
   d. Apply probe to the flank in the prone infant.
   e. Ensure that skin probe is free of contact with bed (Fig. 7.6).

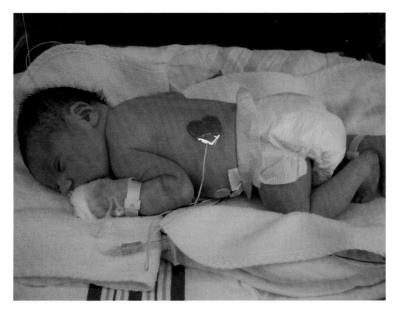

FIG. 7.6. Newborn infant with skin probe free of contact from bed surface.

TABLE 7.2 Potential Pitfalls of Servocontrolled Heating Devices	Skin << Core	Skin > Core	Skin > Core
Increased heater output	Cold stress Shock (vasoconstricted) Hypoxia Acidosis	Dislodged probe (early) Servo fails to shut off Vasodilators (e.g., tolazoline) Shock (vasodilated)	Dislodged probe (late) Servo fails (late)
Decreased heater output	Probe uninsulated (radiant heat)		
Servocontrol malfunction	Fever, overheating		
Internal cold stress	Unheated endotracheal oxygen, exchange transfusion		

Note: Changes in heater output may not be indicated; therefore, it is necessary to intermittently monitor the infant's core temperature (axillary optimal).

2. Application of core probe (Table 7.1)
   a. Choose probe size according to site (i.e., rectum or esophagus).
   b. Esophageal probe
      (1) Does not need lubrication prior to placement, but may need to be warmed to be more pliable prior to insertion.
      (2) Estimate the length of insertion needed to place the tip of the probe in the lower third of the esophagus. Subtract 2 cm from the sum of the distance from the mouth to the tragus of the ear and the distance from the ear to the xiphoid (Fig. 7.4).
      (3) Insert probe through nostril until the desired length is reached.
   c. Rectal probe
      (1) Lubricate probe before placing in rectum.
      (2) Probe should be placed approximately 3 cm beyond anal sphincter; further advancement will increase risk of perforation.
   d. Do not force either probe.
3. Connect the probe to the monitor.
4. Monitor energy output changes.
5. Reposition or replace the probe if temperature recorded does not correlate with that recorded using an electronic thermometer. Skin surface temperature will be cooler than core temperature.

H. Complications

1. Tissue trauma caused by core temperature probe
   a. Rectal or colonic perforation
   b. Pneumoperitoneum
   c. Peritonitis
2. Unsafe environmental temperature control caused by unshielded skin probes or loosely adhered probe, when monitoring is used to servoregulate temperature (Table 7.2)

References

1. AAP Committee on Environmental Health. Mercury in the environment: implications for pediatricians. *Pediatrics.* 2001;107:197.
2. Sganga A, Wallace R, Kiehl E, et al. A comparison of four methods of normal newborn temperature measurement. *MCN Am J Matern Child Nurs.* 2000;25:76.
3. Hicks MA. A comparison of the tympanic and axillary temperatures of the preterm and term infant. *J Perinatol.* 1996;16:261.
4. Hissink Muller PC, van Berkel LH, de Beaufort AJ. Axillary and rectal temperature measurements poorly agree in newborn infants. *Neonatology.* 2008;94(1):31. Epub 2008 Jan 4.
5. Craig JV, Lancaster GA, Taylor S, et al. Infrared ear thermometry compared with rectal thermometry in children: a systematic review. *Lancet.* 2002;360:603.
6. Siberry GK, Diener-West M, Schappell E, et al. Comparison of temple temperatures with rectal temperatures in children under two years of age. *Clin Pediatr (Phila).* 2002;41:405.
7. Weir MR, Weir TE. Are "hot" ears really hot? *Am J Dis Child.* 1989;143:763.
8. Haddock B, Vincent P, Merrow D. Axillary and rectal temperatures of full-term neonates: are they different? *Neonatal Netw.* 1986;5:36.
9. Stephen SB, Sexton PR. Neonatal axillary temperatures: increases in readings over time. *Neonatal Netw.* 1987;5:25.
10. Mayfield SR, Bhatia J, Nakamura KT, et al. Temperature measurements in term and preterm neonates. *J Pediatr.* 1984;104:271.
11. Greenbaum EI, Carson M, Kincannon WN, et al. Hazards of temperature taking. *Br Med J.* 1970;3:4.
12. Greenbaum EI, Carson M, Kincannon WN, et al. Mercury vs. electronic thermometers. *Health Devices.* 1972;2:3.
13. Weiss ME, Poelter D, Gocka I. Infrared tympanic thermometry for neonatal temperature assessment. *J Obstet Gynecol Neonatal Nurs.* 1994;23:798.
14. Ferguson GT, Gohrke C, Mansfield L. The advantages of the electronic thermometer. *Hospitals.* 1971;45:62.
15. Merenstein GB. Rectal perforation by thermometer. *Lancet.* 1970;1:1007.
16. Frank JD, Brown S. Thermometers and rectal perforations in the neonate. *Arch Dis Child.* 1978;53:824.
17. Greenbaum EI, Carson M, Kincannon WN, et al. Rectal thermometer-induced pneumoperitoneum in the newborn. *Pediatrics.* 1969;44:539.
18. Belgaumbar TK, Scott K. Effects of low humidity on small premature infants in servocontrol incubators. *Biol Neonate.* 1975;26:348.
19. Friedman M, Baumgart S. Thermal regulation. In: MacDonald MG, Mullett MD, Seshia MMK, eds. *Neonatology: Pathophysiology and Management of the Newborn.* 6th ed. Philadelphia: Lippincott Williams & Wilkins; 2005:445.
20. Dodman N. Newborn temperature control. *Neonatal Netw.* 1987;5:19.

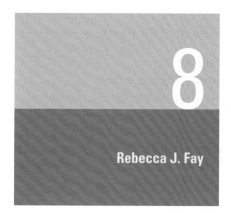

8 Cardiorespiratory Monitoring

Rebecca J. Fay

Cardiac Monitoring

A. Purpose

1. To provide reliable and accurate monitoring of neonatal cardiac activity
   a. Provide trends of heart rate over time
   b. Monitor beat-to-beat heart rate variability (1,2)
2. To allow assessment and surveillance of critically ill neonates
3. To provide early warning of potentially significant changes in heart rate by identification of heart rates above or below preset alarm limits
4. To identify bradycardia (with or without associated apnea) in at-risk infants

B. Background

1. Electrical activity of the heart is detected using impedance technology through skin surface electrodes (3).
2. The low-level electrical signal is amplified and filtered to eliminate interference and artifacts.
3. The electrical signal, defined in millivolts, is displayed as an electrocardiogram (ECG) tracing.
4. R-wave detection from the QRS complex is used to calculate heart rate.
5. The typical three-lead configuration (i.e., leads I, II, III) provides alternative vectors for ECG analysis.

C. Contraindications

None

D. Limitations

1. The three-lead ECG is most useful for long-term continuous cardiac monitoring; more detailed cardiac evaluation (i.e., assessment of hypertrophy or axis) or the identification of abnormal cardiac rhythms may require complete 12-lead ECG with rhythm strip.
2. Close proximity of electrodes in extremely small infants may cause difficulty with signal detection.

E. Equipment

Hardware—Specifications

1. The monitoring system should have the appropriate frequency response and sensitivity to track the fast and narrow QRS complex of the neonate accurately.
2. Heart rate is processed on a beat-to-beat basis with a short updating interval.
3. Default heart rate alarm limits should be tailored to the neonatal population.
   a. Low heart rate (bradycardia) limit of 100 beats/min (Note: Some term infants may have resting heart rates of 80 to 100 beats/min, requiring lower bradycardia alarm settings.)
   b. High heart rate (tachycardia) limit of 175 to 200 beats/min
4. Monitor displays
   a. Cathode-ray tube (CRT)
      (1) Has highest resolution and best definition
      (2) Display can be either color or monochrome
   b. Liquid-crystal display (LCD)
      (1) Flat, thin display monitor
      (2) Resolution may be suboptimal for fast and narrow QRS complex of neonate
      (3) Back-lighting is necessary for viewing in low-light environments
      (4) Unlike CRT, viewing angle is critical
5. Heart rate displayed as alphanumeric part of waveform display or in a separate numerical display window
6. Recorder (optional)
   a. Electronic memory
      (1) Real-time ECG
      (2) Delayed ECG—stored retrospective display used primarily for review of a short time interval prior to the occurrence of an alarm
   b. Printed record of ECG trend information
      (1) Typically used to document selected segments of ECG tracings such as periods associated with alarms or abnormal rhythms
      (2) Monitors may have dedicated printers (often integrated into monitor cases)

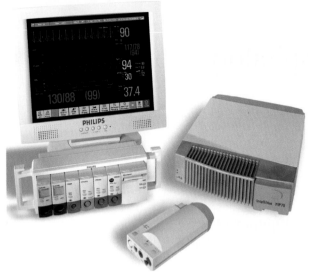

FIG. 8.1. Typical multiparameter neonatal bedside monitor. (Courtesy of Philips Medical Systems.)

(3) Central monitoring stations can provide remote access to information from all networked monitor units with printing capabilities.

7. Units available for both bedside and transport monitoring (Figs. 8.1 and 8.2)
   a. Transport monitors typically smaller and battery-powered
   b. Similar capabilities regarding parameter availability, but monitor-specific

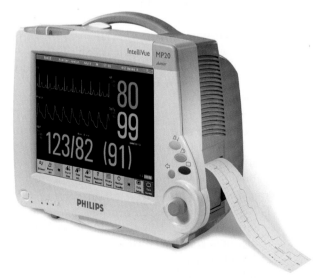

FIG. 8.2. Typical multiparameter neonatal transport monitor with integrated printer. (Courtesy of Philips Medical Systems.)

Consumables—Specifications

1. Disposable neonatal ECG electrodes
   a. Silver–silver chloride electrodes are available in a variety of forms designed specifically for the neonatal population.
      (1) Patient contact surfaces of electrodes are coated in adhesive electrolyte gel, which acts as conductive medium between the patient and the metal lead while preventing direct patient contact with the metal.
      (2) Typical commercially available neonatal leads incorporate silver–silver chloride electrodes directly onto paper, foam, or fabric bodies with integrated lead wires.
      (3) Less commonly, adhesive electrode pads are separate from lead wires, which connect to the electrodes via clips.
      (4) ECG limb plate electrodes may be used rarely, when the application of chest leads would interfere with resuscitation or the performance of other procedures. Use of electrode gel as a conductor at the skin interface (rather than alcohol pads) is imperative in such cases.
   b. Characteristics to consider in electrode selection:
      (1) Adherence to skin of an active infant
      (2) Quality of signal attained
      (3) Minimal skin irritation
      (4) Ease of removal using water or adhesive remover without damage to or removal of skin
      (5) Performance in the warm, moist environment of an infant incubator
      (6) Adhesive–skin interaction under overhead infant warmers
2. Lead wires and patient cable
   a. All cables should be clean and the insulation should be free of nicks or cuts.
   b. Lead wires should lock or snap into the patient cable, preventing easy disconnections.
   c. If using electrodes that attach via clips, use infant/pediatric lead wires with small electrode clips—standard adult-size clips will place too much torsion on the infant electrode, tugging on the skin and possibly peeling off the electrode.

F. Precautions

1. Do not leave alcohol wipes under electrodes as conductors.
2. Do not apply electrodes to broken or bruised skin.
3. Avoid placing electrodes directly on the nipples.
4. Select the smallest appropriate/effective electrode for patient monitoring to minimize skin exposure and limit potential complications from irritation/adhesives.
5. Do not apply electrodes to clear film plastic dressings—dressing will act as an insulator between the skin and the electrode.

6. To avoid skin damage, do not use fingernails to remove electrodes.
7. Secure the patient cable to the patient's environment to prevent excessive traction.
8. Use only monitors that have been checked for safety and performance—usually indicated by a dated sticker on the monitor.
9. Do not use monitors with defects such as exposed wires, broken or dented casing, broken knobs or controls, or cracked display.
10. Monitor alarms should prompt immediate patient assessment.
    a. Note alarm indication (i.e., tachycardia or bradycardia).
    b. Treat patient condition as necessary or correct the source of any false alarm.
    c. If alarm is silenced or deactivated during the course of patient evaluation, it should be reactivated prior to leaving the patient's bedside.

G. Techniques

1. Familiarize yourself with the monitor prior to beginning.
2. *Electrode and lead wire placement:* Although you should refer to the monitor manufacturer's placement instructions, general electrode placement guidelines follow.
    a. *Skin preparation:* Skin should be clean and dry to provide the best electrode-to-skin interface.
        (1) Wipe skin with an alcohol pad and allow to dry thoroughly.
        (2) Avoid the use of tape to secure electrodes—for optimal performance and proper electrical interface, electrodes must adhere directly to skin.
    b. Basic three-lead configuration for electrode placement (for electrodes with integrated lead wires) (Fig. 8.3)
        (1) *Right arm (white):* Right lateral chest at level of the nipple line
        (2) *Left arm (black):* Left lateral chest at level of the nipple line
        (3) *Left leg (red or green):* Left lower rib cage
        (4) Although this configuration allows the use of the same electrodes to monitor both ECG and respiration, optimal ECG signal may be obtained when the right arm lead is at the right midclavicle and the left leg lead is at the xiphoid (4).
    c. If not using electrodes with integrated wires, place electrode pads in basic three-lead configuration as above, then connect lead wires via electrode clips.
        (1) White lead (right arm) to right chest electrode
        (2) Black lead (left arm) to left chest electrode
        (3) Red or green lead (left leg) to left lower rib cage electrode

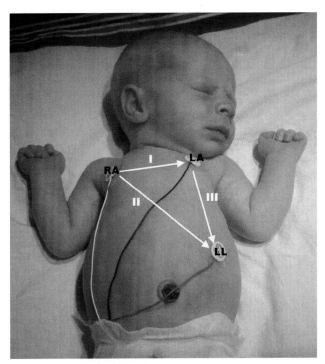

FIG. 8.3. Basic electrode placement and lead vectors for optimal ECG signal detection. Right arm/left arm positions also provide maximal signal for impedance pneumography.

3. Turn monitor on—most monitors will conduct an automatic self-test.
4. Connect the patient cable to the monitor.
5. Select the lead that provides the best signal and QRS size (lead II is usual default) (Fig 8.4).
    a. Ensure that heart rate correlates to QRS complexes seen on display—make sure that the QRS detector is not counting high or peaked T or P waves.
6. Verify that low and high heart rate alarms are set appropriately.

H. Complications

1. Skin lesions (rare)
    a. Irritation from alcohol—may occur with even short-term application to immature skin
    b. Trauma caused by rubbing with excessive vigor during skin preparation
    c. Irritation from incorrectly formulated electrode gel
    d. Secondary effects of skin breakdown
        (1) Cellulitis or abscess formation
        (2) Increased transepidermal water losses
        (3) Hypo- or hyperpigmented marks at sites of prior irritation or inflammation (Fig. 8.5)
2. Erroneous readings caused by artifacts (5) (Table 8.1)
    a. Electrical interference
        (1) Sixty-cycle electrical interference (frequency of typical power lines)

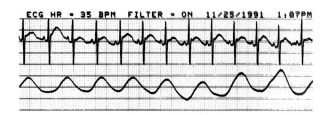

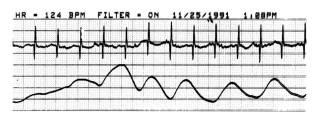

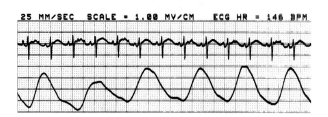

FIG. 8.4. Typical ECG tracings: Lead I (top), lead II (middle), and lead III (bottom).

(2) Interference from other equipment used in the patient's immediate environment

(3) Electrical spike may be generated when certain types of polyvinyl chloride tubing are mechanically deformed by infusion pump devices—spikes appear as ectopic beats on the monitor (rare) (6).

    b. Decreased signal amplitude with motion artifact

    c. Poor electrode contact or dried electrode gel

    d. Incorrect vectors because of inaccurate lead placement (Fig. 8.6)

    e. Inappropriate sensitivity settings

3. Monitor or cable failure

    a. Hardware or software failure

    b. Cable disconnection

4. Alarm failure

    a. False alarms (either tachycardia or bradycardia) resulting from inaccurate interpretation of heart rate

    b. Inappropriate alarm parameters for patient

Respiratory Monitoring

A. Purpose

1. Reliable and accurate monitoring of neonatal respiratory activity

    a. Trending of respiratory activity over time

    b. Detection of apnea

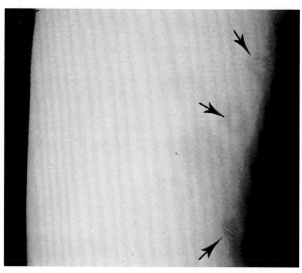

FIG. 8.5. Residual hyperpigmented marks on the extremities present more than 1 year after application of ECG leads for cardiorespiratory monitoring.

2. Assessment and surveillance of critically ill neonates

3. To provide early warning of potentially significant changes in respiratory rate by identifying respiratory rates above or below preset alarm limits

B. Background

1. Measurement of transthoracic impedance is the most commonly used method for determining respiratory rate (7).

    A low-level, high-frequency signal is passed through the patient's chest via surface electrodes.

TABLE 8.1	Steps to Minimize Artifact Interference

Problem	Treatment
Poor electrode contact/ connection	1. Gently clean skin with alcohol wipe and allow to dry prior to electrode reapplication. 2. Check electrode/cable connections.
Dried electrode	Replace
Equipment interference	1. Systematically turn off one piece of adjacent equipment at a time while observing monitor for improvement in signal quality. 2. After source of interference is identified, increase distance between that equipment and patient while rerouting power cords and cables as necessary. 3. If above maneuver is unsuccessful, replace equipment.
60-Hz interference	1. Follow procedure for poor electrode contact. 2. Replace patient cable. 3. If 1 and 2 are unsuccessful, try an alternate monitor.

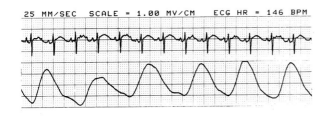

25 MM/SEC SCALE = 1.00 MV/CM ECG HR = 146 BPM

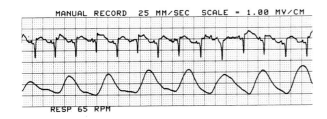

MANUAL RECORD 25 MM/SEC SCALE = 1.00 MV/CM

RESP 65 RPM

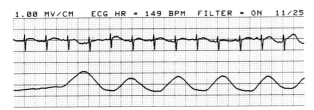

1.00 MV/CM ECG HR = 149 BPM FILTER = ON 11/25

FIG. 8.6. Normal P-, QRS-, and T-wave detection. **Top:** Lead II tracing with electrodes properly placed. Note normal P-, QRS-, and T-wave detection. **Middle:** Lead II tracing with electrodes close together on anterior chest wall. Note altered QRS- and decreased T-wave amplitude. **Bottom:** Lead II tracing with electrodes placed lateral on the abdomen. Note decreased wave amplitude and flattened P wave.

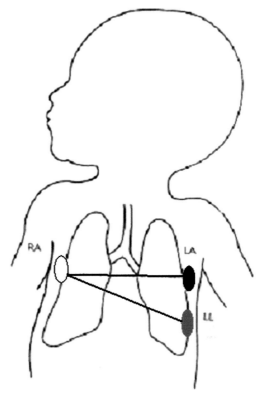

FIG. 8.7. Transthoracic impedance pneumography: Diagrammatic representation of the path of the high-frequency signal between chest wall electrodes. Most monitors transmit signal right arm (white) → left arm (black), less commonly right arm (white) → left leg (red).

(1) Typically utilizes the same electrodes as are used for cardiac monitoring

(2) Signal path usually from right arm (white) to left arm (black) electrodes, although some monitors may use right arm (white) to left leg (red or green) (Fig. 8.7)

b. Impedance to the high-frequency signal is measured.

(1) Impedance is the electrical resistance to the signal.

(2) Changes in lung inflation cause an alteration in the density of the chest cavity, which is detected as a change in impedance.

(3) Changes in impedance modulate a proportional change in the amplitude of the high-frequency signal.

c. The change in impedance, as seen by the modulation of the high-frequency signal, is detected and quantified by the monitor and recorded as breaths per minute.

d. The monitor has an impedance threshold limit below which changes in impedance are not counted as valid respiratory activity—cardiac pumping with associated changes in pulmonary blood flow will also cause changes in thoracic impedance (usually much smaller changes than those associated with respiration).

C. Contraindications

None

D. Equipment

Hardware—Specifications

1. Equipment is the same as that for cardiac monitoring; multiparameter monitors incorporate both cardiac and respiratory monitoring into single units.

2. Respiratory monitoring parameters

a. Low-level threshold (for impedance) for breath validation should not be below 0.2 to minimize cardiogenic artifact.

b. Coincidence alarm with rejection applies when respiratory rate being detected is equal to the heart rate activity being detected by the cardiac portion of the system.

c. Default limits should be tailored to the neonatal population.

(1) Adjustable apnea time-delay setting (length of apnea in seconds before alarming)

(2) Typical apnea time delay is 15 to 20 seconds.

Consumables—Specifications

Same as for cardiac monitor

E. Precautions

1. Include previously discussed precautions for cardiac monitoring

2. Muscular activity may be interpreted as respiration, resulting in failure to alarm during an apneic episode (see G3a following).

F. Technique

1. Same as for cardiac monitor

2. Ensure that the respiratory waveform correlates to the true initiation of inspiration.

3. Move right and left arm electrodes up toward the axillary area if detection of respiration is poor due to shallow breathing.

4. Set desired low and high respiratory rate and apnea delay alarm limits.

G. Complications

1. Skin lesions (see H1 under Cardiac Monitoring)

2. Monitor or cable failure
   a. Hardware or software failure
   b. Cable disconnection

3. Alarm failure
   a. False-positive "respiratory" signal in the absence of effective ventilation
      (1) Chest wall movement with airway obstruction (obstructive apnea)
      (2) Nonrespiratory muscular action (i.e., stretching, seizure, or hiccups) producing motion artifact (Fig. 8.8)
   b. False apnea alarm despite normal respiratory activity
      (1) Improper sensitivity not detecting present respiratory activity
      (2) Incorrect electrode placement
      (3) Loose electrodes
   c. Inappropriate alarm parameters for patient

4. Accurate assessment of respiratory rate not practical when using high-frequency ventilatory modes

Cardiorespirograph Monitoring

A. Definition

1. Graphical representation of heart rate and respiratory rate over time

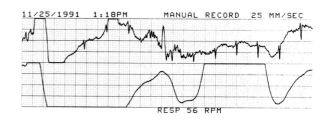

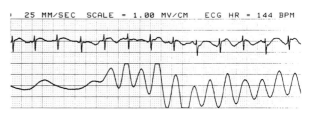

FIG. 8.8.   Tracings of artifacts affecting ECG/respiratory tracings. **Top:** Loose electrode affected by motion. **Bottom:** Motion artifact caused by patient's moving arm coming in contact with chest electrodes (note change in respiratory frequency signal).

B. Purpose

1. Monitoring of infants for identification and quantification of heart rate and respiratory activity, with detection of apnea, periodic breathing, and bradycardia

2. Identification of chronologic relationships between bradycardia and apnea

3. Many systems also provide continuous S_aO_2 information to allow correlation with desaturation events.

C. Background

1. Heart rate is plotted graphically as beats per minute (*y*-axis) versus time (*x*-axis).

2. Respiratory waveform is compressed to allow display of time range.

3. Short-term trending allows constant updating as the oldest information is displaced (typically based on a 2-minute window of time).

4. Time relationship between heart rate and respiratory activity is maintained.
   a. Allows for visualization of entire apneic episodes and identification of precipitating factors (e.g., a drop in respiratory rate may precede bradycardia)

5. Inclusion of S_aO_2 allows identification of temporal relationship for desaturation events (S_aO_2 is plotted in the same fashion as the heart rate on a second *y* axis)

D. Contraindications

None

E. Equipment
Standard features of most neonatal monitors

Emerging Technologies

A. Background
Given the known limitations and potential complications of current methods for cardiac/respiratory monitoring in neonates (i.e., ECG and impedance technologies), research continues to find alternate techniques for monitoring with similar or improved reliability.

B. Techniques under Review
1. Wireless monitoring using photoplethysmography (8)
   a. Utilizes optical probe to detect/record heart and/or respiratory rates
   b. Can eliminate the need for skin electrodes and wires utilizing abdominal belt/band and electronic data receiver
   c. Preliminary data suggest similar data reliability to traditional electrode-based cardiac/respiratory monitoring systems
2. Piezoelectric transducer sensors (9)
   a. Sensors placed in proximity to infant (i.e., under infant) detect an acoustic cardiorespiratory signal from which heart rate and breathing rate are calculated.
   b. Minute movements made by the body are monitored via a transducer that converts the body movements into electrical signals to report the presence or absence of respiration and normal heart rate.
   c. Preliminary data suggest the noninvasive device avoids skin irritation while providing accurate monitoring.
3. May be affected by "noise" from nearby equipment

C. Implications
Although preliminary reports regarding such alternative monitoring devices are encouraging, additional research regarding reliability and safety will be required before such applications gain widespread acceptance.

The views expressed in this article are those of the author(s) and do not necessarily reflect the official policy or position of the Department of the Navy, Department of Defense, or the United States Government.

I am a military service member. This work was prepared as part of my official duties. Title 17 U.S.C. 105 provides that 'Copyright protection under this title is not available for any work of the United States Government.' Title 17 U.S.C. 101 defines a United States Government work as a work prepared by a military service member or employee of the United States Government as part of that person's official duties.

The monitoring of vital signs in neonates provides an important indicator of overall well-being. Progress in computer technology has facilitated the development of bedside monitors that can integrate multiple monitoring parameters into a single system. This chapter covers the fundamentals of cardiac and respiratory monitoring.

References

1. Cabal LA, Siassi B, Zanini B, et al. Factors affecting heart rate variability in preterm infants. *Pediatrics.* 1980;65:50.
2. Valimaki IA, Rautaharju PM, Roy SB, et al. Heart rate patterns in healthy term and premature infants and in respiratory distress syndrome. *Eur J Cardiol.* 1974;1:411.
3. Di Fiore JM. Neonatal cardiorespiratory monitoring techniques. *Semin Neonatol.* 2004;9:195.
4. Baird TM, Goydos JM, Neuman MR. Optimal electrode location for monitoring the ECG and breathing in neonates. *Pediatr Pulmonol.* 1992;12:247.
5. Jacobs MK. Sources of measurement error in noninvasive electronic instrumentation. *Nurs Clin North Am.* 1978;13:573.
6. Sahn DJ, Vaucher YE. Electrical current leakage transmitted to an infant via an IV controller: an unusual ECG artifact. *J Pediatr.* 1976;89:301.
7. Hintz SR, Wong RJ, Stevenson DK. Biomedical engineering aspects of neonatal monitoring. In: Martin RJ, Fanaroff AA, Walsh MC, eds. *Fanaroff and Martin's Neonatal-Perinatal Medicine: Diseases of the Fetus and Infant.* 8th ed. Philadelphia: Mosby; 2006:609.
8. Adu-Amankwa NA, Rais-Bahrami K. Wireless Cardio Respiratory Monitor for Neonates. Abstract presentation at American Academy of Pediatrics National Conference & Exhibition October 1, 2010.
9. Sato S, Ishida-Nakajima W, Ishida A, et al. Assessment of a new piezoelectric transducer sensor for noninvasive cardiorespiratory monitoring of newborn infants in the NICU. *Neonatology.* 2010; 98(2):179.

Blood Pressure Monitoring

M. Kabir Abubakar

Accurate blood pressure (BP) monitoring is essential for the optimal management of critically ill infants in intensive care. The recognition and treatment of abnormal BP states has significant prognostic implication (1–4). Successful BP monitoring should be easy to set up, reliable, and give continuous information or enable measurements to be made at frequent intervals with minimal disturbance to the baby. Neonatal BP monitoring may be performed by noninvasive or invasive methods.

Noninvasive (Indirect) Methods

Noninvasive BP measurement can be done using

1. Auscultatory measurement (manual noninvasive) or
2. Oscillatory arterial BP measurement (automatic noninvasive)

Auscultatory Measurement (Manual Noninvasive)

Utilized for intermittent BP measurements; is simple and inexpensive.

A. Background

1. This technique uses a BP cuff, insufflator, manometer, and stethoscope.
2. The sphygmomanometer uses a pneumatic cuff to encircle the upper arm or leg and a pressure gauge (manometer) to register the pressure in the cuff.
3. There are two types of manometers
   a. Mercury (mercury column)
   b. Aneroid (mechanical air gauge)
4. The encircling pneumatic cuff is inflated to a pressure higher than the estimated systolic pressure in the underlying artery. The cuff pressure compresses the artery and stops blood flow.
5. A stethoscope placed distal to the cuff, over the occluded artery, will pick up the Korotkoff sounds as the cuff is deflated and the pressure of the cuff decreases to the point at which blood flow resumes through the artery.

6. Korotkoff sounds are the noise generated by blood flow returning to the compressed artery and originate from a combination of turbulent blood flow and oscillations of the arterial wall. The sounds have been classified into five phases:
   a. Phase I: Appearance of clear tapping sounds corresponding to the appearance of a palpable pulse
   b. Phase II: Sounds become softer and longer
   c. Phase III: Sounds become crisper and louder
   d. Phase IV: Sounds become muffled and softer
   e. Phase V: Sounds disappear completely. The fifth phase is thus recorded as the last audible sound.
7. An 8- to 9-MHz Doppler device can be used in place of a stethoscope. This device will detect only systolic BP levels.

B. Indications

1. Measurement of BP in larger stable infants or when invasive BP measurement is not required or is unavailable
2. When only intermittent BP measurements are required

C. Contraindications

1. Severe edema in the limb to be measured will muffle the Korotkoff sounds.
2. Decreased perfusion, ischemia, infiltrate or injury in limb
3. Peripheral venous/arterial catheter in limb

D. Limitations

1. Provides only intermittent BP measurements
2. Manual measurement cumbersome or impossible in small infants
3. Accuracy depends on ability to recognize Korotkoff sounds and may be user-dependent.
4. Pressure may not be detectable in low-perfusion states or shock. Do not assume that it is simply an equipment problem; use clinical correlation.
5. Pressure is not detectable or is inaccurate when the baby is actively moving or agitated.
6. Measures only systolic and diastolic BP; mean BP measurement not available

TABLE 9.1	Sources of Error in Indirect Blood Pressure Measurements	
Problem	**Effect on Blood Pressure**	**Precaution**
Defective manometer 1. Air leaks 2. Improper valve function 3. Dry, degraded or cracked tubing 4. Loss of mercury	Falsely low values	1. Check level of mercury at zero cuff pressure 2. Check for cleared definition of meniscus 3. Verify that pressure holds when tightened. Check tubing for cracks
Inappropriate cuff size 1. Too narrow 2. Too wide	1. Falsely high values 2. Falsely low values	*Verify appropriately sized cuff*
Cuff applied loosely	Falsely high values owing to ballooning of bag and narrowing of effective surface	*Apply cuff snugly*
Cuff applied too tightly	Inaccurate reading owing to impedance of flow through artery	Apply cuff snugly without undue pressure
Rapid deflation of cuff	1. Falsely low values owing to inaccurate detection of beginning of sounds or 2. Falsely high values owing to inadequate equilibration between cuff pressure and manometer pressure	*Deflate cuff at rate of 2–3 mm Hg/s*
Active or agitated patient	Variable	Recheck when patient is quiet

7. Can be used only to measure pressure in the upper arm or thigh
8. The Korotkoff sound method tends to give values for systolic pressure that are lower than the true intra-arterial pressure, and diastolic values that are higher.
9. Inaccurate measurements (Table 9.1)

E. Equipment

1. Neonatal cuff (Table 9.2). Select a cuff that will fit comfortably around the upper arm or thigh; the inflatable bladder should completely encircle the extremity without overlapping. The width should be 90% of the limb circumference at the midpoint (5).
2. Mercury manometer or aneroid-type gauge
3. Appropriate-sized stethoscope with diaphragm or Doppler system

TABLE 9.2	Neonatal Cuff
Cuff No. (Size)	**Limb Circumference (cm)**
1	3–6
2	4–8
3	6–11
4	7–13
5	8–15

From American Academy of Pediatrics Task Force Pressure Control: Report. *Pediatrics.* 1977;59:797, with permission.

F. Precautions (Table 9.1)

1. Carefully select the appropriate cuff size, because incorrect size can significantly alter the BP recorded (6).
   a. Cuff too small: BP will be higher than actual BP.
   b. Cuff too large: BP will be lower than actual BP.
2. Check functional integrity of manometer
3. Check integrity of cuff for leaks
4. Check speed of cuff deflation: If deflation is too rapid, accuracy may be compromised.
5. Patient must be quiet and still during measurements.
6. For optimal infection control, use disposable cuff for each patient.

G. Technique

1. Place the infant supine, with the limb fully extended and level with the heart.
2. Measure the limb circumference and select the appropriate size cuff for the limb.
   a. Neonatal cuffs are marked with the size range (Table 9.2).
   b. When the cuff is wrapped around the limb, the end of the cuff should line up with the range mark (Fig. 9.1).
   c. If the end of the cuff falls short of the range mark, the cuff size is too small.
   d. If the end of the cuff falls beyond the range mark, the cuff size is too large.
3. Apply the cuff snugly to the bare limb, above the elbow or knee joint.

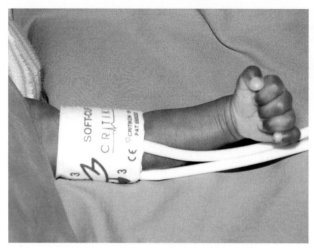

FIG. 9.1.   Cuff of correct size applied to upper arm.

4. Place the stethoscope or Doppler over the brachial artery for the upper arm or above the popliteal artery for the thigh.
5. Inflate the cuff rapidly to a pressure 15 mm Hg above the point at which the brachial pulse disappears.
6. Deflate the cuff slowly.
7. The pressure at which a sound is first heard is the systolic pressure (Korotkoff I). The pressure at which silence begins corresponds to the diastolic pressure (Korotkoff V). The pressure should be measured to the nearest 2 mm Hg.

In patients in whom the sounds do not disappear, the point at which the sounds change abruptly to a muffled tone can be accepted as an approximation of the diastolic pressure but will be slightly higher than true diastolic pressure.

H. Complications
1. Perfusion in the limb may be compromised if the cuff is not completely deflated.
2. Prolonged or repeated cuff inflation has been associated with ischemia, purpura, and/or neuropathy.

3. Cuff inflation will interfere with pulse oximetry measurement in the same limb.
4. Nosocomial infection may result from using the same cuff for more than one patient.

Oscillometric Measurement of Arterial Blood Pressure (Automatic Noninvasive)

A. Background
The oscillometric or noninvasive blood pressure (NIBP) monitoring technique offers a method for measuring all arterial blood pressure parameters (systolic, diastolic, mean, heart rate) (7–15). The underlying principle of this method is that the arterial wall oscillates when blood flows in pulsatile fashion through a vessel. These oscillations are transmitted to a cuff placed around the limb. As the pressure within the cuff is reduced, the pattern of oscillations changes (Fig. 9.2). When arterial pressure is just above the cuff pressure, there is a rapid increase in the amplitude of the oscillations and this is taken as systolic pressure. The point at which the amplitude of the oscillations is maximal coincides with the mean arterial pressure. Diastolic pressure is recorded when there is a sudden decrease in oscillations. Although many types of monitors use the same basic technique, the integration of the oscillometric method within an NIBP algorithm may differ substantially between manufacturers.

1. This technique employs a BP cuff interfaced to a computerized BP monitor.
2. A pneumatic cuff is used in the same fashion as with the auscultatory technique.
3. The monitor employs a miniature computer-controlled air pump and a bleed valve to control inflation and deflation of the cuff.
4. A pressure transducer interfaced to the cuff tubing senses the inflation pressure of the cuff and oscillations transmitted to the cuff by the underlying artery.

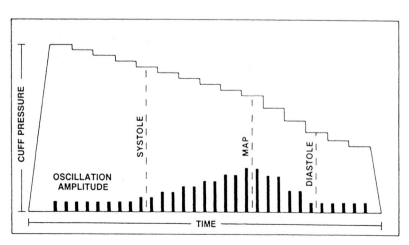

FIG. 9.2.   Determination sequence for oscillometric measurement.

5. The system will inflate the cuff to a level above the point at which no pulsations are detected.

6. As the cuff is being deflated to the level of the systolic pressure, oscillations from the arterial wall are transmitted to the cuff. A transducer measures static pressure and pressure oscillations received and transmitted by the cuff

7. The systolic pressure is assigned the value of the cuff pressure at the time oscillations were initially detected.

8. Mean arterial pressure is generally the lowest cuff pressure with the greatest average oscillation amplitude. The diastolic value is determined by the lowest cuff pressure when there is a sudden decrease in oscillations.

9. Heart rate values are calculated by computing the mean value of the time interval between pulsations.

10. Higher detection sensitivity allows this technique to be used on parts of the extremities where auscultatory methods are not possible (i.e., forearm and lower leg).

B. Indications

1. Measurement of BP in stable infants or when invasive BP measurement is not required or is unavailable

2. When only intermittent BP measurements are required

C. Contraindications

1. Severe edema in the limb to be measured; will affect result

2. Decreased perfusion, ischemia, infiltrate or injury in limb

3. Peripheral venous/arterial catheter in place in limb

D. Limitations

1. Provides only intermittent BP measurements

2. Pressure may not be detectable in low-perfusion state or shock. Do not assume that it is simply an equipment problem; use clinical correlation.

3. Pressure is not detectable or may be inaccurate in neonates who are restless or having seizures.

4. Inaccurate measurements (Table 9.1)

E. Equipment

1. Neonatal NIBP monitor—display should include systolic, diastolic, mean, and heart rate values (Fig. 9.3)

2. Neonatal cuff (designed for use with the specific monitor)—cuff may be single-tube or double-tube type, provided the appropriate adapter is used. Neonatal cuff sizes range from 1 to 5 (Table 9.2).

F. Precautions

1. Incorrect cuff size can significantly alter the BP value obtained; therefore, careful selection of cuff size is very important.

   a. An oversized cuff will yield lower BP values; an undersized cuff will produce higher BP values.

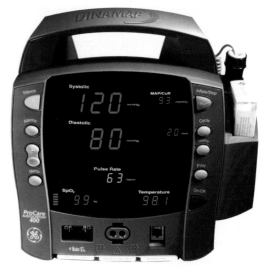

FIG. 9.3. Oscillometric BP monitor. (Courtesy of GE Healthcare.)

2. Patient must be still during measurements.

3. For optimal infection control, cuffs should be for single-patient use only.

4. Oscillometric BP measurement may lose accuracy in very hypotensive states; this needs to be taken into consideration in such patients (16,17).

G. Technique

1. Become familiar with the monitor and the equipment to be used. Be aware of the normal BP changes with gestational and postnatal age (18).

2. Measure the circumference of the extremity where the cuff is to be applied. Select the appropriately sized cuff for the limb (Fig. 9.1).

3. Apply the cuff snugly to the limb. The cuff can be applied over a thin layer of clothing if necessary; however, a bare limb is recommended.

4. Attach the monitor air hoses to the cuff. The limb from which pressure is to be measured should be level with the heart.

5. Turn the monitor on and ensure that it passes the power-on self-test before proceeding.

6. Press the appropriate button to start a blood pressure determination cycle.

7. If the values obtained from the initial cycle are questionable, repeat the measurement.

   Multiple readings with similar values yield the optimal assurance of accuracy.

8. If readings are still questionable after repeating the cycle, reposition the cuff and repeat the measurement.

9. Periodic inspection of the cuff and extremity is critical to avoid problems such as cuff detachment or shift in extremity position.

10. Most NIBP systems can be programmed by the user to measure BP automatically at user-determined intervals. The interval between measurements should be long

enough to ensure adequate circulation and minimize trauma to the limb and skin distal to the cuff.

11. In infants with suspected congenital heart disease, BP should be measured in all four extremities or at least the right arm and a leg for pre- and postductal comparison.

H. Complications

1. Perfusion in the limb may be compromised if the cuff is not completely deflated.
2. Repeated continuous cycling may cause ischemia, purpura, and/or neuropathy in the extremity.
3. Cuff inflation will interfere with pulse oximetry measurement and IV infusion in the same limb.
4. Nosocomial infection may arise from using the same cuff for more than one patient.

Continuous Blood Pressure Monitoring (Invasive)

A. Purpose

Intra-arterial direct continuous BP monitoring is considered to be the "gold standard" for measuring BP. It has the added advantage of permitting access for repeated arterial blood sampling in critically ill neonates.

B. Background

1. BP measurement is obtained from the vascular system via a catheter that has been introduced into an artery, either the umbilical artery in the neonate or a peripheral artery (Chapters 29 and 31).
2. The pressure waveform of the arterial pulse is transmitted by a column of fluid to a pressure transducer where it is converted to an electrical signal, which is transformed into a visual display by a microprocessor.
3. A BP transducer is a device that converts mechanical forces (pressure) to electrical signals. There are two major types of transducers
   a. *Strain gauge pressure transducer:* Composed of metal strands or foil that is either stretched or released by the applied pressure on the diaphragm
      (1) Applied pressure causes a proportional and linear change in electrical resistance.
      (2) Problems associated with strain gauges include drift due to temperature changes (departure from the real signal value), fragility, and cost.
   b. *Solid-state pressure transducer (semiconductor):* Composed of a silicon chip that undergoes electrical resistance changes because of the applied pressure
      (1) Lower cost, accurate, and disposables
      (2) Because of the miniature integration on the silicone chip, the circuitry necessary to minimize temperature drift is incorporated in the device.

4. Miniature transducer-tipped catheters are available that do not depend on fluid-filled lines for the transmission of pressure. Microtransducer catheters in general have better fidelity characteristics, but at a much higher cost than conventional fluid-filled systems and are currently not generally available for neonatal use

5. The standard medical BP transducer output rating is 5 μV/V/mm Hg. The pressure monitor processes the electrical signal generated by the transducer and converts it to BP units in either millimeters of mercury or kilopascals, including generation of systolic, diastolic, and mean values. The monitor provides a user-friendly numerical and graphical display allowing beat-to-beat measurement of pressure and also allows analysis of the waveform. Analysis can be clinical (e.g., morphology, determining the position of the dicrotic notch or "swing" that can give information regarding filling status and cardiac output) or computerized.

C. Indications

To continuously monitor intravascular pressure
1. In very small or unstable infants, particularly those with severe hypotension, on inotropic support
2. During major procedures that could cause or exacerbate intravascular instability
3. To monitor infants on ventilator support or extracorporeal membrane oxygenation
4. Allow frequent arterial blood sampling.

D. Contraindications

None absolute, except for those specific to catheter placement

E. Limitations

1. The pulse pressure waveform measured in the periphery is narrower and taller than that in the proximal aorta. Thus, systolic BP in the peripheral arteries can be higher than that in proximal aorta. This amplification is greater in patients with increased vascular tone or on inotropic therapy.
2. Very small-diameter catheters may result in underreading of systolic BP.

F. Equipment

There are five components of the intra-arterial BP monitoring system (Figs. 9.4 and 9.5). Commercial pressure monitoring kits have most components integrated.

1. *Intra-arterial catheter:* May be an umbilical arterial catheter (Chapter 29) or peripheral arterial catheter (Chapter 31).
2. *Pressure monitoring tube:* Fluid-filled tubing to couple arterial cannula to the pressure transducer. This tubing should be short (not exceed 100 to 120 cm from the transducer to the patient connection) and stiff (low

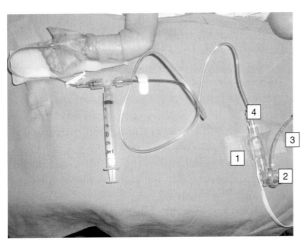

FIG. 9.4. Representative disposable BP transducer setup. *(1)* Pressure transducer; *(2)* integral continuous flush device; *(3)* infusion port (connects to infusion pump); *(4)* high-pressure tubing.

compliance to reduce damping of pressure wave). A three-way tap is incorporated in the tubing to allow the system to be zeroed and blood samples taken.

3. Pressure transducer with cable to signal processor
4. Neonatal physiologic monitor (multiparameter monitoring system)
   a. Minimum configuration should have the capability of displaying systolic, diastolic, and mean pressures and heart rate.
   b. It should have provision for high and low alarm settings.
5. Mechanical infusion device (infusion pump) with syringe and tubing to deliver heparinized saline (0.5 to

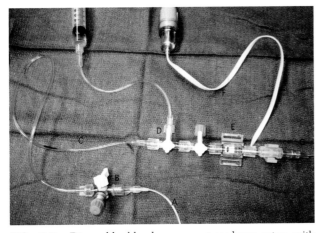

FIG. 9.5. Disposable blood pressure transducer setup with closed loop system for sampling. **A:** Umbilical arterial catheter. **B:** Stopcock with special valve to draw blood samples. **C:** High pressure tubing. **D:** Stopcock attached to heparinized saline flush syringe. **E:** Stopcock for zeroing transducer. **F:** Pressure transducer. **G:** Transducer cable. **H:** Tubing with continuous heparinized saline infusion from infusion pump.

1 U heparin/mL of fluid) at 0.5 to 1 mL/h. Pressurized IV bag should not be used.

6. Some disposable pressure-monitoring kits offer closed-loop systems for sampling (Fig. 9.5)
   a. The system employs a mechanism for aspirating and holding a fixed amount of blood in the pressure tubing rather than in a syringe.
   b. The distal end is equipped with a small chamber with a rubber septum that allows a self-guiding short blunt syringe adapter to penetrate and aspirate blood for the sample.
   c. The initial volume pulled back is sufficient to ensure that the blood drawn into the sample chamber is greater than the catheter/distal tubing volume and is not diluted by the fluid being infused. The absence of stopcocks at the distal end eliminates a possible site for contamination. In addition, the blood pulled back is conserved, and the amount of fluid used to flush the sample line is reduced.

G. Technique

For catheter placement, see Part 5 of the book, "Vascular Access"

1. Familiarize yourself with the bedside monitor and the pressure zero/calibration procedure. To maintain accuracy the pressure transducer is exposed to atmospheric pressure to calibrate the reading to zero. This is done in several ways depending on the particular transducer.
2. If using discrete components, assemble the pressure-monitoring circuit, maintaining the sterile integrity.
   a. A basic circuit configuration will consist of a transducer dome, flush device, stopcock, pressure tubing, and an optional arterial extension set (short length of pressure tubing, <12 inches in length, inserted between the catheter and the pressure tubing).
   b. Ensure that all the Luer-lock connections are tight and free of any defects.
   c. If possible, avoid the use of IV tubing components in the pressure-monitoring circuit.
3. Set up the infusion pump that will be used for the continuous infusion through the flush device. Continuous flush devices limit flow rates to 3 or 30 mL/h, depending on the model (19–21). For neonatal arterial lines, the infusion pump supplying the flush device should be set to 0.5 to 3 mL/h and should never exceed the flow rating of the flush device. When pump flow exceeds the flush device rating, it will cause an occlusion alarm in most IV pumps. A pump flow rate of 1 mL/h is recommended for most arterial lines.
4. For circuit priming, use the solution that will be used for the continuous infusion. Prime the circuit slowly to avoid trapping air bubbles in the flush device inlet.

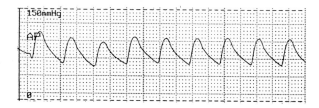

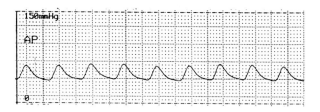

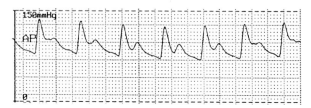

FIG. 9.6. Arterial pressure waveforms: normal arterial waveform (**top**); dampened arterial waveform (**middle**); arterial waveform with spike caused by catheter whip or inappropriate tubing (**bottom**). (Note that figure demonstrates waveform appearance only and not actual pressure values.)

Ensure that the entire circuit and all the ports are fluid filled and bubble-free.

5. If using disposable transducers, connect the reusable interface cable to the transducer and to the monitor. Turn the monitor on.
6. Secure the transducer at the patient's reference level, defined as the midaxillary line (heart level). If using transducer holders, level the reference mark on the holder at the patient's reference level.
7. Connect the distal end of the circuit to the patient's catheter, ensuring that the catheter hub is filled with fluid and is bubble-free.
8. Start the infusion pump. The pump rate cannot exceed the flow rate of the flush device.
9. Open the stopcock connected to the transducer to air (shut off to the patient, open to atmosphere).
10. Zero/calibrate the monitor according to the manufacturer's instructions.
11. Close the stopcock connected to the transducer (open to the patient).
12. Set the monitor pressure waveform scale to one that accommodates the entire pressure wave.
13. Observe the waveform obtained. If the wave appears to be damped (flattened, poorly defined, with slow rise time), check the circuit for air bubbles starting at the

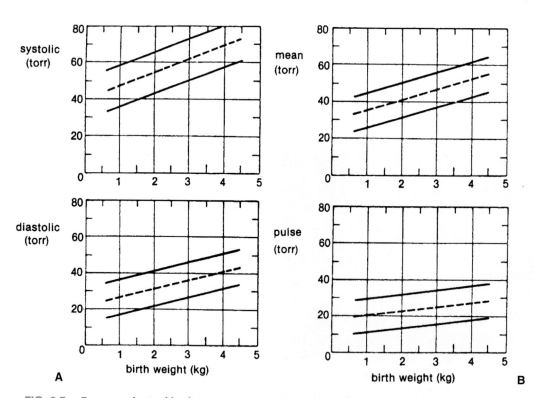

FIG. 9.7. Pressures obtained by direct measurement through umbilical artery catheter in healthy newborn infants during first 12 hours of life. Broken lines represent linear regressions; solid lines represent 95% confidence limits. **A:** Systolic pressure (**top**) and diastolic pressure (**bottom**). **B:** Mean aortic pressure (**top**) and pulse pressure (systolic–diastolic pressure amplitude) (**bottom**). (From Versmold HT, Kitterman JA, Phibbs RH, et al. Aortic blood pressure during the first 12 hours of life in infants with birth weight 610 to 4,220 grams. *Pediatrics.* 1981;67:611, with permission of American Academy of Pediatrics.)

distal end (Fig. 9.6). If no air bubbles are detected, then gently flush the catheter.

14. Once a stable pressure reading is obtained, set the alarm limits. Mean arterial pressure value is optimally used to set alarm limits (Fig. 9.7).
15. Zero the transducer every 8 hours.
16. When blood samples are drawn from the line, flushing should be done gently with a syringe using a minimal amount of heparinized saline solution.

H. Complications (Table 9.3)

1. Defective transducer
2. Cracked Luer-lock connections, causing leaks, low pressure readings, or blood to back up in the line
3. Air bubbles in the line
4. Malfunctioning infusion pump not providing continuous flush, causing the line to clot off
5. Defective reusable transducer interface cable (disposable transducer system)
6. Erroneous readings caused by the transducer not being properly set at the patient's reference level. Lower readings occur when the transducer is high; higher readings occur when the transducer is lower than the patient's reference level.
7. Problems associated with catheters
8. Tip of the catheter lodging against the wall of the vessel (will cause the pressure wave to flatten and the pressure to rise slowly as a result of the continuous infusion)
9. Transducer not zeroed to atmosphere (static pressure trapped by stopcock valve and a syringe stuck in the port that should be opened to air). This will cause lower or negative pressure readings.
10. Loss of blood if stopcock is left open and third port is not capped.
11. Fluid overload if a pressurized IV bag is used instead of an infusion pump and the fast flush mode is used to clear the line (20)

TABLE 9.3 Trouble-shooting for Intravascular Pressure Monitoring			
Problem	**Cause**	**Prevention**	**Treatment**
Damped pressure tracing	Catheter tip against vessel wall	Usually unavoidable	Reposition catheter while observing waveform
	Partial occlusion of catheter tip by clot	Use continuous infusion of normal saline or ½ normal saline with 0.5–1 U heparin/mL of fluid	Remove line if possible. If line removal is not an option, then aspirate clot with syringe and flush with heparinized saline
	Clotting in stopcock or transducer, or blood in system	Flush catheter carefully after blood withdrawal and re-establish continuous infusion; back-flush stopcocks to remove blood	Change components
Abnormally high or low readings	Change in transducer level. A 10 cm change in height will alter the pressure reading by 7.5 mm Hg. Note: If the cannula is inserted into the radial artery, raising the hand will not effect the measurement as long as the transducer is maintained level with the heart[a].	Maintain the transducer at the same level as the patient's heart	Recheck patient and transducer positions
	Leaks in transducer system	Assemble transducer carefully, ensuring that dome is attached snugly; use Luer-lock fittings and disposable stopcocks	Check all fittings, transducer dome, and stopcock connections
	External vascular compression	Secure catheter firmly without putting tape circumferentially on extremity	Loosen tape, securing catheter in place
	Strained transducer	Attention to stopcocks when aspirating to module	Replace transducer
	High intrathoracic pressure secondary to mechanical ventilation; reduces venous return and cardic output	Be aware of problem	Use minimal amount of mean airway pressure required to achieve optimal ventilation
Damped pressure without improvement after flushing	Air bubbles in transducer connector tubing	Flush transducer and tubing carefully when setting up system and attaching to catheter; handle system carefully	Check system, rapid flush, attach syringe to transducer, and aspirate bubble
No pressure reading available	Transducer not open to catheter or settings on monitor amplifiers incorrect–still on zero, cal, or off	Follow routine, systematic steps for setting up system and pressure measurements	Check system–stopcocks, monitor, and amplifier setup

[a]From Ward M, Langton JA. Blood pressure measurement. *Cont Edu Anaesth Crit Care Pain.* 2007;7(4):122–126. © 2007 Oxford University Press.

References

1. Nuntnarumit P, Yang W, Bada-Ellzey HS. Blood pressure measurements in the newborn. *Clin Perinatol.* 1999;26(4):981.
2. Fanaroff JM, Fanaroff AA. Blood pressure disorders in the neonate: hypotension and hypertension. *Semin Fetal Neonatal Med.* 2006;11(3):174. Epub 2006 Mar 3.
3. Engle WD. Blood pressure in the very low birth weight neonate. *Early Hum Dev.* 2001;62(2):97.
4. de Boode WP. Clinical monitoring of systemic hemodynamics in critically ill newborns. *Early Hum Dev.* 2010;86(3):137.
5. Ogedegbe G, Pickering T. Principles and techniques of blood pressure measurement. *Cardiol Clin.* 2010;28(4):571.
6. Moss AJ. Indirect methods of blood pressure measurement. *Pediatr Clin North Am.* 1978;25:3.
7. Pickering TG, Hall JE, Appel LJ, et al. Subcommittee of Professional and Public Education of the American Heart Association Council on High Blood Pressure Research. Recommendations for blood pressure measurement in humans and experimental animals: Part 1: blood pressure measurement in humans: a statement for professionals from the Subcommittee of Professional and Public Education of the American Heart Association Council on High Blood Pressure Research. *Hypertension.* 2005;45(1):142.
8. Sadove MS, Schmidt G, Wu H-H, et al. Indirect blood pressure measurement in infants: a comparison of four methods in four limbs. *Anesth Analg.* 1973;52:682.
9. Ramsey M III. Automatic oscillometric noninvasive blood pressure: theory and practice. In: Meyer-Sabellak W, ed. *Blood Pressure Measurements.* Darmstadt: Steinkopff Verlag; 1990:15.
10. Kimble KJ, Darnall RA Jr, Yelderman M, et al. An automated oscillometric technique for estimating mean arterial pressure in critically ill newborns. *Anesthesiology.* 1981;54:423.
11. Friesen RH, Lichtor JL. Indirect measurement of blood pressure in neonates and infants utilizing an automatic noninvasive oscillometric monitor. *Anesth Analg.* 1981;60:742.
12. Park MK, Menard SM. Accuracy of blood pressure measurement by the Dinamap monitor in infants and children. *Pediatrics.* 1987;79:907.
13. Takci S, Yigit S, Korkmaz A, et al. Comparison between oscillometric and invasive blood pressure measurements in critically ill premature infants. *Acta Paediatr.* 2012;101(2):132.
14. Dannevig I, Dale HC, Liestol K, et al. Blood pressure in the neonate: three non-invasive oscillometric pressure monitors compared with invasively measured blood pressure. *Acta Paediatrica* 2005;94(2):191.
15. Meyer S, Sander J, Gräber S, et al. Agreement of invasive versus non-invasive blood pressure in preterm neonates is not dependent on birth weight or gestational age. *J Paediatr Child Health.* 2010;46(5):249.
16. Weindling AM. Blood pressure monitoring in the newborn. *Arch Dis Child.* 1989;64:444.
17. Weindling AM, Bentham J. Blood pressure in the neonate. *Acta Paediatr.* 2005;94(2):138.
18. Lee J, Rajadurai VS, Tank KW. Blood pressure standards for very low birth weight infants during the first days of life. *Arch Dis Child Fetal Neonat Ed.* 1999;81:F168.
19. Morray J, Todd S. A hazard of continuous flush systems for vascular pressure monitoring in infants. *Anesthesiology.* 1983;38:187.
20. Barbeito A, Mark JB. Arterial and central venous pressure monitoring. *Anesthesiol Clin.* 2006;24(4):717.
21. Pinsky MR, Payen D. Functional hemodynamic monitoring. *Crit Care.* 2005;9(6):566.

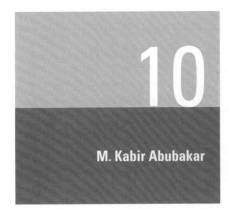

10 Continuous Blood Gas Monitoring

M. Kabir Abubakar

Blood gas monitoring is essential for the management of critically ill patients. Arterial blood gas measurement is the gold standard for assessing gas exchange and acid base status in critical care, but is invasive and provides only intermittent data. Noninvasive methods, including pulse oximetry, transcutaneous blood gas measurement, and capnometry, have been developed to supplement arterial blood gas measurement and provide real-time continuous monitoring in critically ill neonates.

Pulse Oximetry

Pulse oximetry is the most common method of continuous oxygen monitoring in clinical care. It is noninvasive, easy to use, readily available, and able to provide continuous monitoring of arterial oxygen saturations and heart rate.

A. Definitions

1. Arterial oxyhemoglobin saturation measured by arterial blood gas analysis is referred to as SaO_2.
2. Arterial oxyhemoglobin saturation measured noninvasively by pulse oximetry is referred to as SpO_2.

B. Background

1. Principles of oxygen transport
   a. Approximately 98% of the oxygen in the blood is bound to hemoglobin.

      The amount of oxygen content in the blood is related directly to the amount of hemoglobin in the blood, amount of oxygen bound to the hemoglobin and to the partial pressure of unbound, dissolved oxygen in the blood (PaO_2) (1). The relationship of arterial PO_2, in near-term infants, to percent saturation measured by pulse oximeter is shown in Fig. 10.1.
   b. The relationship between blood PaO_2 and the amount of oxygen bound to hemoglobin is presented graphically as an oxygen–hemoglobin affinity curve (Fig. 10.2). Percent oxygen saturation is calculated using the formula

$$\frac{Oxyhemoglobin}{Oxhyhemoglobin + Deoxyhemoglobin} \times 100$$

2. Principles of pulse oximetry
   a. Based on the principles of spectrophotometric oximetry and plethysmography (2)
   b. Arterial saturation and pulse rate are determined by measuring the absorption of selected wavelengths of light

      Oxygenated hemoglobin (oxyhemoglobin) and reduced hemoglobin (deoxyhemoglobin) absorb light as known functions of wavelengths. By measuring the absorption levels at different wavelengths of light, the relative percentages of these two constituents and SpO_2 are calculated.
   c. A sensor composed of two light-emitting diodes (LEDs) as light sources and one photodetector as a light receiver is employed. The photodetector is an electronic device that produces a current proportional to the incident light intensity (2,3).

      There are two methods of sending light through the measuring site: transmission and reflectance. In the transmission method, the emitter and photodetector are opposite of each other with the measuring site in between. In the reflectance method, the emitter and photodetector are next to each other on the measuring site. The light bounces from the emitter to the detector across the site. The transmission method is the most common type used and is discussed here.
   (1) One LED emits red light with an approximate wavelength of 660 nm.

      Red light is absorbed selectively by deoxyhemoglobin.
   (2) The other LED emits infrared light with an approximate wavelength of 925 nm.

      Infrared light is absorbed selectively by oxyhemoglobin.

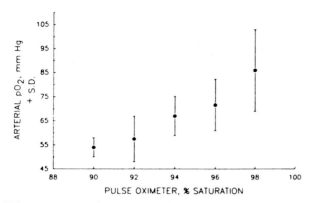

FIG. 10.1. Arterial PO$_2$ versus pulse oximeter percent saturation in near-term newborn infants in whom pulse saturation was fixed by adjusting F$_i$O$_2$ first and then measuring PaO$_2$. Values are means ± SD. (From Brockway J, Hay WW Jr. Ability of pulse O$_2$ saturations to accurately determine blood oxygenation. *Clin Res.* 1988; 36:227A, with permission.)

d. The different absorption of the wavelengths when transmitted through tissue, pulsatile blood, and non-pulsatile blood are utilized (Fig. 10.3).

(1) The photodetector measures the level of light that passes through without being absorbed.

(2) During the absence of pulse (diastole), the detector establishes baseline levels for the wavelength absorption of tissue and nonpulsatile blood.

(3) With each heartbeat, a pulse of oxygenated blood flows to the sensor site.

(4) Absorption during systole of both the red and the infrared light is measured to determine the percentage of oxyhemoglobin.

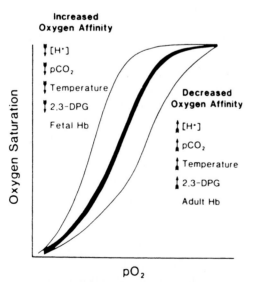

FIG. 10.2. Factors affecting hemoglobin–oxygen affinity. 2,3-DPG, 2,3-diphosphoglycerate. (From Hay WW Jr. Physiology of oxygenation and its relation to pulse oximetry in neonates. *J Perinatol.* 1987;7:309, with permission.)

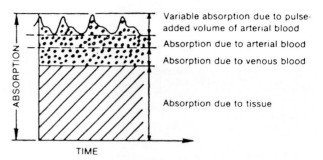

FIG. 10.3. Tissue composite showing dynamic as well as static components affecting light absorption. (From Wukitch MW, Petterson MT, Tobler DR, et al. Pulse oximetry: analysis of theory, technology and practice. *J Clin Monit.* 1988;4:290, with permission.)

(5) Because the measurements of the change in absorption are made during a pulse (systole), these pulses are counted and displayed as heart rate.

C. Indications

1. Noninvasive continuous or intermittent arterial oxygen saturation and heart rate monitoring

2. To monitor oxygenation in infants suffering from conditions associated with
   a. Hypoxia
   b. Apnea/hypoventilation
   c. Cardiorespiratory disease
   d. Bronchopulmonary dysplasia

3. To monitor response to therapy
   a. Resuscitation
      Pulse oximetry is a necessary adjunct to monitoring in the delivery room. With the use of pulse oximetry, SpO$_2$ values can be obtained within 1 minute after birth (4–8) (Fig. 10.4).
   b. Monitoring effectiveness of bag and mask ventilation or during placement of an endotracheal tube

4. To monitor side effects of other therapy
   a. Endotracheal tube suctioning
   b. Positioning for laryngoscopy, spinal tap, etc.

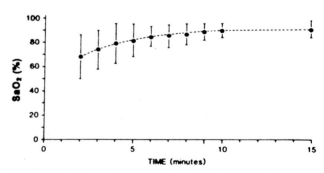

FIG. 10.4. Mean arterial oxygen saturation (S$_a$O$_2$) values measured by pulse oximetry from the time of cord clamping. Values are means ± SD. (From House JT, Schultetus RR, Gravenstein N. Continuous neonatal evaluation in the delivery room by pulse oximetry. *J Clin Monit.* 1987;3:96, with permission.)

5. For extremely low-birthweight infants <1,000 g (9–11)

   It is optimal to use pulse oximetry for oxygen monitoring in the very low-birthweight infant because of its noninvasiveness. Pulse oximetry can be used reliably in very low-birthweight infants with acute as well as chronic lung disease (9–11).

6. Pulse oximetry also offers an advantage for precise fraction of inspired oxygen (F_iO_2) control during neonatal anesthesia because of the short response time to changes in SpO_2 (10).

D. Limitations

1. Decreased accuracy when arterial saturation is <65%

   Pulse oximetry will overestimate SpO_2 at this level; therefore, blood gas confirmation is imperative (9–11).

2. Not a sensitive indicator for hyperoxemia (10)

   Pulse oximeter accuracy does not allow for precise estimation of PO_2 at saturations >90%. Small changes in O_2 saturation (1% to 2%) may be associated with large changes in PO_2 (6 to 12 mm Hg) (10).

3. Because pulse oximeters rely on pulsatile fluctuations in transmitted light intensity to estimate SpO_2, they are all adversely affected by movement (9–11)

   In some cases, the pulse oximeter may calculate an SpO_2 value for signals caused by movement, or it may reject the signal and not update the display. Usually, the heart rate output from the oximeter will reflect the detection of nonarterial pulsations, indicating either "0" saturation or "low-quality signal" (3). Advances in microprocessor technology have led to improved signal processing, which makes it possible to minimize motion artifact and monitor saturation more accurately during motion or low-perfusion states. (10)

4. Significant levels of carboxyhemoglobin or methemoglobin can yield erroneous readings (carboxyhemoglobin absorbs light at the 660-nm wavelength) (10). However, carboxyhemoglobin levels of <3% will not affect the accuracy of the instrument.

5. SpO_2 may be overestimated in darkly pigmented infants.

   Some oximeters will give a message such as "insufficient signal detected" if a valid signal is not obtained (10–13)

6. Erroneous readings can occur in the presence of high fetal hemoglobin (14)

   A smaller effect on accuracy is noted when fetal hemoglobin levels are <50% (14). With a predominance of fetal hemoglobin, an SpO_2 of >92% may be associated with hyperoxemia (14). However, whereas saturations may appear adequate, PO_2 may be low enough to produce increased pulmonary vascular resistance (SpO_2/PO_2 curve shift to the left).

   Infants with chronic lung disease and prolonged oxygen dependence are older and have less fetal hemoglobin; therefore, SpO_2 readings obtained from these patients may be more accurate than those obtained from neonates with acute respiratory disorders at an earlier age (14). The same situation exists in infants who have undergone exchange transfusion because of decreased levels of fetal hemoglobin.

7. Light sources that can affect performance include surgical lights, xenon lights, bilirubin lamps, fluorescent lights, infrared heating lamps, and direct sunlight.

   Although jaundice does not account for variability in pulse oximeter accuracy (15), phototherapy can interfere with accurate monitoring. Therefore, appropriate precautions should be taken, such as covering the probe with a relatively opaque material (1).

8. Do not correlate SpO_2 values with laboratory hemoximeters (15).

   Most laboratory oximeters measure fractional oxygen saturation (all hemoglobin including dysfunctional hemoglobin) as opposed to functional oxygen saturation (oxyhemoglobin and deoxyhemoglobin excluding all dysfunctional hemoglobin).

   Use of normal adult values for hemoglobin, 2,3-diphosphoglycerate, and, in some cases, PCO_2 can lead to errors in the algorithm to calculate SpO_2 with some blood gas analysis instruments (15).

9. Although pulse oximeters can detect hyperoxemia, it is important that type-specific alarm limits are set (16).

   To avoid hyperoxemia, a minimal sensitivity of at least 95% is required.

10. Pulse oximeters rely on detecting pulsatile flow in body tissues; therefore, a reduction in peripheral pulsatile blood flow produced by peripheral vasoconstriction results in an inadequate signal for analysis.

11. Pulse oximeters average their readings over several seconds depending on oximeter type and internal settings. Oximeters with a long averaging time may not be able to detect acute and transient changes in SpO_2.

12. Venous congestion may produce venous pulsations, which can produce low readings.

13. The pulse oximeter only provides information about oxygenation. It does not give any indication of the patient's carbon dioxide elimination.

In summary, it is optimal to make some correlation between SpO_2 and PaO_2 throughout a reasonable range of SpO_2 (lower, 85% to 88%; higher, 95% to 97%) before relying completely on SpO_2 for oxygen and/or respirator management (14,16).

E. Equipment

1. Manufacturer-specific sensor and monitor (Fig. 10.5) with
   a. Display of SpO_2 and pulse rate and a pulse indicator
   b. Adjustable alarm limits for SpO_2 and pulse rate
   c. Battery-powered operation
2. Neonatal sensor, either disposable or reusable
   a. Disposable sensors have become the standard for infection and quality control.

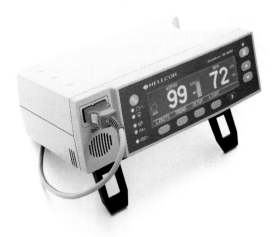

FIG. 10.5. Pulse oximeter. Vertical column indicates pulse. (Courtesy of Nellcor, Pleasanton, California.)

b. Disposable neonatal sensors are available in different sizes, depending on the site to be used.

F. Precautions

1. Use only with detectable pulse.

   Cardiopulmonary bypass with nonpulsating flow, inflated blood pressure cuff proximal to the sensor, tense peripheral edema, hypothermia, low-perfusion state secondary to shock or severe hypovolemia, and significant peripheral vasoconstriction may interfere with obtaining accurate readings (9)

2. Assess the sensor site every 8 hours to be certain that the adherent bandage is not constricting the site and that the skin is intact.

3. Whenever possible, the SpO_2 sensor should not be on the same extremity as the blood pressure cuff.

   When the cuff is inflated, the SpO_2 sensor will not detect a pulse, will not update SpO_2 values, and will alarm. Use of ace bandages on the extremities to increase central venous return may also interfere with the function of the sensor.

4. *Malpositioned sensor:* When a probe is not placed symmetrically, it can allow some light from the LED emitters to reach the photodetector in the sensor without going through the tissue at the monitoring site and will therefore produce falsely low readings. This is called the penumbra effect.

5. To avoid possible transfer of infection, do not share pulse oximetry probes between patients.

G. Technique

1. Familiarize yourself with the system before proceeding.
2. Select an appropriate sensor and apply it to the patient.
   a. Finger, toe, lateral side of the foot, or across the palm of the hand. (Placing the sensor in a position matching that of the peripheral arterial line, if present, may avoid discrepancies caused by intracardiac or ductal shunts when trying to correlate SpO_2 with arterial PO_2.)
   b. For neonates 500 g to 3 kg, anterolateral aspect of a foot (Fig. 10.6) (1).
   c. For infants weighing >3 kg, use the palm, thumb, great toe, or index finger (1).
   d. Align the LEDs (light source) and the detector so they are directly opposite each other.
   e. Reusable sensors should be applied with nonadhesive elastic wrap.

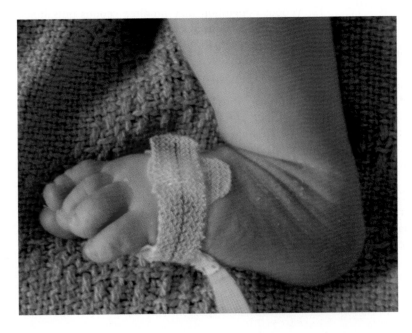

FIG. 10.6. Disposable sensor applied to foot.

f. Tighten sensor snugly to the skin but not so as to impede circulation. The probe should then be left in place for several seconds until extremity movement stops and the signal is stable.

g. Secure the sensor to the site to prevent tugging or movement of the sensor independent of the body part.

h. Cover the sensor to reduce the effect of intense light levels, direct sunlight, or phototherapy.

3. Attach the sensor to the system interconnecting cable and turn on the monitor. (Attaching the sensor to the baby before connecting the cable to the monitor that is already turned on will shorten the time taken for data acquisition and display of SpO_2 information.) (6)

4. Calibration of the system is not required (internal auto-calibration).

5. After a short interval, if all connections are correct, the monitor will display the pulse detected by the sensor. If the pulse level is adequate, it will display SpO_2 and pulse rate. If the pulse indicator is not synchronous with the patient's pulse rate, reposition the probe. After repositioning the sensor, if the pulse detector is still not indicating properly, change the sensor site.

6. Once reliable operation is achieved, set the high and low alarm limits.

   a. Although pulse oximeters can detect hyperoxemia, it is important that type-specific alarm limits are set and a low specificity is accepted (16,17). Alarm limits are determined by gestational age, presence of acute or chronic lung disease, cardiac disease, and risk of retinopathy of prematurity (18).

   b. The optimal alarm limit, defined as having a sensitivity of 95% or more, associated with maximal specificity, will differ depending on which particular monitor is used.

      Note that SpO_2 is a more sensitive indicator of hypoxemia and decreased tissue oxygenation than is PaO_2. Lower alarm limits should be individualized to alert the user when the oxygenation requirements of the given patient are not satisfied.

H. Complications

1. Management based on erroneous readings caused by a misapplied sensor or conditions affecting instrument performance.

2. Limb ischemia if sensor applied too tightly, particularly in an edematous limb.

Transcutaneous Blood Gas Monitoring

Transcutaneous measurements of oxygen and carbon dioxide are useful in the neonatal intensive care unit because they provide continuous and relatively noninvasive estimation of these parameters to supplement arterial blood gas measurements.

A. Definitions

1. Transcutaneous measurement of oxygen is referred to as $P_{tc}O_2$.

2. Transcutaneous measurement of carbon dioxide is referred to as $P_{tc}CO_2$.

B. Purpose

1. Noninvasive blood gas monitoring of PO_2 and PCO_2

2. Trending of PO_2 and PCO_2 over time

C. Background

1. Transcutaneous monitoring measures skin-surface PO_2 and PCO_2 to provide estimates of arterial partial pressure of oxygen and carbon dioxide. The devices increase tissue perfusion by heating the skin and then electrochemically measuring the partial pressure of oxygen and carbon dioxide.

2. Accomplished by two electrodes contained in a heated block that maintains the electrodes and the skin directly beneath it at a constant temperature (19) (Fig. 10.7)

   a. Arterialized capillary oxygen levels are more accurately measured by heating the skin to establish hyperemia directly beneath the sensor.

   b. The electrodes are covered with an electrolyte solution and sealed with a semipermeable plastic membrane.

3. A modified Clark electrode is used to measure oxygen.

   a. It produces an electrical current that is proportional to PO_2.

   b. Measured current is converted to PO_2 and then corrected for temperature.

4. A Severinghaus electrode is used to measure CO_2.

   a. pH-sensitive glass electrode

   b. CO_2 diffuses from the skin surface through the membrane. The CO_2 changes the pH of the electrolyte solution bathing the electrode.

   c. The measured pH is converted to PCO_2 and then corrected for temperature.

      Conversion of electric current and pH to PO_2 and PCO_2, respectively, is based on conversion equations adjusted by a two-point calibration. This is part of the setup and calibration process.

D. Indications

1. To approximate arterial PaO_2 and $PaCO_2$ for respiratory management (19)

   a. To monitor the effect of therapeutic ventilatory maneuvers particularly in infants who have combined oxygenation and ventilation problems

   b. For stabilization and monitoring during transport

2. To reduce the frequency of arterial blood gas analysis (19,20)

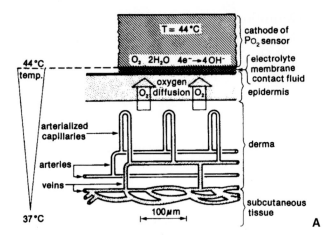

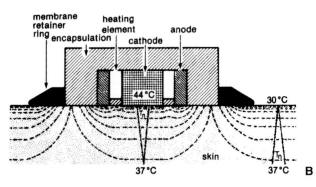

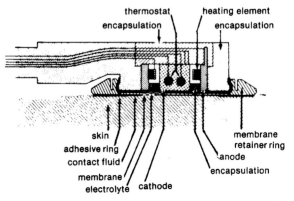

FIG. 10.7. A: Principle of cutaneous PO_2 measurement by heated oxygen sensor. **B:** Temperature profile of cutaneous tissue. **C:** Cross section of cutaneous oxygen sensor. (Courtesy of Kontron Medical Instruments, Ergolding, Germany.)

3. To determine by a noninvasive and continuous method the regional arterial oxygen tension (19,20)
4. To infer regional arterial blood flow (e.g., in the lower limbs of infants with duct-dependent coarctation of the aorta) (19,20)

E. Contraindications

1. Skin disorders (e.g., epidermolysis bullosa, staphylococcal scalded skin syndrome)

2. Relative contraindications
   a. The extremely low-birthweight infant (19,20)
   b. Severe acidosis
   c. Significant anemia
   d. Decreased peripheral perfusion
   e. $P_{tc}O_2$ may underestimate PaO_2 (19,20)

F. Equipment—Specifications

1. Transcutaneous monitor components
   a. Dual electrode
   b. Electrode cleaning kit
   c. Electrolyte and membrane kit
   d. Contact solution
   e. Double-sided adhesive rings
   f. Calibration gas cylinders with delivery apparatus
2. Digital display shows values for $P_{tc}O_2$, $P_{tc}CO_2$, and site of sensor (Fig. 10.8).
   Monitor with controls for both high and low alarm limits, and for electrode temperature. The monitor may also have a site placement timer that will alarm as an indication to change the site of the electrode.

G. Precautions

1. Be aware that
   a. Equilibration requires approximately 20 minutes after the electrode is placed, with the response time for $P_{tc}O_2$ being much faster than that for $P_{tc}CO_2$. Therefore, management changes based on transcutaneous values should be guided by values that have been consistent for at least 5 minutes.
   b. Periodic correlation with PO_2 from appropriate arterial sites is recommended (19,20)
   c. $P_{tc}O_2$ may underestimate PaO_2 in the infant with hyperoxemia ($PaO_2 >100$ mm Hg), with reliability of $P_{tc}O_2$ measurement decreasing as PaO_2 increases (19,20)
   d. $P_{tc}O_2$ may underestimate PaO_2 in older infants with bronchopulmonary dysplasia (21,22).
   e. Pressure on the sensor (e.g., infant lying on sensor) may restrict blood supply, resulting in falsely low $P_{tc}O_2$ values.
   f. Manufacturers' parts are not interchangeable. Only supplies of the same brand and designated for the monitor should be used.
2. To avoid skin burns, change electrode location *at least* every 4 hours.
3. $P_{tc}O_2$ may underestimate PaO_2 in the presence of
   a. Severe acidosis
   b. Severe anemia
   c. Decreased peripheral perfusion

H. Technique

1. Familiarize yourself with the system before proceeding.

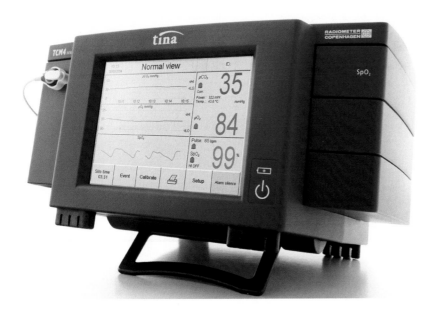

FIG. 10.8. Combined transcutaneous PO_2/PCO_2 and SpO_2 monitor. (Courtesy of Radiometer.)

2. Perform routine electrode maintenance, if there is any question as to the status of the electrode.
   a. Remove the membrane, rinse the electrode with deionized water, and dry with a soft lint-free tissue or gauze.
   b. Clean the electrode using the solution provided in the cleaning kit; abrasive compounds or materials should never be used (they will permanently damage the electrode).
   c. Rinse the electrode with deionized water, and dry with lint-free tissue.
   d. Apply the electrolyte solution.
   e. Place a new membrane on the electrode. Avoid finger contact, and always handle the membrane inside its protective package or with plastic tweezers.
3. Perform two-point gas calibration using the device-specific apparatus, as per manufacturer's instruction.
4. Use an alcohol pad to clean and degrease the skin site where the sensor is to be placed.
5. Apply double-sided adhesive ring to the sensor.
6. Apply one drop of contact solution to the skin site.
7. Peel the protective backing from the adhesive ring, place the sensor on the skin over the contact solution, and press the sensor to the skin.
   a. For best results, place the sensor on a location with good blood flow.
      (1) Appropriate sites include the lateral abdomen, anterior or lateral chest, volar aspect of the forearm, inner upper arm, inner thigh, or posterior chest (Fig. 10.9) (21)
      (2) Although large differences between pre- and postductal PaO_2 values are uncommon in premature infants with hyaline membrane disease, preductal location of the electrode is optimal for prevention of hyperoxemia (22)
   b. Choose a site devoid of hair.
   c. Avoid bony prominences.
   d. Avoid areas with large surface blood vessels (Fig. 10.9).
8. Secure the sensor cable to prevent tugging of the electrode when the cable is manipulated.
9. Allow 15 to 20 minutes for site equilibration before taking readings.
10. Note the time at which the sensor was placed on the skin, so that the site can be changed after a 4-hour period (maximum site time). When changing the sensor site
    a. Use an alcohol pad to help loosen the adhesive and peel gently from the skin.
    b. Inspect the skin site for signs of sensitivity to heat or to the adhesive. In the event of skin irritation, either lower the sensor temperature or change the site more frequently; mild erythema after sensor removal is typical.

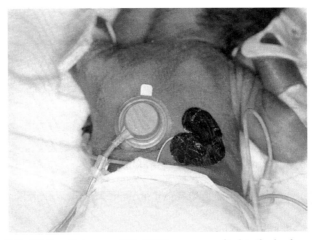

FIG. 10.9. Cutaneous PO_2/PCO_2 sensor applied to the back.

TABLE 10.1	Poor Correlation of $P_{tc}O_2$ and PaO_2		
Problem	**Technical Solution**		**Clinical**
$P_{tc}O_2 < PaO_2$ 1. Improper calibration 2. Insufficient warm-up period after electrode application 3. Insufficient heating temperature	1. Recalibrate 2. Allow longer warm-up period 3. Increase heating temperature		Presence of shock Use with high-dose dopamine Obstructive heart disease with hypoperfusion Edema Severe hypothermia
$P_{tc}O_2 > PaO_2$ 1. Improper calibration 2. Reading taken immediately after electrode application 3. Air bubble beneath membrane or leak to atmosphere 4. Excessive heating temperature	1. Recalibrate 2. Allow longer warm-up period 3. Reapply electrode 4. Attempt calibration at lower temperature		Right-to-left ductal shunt with preductal electrode and postductal arterial sample

c. Peel adhesive ring off the sensor.

d. Flush the membrane surface with deionized water.

e. Gently blot excess water and dry the sensor.

f. Recalibrate if instructed to do so by the manufacturer's guidelines.

Most manufacturers recommend recalibration every 4 to 8 hours.

11. Remember that response time for gas measurements is slow and values will not always immediately reflect physiologic changes.
    a. Average 90% response time for O_2 is 15 to 20 seconds.
    b. Average 90% response time for CO_2 is 60 to 90 seconds.

12. Complications

13. Skin blisters or burns (23)

14. Management based on erroneous readings if the unit was not calibrated properly or site precautions were not adhered to (Table 10.1)

Continuous Umbilical Artery PO_2 Monitoring (24,25)

The following method for monitoring PO_2 and the subsequent method for monitoring blood gases are included for completeness. The editors are not aware of any current commercial source of the required equipment in the United States.

A. Purpose

1. Continuous arterial PO_2 monitoring from the umbilical artery

    Continuous PaO_2 monitoring through the umbilical artery offers a means for determining precise data on a continuous basis.

2. Trending of PaO_2 over time

B. Background

1. Dual-purpose biluminal catheter
    a. A miniature polarographic bipolar oxygen electrode is incorporated into the tip of a bilumen umbilical catheter.
    b. The small lumen contains the wires for the electrode.
    c. The larger lumen can be used for blood sampling, infusion, blood pressure monitoring, and sampling for instrument calibration.
    d. The electrode is covered by a gas-permeable membrane, under which is a layer of dried electrolyte. The probe is packed dry and is then activated before use. Water vapor from the activating (hydrating) solution diffuses through the membrane to form a thin layer of liquid electrolyte on the surface of the electrode.
    e. While it is in the artery, the electrode will produce an electrical current proportional to the PO_2 in the blood.
    f. The device is calibrated to the PO_2 value obtained from a blood sample drawn from the catheter.

C. Contraindications

1. Previous history of or evidence of compromise to the vascular supply of the lower extremities or the buttock area
2. History of previous complications related to an umbilical arterial line
3. Peritonitis
4. Necrotizing enterocolitis
5. Omphalitis
6. Omphalocele

D. Equipment

Previously commercially available monitoring systems have been withdrawn from the market recently because of high production costs.

E. Precautions

See also Chapter 29.

1. This specialized catheter is stiffer and has a wider outer diameter than other umbilical artery catheters. There is the theoretical possibility of a higher rate of failure to insert the catheter and potential increase in rates of vascular spasm and thrombosis.
2. Failure to insert this catheter does not imply that insertion of other arterial catheters will be unsuccessful.
3. The electrode may fail to activate or may lose activation.
4. The catheter should be removed slowly to ensure that physiologic vasospasm occurs with removal.

F. Technique

1. Use sterile procedure.
2. Prepare the catheter according to the manufacturer's instructions.
3. 4 Fr catheters are recommended for infants weighing <1,500 g.
4. The technique for placement/insertion is the same as that used for the placement of conventional umbilical artery catheters (see Chapter 29).
5. Verify catheter position by radiography.
6. Draw blood sample for calibration.
7. Calibrate the monitor according to the manufacturer's instructions.

G. Complications

Same as for umbilical artery catheterization. See Chapter 29.

Continuous Umbilical Artery PO_2, PCO_2, pH, and Temperature Blood Gas Monitoring (26–32)

A. Purpose

1. Continuous arterial blood gas monitoring from the umbilical artery
   Continuous blood gas monitoring through the umbilical artery offers a means for determining precise data on a continuous basis.
2. Trending of blood gas data over time

B. Background

1. A very thin, multiparameter, single-use disposable fiberoptic sensor
   a. Measures pH, PCO_2, PO_2, and temperature directly
   b. Introduced into the bloodstream via the umbilical artery catheter
   c. Port allows blood sampling, blood pressure monitoring, and drug infusion
2. Calculated parameters include bicarbonate, base excess, and oxygen saturation.

3. Delivers continuous ventilation, oxygenation, and acid balance information, while also conserving blood volume by reducing blood sampling

C. Contraindications

1. Previous history or evidence of compromise to the vascular supply of the lower extremity or the buttock area
2. History of previous complications related to an umbilical arterial line
3. Peritonitis
4. Necrotizing enterocolitis
5. Omphalitis
6. Omphalocele

D. Equipment

Previously commercially available monitoring systems have been withdrawn from the market recently because of high production costs.

E. Precautions

1. The fiberoptic sensor may fail as a result of excessive kinking during sensor insertion into the umbilical artery catheter.
2. The sensor should be removed slowly to ensure that there is no microthrombus release if heparinization of the catheter was suboptimal.
3. See also Chapter 29.

F. Technique

1. Use sterile procedure.
2. Insert umbilical artery catheter (see Chapter 29).
3. Verify catheter position by radiography.
4. Calibrate sensor following the manufacturer's instructions.
5. Introduce the sensor into the umbilical artery catheter following the manufacturer's instructions.

G. Complications

Same as for umbilical artery catheterization; see Chapter 29.

References

1. Hay WW. Physiology of oxygenation and its relation to pulse oximetry in neonates. *J Perinatol.* 1987;7:309.
2. Dziedzic K, Vidyasagar D. Pulse oximetry in neonatal intensive care. *Clin Perinatol.* 1989;16:177.
3. Barrington KJ, Finer NN, Ryan CA. Evaluation of pulse oximetry as a continuous monitoring technique in the neonatal intensive care unit. *Crit Care Med.* 1988;16:1147.
4. Di Fiore JM. Neonatal cardiorespiratory monitoring techniques. *Semin Neonatol* 2004;9(3):195.
5. Davis PG, Dawson JA. New concepts in neonatal resuscitation. *Curr Opin Pediatr.* 2012;24:147.
6. Dawson JA, Davis PG, O'Donnell CP, et al. Pulse oximetry for monitoring infants in the delivery room: a review. *Arch Dis Child Fetal Neonatal Ed.* 2007;92(1):F4.
7. Kattwinkel J, Perlman JM, Aziz K, et al. Neonatal resuscitation: 2010 American Heart Association Guidelines for Cardiopulmonary Resuscitation and Emergency Cardiovascular Care. *Pediatrics.* 2010;126(5):e1400.

8. Perlman JM, Wyllie J, Kattwinkel J, et al. Neonatal resuscitation: 2010 International Consensus on Cardiopulmonary Resuscitation and Emergency Cardiovascular Care Science with Treatment Recommendations. *Pediatrics.* 2010;126(5):e1319.

9. Workie FA, Rais-Bahrami K, Short BL. Clinical use of new-generation pulse oximeters in the neonatal intensive care unit. *Am J Perinatol.* 2005;22(7):357.

10. Hay WW Jr, Rodden DJ, Collins SM, et al. Reliability of conventional and new pulse oximetry in neonatal patients. *J Perinatol.* 2002;22(5):360.

11. Soubani AO. Noninvasive monitoring of oxygen and carbon dioxide. *Am J Emerg Med.* 2001;19(2):141.

12. Bohnhorst B, Peter CS, Poets CF. Pulse oximeters' reliability in detecting hypoxemia and bradycardia: comparison between a conventional and two new generation oximeters. *Crit Care Med.* 2000;28(5):1565.

13. Emery JR. Skin pigmentation as an influence on the accuracy of pulse oximetry. *J Perinatol.* 1987;7:329.

14. Anderson JV. The accuracy of pulse oximetry in neonates: effects of fetal hemoglobin and bilirubin. *J Perinatol.* 1987;7:323.

15. Hay WW, Brockway J, Eyzaguirre M. Neonatal pulse oximetry: accuracy and reliability. *Pediatrics.* 1989;83:717.

16. Bucher H-U, Fanconi S, Baeckert P, et al. Hyperoxemia in newborn infants: detection by pulse oximetry. *Pediatrics.* 1989;84:226.

17. Shiao SY, Ou CN. Validation of oxygen saturation monitoring in neonates. *Am J Crit Care.* 2007;16(2):168.

18. Saugstad OD, Aune D. In search of the optimal oxygen saturation for extremely low birth weight infants: a systematic review and meta-analysis. *Neonatology.* 2011;100:1.

19. Sandberg KL, Brynjarsson H, Hjalmarson O. Transcutaneous blood gas monitoring during neonatal intensive care. *Acta Paediatr* 2011;100(5):676.

20. Tobias JD. Transcutaneous carbon dioxide monitoring in infants and children. *Paediatr Anaesth.* 2009;19(5):434.

21. Palmisano BW, Severinghaus JW. Transcutaneous PCO_2 and PO_2: a multicenter study of accuracy. *J Clin Monit.* 1990;6:189.

22. Pearlman SA, Maisels MJ. Preductal and postductal transcutaneous oxygen tension measurements in premature newborns with hyaline membrane disease. *Pediatrics.* 1989;83:98.

23. Golden SM. Skin craters—a complication of transcutaneous oxygen monitoring. *Pediatrics.* 1981;67:514.

24. Fink SE. Continuous PaO_2 monitoring through the umbilical artery. *Neonat Intensive Care.* 1990;3:16.

25. Durand DJ, Mickas NA. Blood gases: technical aspects and interpretation. In: Goldsmith JP, Karotkin EH, eds. *Assisted Ventilation of the Neonate.* 5th ed. St. Louis: Elsevier Saunders, 2011:292.

26. Weiss I, Fink S, Harrison R, et al. Clinical use of continuous arterial blood-gas monitoring in the pediatric intensive care unit. *Pediatrics.* 1999;103:440.

27. Coule LW, Truemper EJ, Steinhart CM, et al. Accuracy and utility of a continuous intra-arterial blood-gas monitoring system in pediatric patients. *Crit Care Med.* 2001;29:420.

28. Meyers PA, Worwa C, Trusty R, et al. Clinical validation of a continuous intravascular neonatal blood gas sensor introduced through an umbilical artery catheter. *Respir Care.* 2002;47(6):682.

29. Rais-Bahrami K, Rivera O, Mikesell GT, Short BL. Continuous blood gas monitoring using an in-dwelling optode method: comparison to intermittent arterial blood gas sampling in ECMO patients. *J Perinatol.* 2002;22(6):472.

30. Rais-Bahrami K, Rivera O, Mikesell GT, Short BL. Continuous blood gas monitoring using an in-dwelling optode method: clinical evaluation of the Neotrend® sensor using a Luer stub adaptor to access the umbilical artery catheter. *J Perinatol.* 2002;22(5):367.

31. Ganter M, Zollinger A. Continuous intravascular blood gas monitoring: development, current techniques, and clinical use of a commercial device. *Br J Anaesth.* 2003;91(3):397.

32. Tobias JD, Connors D, Strauser L, et al. Continuous pH and PCO_2 monitoring during respiratory failure in children with the Paratrend 7 inserted into the peripheral venous system. *J Pediatr.* 2000;136(5):623.

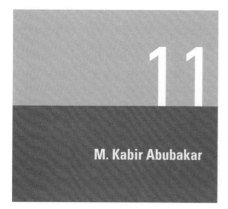

11

End-Tidal Carbon Dioxide Monitoring

M. Kabir Abubakar

Capnography

Capnography or end-tidal carbon dioxide ($P_{et}CO_2$) monitoring is the continuous and noninvasive measurement of CO_2 in exhaled respiratory gas. It is a useful adjunct tool in the management of ventilated infants, providing information about CO_2 production, pulmonary perfusion, alveolar ventilation, respiratory patterns, and the elimination of CO_2 from the lungs. If ventilation and perfusion are well matched, $P_{et}CO_2$ will approximate $PaCO_2$.

A. Definitions

1. Capnography is the continuous analysis and graphical representation over time of CO_2 concentrations in exhaled respiratory gases. A capnograph is the measuring instrument that displays the waveform or the capnogram.
2. Capnometry refers to numerical measurement or analysis of CO_2 concentrations. A capnometer is a device that measures and displays the breath-to-breath numeric values of CO_2.

B. Purpose

1. Noninvasive continuous analysis and recording of CO_2 during tidal breathing (1)
2. $P_{et}CO_2$ monitoring (2)
3. Confirmation of endotracheal tube placement (3)

C. Background

1. *CO_2 may be measured in a gas sample by several techniques. Infrared and colorimetric technology are the most commonly used methods in clinical practice:*
   a. *Infrared technology:* The most commonly used technique in capnography. CO_2 absorbs specific wavelengths of infrared light. The amount of CO_2 in a gas sample can be determined by comparing the measured absorbance of infrared light by that gas with the absorbance of a known standard.
   b. *Colorimetry:* Used primarily for small disposable $P_{et}CO_2$ detectors for verification of endotracheal tube placement. A pH-sensitive nontoxic chemical indicator strip is housed in a clear dome; the strip changes color from purple to yellow in the presence

of exhaled CO_2; the color change is reversible and changes from purple to yellow with each exhaled breath in correctly intubated patients.
   c. Molecular correlation spectrography
   d. Raman spectrography
   e. Mass spectrography
   f. Photoacoustic spectrography
2. *Capnographic devices incorporate one of two types of analyzers:* Mainstream and sidestream (4–7)
   a. With a mainstream analyzer, the sensor is attached directly to an optical adapter that is in line with the endotracheal tube (Fig. 11.1).
   b. With a sidestream analyzer, a low–dead-space adapter is placed in line with the endotracheal tube and gas is aspirated continuously to the analyzer for measurement (Fig. 11.2).

D. Indications

1. Evaluation of the exhaled CO_2, specifically $P_{et}CO_2$, which is the maximum partial pressure of CO_2 exhaled during a tidal breath just prior to the beginning of inspiration (designated $P_{et}CO_2$) (4–10).
2. Monitoring the severity of pulmonary disease and evaluating response to therapy, particularly therapy intended to change the ratio of dead space to tidal volume (11) or to improve the matching of ventilation to perfusion (V/Q) (12)
3. Accurate and continuous graphic reflection of CO_2 elimination when weaning ventilator support (4,13)
4. Continued monitoring of the integrity of the ventilatory circuit (14)
5. Use of capnography in combination with pulse oximetry can allow for additional monitoring to detect airway obstruction or subclinical degrees of respiratory depression in the sedated patient (5).
6. Verifying that tracheal rather than esophageal intubation has taken place (3,15,16)

E. Contraindications

There are no absolute contraindications to capnography in the mechanically ventilated infant, but consideration should be given to the amount of dead space and weight that will be added to the breathing circuit by these devices.

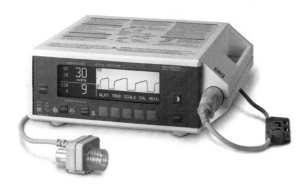

FIG. 11.1. Mainstream capnographic monitor unit and clip-on sensor assembly. (Courtesy of Respironics, Inc., Murrysville, Pennsylvania.)

F. Limitations (4,17,18)

1. The composition of the respiratory gas mixture may affect the capnogram; the infrared spectrum of CO_2 has some similarities to the spectra for both oxygen and nitrous oxide (most available capnographs have a correction factor already incorporated into the calibration).

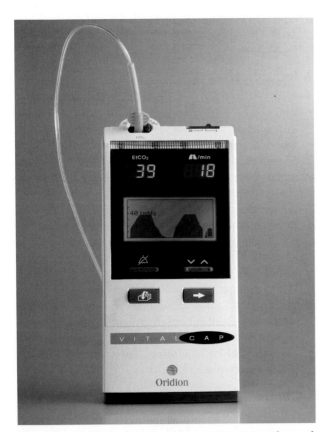

FIG. 11.2. Sidestream capnographic monitor unit with sample line. Note $P_{et}CO_2$ value and wave. (Courtesy of Oridion Capnography, Needham, Massachusetts.)

2. Rapid changes in respiratory rate and tidal volume may lead to measurement error, depending on the frequency response of the capnograph; different capnographs may have different frequency responses.
3. Contamination of either the monitor or the sampling system by secretions, blood, or condensation may lead to inaccurate results.
4. Large dead space affects $P_{et}CO_2$ measurements. The difference between $P_{et}CO_2$ and $PaCO_2$ increases as dead-space volume increases and may vary within the same patient over time.
5. The $P_{et}CO_2$ adapter can add to the dead space and resistance of the respiratory circuit, particularly in small infants.
6. $P_{et}CO_2$ measurements may not provide an accurate correlation with $PaCO_2$ in small preterm infants with nonhomogenous lung disease and, therefore, cannot be substituted for $PaCO_2$ analyses in preterm infants during this critical period (19,20).
7. Acute pulmonary hypoperfusion during cardiac surgery may be associated with a sudden decrease in $P_{et}CO_2$ and mimic accidental endotracheal extubation (21).

G. Equipment

1. Use adaptors specifically designed for neonatal application.
2. For mainstream capnography, an airway adapter is needed, along with a reusable sensor attachment.
3. For sidestream capnography, an airway adapter with sampling tube is used (Fig. 11.3).
4. Sidestream technology can be used with nasal prongs in spontaneously breathing patients.
5. Capnograph or capnometer

H. Precautions

1. In the mainstream adapter, prevent condensation in the airway adapter.
2. In the sidestream adapter, prevent fluid (water) buildup in the sampling tube.
3. For both mainstream and sidestream, when adding bulk to the endotracheal tube, extra attention should be given to properly securing the position of the tube.
4. Tidal volume measurements may be affected if the $P_{et}CO_2$ adapter is placed between the endotracheal tube and the ventilator flow sensor.

I. Technique

1. Familiarize yourself with the system before proceeding.
2. Follow manufacturer's instructions for equipment calibration
3. Attach the adapter in line with the endotracheal tube and the ventilator T piece (both sidestream and mainstream) (Fig. 11.4).
4. For mainstream capnography, connect the sensor to the airway adapter.

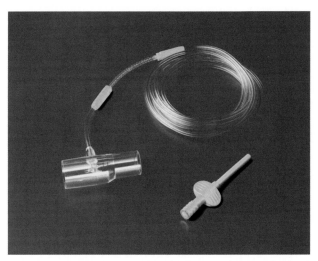

FIG. 11.3. Infant sidestream low–dead-space adapter with sample tubing. (Courtesy of Oridion Capnography, Needham, Massachusetts.)

5. For sidestream capnography, connect the sampling tube to the analyzer.

J. Complications

1. With mainstream analyzers, the use of too large an airway tube adapter together with the weight of the probe may introduce an excessive amount of bulk and weight to the endotracheal tube increasing the risk of tube kinking or dislodgement.
2. With sidestream capnography, a low–dead-space adapter allows for less bulk and weight; however, care must be taken not to pull excessively on the sample line that is connected to the measurement instrument (6,7)

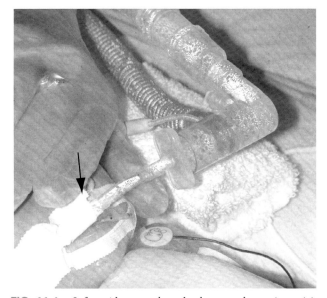

FIG. 11.4. Infant sidestream low–dead-space adapter (*arrow*) in line with endotracheal tube.

Colorimetric Carbon Dioxide Measurement

Colorimetry provides a quick qualitative measure of CO_2 in a gas sample. This method uses a pH-sensitive chemical indicator (similar to a litmus paper) in a plastic housing that is attached between the endotracheal tube and the ventilator circuit or positive-pressure delivery device. The pH-sensitive indicator changes color when exposed to CO_2 (usually from purple to yellow, depending on the device). The response time is sufficiently fast to detect exhaled CO_2 within 1 or 2 breaths.

A. Indications

1. For confirmation of endotracheal tube placement
2. International consensus statements on neonatal resuscitation recommend that endotracheal tube placements be verified by using clinical signs and detection of exhaled CO_2 (22)

B. Procedure

1. Immediately following endotracheal intubation, attach calorimetric CO_2 detector to endotracheal tube adaptor and continue positive-pressure ventilation with T-piece resuscitator or Ambu bag.
2. Within 1 to 2 breaths, the indicator color should change from purple to yellow with every exhalation if the tube is within the trachea and not in the esophagus. Some CO_2 detectors have a small plastic strip that needs to be removed for the gas to flow through.
3. Remove the CO_2 detector before attaching the ventilator circuit.

C. Limitations

1. This device is not very sensitive when CO_2 output is low, as may be the case in patients with cardiac arrest and minimal CO_2 excretion and in very preterm infants during initial resuscitation (3,22,23)

References

1. Walsh BK, Crotwell DN, Restrepo RD. Capnography/Capnometry during mechanical ventilation: *Respir Care.* 2011; 56(4):503.
2. Galia F, Brimioulle S, Bonnier F, et al. Use of maximum end-tidal CO(2) values to improve end-tidal CO(2) monitoring accuracy. *Respir Care.* 2011;56(3):278.
3. Wyllie J, Carlo WA. The role of carbon dioxide detectors for confirmation of endotracheal tube position. *Clin Perinatol* 2006 ;33(1):111.
4. Rozycki HJ, Sysyn GD, Marshall MK, et al. Mainstream end-tidal carbon dioxide monitoring in the neonatal intensive care unit. *Pediatrics.* 1998;101:648.
5. Lightdale JR, Goldmann DA, Feldman HA, et al. Microstream capnography improves patient monitoring during moderate sedation: a randomized, controlled trial. *Pediatrics.* 2006;117(6):e1170.
6. Kugelman A, Zeiger-Aginsky D, Bader D, et al. A novel method of distal end-tidal CO_2 capnography in intubated infants: comparison with arterial CO_2 and with proximal mainstream end-tidal CO_2. *Pediatrics.* 2008;122(6):e1219.

7. Lopez E, Mathlouthi J, Lescure S, et al. Capnography in spontaneously breathing preterm infants with bronchopulmonary dysplasia. *Pediatr Pulmonol.* 2011;46(9):896.

8. Bhat YR, Abhishek N. Mainstream end-tidal carbon dioxide monitoring in ventilated neonates. *Singapore Med J.* 2008;49(3):199.

9. Wu CH, Chou HC, Hsieh WS, et al. Good estimation of arterial carbon dioxide by end-tidal carbon dioxide monitoring in the neonatal intensive care unit. *Pediatr Pulmonol.* 2003;35:292.

10. Trevisanuto D, Giuliotto S, Cavallin F, et al. End-tidal carbon dioxide monitoring in very low birth weight infants: Correlation and agreement with arterial carbon dioxide. *Pediatr Pulmonol.* 2012:47:367.

11. McSwain SD, Hamel DS, Smith PB, et al. End-tidal and arterial carbon dioxide measurements correlate across all levels of physiologic dead space. *Respir Care.* 2010;55(3):288.

12. Frankenfield DC, Alam S, Bekteshi E, et al. Predicting dead space ventilation in critically ill patients using clinically available data. *Crit Care Med.* 2010;38(1):288.

13. Morley TF, Giamo J, Maroszan E, et al. Use of capnography for assessment of the adequacy of alveolar ventilation during weaning from mechanical ventilation. *Am Rev Respir Dis.* 1993;148:339.

14. Hamel DS, Cheifetz IM. Do all mechanically ventilated pediatric patients require continuous capnography? *Respir Care Clin N Am.* 2006;12(3):501.

15. Gowda H. Should carbon dioxide detectors be used to check correct placement of endotracheal tubes in preterm and term neonates? *Arch Dis Child.* 2011;96(12):1201.

16. Langhan ML, Auerbach M, Smith AN, et al. Improving Detection by Pediatric Residents of Endotracheal Tube Dislodgement with Capnography: A Randomized Controlled Trial. *J Pediatr.* 2012. [Epub ahead of print]

17. Sullivan KJ, Kissoon N, Goodwin SR. End-tidal carbon dioxide monitoring in pediatric emergencies. *Pediatr Emerg Care.* 2005;21(5):327.

18. Molloy EJ, Deakins K. Are carbon dioxide detectors useful in neonates? *Arch Dis Child Fetal Neonatal Ed.* 2006;91(4):F295.

19. Aliwalas LL, Noble L, Nesbitt K, et al. Agreement of carbon dioxide levels measured by arterial, transcutaneous and end tidal methods in preterm infants < or = 28 weeks gestation. *J Perinatol.* 2005;25(1):26.

20. Lopez E, Grabar S, Barbier A, et al. Detection of carbon dioxide thresholds using low-flow sidestream capnography in ventilated preterm infants. *Intensive Care Med.* 2009;35(11):1942.

21. Misra S, Koshy T, Mahaldar DA. Sudden decrease in end-tidal carbon dioxide in a neonate undergoing surgery for type B interrupted aortic arch. *Ann Card Anaesth.* 2011;14:206.

22. Kattwinkel J, Perlman JM, Aziz K, et al. Neonatal Resuscitation: 2010 American Heart Association Guidelines for Cardiopulmonary Resuscitation and Emergency Cardiovascular Care. *Pediatrics.* 2010;126:e1400.

23. Schmolzer GM, Poulton DA, Dawson JA, et al. Assessment of flow waves and colorimeteric CO_2 detector for endotracheal tube placement during neonatal resuscitation. *Resuscitation.* 2011;82:307.

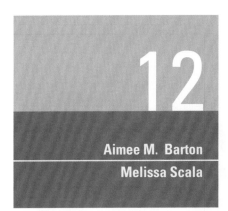

12 Transcutaneous Bilirubin Monitoring

Aimee M. Barton

Melissa Scala

A. Background

1. Jaundice occurs in most newborn infants. A high level of unconjugated bilirubin is potentially toxic to the nervous system, causing bilirubin encephalopathy and kernicterus (1).
2. A systematic assessment of all newborn infants for the risk of severe hyperbilirubinemia should be undertaken prior to discharge, and appropriate follow-up should be provided. This assessment may be performed by measuring total serum bilirubin (TSB) or transcutaneous bilirubin (TCB) (2,3).
3. Visual assessment of jaundice, although clinically important, may not be accurate (4,5).
4. Transcutaneous bilirubinometers measure the yellowness of reflected light from the skin and subcutaneous tissues to provide an objective *noninvasive* measurement of the degree of neonatal jaundice and thereby predict the approximate TSB.
5. Transcutaneous bilirubinometers are predominantly used for *screening* for significant hyperbilirubinemia in term and near-term newborn infants.
6. Two transcutaneous bilirubinometers are currently used in the United States. Although these instruments use different technologies and algorithms, their underlying principles of operation are similar. Both bilirubinometers provide TCB measurements that correlate well with TSB values at levels <15 mg/dL, in term and late preterm newborn infants; but wider variations have been noted at higher bilirubin levels (6,7).
   a. Konica Minolta/Air-Shields JM-103 Jaundice Meter (Dräger Medical, Telford, Pennsylvania) (5,8) (Fig. 12.1)
   b. BiliChek Noninvasive Bilirubin Analyzer (Children's Medical Ventures/Respironics, Norwell, Massachusetts) (5,7) (Fig. 12.2).
   c. Two other transcutaneous bilirubinometers, the Bilitest BB77 (Bertocchi SRL Elettromedicali, Cremona, Italy) and BiliMed (Medick SA, Paris, France) are used in Europe, but are not approved for use in the United States (9,10).

B. Indications

1. TCB may be obtained
   a. As part of routine predischarge assessment between 1 and 4 days of life in term and near-term newborn infants, to assess the risk of development of severe hyperbilirubinemia, by using the hour-specific bilirubin nomogram (Figs. 12.3 and 12.4) (2,3,11). The American Academy of Pediatrics recommends routine predischarge bilirubin screening of all newborns.
   b. For repeated noninvasive measurement of progression of jaundice in term or near-term newborn infants.
   c. When clinical jaundice is noted in the first 24 hours of life
   d. When jaundice appears excessive for the infant's age
2. TSB (in addition to other studies to determine underlying pathology) should be obtained when (2,3)
   a. Infant is receiving phototherapy or the TSB is rising rapidly
   b. TSB value approaching exchange transfusion levels or not responding to phototherapy
   c. Infant has an elevated direct bilirubin level
   d. Jaundice is present at or beyond age 3 weeks
   e. In sick or premature (<35 weeks' gestation) infants

C. Limitations

1. TCB measurement is a *screening tool* and should not be used for treatment decisions, but rather to select those infants who should undergo TSB measurement (1).
2. The two large studies evaluating the BiliChek device and the JM-103 device included few patients with TSB values >15 mg/dL. The accuracy of TCB measurement in this range has not been evaluated adequately (6,7).
3. All TCB devices are not the same. Significant variations can occur among instruments (9). New instruments should be compared with hospital laboratory measurements.
4. TCB measurements become less accurate if the infant is being treated with phototherapy or has received an

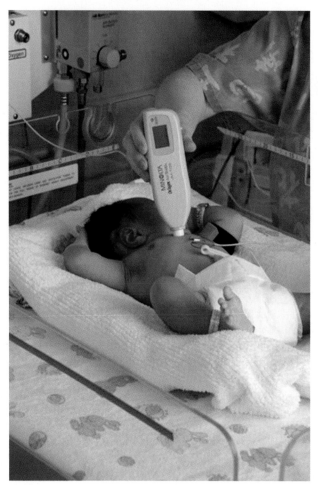

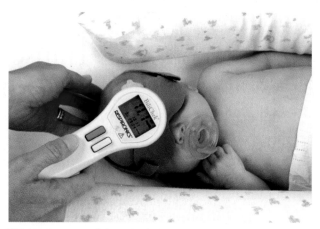

FIG. 12.2. Use of the BiliChek Noninvasive Bilirubin Analyzer on the forehead. (Photo provided by Children's Medical Ventures/ Respironics.)

exchange transfusion and should not be used within 24 hours of either of these therapies (2,5,12–14).

a. Phototherapy alters the chemical structure of bilirubin in the subcutaneous tissues, making it more water-soluble. Measurement of TCB in infants undergoing phototherapy is not reliable because the large decrease in subcutaneous bilirubin may not yet be reflected in the serum (13,14). Correlation coefficients have been found to decrease to as low as 0.33 in infants undergoing phototherapy for longer than 48 hours (13).

FIG. 12.1. Use of the Konica Minolta/Air-Shields JM-103 Jaundice Meter on the sternum. (Photo provided by Dräger Medical.)

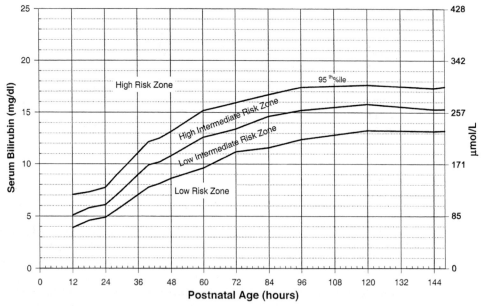

FIG. 12.3. Nomogram for designation of risk in 2,840 well newborns at 36 or more weeks' gestational age with birth weight of 2,000 g or more or 35 or more weeks' gestational age and birth weight of 2,500 g or more based on hour-specific serum bilirubin values (2,8). (Reproduced with permission from *Pediatrics*, Vol. 114, Page 301, Copyright © 2004 by the AAP.)

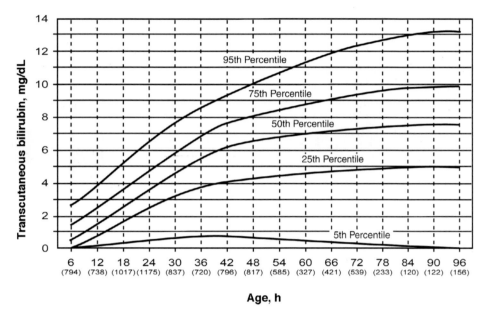

FIG. 12.4.   Nomogram showing smoothed curves for the 5th, 25th, 50th, 75th and 95th percentiles for TCB measurements among healthy newborns (gestational age ≥35 weeks). A total of 9,397 TCB measurements were obtained for 3,894 newborns. The number of infants studied at each interval is shown in parentheses. (Reproduced with permission from *Pediatrics*, Vol. 117(4), Pages 1169–1173, Copyright © 2006 by the AAP.)

b. The use of a photo-opaque patch on the forehead to shield the skin may allow for continued measurement TCB levels in term infants undergoing phototherapy. Good agreement has been shown between serum bilirubin levels and TCB measured from the patched area, and is most effective in following trends in bilirubin values in infants undergoing phototherapy (12).

5. Measurements should not be made on skin that is bruised, covered with hair, or has a birthmark. Localized edema and poor tissue perfusion may also alter TCB readings (15).

6. TCB measurements may decrease the need for multiple TSB measurements in late preterm infants; little information is available in very preterm infants, in whom measurements may be less reliable (12,14,15).

D. Equipment

TCB monitors currently in use in the United States include:

1. Konica Minolta/Air-Shields JM-103 Jaundice Meter (Dräger Medical, Telford, Pennsylvania) (Figs. 12.1 and 12.5)
   a. Determines the yellowness of subcutaneous tissue by measuring the difference between optical densities for light in the blue and green wavelengths
   b. Measurement probe has two optical paths
   c. By calculating the difference between the optical densities, the parts common to the epidermis and

dermis are deducted. As a result, the difference can be obtained for subcutaneous tissue only.
   d. Theoretically allows for measurement of degree of yellowness of skin and subcutaneous tissue with minimal influence of melanin pigment and skin maturity
   e. Linear correlation of this measurement with TSB allows for conversion to TSB by the meter, which is indicated digitally.

2. BiliChek Noninvasive Bilirubin Analyzer (Children's Medical Ventures/Respironics, Norwell, Massachusetts) (Figs. 12.2 and 12.6)
   a. Noninvasive device consisting of light source, microspectrophotometer, fiberoptic probe, and microprocessor control circuit
   b. Uses entire spectrum of visible light reflected by the skin
   c. White light is transmitted into the skin and the reflected light is collected for analysis.
   d. Algorithms take into account the effect of hemoglobin, melanin, and dermal thickness.
   e. Absorption of light due to bilirubin in the capillary bed and subcutaneous tissue is isolated by spectral subtraction.

E. Special Circumstances/Considerations

1. Hospital protocols should include the conditions under which TCB and TSB levels are to be obtained (1). Protocols for training and recertification of TCB users should be in place.

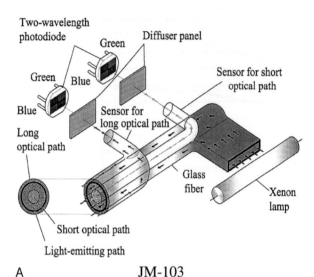

A   JM-103

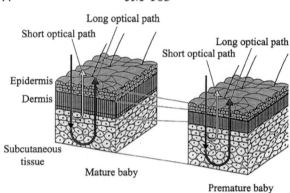

B   JM-103

FIG. 12.5. Measurement principle of Konica Minolta/Air-Shields JM-103 Jaundice Meter. (Reproduced with permission from *J Perinat Med.*, Vol. 31, Pages 81–88, Copyright © 2003 by Walter de Gruyter GmbH & Co. KG Berlin, New York.)

2. Only TSB measurements should be performed in infants with severe enough jaundice to warrant exchange transfusion (7).
3. TCB is less accurate in infants undergoing phototherapy; therefore, serum levels are preferred for monitoring bilirubin values in such infants (2,5,11,13).
4. Race/skin color: TCB readings obtained by the BiliChek have been found to correlate with TSB values in white, black, Asian, Hispanic, indigenous African, and Indian infants (7,13,16). In black infants, TCB readings obtained by the JM-103 correlate less closely with TSB values, with the TCB generally being greater than the TSB (6).

F. Techniques

1. Calibrate the TCB device according to manufacturer specifications. New devices should be correlated with serum samples before use.

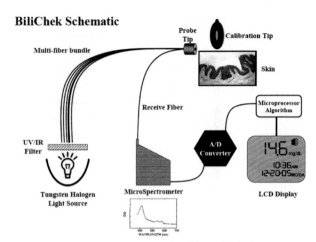

BiliChek Schematic

FIG. 12.6. Measurement principle of the BiliChek Noninvasive Bilirubin Analyzer. (Reproduced with permission of Children's Medical Ventures/Respironics.)

2. Measure TCB by pressing the trigger button and gently pressing the tip to the infant's forehead or sternum until the device indicates that reading is complete.
   a. Some studies have shown that TCB measurements from the sternum correlated slightly better with TSB levels than TCB measurements from the forehead, possibly as a result of the exposure of the forehead to ambient light. Other studies indicate both sites to be equivalent (6,17).
   b. Measurements must be taken in a consistent manner with regard to placement of the probe and amount of pressure applied to the device. Interoperative and intraoperative variability may be minimized with proper training (6).
   c. Measurement of the TCB using the BiliChek system takes approximately 20 to 80 seconds. This time is required for the monitor to make five measurements that are averaged to provide one TCB value. The JM-103 takes approximately 10 seconds to obtain its dual measurements and calculate the TCB value.
3. Repeated use of the disposable probes is not recommended.

G. Complications

No complications have been reported from the use of TCB monitors, except for the risk of inappropriate use and the possibility of underestimation of the level of jaundice.

H. Effectiveness

TCB measurement has been shown to decrease the number of heel pricks in some studies but has not changed the length of hospital stay or number of newborns requiring phototherapy. TCB monitoring has been shown to reduce the number of infants readmitted for phototherapy (18).

References

1. American Academy of Pediatrics Subcommittee on Hyperbilirubinemia. Neonatal jaundice and kernicterus. *Pediatrics.* 2001;108(3):31.
2. American Academy of Pediatrics Subcommittee on Hyperbilirubinemia. Management of hyperbilirubinemia in the newborn infant 35 or more weeks of gestation. *Pediatrics.* 2004; 114:297.
3. Maisels MJ, Bhutani VK, Bogen D, et al. Hyperbilirubinemia in the Newborn Infant >/= 35 weeks' gestation: an update with clarifications. *Pediatrics.* 2009;124;1193.
4. Szabo P, Wolf M, Bucher HU, et al. Detection of hyperbilirubinaemia in jaundiced full-term neonates by eye or bilirubinometer? *Eur J Pediatr.* 2004;163(12):722.
5. Maisels MJ. Transcutaneous bilirubinometry. *NeoReviews.* 2006; 7(5):e217.
6. Maisels MJ, Ostrea EM, Touch S, et al. Evaluation of a new transcutaneous bilirubinometer. *Pediatrics.* 2004;113:1628.
7. Bhutani VK, Gourley GR, Adler S, et al. Noninvasive measurement of total serum bilirubin in a multiracial predischarge newborn population to assess the risk of severe hyperbilirubinemia. *Pediatrics.* 2000;106:e17.
8. Yasuda S, Itoh S, Isobe K, et al. New transcutaneous jaundice device with two optical paths. *J Perinat Med.* 2003;31:81.
9. De Luca D, Zecca E, Corsello M. Attempt to improve transcutaneous bilirubinometry: a double-blind study of Medick BiliMed versus Respironics Bilicheck. *Arch Dis Child Fetal Neonatal Ed.* 2008;93:F135.
10. Bertini G, Pratesi S, Consenza E, et al. Transcutaneous bilirubin measurement: evaluation of Bilitest. *Neonatology.* 2008;93: 101.
11. Bhutani VK, Johnson L, Sivieri EM. Predictive ability of a predischarge hour-specific serum bilirubin for subsequent significant hyperbilirubinemia in healthy term and near-term newborns. *Pediatrics.* 1999;103(1):6.
12. Zecca E, Barone G, DeLuca D, et al. Skin bilirubin measurement during phototherapy in preterm and term newborn infants. *Early Human Development.* 2009;85:537.
13. Mahajan G, Kaushal RK, Sankhyan N, et al. Trancutaneous bilirubinometer in assessment of neonatal jaundice in Northern India. *Indian Pediatr.* 2005;42:41.
14. Nanjundaswamy S, Petrova A, Mehta R, et al. Transcutaneous bilirubinometry in preterm infants receiving phototherapy. *Am J Perinatol.* 2005;22(3):127.
15. Willems WA, van den Berg LM, de Wit H, et al. Transcutaneous bilirubinometry with the Bilicheck® in very premature newborns. *J Mat Fetal Neonatal Med.* 2004;16:209.
16. Slusher TM, Angyo IA, Bode-Thomas F, et al. Transcutaneous bilirubin measurements and serum total bilirubin levels in Indigenous African infants. *Pediatrics.* 2004;113:1636.
17. Ebbesen F, Rasmussen LM, Wimberley PD. A new transcutaneous bilirubinometer, BiliChek®, used in the neonatal intensive care unit and the maternity ward. *Acta Paediatr.* 2002;91:203.
18. Peterson JR, Okorodudu AO, Mohammad AA, et al. Association of trancutaneous bilirubin testing in hospital with decreased readmission rate for hyperbilirubinemia. *Clinical Chem.* 2005;51: 540.

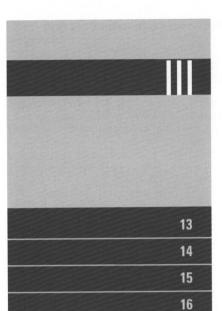

III Blood Sampling

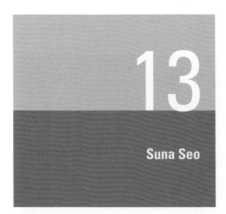

Vessel Localization

Suna Seo

Transillumination

A. Indication

Failure to locate an accessible artery or vein under normal lighting conditions for
1. Puncture for sampling (1–3)
2. Vessel cannulation (4,5)

B. Contraindications

None

C. Precautions

Verify that the light source equipment has an intact heat-absorbing glass and infrared and UV filters (6).

D. Equipment

1. Transillumination source
   a. High-intensity cold source with a fiberoptic cable (Fig. 13.1)
   b. Light-emitting diode (LED) (Fig. 13.2) (4,5)
   c. Otoscope light may be used in some instances (Fig. 13.3) (1)
2. Alcohol swab
3. Sterile glove or disposable plastic covers

E. Technique

1. Clean end of light source with an alcohol swab. Cover with sterile glove or disposable plastic cover.
2. Dim light in room. Some residual light is necessary to visualize operating field.
3. Set light source at low intensity and increase as needed for visualization.
4. Position probe to transilluminate vessel.
5. Identify vessel as a dark, linear structure (Figs. 13.4 and 13.5).
6. Compensate for distortion if light is not directly opposite the puncture site.

7. Do not maintain contact between light source and extremity for long periods of time.

F. Complications

1. Thermal burns from light probe (Figs. 13.6 and 13.7) (6–10)
2. Contamination from breach of sterile technique

Ultrasonography

A. Background

The use of portable ultrasound (US) as an adjunct tool for neonatal percutaneously inserted central catheter (PICC) placement has increased with the advent of smaller neonatal probes, and growing knowledge and experience of US (11).

B. Indication

To locate artery or vein for vessel cannulation (11–13)

C. Contraindications

None

D. Precautions

The difference between veins and arteries can be subtle in neonates. Veins are usually collapsible and arteries are pulsatile (12).

E. Equipment

1. High-frequency (>10 MHz) small (<30 mm width) linear US probe
2. Doppler function (screening for thrombosis and occlusion)
3. Zoom function
4. Sterile gel
5. Sterile probe cover

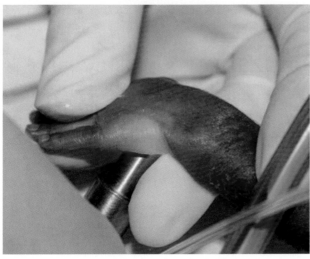

FIG. 13.1. Fiberoptic transilluminator placed on the palmar surface to visualize veins on the dorsum of hand.

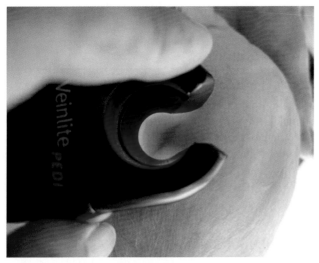

FIG. 13.2. LED transilluminator positioned to visualize a scalp vein. (Courtesy of Veinlite by Translite, Sugar Land, Texas.)

FIG. 13.3. Otoscope placed on the palmar surface to visualize cephalic vein.

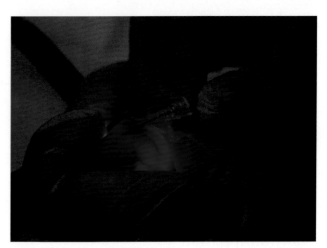

FIG. 13.4. Transilluminator placed on the palmar surface to visualize the veins on the dorsum during IV insertion.

F. Technique

1. Place a sterile cover over the probe, and use sterile lubricant on the probe
2. Use your nondominant hand to hold and position the US probe (Fig. 13.8)

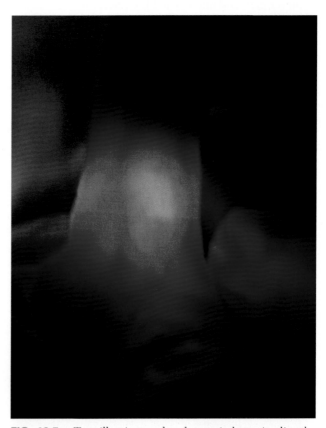

FIG. 13.5. Transilluminator placed posteriorly to visualize the posterior tibial artery.

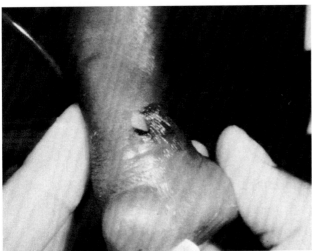

FIG. 13.6. Burn from transilluminator.

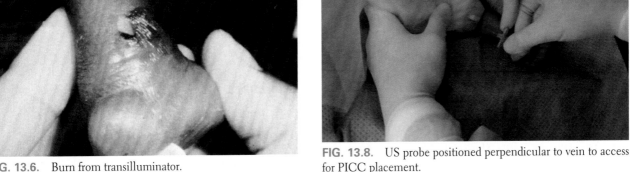

FIG. 13.8. US probe positioned perpendicular to vein to access for PICC placement.

3. Optimize probe orientation, placing the target vessel in the center of the screen.
   a. Short-axis or transverse view: Probe is placed transverse to the direction of the vessel, which is seen in cross-section (Fig. 13.9).
   b. Long-axis or sagittal view: Probe follows the direction of the vessel, which is seen in its length. Following the vein's path, identify valves, stenosis, or thrombosis.

   c. Out-of-plane where the needle crosses the US beam perpendicularly
   d. In-plane where the needle stays in the US beam
4. Position the handheld transducer probe perpendicular to a vein.
5. The needle tip should always be in the field of view during the procedure.

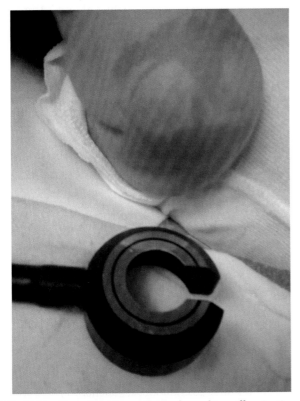

FIG. 13.7. Superficial burn after prolonged transillumination.

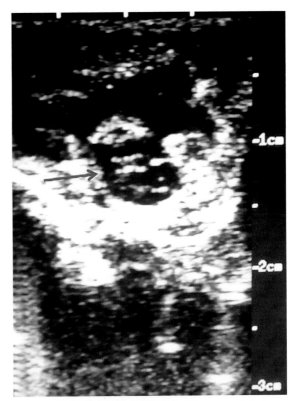

FIG. 13.9. Transverse view with cross-section of the vessel visualized.

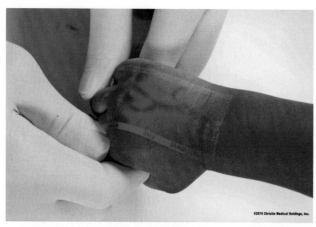

FIG. 13.10.   Near-infrared light image showing the dorsal venous arch. (Courtesy of Christie Medical Holdings, Inc., Memphis, Tennessee.)

G. Complications

None

Near-Infrared Visualization

A. Background

The infrared light source emits a harmless, near-infrared light, which is absorbed by the blood. Tissues surrounding the blood reflect the light and this image is captured by a digital video camera and processed. A green LED adds contrast to the image, which is then directly projected onto the surface of the skin in real time. This device requires no patient contact and has no heat, radiation or laser–eye safety issues (15,16).

B. Indication

1. To locate an accessible artery or vein for
   a. Phlebotomy
   b. Vessel cannulation

C. Contraindications

None

D. Equipment

Direct projection vascular imaging device

E. Technique

1. Position the head unit at 90 degrees and approximately 13 inches (33 cm) above the target location
2. Focus the device
3. Switch to and utilize alternate modes
   a. Universal (Fig. 13.10)
   b. Inverse
   c. Resize
   d. Fine Detail

References

1. Goren A, Laufer J, Yativ N, et al. Transillumination of the palm for venipuncture in infants. *Pediatr Emerg Care.* 2001;17(2):130.
2. Mattson D, O'Connor M. Transilluminatior assistance in neonatal venipuncture. *Neonatal Netw.* 1986;5:42.
3. Dinner M. Transillumination to facilitate venipuncture in children. *Anesth Analg.* 1992;74:467.
4. Hosokawa K, Kato H, Kishi C, et al. Transillumination by light-emitting diode facilitates peripheral venous cannulations in infants and small children. *Acta Anaesthesiol Scand.* 2010;54:957.
5. John J. Transillumination for vascular access: old concept, new technology. *Pediatr Anesth.* 2007;17:189.
6. Sumpelmann R, Osthaus W, Irmler H, et al. Prevention of burns caused by transillumination for peripheral venous access in neonates. *Pediatr Anesth.* 2006;16:1094.
7. Perman M, Kauls L. Transilluminator burns in the neonatal intensive care unit: a mimicker of more serious disease. *Pediatr Dermatol.* 2007;24:168.
8. Keroack MA, Kotilainen HR, Griffin BE. A cluster of atypical skin lesions in well-baby nurseries and a neonatal intensive care unit. *J Perinatol.* 1996;16:370.
9. Sajben FP, Gibbs NF, Friedlander SF. Transillumination blisters in a neonate. *J Am Acad Dermatol.* 1999;41:264.
10. Withey SJ, Moss ALH, Williams GJP. Cold light, heat burn. *Burns.* 2000;26:414.
11. Pettit J. Technological advances for PICC placement and management. *Adv Neonatal Care.* 2007;7:122.
12. Detaille T, Pirotte T, Veyckemans F. Vascular access in the neonate. *Best Pract Res Clin Anaesthesiol.* 2010;24:403.
13. Fidler HL. The use of bedside ultrasonography for PICC placement and insertion. *Adv Neonatal Care.* 2011;11:52.
14. Moureau NL. Using ultrasound to guide PICC insertion. *Nursing.* 2003;33:20.
15. Hess HA. A biomedical device to improve pediatric vascular access success. *Pediatr Nurs.* 2010;36:259.
16. Perry AM, Caviness AC, Hsu D. Efficacy of a near-infrared light device in pediatric intravenous cannulation: a randomized controlled trial. *Pediatr Emerg Care.* 2011;27(1):5.

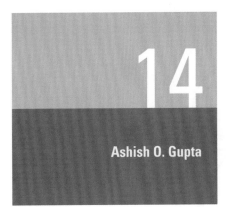

Venipuncture

Ashish O. Gupta

A. Indications

1. Blood sampling
   a. Routine laboratory tests, particularly if the volume of blood required is larger than can be obtained by capillary sampling.
   b. Blood culture
   c. Central hematocrit
   d. Preferred (over capillary sample) for certain studies (1,2)
      (1) Ammonia, lactate or pyruvate level (arterial optimal)
      (2) Drug levels
      (3) Cross-matching blood
      (4) Hemoglobin/hematocrit
      (5) Karyotype
      (6) Coagulation studies
2. Administration of medications

B. Contraindications

1. Use of deep vein in presence of coagulation defect
2. Local infection and/or inflammation at puncture site
3. Femoral or internal jugular vein (see G)
4. External jugular vein in infants with respiratory distress, intracranial hemorrhage, or raised intracranial pressure

C. Precautions

1. Observe universal precautions.
2. When sampling from neck veins, place infant in head-down position to avoid cranial air embolus. Do not use neck veins in infants with intracranial bleeding or increased intracranial pressure.
3. Remove tourniquet before removing needle (to minimize hematoma formation).
4. Apply local pressure with dry gauze to produce hemostasis (usually 2 to 3 minutes).
5. Avoid using alcohol swab to apply local pressure (painful, impairs hemostasis).

D. Special Considerations for Neonates

1. Conserve sites to preserve limited venous access by using distal sites first whenever possible.
2. Use small needle or scalp vein butterfly. A 23-gauge needle is the best. Hemolysis or clotting may occur with a 25-gauge or smaller needle.
3. Choice of veins in order of preference (Fig. 14.1)
   a. Basilic, cephalic, or cubital veins in the antecubital fossa
   b. Greater saphenous vein at the ankle
   c. Dorsum of hands
   d. Dorsum of feet
   e. Vein in center of the volar aspect of the wrist
   f. Proximal greater saphenous vein
   g. Scalp
   h. Neck
4. Pain control
   a. Lidocaine–prilocaine topical anesthetic cream applied 30 minutes prior to procedure, if time allows (3,4).
   b. Oral sucrose solution (12% to 25%) provides quick and effective pain control for venipuncture (4,5).
   c. Heel lancing can be more painful and require more punctures than venipuncture in infants (3,6).

E. Equipment

1. Gloves
2. A 23-gauge venipuncture needle (Fig. 14.2).
3. Syringe with volume just larger than sample to be drawn
4. Alcohol swabs
5. Gauze pads
6. Appropriate containers for specimens
7. For blood culture
   a. Povidone–iodine solution preparation (three swabs)
   b. Sterile gloves
   c. Blood culture bottle(s)
   d. Transfer needle
8. Tourniquet or sphygmomanometer cuff

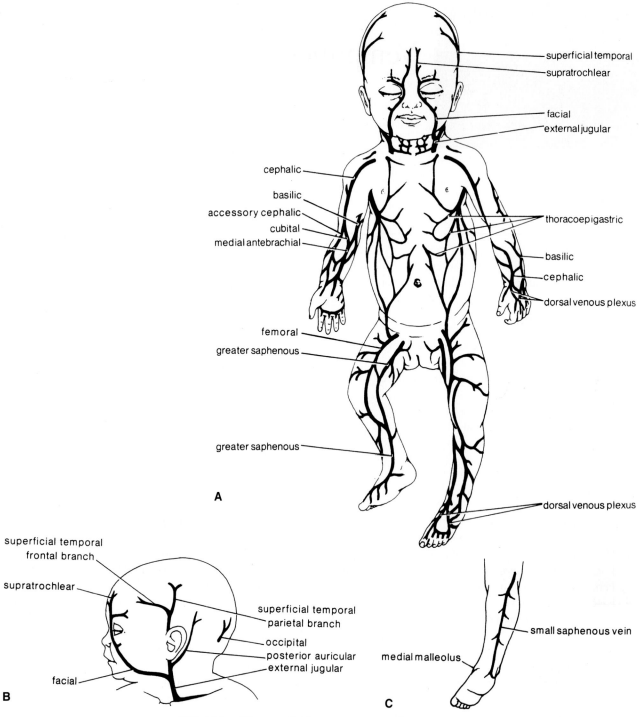

superficial temporal
supratrochlear

facial
external jugular

cephalic

basilic

accessory cephalic

cubital

medial antebrachial

thoracoepigastric

basilic

cephalic

dorsal venous plexus

femoral

greater saphenous

greater saphenous

A

dorsal venous plexus

superficial temporal
frontal branch

supratrochlear

superficial temporal
parietal branch

occipital

posterior auricular

external jugular

facial

B

small saphenous vein

medial malleolus

C

FIG. 14.1. The superficial venous system in the neonate.

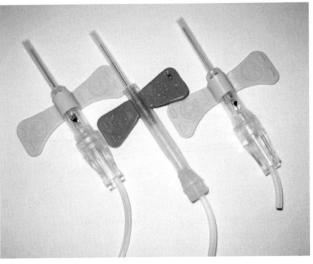

FIG. 14.2. Safety-engineered needles for venipuncture.

F. Technique

General Venipuncture

1. Locate the appropriate vessel. Use transillumination if necessary (see Chapter 13). Warm extremity with heel warmer or warm washcloth if circulation is poor.
2. Apply anesthetic cream if time permits, and/or administer sucrose solution if possible.
3. Restrain infant appropriately.
4. Prepare area with antiseptic (see Chapter 5).
5. Occlude vein proximally using either
   a. Blood pressure cuff inflated to level between systolic and diastolic pressure
   b. Rubber band (loop two bands together, tied as in Fig. 14.3)

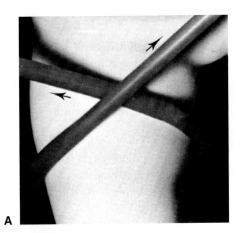

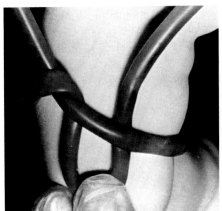

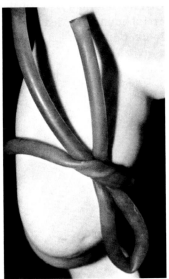

FIG. 14.3. Correct application of a tourniquet for quick release.

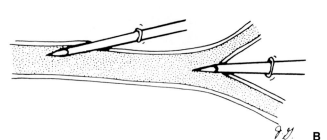

A   **B**

FIG. 14.4.   **A:** Venipuncture technique. Note position of fingers with forefinger occluding vein proximally. **B:** Needle penetrating skin a short distance from site of venipuncture.

   c. Using forefinger and thumb to encircle the extremity or use forefinger and middle finger as a tourniquet (Fig. 14.4A)
6. Remove occlusion device and replace to promote optimal vein distension.
7. Syringe collection: Check syringe function and attach to needle. Penetrate skin first and position for entry of vein (Fig. 14.4A,B).
   a. Angle of entry 15 to 30 degrees
   b. Bevel up preferred for optimal blood flow (less chance of needle occlusion by vein wall)
   c. Direction of entry against the direction of blood flow
   d. If possible, insert needle at area where vessel bifurcates to avoid "rolling" of veins.
8. Collect sample by gentle suction
   a. To prevent occlusion by vein wall
   b. To avoid hemolysis
9. Release tourniquet.
10. Remove needle and apply local pressure with dry gauze for 1 to 3 minutes or until complete hemostasis.

Drip Technique

1. Cut the extension tubing of the 23-guage butterfly needle catheter at 1 to 2 cm length (Fig. 14.2).
2. Follow steps 1 to 6, as above.
3. Insert the needle in the vein as in step 7, but without a syringe attached to the needle.
4. Collect the drops of blood directly into specimen container (Fig. 14.5).
5. Short sterile hypodermic needles (23 or 24 gauge) may also be used to collect blood samples by the drip method but are sometimes less successful because the blood may pool at the hub of the needle and clot.
6. Drip method cannot be used for blood culture or coagulation studies (6).

Scalp Vein

1. Shave adequate area of frontal or parietal scalp.
2. Use scalp vein needle set or 23-gauge butterfly.
3. Occlude vein proximally with finger.
4. Feel for a pulse to avoid entering an artery.
5. Use a shallow angle (15 to 20 degrees).
6. See F, "General Venipuncture."

Proximal Greater Saphenous Vein (7)

1. Use only in older infants or in term neonates without evidence of coagulopathy.
2. Have assistant hold infant's thighs abducted with knees and hips slightly flexed.
3. Locate femoral triangle (Fig. 14.6A).
   a. **Proximal boundary:** Inguinal ligament
   b. **Lateral boundary:** Medial border of sartorius muscle
   c. **Medial boundary:** Lateral border of adductor longus muscle

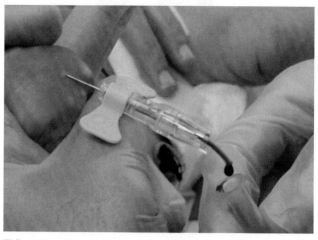

FIG. 14.5.   Drip technique of blood collection.

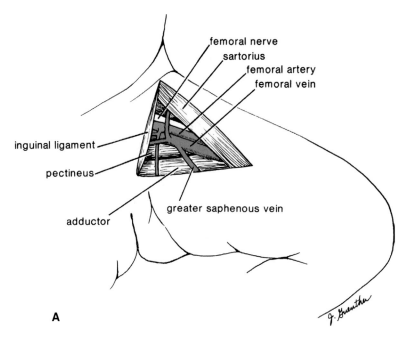
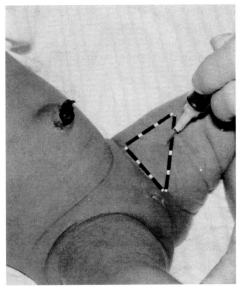

FIG. 14.6. **A:** Anatomy of the femoral triangle as defined in the text. (Adapted from Plaxico DT, Bucciarella RL. Greater saphenous vein venipuncture in the neonate. *J Pediatr.* 1978;93:1025, with permission.) **B:** Position of the femoral triangle on the abducted thigh.

4. Enter skin and then vein at point medial to the arterial pulsation, approximately two-thirds along the line from inguinal ligament to apex of triangle (Fig. 14.6B).
   a. Use relatively steep angle (45 to 60 degrees).
   b. After entering skin, advance 1 to 4 mm while applying gentle suction until blood return is achieved.
5. See F, "General Venipuncture."

External Jugular Vein

1. Position infant in head-down position with head extended and rotated away from selected vessel (Fig. 14.7).

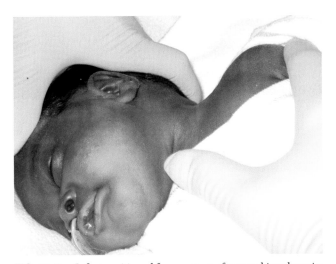

FIG. 14.7. Infant positioned for puncture of external jugular vein.

2. Prepare skin over sternocleidomastoid muscle with antiseptic.
3. Flick infant's heel to induce crying and optimize vein distension.
4. Visualize external jugular vein running from angle of jaw to posterior border of sternocleidomastoid in its lower third.
5. Puncture vessel where it runs across the anterior border of the sternocleidomastoid muscle.
6. See F, "General Venipuncture."

G. Complications (8–11)

1. Hemorrhage with
   a. Coagulation defect
   b. Puncture of deep vein
2. Venous thrombosis or embolus, limb ischemia, and arteriovenous fistula with puncture of large, deep vein (9)
3. Laceration of adjacent artery
4. During femoral vein puncture
   a. Reflex arteriospasm of femoral artery with gangrene of extremity (10)
   b. Penetration of peritoneal cavity
   c. Septic arthritis of hip (11)
   d. Arteriovenous fistula (9)
5. During internal jugular puncture
   a. Laceration of carotid artery
   b. Pneumothorax/subcutaneous emphysema

c. Interference with ventilation due to positioning
d. Raised intracranial pressure to head-down position aggravating intraventricular hemorrhage

6. During scalp vein puncture
   a. Laceration of artery
   b. Corneal abrasion or other eye damage if rubber band used improperly

References

1. Baral J. Use of a simple technique for the collection of blood from premature and full-term babies. *Med J Aust.* 1968;1:97.
2. Kayiran SM, Ozbek N, Turan M, et al. Significant differences between capillary and venous complete blood counts in the neonatal period. *Clin Lab Haematol.* 2003;25:9.
3. Shah VS, Ohlsson A. Venepuncture versus heel lance for blood sampling in term neonate. *Cochrane Database Syst Rev.* 2011;(10):CD001452.
4. Biran V, Gourrier E, Cimerman P, et al. Analgesic effects of EMLA cream and oral sucrose during venepuncture in preterm infants. *Pediatrics.* 2011;128(1):e63.
5. Stevens B, Yamada J, Ohlsson A. Sucrose for analgesia in newborn infants undergoing painful procedures. *Cochrane Database Syst Rev.* 2004;(3):CD001069.
6. Ogawa S, Ogihara T, Fujiwara E, et al. Venepuncture is preferable to heel lance for blood sampling in term neonate. *Arch Dis Child Fetal Neonatal Ed.* 2005;90(5):F432.
7. Plaxico DT, Bucciarelli RL. Greater saphenous vein venipuncture in the neonate. *J Pediatr.* 1978;93:1025.
8. Ramasethu J. Complications of vascular catheters in the neonatal intensive care unit. *Clin Perinatol.* 2008;35:199.
9. Gamba P, Tchaprassian Z, Verlato F, et al. Iatrogenic vascular lesions in extremely low birth weight and low birth weight neonates. *J Vasc Surg.* 1997;26(4):643.
10. Kantr RK, Gorton JM, Palmieri K, et al. Anatomy of femoral vessels in infants and guidelines for venous catheterizations. *Pediatrics.* 1989;33:1020.
11. Asnes RS, Arendar GM. Septic arthritis of the hip: a complication of venipuncture. *Pediatrics.* 1966;38:837.

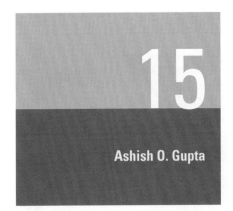

15 Arterial Puncture

Ashish O. Gupta

A. Indications (1,2)

1. Sampling for arterial blood gas determination
2. Sampling for routine laboratory test when venous and capillary sampling are not suitable or unobtainable
3. Sampling for ammonia, lactate, or pyruvate level
4. To obtain a large quantity of blood

B. Contraindications

1. Coagulation defects, thrombocytopenia
2. Circulatory compromise in the extremity
3. Inappropriate artery
   a. Femoral artery
   b. Use of radial artery if collaterals are inadequate (see Allen test below)
   c. Ulnar artery (poor collaterals)
4. Infection and/or inflammation in sampling area
5. When cannulation of that vessel is anticipated
6. Use of peripheral arteries on the ipsilateral arm in an infant with congenital heart disease requiring a shunt via the subclavian artery

C. Precautions

1. Perform arterial sampling only when venous or capillary sampling is inappropriate or unobtainable.
2. Use smallest possible (23- to 27-gauge) needle to minimize trauma to vessel and to prevent hematoma formation.
3. Avoid laceration of the artery caused by puncturing both sides of arterial wall in exactly opposite locations.
4. Remove excess heparin and air bubble from the blood gas syringe. If a small bubble gets into the sample, point the top of the syringe up, expel the air bubble immediately, and cap syringe.
5. Guarantee hemostasis at the end of the procedure. Pressure must be applied even if an attempt is unsuccessful or results in an inadequate sample.
6. Check distal circulation after puncture.
   a. Arterial pulse
   b. Capillary refill time
   c. Color and temperature
7. Take action to reverse arteriospasm, if necessary. (See Chapter 34.)

D. Selection of Arterial Site

1. Peripheral site preferred.
2. Radial artery preferred if ulnar collateral intact.
3. Posterior tibial artery satisfactory.
4. Dorsalis pedis artery is often small or absent, but may be accessible in some infants.
5. Brachial artery *only* if indication is urgent *and peripheral arterial or umbilical artery access is not available* because of risk of injury to the adjacent median nerve, and the risk of ischemia due to the absence of collaterals at this site (3).
6. Temporal artery should be avoided because of risk of neurologic damage (4,5).
7. Ulnar artery should be avoided because of the risk of impaired circulation to the hand due to poor collateral circulation or damage to the ulnar or the median nerve.

E. Equipment

1. Sterile gloves
2. Sterile needle
   a. A 23- to 25-gauge venipuncture needle, preferably a safety-engineered needle
   b. A butterfly needle with extension tubing is often easier to use
3. Appropriate syringes, including a preheparinized blood gas syringe
4. Povidone–iodine solution and alcohol prep pads or wipes for minor skin preparation
5. Gauze pads
6. High-intensity fiberoptic light for transillumination (optional) and a sterile glove to cover (see Chapter 13)
7. Oral sucrose solution (24% to 25%) or eutectic mixture of local anesthetics for pain control, if possible (6,7).

F. Technique (See Procedures Website for Video)

General Principles (1,2)

1. Transillumination may assist location of vessel (8) (see Fig. 13.5).
2. Clean the site with povidone–iodine and alcohol.
3. Position needle for arterial puncture against direction of blood flow.
   a. Keep angle of entry shallow for superficial vessels at 15 to 30 degrees; use 45-degree angle for deeper artery.
   b. Penetrate the skin first slightly proximal to the best point of pulsation, and then puncture artery to minimize trauma to vessel, keeping bevel of needle up.
   c. Apply gentle suction on syringe as soon as blood flow is observed; maintain needle in same position until all blood samples have been collected.
   d. If no blood flow is obtained or blood flow ceases, adjust depth of penetration or the angle of the needle. If resistance is encountered, withdraw needle cautiously until blood returns. Be patient and gentle—artery may spasm when needle is introduced, or with multiple attempts.
   e. Use fresh needle and repeat skin preparation if withdrawal from skin is necessary.
4. Apply firm, local pressure for 1 to 3 minutes to achieve complete hemostasis.
5. Inspect fingers for circulatory compromise (9,10).

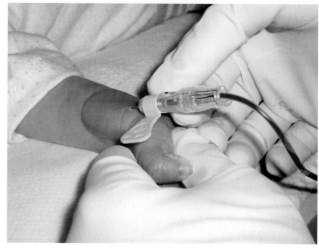

FIG. 15.1.   Radial artery puncture.

Radial Artery Puncture (2) (Fig. 15.1)

1. Slightly extend supine wrist, avoiding hyperextension, which may occlude the vessel.
2. Locate radial and ulnar arteries at proximal wrist crease (Fig. 15.2).
   a. Radial artery is lateral to flexor carpi radialis tendon.
   b. Ulnar artery is medial to flexor carpi ulnaris tendon.

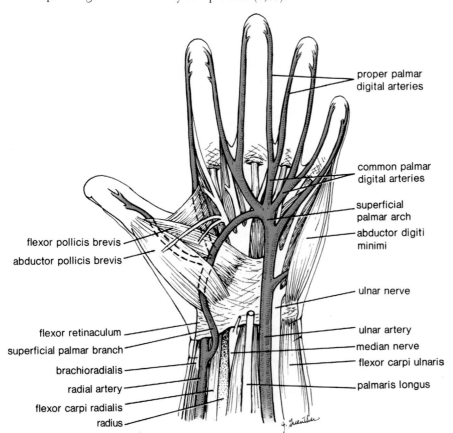

proper palmar digital arteries

common palmar digital arteries

superficial palmar arch

abductor digiti minimi

ulnar nerve

ulnar artery

median nerve

flexor carpi ulnaris

palmaris longus

flexor pollicis brevis

abductor pollicis brevis

flexor retinaculum

superficial palmar branch

brachioradialis

radial artery

flexor carpi radialis

radius

FIG. 15.2.   Anatomy of the major arteries of the wrist and hand.

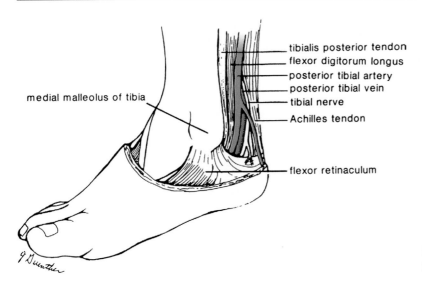

medial malleolus of tibia

tibialis posterior tendon
flexor digitorum longus
posterior tibial artery
posterior tibial vein
tibial nerve
Achilles tendon

flexor retinaculum

FIG. 15.3. Anatomic relations of the posterior tibial artery.

3. The effectiveness of the modified Allen test (described below) for assessing the adequacy of collateral supply to the hand has not been adequately studied in neonates and suffers from poor interobserver reliability. Transillumination is a valuable adjunct and use of ultrasound has also been reported (11).
   a. Elevate infant's hand.
   b. Occlude both radial and ulnar arteries at wrist.
   c. Massage palm toward wrist.
   d. Release occlusion of ulnar artery only.
   e. Look for color to return to hand in <10 seconds, indicating adequate collateral supply.

   f. Do not puncture radial artery if color return takes more than 15 seconds.
4. Puncture the skin at the level of proximal crease and penetrate artery at 15 to 30 degrees with bevel up.
5. See F, "General Principles."

Posterior Tibial Puncture

1. Locate artery by palpation or transillumination between Achilles tendon and medial malleolus (Fig. 15.3; see also Fig. 13.5). Puncture the artery just posterior to medial malleolus.
2. See F, "General Principles."

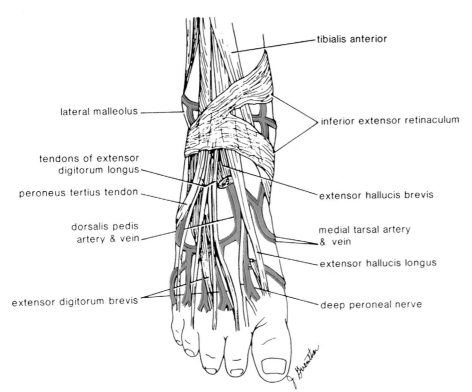

tibialis anterior

lateral malleolus

inferior extensor retinaculum

tendons of extensor digitorum longus

peroneus tertius tendon

extensor hallucis brevis

dorsalis pedis artery & vein

medial tarsal artery & vein

extensor hallucis longus

extensor digitorum brevis

deep peroneal nerve

FIG. 15.4. Anatomic relations of the dorsalis pedis artery.

Dorsalis Pedis Puncture

1. Locate artery by palpation or transillumination on dorsum of foot between extensor hallucis longus and extensor digitorum longus tendons (Fig. 15.4). It can be located between the first and second metatarsal in the dorsal midfoot between the first and second toes.
2. See F, "General Principles."

Brachial Artery Puncture

1. Locate the artery by palpation or transillumination along the medial margin of the biceps muscle at the bend of elbow and enter the artery at or above the level of anterior cubital fossa.
2. See F, "General Principles."

G. Complications (10)

See Chapter 34 for complications of arterial cannulation.

1. Distal ischemia from arteriospasm, thrombosis, or embolism
2. Infection (rare)
   a. Osteomyelitis (12)
   b. Infected hip joint after femoral puncture (12)
3. Hemorrhage or hematoma
4. Nerve damage (13)
   a. Median nerve (brachial artery puncture)
   b. Posterior tibial nerve
   c. Femoral nerve
5. Extensor tendon sheath injury, resulting in "false cortical thumb" (14)
6. Pseudoaneurysm following brachial artery puncture (15)

References

1. Smith AD. Arterial blood sampling in neonates. *Lancet.* 1975; 1:254.
2. Shaw JC. Arterial sampling from the radial artery in premature and full-term infants. *Lancet.* 1968;2:389.
3. Okeson GC, Wulbrecht PH. The safety of brachial artery puncture for arterial blood sampling. *Chest.* 1998;114:748.
4. Bull MJ, Schreiner RL, Garg BP, et al. Neurologic complications following temporal artery catheterization. *J Pediatr.* 1980;96:1071.
5. Simmons MA, Levine RL, Lubchenco LO, et al. Warning: serious sequelae of temporal artery catheterization. *J Pediatr.* 1978; 92:284.
6. Acharya AB, Annamali S, Taub NA, et al. Oral sucrose analgesia for preterm infant venipuncture. *Arch Dis Childhood Fetal Neonatal Ed.* 2004;89:F17.
7. Stevens B, Yamada J, Ohlsson A. Sucrose for analgesia in newborn infants undergoing painful procedures. *Cochrane Database Syst Rev.* 2004;(3):CD001069.
8. Wall PM, Kuhns LR. Percutaneous arterial sampling using transillumination. *Pediatrics.* 1977;59:1032.
9. Noreng MF. Blood flow in the radial artery before and after arterial puncture. *Acta Anaesthesiol Scand.* 1986;30:281.
10. Gillies ID, Morgan M, Sykes MK, et al. The nature and incidence of complications of peripheral artery puncture. *Anaesthesia.* 1979;34:506.
11. Barone JE, Madlinger RV. Should an Allen test be performed before radial artery cannulation? *J Trauma.* 2006;61:468.
12. Nelson DL, Hable KA, Matsen JM. *Proteus mirabilis* osteomyelitis in two neonates following needle puncture. Successful treatment with ampicillin. *Am J Dis Child.* 1973;125:109.
13. Pape KE, Armstrong DL, Fitzhardinge PM. Peripheral median nerve damage secondary to brachial arterial blood gas sampling. *J Pediatr.* 1978;93:852.
14. Skogland RR, Giles EJ. The false cortical thumb. *Am J Dis Child.* 1986;140:375.
15. Landau D, Schreiber R, Szendro G, et al. Brachial artery pseudoaneurysm in a premature infant. *Arch Dis Child Fetal Neo Ed.* 2003;88:F152.

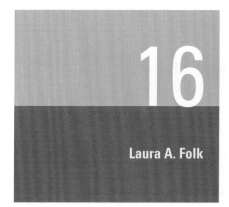

16 Capillary Blood Sampling

Laura A. Folk

A. Purpose

To obtain capillary blood samples that provide accurate laboratory results with minimal discomfort and potential for injury/infection

B. Background

Capillary heel blood sampling is an easily mastered, minimally invasive technique that, when performed with proper technique and equipment, provides laboratory results within acceptable tolerances compared with samples from arterial catheters (1). The advantage of capillary sampling is that repeated testing may be carried out, and peripheral veins may be saved for IV access.

C. Indications

1. Capillary blood gas sampling
2. Routine laboratory analysis (standard hematology, chemistries, toxicology/drug levels) requiring a limited amount of blood in which minimal cell lysis does not alter results
3. Newborn metabolic screen

D. Contraindications

1. Edema, because interstitial fluid dilutes the sample and gives inaccurate results
2. Injury or anomalies that preclude putting pressure on the foot
3. Areas that are bruised or injured by multiple previous heelsticks
4. Poor perfusion
5. Local infection

E. Limitations

1. Venous or arterial blood rather than capillary samples should be used for
   a. Blood cultures, which require sterile technique
   b. Tests in which even a minimal amount of hemolysis will compromise results
   c. Special tests such as coagulation studies (newer coagulation tests that require only a few drops of blood are still not widely available)
   d. Laboratory tests that require more than 1.5 mL of blood

F. Equipment

1. Gloves
2. Heel-warming device or a warm towel (see G)
3. Antiseptic (Betadine/saline or alcohol swab)
4. Pad or other means of protecting bed linens
5. Heel-lancing device (see G). Use appropriate size for infant (Table 16.1).
6. Specimen collector as appropriate
   a. Serum separators
   b. Hematology tubes
   c. Capillary blood gas tube
   d. Newborn metabolic screen filter paper
7. Capillary tubes for blood transfer to lab tubes if appropriate
8. Small adhesive bandage or gauze wrap

G. Heel-Lancing Devices and Heel Warmers

1. **Automated heel-lancing device:** Encased, spring-loaded, retractable blade that provides a controlled and consistent width and depth of incision for blood testing
   a. Incision depths range from 0.65 to 2 mm for micro-preemies through toddlers (Tenderfoot, International Technidyne Corporation, Edison, New Jersey) and from 0.85 to 1 mm for preemies and newborns (BD Quickheel Lancet, BD Vacutainer Systems, Franklin Lakes, New Jersey) (Table 16.1).
   b. The controlled depths avoid damage to the calcaneus (2,3) while providing greater yield with less pain, hemolysis, and laboratory-value error (4–7). The shallower devices can be used to obtain small

TABLE 16.1	Examples of Automated Heel-Lancing Products Based on Infant Size	
Infant Size	**Available Products**	**Incision Depth/Length**
<1,000 g	Tenderfoot Micro-preemie	0.65 mm/1.40 mm
Low-birthweight and preemie >1,000 g	Tenderfoot Preemie/BD Quickheel Preemie	0.85 mm/1.75 mm
Term to 3–6 mo	Tenderfoot Newborn/BD Quickheel Infant	1.0 mm/2.50 mm
6 mo–2 y	Tenderfoot Toddler	2.0 mm/3.00 mm

samples from larger infants who require frequent point-of-care glucose testing (8).

c. Nonautomated (manual) stylet-type lancets and spring-loaded needle-puncture devices designed for adult glucose testing are not appropriate for infants (7).

2. **Heel warmer:** Chemically activated packet to heat heel prior to capillary testing. If heel warming is used, a commercial prepackaged unit provides controlled temperature. The warmer should be applied for 5 minutes and then removed prior to heelstick.

H. Precautions

1. Site
   a. Do not use the end of the heel. The calcaneum is superficial at this site, and there is an increased risk of osteomyelitis (2).
   b. Do not use fingertips, toes, or earlobes of babies.
2. Hand position
   Do *not* squeeze the heel. Squeezing the heel results in greater pain, lower blood yield, and increased cell lysis.
3. Collection
   a. If using capillary tubes for blood transfer, it is essential to determine whether the tube contains substances such as anticoagulants, which may have the potential to interfere with lab results. Do not use tubes containing anticoagulants for newborn metabolic screens.
   b. Scoop-shaped collectors provided with mini–lab tubes are used to guide blood drops to the specimen tube. Avoid repeated "scooping" along the surface of the foot. Microclots that form in blood on the skin can alter lab results.

I. Technique

1. Identify site; the preferred areas for capillary heel testing are the outer aspects of the heel (Fig. 16.1).
   a. Vary sites to prevent bruising and skin damage.
   b. The plantar surface can be used in term and late preterm term infants if the preferred areas are compromised by previous frequent testing (Fig. 16.2). The skin-to-calcaneal perichondrium distance is at

least 3 mm in most term babies and in 91% of babies at 33 to 37 weeks' gestation, but is at least 3 mm in only about 60% of babies <33 weeks' gestation (2).

2. Apply heel warmer or warm towel for 5 minutes. Remove just before procedure.
3. Provide comfort measures: Facilitated tucking/swaddling and the use of pacifiers combined with administration of a concentrated sucrose solution results in less measurable pain and faster resolution of discomfort in the infant following the procedure (9,10) (Fig. 4.1). Kangaroo Care 30 minutes prior to and during procedure has shown a reduction in pain scores for stable premature infants; however, the long-term association of maternal contact during painful stimulus has not been studied. (11,12)
4. Wash hands and put gloves on.
5. Cleanse site with Betadine followed with saline wipe or alcohol wipe.
6. Position hand with fingers along the calf and thumb at ball of foot to stabilize. Apply pressure along calf toward heel (Fig. 16.3).
7. Prepare automated device by removing release clip.
8. Place automated device on site and activate.
9. Apply pressure to leg with counterpressure to ball of foot and allow blood drop to form.
10. Wipe away first drop of blood with gauze or clean wipe.
11. Using capillary action, fill blood gas tube, holding tube horizontally (Fig. 16.4).

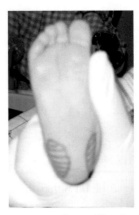

FIG. 16.1.   Appropriate sites for capillary heelstick sampling are along the sides of the heels.

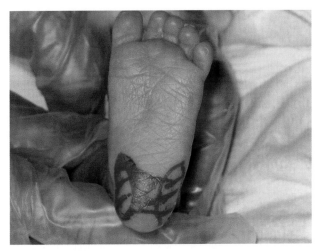

FIG. 16.2. Alternative site for capillary heelstick sampling. If frequent sampling has rendered the sides of the heels unsuitable, the plantar surface between them can be used. Do not incise the end of the heel.

12. Release pressure, allowing capillaries to refill.
13. Guide blood drops into tube or collect with capillary tube for transfer to laboratory tube.
14. If blood stops flowing, wipe site to remove clot with alcohol swab, gauze, or clean wipe; ensure time for capillary refill; and then reapply pressure to leg. If blood does not flow, choose another site and repeat procedure or consider venipuncture.
15. When samples have been collected, apply pressure to puncture site and wrap with gauze or apply adhesive bandage.
16. Continue comfort measures.

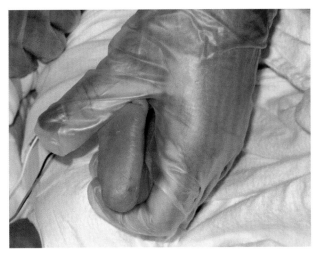

FIG. 16.3. Position for hand and automated lancing device. Position heel in the apex of the angle of the thumb and forefinger with fingers along the calf and thumb along the ball of the foot. Place automated lancing device in appropriate position. Apply pressure along the calf with counterpressure by the thumb. Do not squeeze the heel.

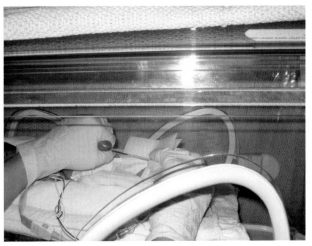

FIG. 16.4. Capillary blood gas sampling.

J. Specimen Handling

1. Collect blood gas sample first, then hematology samples, and then chemistry/toxicology samples.
2. Ensure that blood gas samples are free of air bubbles.
   a. Place the tube horizontally so that the blood is drawn by capillary action and does not collect air bubbles that can alter results. Apply caps to ends of tube.
   b. Capillary blood gas samples should be analyzed within 10 minutes or should be kept horizontally on ice for up to 1 hour, and the tube must be rolled prior to analysis. Consult institution laboratory for guidance on blood gas sample storage and transport.
3. Flick side of hematology microtube during collection process to activate anticoagulant and prevent clotting.
4. *Newborn metabolic screen*: Specific collection guidelines (13)
   a. Minimum 24 to 48 hours after birth
   b. Integrity of collection medium: Avoid touching filter paper, as oils from finger can compromise results.
   c. Single (no overlapping) drops on filter paper. Position infant so that incision is in the dependent position, allowing a large drop of blood to form. Blood should drop freely onto designated circle on filter paper. Repeat for each circle.
   d. Do not apply blood using capillary tubes that contain anticoagulants or other materials that can interfere with lab results.

K. Complications

1. Pain
2. Infection (cellulitis, abscess, perichondritis, osteomyelitis) (Fig. 16.5) (14,15)
3. Tissue loss and scarring
4. Calcified nodules (16)

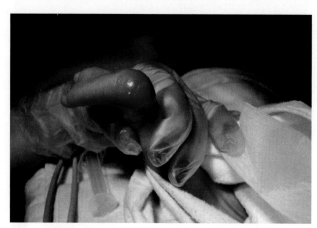

FIG. 16.5. Cellulitis of heel—complication of capillary heel-stick sampling.

L. Inaccurate Laboratory Results

1. Hyperkalemia secondary to excessive hemolysis
   a. Use proper technique and procedures to minimize cell lysis.
2. Erroneous blood gas results
   a. Ensure that sample is free of air bubbles.
   b. Avoid delay in analysis.
   c. Use proper technique and procedures to minimize cell lysis.

References

1. Johnson K, Cress G, Connolly N, et al. Neonatal laboratory blood sampling: comparison of results from arterial catheters with those from an automated capillary device. *Neonatal Network.* 2000; 19(1):27.
2. Arena J, Emparanza J, Nogues A, et al. Skin to calcaneus distance in the neonate. *Arch Dis Child Fetal Neonatal Ed.* 2005;90(4):F328.
3. Vertanen H, Fellman V, Brommels M, et al. An automated incision device for obtaining blood samples from the heels of preterm infants causes less damage than a conventional manual lancet. *Arch Dis Child Fetal Neonatal Ed.* 2001;84(1):F53.
4. Shepherd AJ, Glenesk A, Niven CA, et al. A Scottish study of heel-prick blood sampling in newborn babies. *Midwifery.* 2005; 7(2):158.
5. Kellan B, Waller J, McLaurin C, et al. Tenderfoot preemie vs a manual lancet: a clinical evaluation. *Neonatal Network.* 2001; 20(7):31.
6. Kazmierczak SC, Robertson AF, Briley KP. Comparison of hemolysis in blood samples collected using an automatic incision device and a manual lancet. *Arch Pediatr Adolesc Med.* 2002;156(11):1072.
7. Shah V, Taddio A, Kulasekaran K, et al. Evaluation of a new lancet device (BD QuickHeel) on pain response and success of procedure in term neonates. *Arch Pediatr Adolesc Med.* 2003;157(11):1075.
8. Noerr B. State of the science: neonatal hypoglycemia. *Adv Neonatal Care.* 2001;1(1):4.
9. Gibbins S, Stevens B. The influence of gestational age on the efficacy and short-term safety of sucrose for procedural pain relief. *Adv Neonatal Care.* 2003;3(5):241.
10. Coleman M, Solarin K, Smith C. Assessment and management of pain and distress in the neonate. *Adv Neonatal Care.* 2002; 2(3):123.
11. Cong X, Ludington-Hoe SM, McCain G, et al. Kangaroo care modifies preterm infant heart rate variability in response to heel stick pain: pilot study. *Early Human Dev.* 2009;85(9):561.
12. Ludington-Hoe SM, Hosseini R, Torowicz DL. Skin-to-skin contact (Kangaroo Care) analgesia for preterm infant heel stick. *AACN Clin Issues.* 2005;16(3):373.
13. Bryant K, Horns K, Longo N, et al. A primer on newborn screening. *Adv Neonatal Care.* 2004;4(5):306.
14. Abril Martin JC, Aguilar Rodriguez L, Albinana Cilvetti J. Flatfoot and calcaneal deformity secondary to osteomyelitis after heel puncture. *J Pediatr Orthop.* 1999;8:122.
15. Lauer BA, Altenburgher KM. Outbreak of staphylococcal infections following heel puncture for blood sampling. *Am J Dis Child.* 1981;135:277.
16. Williamson D, Holt PJ. Calcified cutaneous nodules on the heels of children: a complication of heelsticks as a neonate. *Pediatr Dermatol.* 2001;18:138.

IV Miscellaneous Sampling

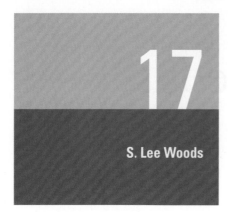

Lumbar Puncture

S. Lee Woods

A. Indications (1–3)

1. To diagnose central nervous system (CNS) infections (meningitis, encephalitis), including congenital infections (TORCH—toxoplasmosis, other infections [usually implying syphilis], rubella, cytomegalovirus, and herpes simplex) as well as bacterial and fungal infections

   Routine inclusion of lumbar puncture (LP) in the initial sepsis evaluation of newborn infants (in the first 7 days of life) is controversial (4–8). Meningitis occurs less frequently in this population than in older newborns, and the majority of cases of meningitis occur in infants with positive blood cultures. The procedure may be poorly tolerated by newborns with cardiorespiratory compromise (9–11). LP is indicated if early bacteremia is documented or if signs of CNS involvement are present (seizures, coma, focal neurologic abnormality). LP is also indicated in the evaluation for acquired infection in the later neonatal period, when the incidence of meningitis is significant. In one review (8), as many as one-third of very low-birthweight infants who had late-onset meningitis (after 3 days of life) did so in the absence of positive blood culture.
2. To monitor efficacy of antimicrobial therapy in the presence of CNS infection by examining cerebrospinal fluid (CSF) cell count, microbiology, and drug levels (12,13).
3. To drain CSF in communicating hydrocephalus associated with intraventricular hemorrhage (1–3,14)

   For effective treatment of posthemorrhagic hydrocephalus by this means, there must be communication between the lateral ventricles and the lumbar subarachnoid space, and an adequate volume of CSF (10 to 15 mL/kg) must be obtained. Communication is demonstrated by an immediate decrease in ventricular size or change in anterior fontanelle or head circumference following LP. Efficacy and safety of serial LPs in the temporary amelioration or long-term improvement of posthemorrhagic hydrocephalus are controversial (14–18). Potential risks of repeated LPs must be weighed against possible benefits.
4. To aid in the diagnosis of metabolic disease (1,2,19)

5. To diagnose intracranial hemorrhage

   The finding of increased red blood cells and protein content in the CSF or xanthochromia of centrifuged fluid suggests intracranial hemorrhage. The definitive diagnosis and determination of the site of hemorrhage (subdural, subarachnoid, intraparenchymal, intraventricular) are best made by neuroimaging techniques such as CT or MRI.
6. To diagnose CNS involvement with leukemia
7. To inject chemotherapeutic agents
8. To instill contrast material for myelography

B. Contraindications (1–3,20,21)

1. Increased intracranial pressure (ICP)

   Increased ICP may occur with bacterial meningitis or intracranial mass lesions. In the neonate with open cranial sutures, this rarely results in signs of transtentorial or cerebellar herniation. However, herniation can occur after LP in the presence of elevated ICP, even when the sutures are open. If signs of significant increased ICP exist (rapidly declining or severely depressed level of consciousness, abnormal posturing, cranial nerve palsies, tense anterior fontanelle, abnormalities in heart rate, respirations, or blood pressure without other cause), CT or MRI should be performed before LP. Papilledema is a late sign and is rarely present in the neonate, regardless of the degree of increased ICP.
2. Uncorrected thrombocytopenia or bleeding diathesis
3. Infection in the skin or underlying tissue at or near the puncture site
4. Lumbosacral anomalies
5. Cardiorespiratory instability, which may be exacerbated by the procedure

C. Equipment

Except for the face mask, all equipment must be sterile. Prepackaged lumbar puncture kits are available.

1. Gloves and mask
2. Cup with iodophor antiseptic solution

3. Gauze swabs
4. Towels or transparent aperture drape
5. Spinal needle with short bevel and stylet, 20 or 22 gauge × 1.5 inches
6. Three or more specimen tubes with caps
7. Adhesive bandage

D. Precautions

1. Monitor vital signs and oxygen saturation. Increased supplemental oxygen during the procedure can prevent hypoxemia (22). Airway compromise can be reduced by avoiding the fully flexed lateral decubitus position and direct flexion of the neck (9–11). Flexing the hips to only 90 degrees avoids abdominal compression and the potential for aspiration.
2. Use strict aseptic technique as for a major procedure (see Chapter 5).
3. Always use a needle with stylet to avoid development of intraspinal epidermoid tumor (23).
4. To prevent traumatic tap caused by overpenetration, insert the needle slowly while removing the stylet at frequent intervals to detect CSF as soon as the subdural space is entered (24–27). Use of local anesthetic may also help reduce the incidence of traumatic tap (26,27).
5. Never aspirate CSF with a syringe. Even a small amount of negative pressure can increase the risk of subdural hemorrhage or herniation.

6. Palpate landmarks accurately to prevent puncture above the L2–L3 interspace (lower interspace should be used for preterm infants; see discussion under E2).

E. Technique (20,21) (See Procedures Website for Video)

1. Have an assistant restrain the infant in the lateral decubitus or sitting position, with spine flexed (Figs. 17.1 and 17.2). Avoid flexion of the neck, as this increases the chance of airway compromise.
2. Palpate the interspace that falls immediately above or below an imaginary line drawn between the iliac crests (L3–L4 and L4–L5 interspaces, preferred sites for LP) (Fig. 17.3).

   The termination of the spinal cord relative to the spine changes during fetal development and early infancy (28–30). The normal adult termination, between the middle of T12 and the lower portion of L3 vertebrae, is not achieved until 2 months postterm (30). Between 25 and 40 weeks' gestation, the cord termination gradually ascends from L4 to L2 (30). This should be taken into account, and the lower L4–L5 interspace used for lumbar puncture in significantly preterm infants, to avoid possible cord penetration (28).
3. Prepare as for major procedure (see Chapter 5). Put mask on. Wash hands thoroughly and wear sterile gloves.

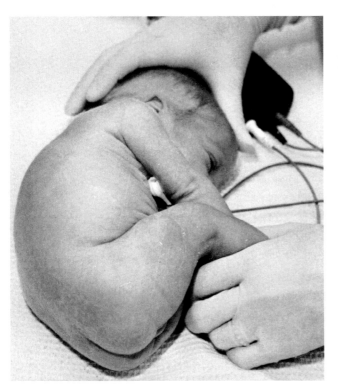 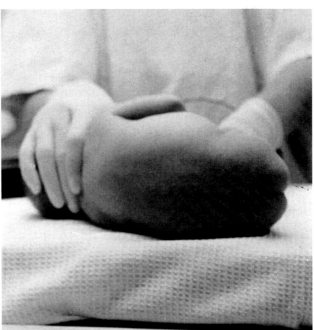

FIG. 17.1. Restraining infant for LP in the lateral recumbent position. Neck should not be flexed.

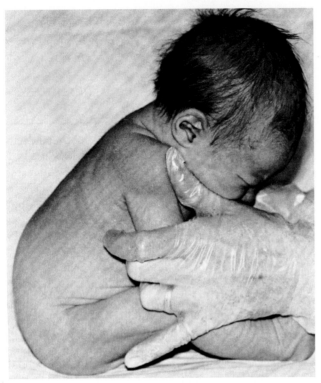

FIG. 17.2. Restraining infant for LP in the sitting position.

4. Clean the lumbar area three times with antiseptic.
   a. Begin at the desired interspace and wash in enlarging circles to include the iliac crests.
   b. Allow antiseptic to dry or blot excess with sterile gauze.

5. Drape, leaving the puncture site and infant's face exposed. A transparent aperture drape is recommended because it does not obstruct the view of the patient.

   Use of local anesthetic cream prior to cleaning the area may be helpful in reducing pain during LP (31–33). Use of local anesthetic does not reduce physiologic instability, but may reduce struggling by the infant during the procedure (34,35) and the incidenc of traumatic tap (26,27).

6. Insert the needle in the midline into the desired interspace.
   a. Aim slightly cephalad (on a plane with the umbilicus) to avoid the vertebral bodies (Fig. 17.4).
   b. If resistance is met, withdraw the needle slightly and redirect more cephalad.
   c. Hold a finger on the vertebral process above the interspace to aid in locating the puncture site if the infant moves.

7. Advance the needle slowly to a depth of approximately 1 to 1.5 cm in a term infant, less in a preterm infant, until the epidermis and dermis are traversed.
   a. As the needle is further advanced, remove the stylet frequently to check for fluid. Replace the stylet before advancing the needle.
   b. A change in resistance can often be felt as the needle passes through the ligamentum flavum and dura (Fig. 17.5). This may be more difficult to appreciate in a young infant than in an older child.
   c. Wait for fluid after removing the stylet, as the flow may be slow.
   d. If no fluid is obtained, rotate the needle to reorient the bevel. If no fluid is obtained, replace the stylet,

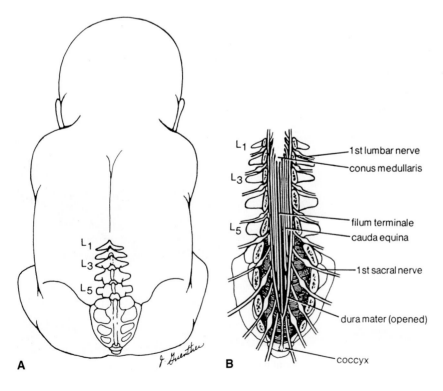

FIG. 17.3. **A:** Externally palpable anatomic landmarks. **B:** Vertebral bodies removed to show anatomy of spinal cord in lumbosacral area in relation to external landmarks.

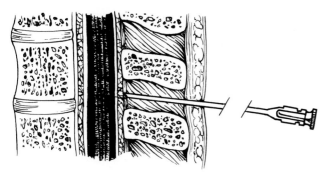

FIG. 17.4. Inserting spinal needle in slightly cephalad direction to avoid vertebral bodies.

remove the needle, and try one interspace above or below, using a new needle for each attempt.

8. Collect CSF for diagnostic studies. Allow CSF to flow passively into the collection tubes; never aspirate with a syringe. Accurate opening pressure measurement is possible in a quiet infant.
   a. Collect 1 mL of CSF in each of three to four tubes.
   b. Send first sample for bacterial culture.
   c. Send last sample for cell count, unless fluid becomes visibly more bloody during the tap.
   d. Send the remainder for desired chemical and microbiologic studies.
   e. Look for clearing of fluid in successive collections in the event of a traumatic tap.

9. For myelography or instillation of chemotherapeutic agents, it is not necessary to remove CSF.

10. For treatment of hydrocephalus, remove 10 to 15 mL/kg of CSF, or collect until CSF flow ceases (up to 10 minutes).

11. Replace the stylet before removing the needle to prevent entrapment of spinal nerve roots in the extradural space. Remove the needle, and place an adhesive bandage over the puncture site.

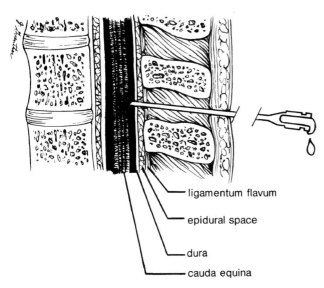

- ligamentum flavum
- epidural space
- dura
- cauda equina

FIG. 17.5. Needle has penetrated the dura, and stylet has been removed to allow free flow of spinal fluid.

F. Complications (1,2,36)

In older children and adults, headache is the most common complication following LP, occurring in up to 40% of patients (36). There is no clear evidence that headache occurs in infants. In neonates, the most common complication is transient hypoxemia from positioning for the procedure (9–11). In some reports, this is seen in a majority of cases and depends on the method of positioning used. Also common, occurring in up to one-third of LPs in neonates (26,27), is contamination of the CSF sample with blood from puncture of the epidural venous plexus on the posterior surface of the vertebral body (traumatic tap). Other potential complications listed below are rare, occurring in about 0.3% of LPs (36).

1. Hypoxemia from knee–chest position (9–11)
2. Contamination of CSF sample with blood (traumatic tap) (26,27)
3. Aspiration
4. Cardiopulmonary arrest
5. Sudden intracranial decompression with cerebral herniation (37,38)
6. Infection
   a. Meningitis from LP performed during bacteremia (incidence about 0.2%) (39,40)
   b. Discitis (41)
   c. Spinal cord abscess (42)
   d. Epidural abscess (42,43)
   e. Vertebral osteomyelitis (43)
7. Bleeding
   a. Spinal epidural hematoma (44)
   b. Spinal or intracranial subdural hematoma (45,46)
   c. Spinal or intracranial subarachnoid hematoma (46,47)
8. Epidural CSF collection (48–51)
9. Intraspinal epidermoid tumor from epithelial tissue introduced into the spinal canal (23)
10. Spinal cord puncture and nerve damage if puncture site is above the level of cord termination (see discussion in E2 concerning cord termination in preterm infants) (28)
11. Sixth-nerve palsy caused by removal of excessive CSF with resulting traction on the nerve (52)
12. Deformity of the lumbar spine secondary to acute spondylitis (53)

References

1. Lehman RK, Schor NF. Neurologic evaluation. In: Kliegman RM, Stanton BF, St. Geme JW, et al, eds. *Nelson Textbook of Pediatrics.* 19th ed. Philadelphia: Elsevier; 2011:1998.
2. Michelson DJ. Spinal fluid evaluation. In: Swaiman KF, Ashwal S, Ferriero DM, eds. *Pediatric Neurology.* 4th ed. Philadelphia: Mosby; 2006:153.

3. Menkes JH, Moser FG. Neurologic examination of the child and infant. In: Menkes JH, Sarnat HB, Maria BL, eds. *Child Neurology.* 7th ed. Philadelphia: Lippincott Williams & Wilkins; 2006:1.

4. Hamada S, Vearncombe M, McGreer A, et al. Neonatal group B streptococcal disease: incidence, presentation, and mortality. *J Matern Fetal Neonat Med.* 2008;21:53.

5. Ray B, Mangalore J, Harikumar C, et al. Is lumbar puncture necessary for evaluation of early neonatal sepsis? *Arch Dis Child.* 2006;91:1033.

6. Garges HP, Moody MA, Cotton CM, et al. Neonatal meningitis: what is the correlation among cerebrospinal fluid cultures, blood cultures, and cerebrospinal fluid parameters? *Pediatrics.* 2006;117:1094.

7. Malbon K, Mohan R, Nicholl R. Should a neonate with possible late onset infection always have a lumbar puncture? *Arch Dis Child.* 2006;91:75.

8. Stoll BJ, Hansen N, Fanaroff AA, et al. To tap or not to tap: high likelihood of meningitis without sepsis among very low birth weight infants. *Pediatrics.* 2004;113:1181.

9. Abo A, Chen L, Johnston P, et al. Positioning for lumbar puncture in children evaluated by bedside ultrasound. *Pediatrics.* 2010;125: e1149.

10. Weisman LE, Merenstein GB, Steenbarger JR. The effect of lumbar puncture position in sick neonates. *Am J Dis Child.* 1983;137:1077.

11. Gleason CA, Martin RJ, Anderson JV, et al. Optimal position for a spinal tap in preterm infants. *Pediatrics.* 1983;71:31.

12. Greenberg RG, Benjamin DK Jr, Cohen-Wolkowiez M, et al. Repeat lumbar puncture in infants with meningitis in the neonatal intensive care unit. *J Perinatol.* 2011;31:425.

13. Kimberlin DW. Meningitis in the neonate. *Curr Treat Options Neurol.* 2002;4:239.

14. Whitelaw A. Intraventricular hemorrhage and posthemorrhagic hydrocephalus: pathogenesis, prevention and future interventions. *Semin Neonatol.* 2001;6:135.

15. McCrea HJ, Ment LR. The diagnosis, management, and postnatal prevention of intraventricular hemorrhage in the preterm neonate. *Clin Perinatol.* 2008;35:777.

16. Whitelaw A, Evans D, Carter M, et al. Randomized clinical trial of prevention of hydrocephalus after intraventricular hemorrhage in preterm infants: brain-washing versus tapping fluid. *Pediatrics.* 2007;119:e1071.

17. Soul JS, Eichenwald E, Walter G, et al. CSF removal in infantile posthemorrhagic hydrocephalus results in significant improvement in cerebral hemodynamics. *Pediatr Res.* 2004;55:872.

18. Ventriculomegaly Trial Group. Randomized trial of early tapping in neonatal posthaemorrhagic ventricular dilatation: results at 30 months. *Arch Dis Child.* 1994;70:F129.

19. Hoffman GF, Surtees RA, Wevers RA. Cerebrospinal fluid investigations for neurometabolic disorders. *Neuropediatrics.* 1998;29:59.

20. Barone MA. Pediatric procedures. In: McMillan JA, Feigin RD, DeAngelis CD, et al., eds. *Oski's Pediatrics: Principles and Practice.* 4th ed. Philadelphia: Lippincott Williams & Wilkins; 2006:2671.

21. Sigman LJ. Procedures. In: Tschudy MM, Arcara KM, eds. *The Harriet Lane Handbook.* 19th ed. Philadelphia: Elsevier; 2012:57.

22. Fiser DH, Gober GA, Smith CE, et al. Prevention of hypoxemia during lumbar puncture in infancy with preoxygenation. *Pediatr Emerg Care.* 1993;9:81.

23. Ziv ET, Gordon McComb J, Krieger MD, et al. Iatrogenic intraspinal epidermoid tumor: two cases and a review of the literature. *Spine.* 2004;29:E15.

24. Mellick L, Vining M. Maximizing infant spinel tap success. *Pediatr Emerg Care.* 2010;26:687.

25. Murray MJ, Arthurs OJ, Hills MH, et al. A randomized study to validate a midspinal canal depth nomogram in neonates. *Am J Perinatol.* 2009;26:733.

26. Nigrovic LE, Kuppermann N, Neuman MI. Risk factors for traumatic or unsuccessful lumbar puncture in children. *Ann Emerg Med.* 2007;49:762.

27. Baxter AL, Fisher RG, Burke BL, et al. Local anesthetic and stylet styles: factors associated with resident lumber puncture success. *Pediatrics.* 2006;117:876.

28. Tubbs RS, Smyth MD, Wellons JC, et al. Intramedullary hemorrhage in a neonate after lumbar puncture resulting in paraplegia. *Pediatrics.* 2004;113:1403.

29. Wilson DA, Prince JR. MR imaging determination of the location of the normal conus medullaris throughout childhood. *Am J Roentgenol.* 1989;152:1029.

30. Barson AJ. The vertebral level of termination of the spinal cord during normal and abnormal development. *J Anat.* 1970;106:489.

31. Kaur G, Gupta P, Kumar A. A randomized trial of eutectic mixture of local anesthetics during lumbar puncture in newborns. *Arch Pediatr Adolesc Med.* 2003;157:1065.

32. Dutta S. Use of eutectic mixture of local anesthetics in children. *Indian J Pediatr.* 1999;66:707.

33. Taddio A, Ohlsson A, Einarson TR, et al. A systematic review of lidocaine–prilocaine (EMLA) in the treatment of acute pain in neonates. *Pediatrics.* 1998;101:e1.

34. Pinheiro JMB, Furdon S, Ochoa LF. Role of local anesthesia during lumbar puncture in neonates. *Pediatrics.* 1993;91:379.

35. Porter FL, Miller JP, Cole FS, et al. A controlled clinical trial of local anesthesia for lumbar punctures in newborns. *Pediatrics.* 1991;88:663.

36. Evans RW. Complications of lumbar puncture. *Neurol Clin North Am.* 1998;16:83.

37. Shetty AK, Desselle BC, Craver RD, et al. Fatal cerebral herniation after lumbar puncture in a patient with a normal computed tomography scan. *Pediatrics.* 1999;103:1284.

38. Rennick G, Shann F, de Campo J. Cerebral herniation during bacterial meningitis in children. *Br Med J.* 1993;306:953.

39. Domingo P, Mancebo J, Blanch L, et al. Iatrogenic streptococcal meningitis. *Clin Infect Dis.* 1994;19:356.

40. Eng RHK, Seligman SJ. Lumbar puncture-induced meningitis. *JAMA.* 1981;245:1456.

41. Bhatoe HS, Gill HS, Kumar N, et al. Post lumbar puncture discitis and vertebral collapse. *Postgrad Med J.* 1994;70:882.

42. Bertol V, Ara JR, Oliveros A, et al. Neurologic complications of lumbar spinal anesthesia: spinal and paraspinal abscess. *Neurology.* 1997;48:1732.

43. Bergman I, Wald ER, Meyer JD, et al. Epidural abscess and vertebral osteomyelitis following serial lumbar punctures. *Pediatrics.* 1983;72:476.

44. Adler MD, Comi AE, Walker AR. Acute hemorrhagic complication of diagnostic lumbar puncture. *Pediatr Emerg Care.* 2001;17:184.

45. Vos PE, De Boer WA, Wurzer JAL, et al. Subdural hematoma after lumbar puncture: two case reports and review of the literature. *Clin Neurol Neurosurg.* 1991;93:127.

46. Hart IK, Bone I, Hadley DM. Development of neurological problems after lumbar puncture. *Br Med J.* 1988;296:51.

47. Blade J, Gaston F, Montserrat E, et al. Spinal subarachnoid hematoma after lumbar puncture causing reversible paraplegia in acute leukemia. *J Neurosurg.* 1983;58:438.

48. Ng WH, Drake JM. Symptomatic spinal epidural CSF collection after lumbar puncture in a young adult: case report and review of literature. *Childs Nerv Syst.* 2010;26:259.

49. Aronson PL, Zonfrillo MR. Epidural cerebrospinal fluid collection after lumbar puncture. *Pediatr Emerg Care.* 2009;25:467.

50. Koch BL, Moosbrugger EA, Egelhoff JC. Symptomatic spinal epidural collections after lumbar puncture in children. *Am J Neuroradiol.* 2007;28:1811.

51. Amini A, Liu JK, Kan P, et al. Cerebrospinal fluid dissecting into epidural space after lumbar puncture causing cauda equine syndrome: review of literature and illustrative case. *Childs Nerv Syst.* 2006;22:1639.

52. Bryce-Smith R, Macintosh RR. Sixth-nerve palsy after lumbar puncture and spinal analgesia. *Br Med J.* 1951;1:275.

53. Lintermans JP, Seyhnaeue V. Spondolytic deformity of the lumbar spine and previous lumbar punctures. *Pediatr Radiol.* 1977; 5:181.

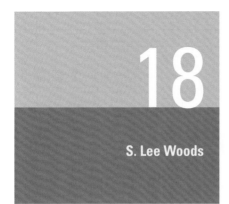

18 Subdural Tap

S. Lee Woods

A. Indications (1–4)

1. To diagnose acute subdural collection over the cerebral convexities (hemorrhage, effusion, empyema) (5–7)

   Computerized tomography (CT) is now generally available and is a safer method for detecting subdural fluid. Subdural tap should be reserved as a diagnostic tool for the infant who is too unstable to be transported for CT scanning.
2. To sample convexity subdural collection for hematologic, microbiologic, and biochemical studies
3. To drain convexity subdural collection to reduce increased intracranial pressure or to prevent the development of craniocerebral disproportion

   Repeated therapeutic subdural taps should not be performed unless the infant is symptomatic or the head size is growing rapidly. Surgical intervention is indicated if subdural taps are not effective in controlling these symptoms (2).

B. Contraindications

1. Clinical instability when risk exceeds potential benefit
2. Uncorrected thrombocytopenia or bleeding diathesis
3. Infection in the skin or underlying tissue at or near the puncture site

C. Equipment

All equipment must be sterile, except safety razor and face mask.

1. Gloves and face mask
2. Cup with iodophor antiseptic solution
3. Gauze swabs
4. Drapes or surgical towels
5. Two short bevel needles, 19 to 22 gauge × 1 inch, with stylets
6. Specimen tubes with caps
7. Adhesive bandage
8. Safety razor

D. Precautions

1. Use strict aseptic technique as for a major procedure (see Chapter 5).
2. Insert the needle as far laterally as possible at the border of the anterior fontanelle or along the coronal suture, at least 1 to 2 cm from the midline, to avoid puncturing the sagittal sinus. Do not direct the needle medially during insertion.
3. Remove the needle if there is not a definite change in resistance on penetrating the dura after insertion to approximately 0.5 to 1 cm.
4. Hold the needle securely at all times to avoid inadvertent movement of the needle tip. Grasp the needle firmly or apply a hemostat at approximately 1 cm from the beveled end of the needle, to prevent inadvertent advancement of the needle into the cerebral cortex.
5. Allow fluid to drain spontaneously. Do not aspirate with a syringe.
6. Limit fluid collected to 15 to 20 mL from each side. Removal of larger volumes can lead to bleeding into the subdural space.
7. If frequent taps are required, vary the puncture site slightly to prevent fistula formation.
8. Following the procedure, apply pressure to the scalp for 2 to 3 minutes to prevent fluid leak from the puncture site or subgaleal fluid collection.

E. Technique (1,8,9)

1. Place the infant supine, with the crown of the head at the table edge. Monitor cardiorespiratory status.
2. Have the assistant restrain the infant and steady the infant's head (Fig. 18.1).
3. Shave the head over a wide area surrounding the anterior fontanelle (Fig. 18.1).
4. Locate the junctions of the coronal sutures and anterior fontanelle.
5. Put on mask. Wash hands thoroughly and put on sterile gloves.

6. Clean the fontanelle and surrounding area three times with antiseptic solution. (See Chapter 5 for aseptic preparation for major procedure.)
   a. Begin at the fontanelle and wash in enlarging circles.
   b. Allow antiseptic to dry. Blot excess with sterile gauze.
7. Cover infant's head with sterile drapes, leaving the anterior fontanelle and the infant's nose and mouth exposed.
8. Locate the coronal suture by palpation at the lateral corner of the anterior fontanelle.

   Generally, anesthesia is not required, but local injection of lidocaine at this time or application of topical anesthetic cream prior to cleaning the area can be used for local anesthesia at the puncture site (1,10–13).
9. Insert the needle slowly through the coronal suture, just lateral to its junction with the anterior fontanelle (see Fig. 18.1).
   a. Hold the needle perpendicular to the skin surface.
   b. Grasp the needle shaft with thumb and index finger, bracing the hand against the infant's head to maintain control of the needle during insertion (Fig. 18.2).
   c. As the needle advances through the skin, pull the scalp slightly to create a Z-like track through the underlying tissue. This will help prevent fluid leakage from the puncture site or into the subgaleal space after removal of the needle.
10. Advance until a "pop" is felt upon penetrating the dura. Remove the stylet (Fig. 18.2).
11. Allow fluid to drain spontaneously into the sterile tubes until flow ceases or a maximum volume of 15 to 20 mL

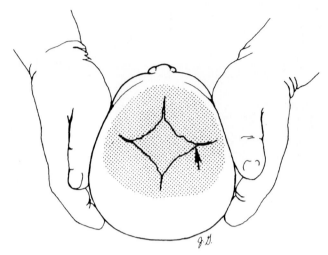

FIG. 18.1. Position and restraint for subdural tap. Stippling demonstrates area to be prepared for procedure. An *arrow* indicates site for needle puncture.

is reached. Send fluid for protein content, cell count, and culture.
12. If no fluid appears, replace the stylet and remove the needle slowly. Do not reattempt procedure on the same side.
13. Repeat the procedure on the opposite side with a new, sterile needle.
14. After removing the needle, apply firm pressure to the puncture site with sterile gauze for 2 to 3 minutes.
15. Dress the puncture site with a small adhesive bandage.

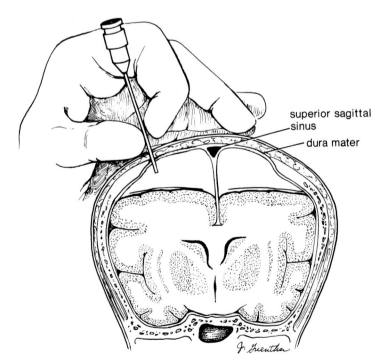

superior sagittal sinus
dura mater

FIG. 18.2. Coronal section of anatomic drawing showing subdural needle penetrating the dura in a patient with bilateral convexity subdural fluid collections. Operator's fingers are placed for maximal stabilization of the needle.

F. Complications (8,9)

1. Subdural bleeding from laceration of the superior sagittal sinus or smaller vessels or from removal of excessive fluid with shift of intracranial contents and rebleeding

2. Development of chronic subdural fluid collection (14,15)

    This complication may develop more frequently in infants treated with subdural tap. In one case series, 41.6% of patients treated with subdural tap developed chronic subdural collections, compared with 13% of those treated with craniotomy (15).

3. Subgaleal fluid or blood accumulation

4. Failure of the procedure to remove clotted subdural blood

5. Infection

    In one small case series, 1 of 12 infants (8%) treated with subdural tap developed subdural empyema after multiple taps (15).

6. Trauma to the underlying cortex caused by inserting the needle too far

7. Fistula formation after repeated taps

References

1. Lehman RK, Schor NF. Neurologic evaluation. In: Kliegman RM, Stanton BF, St. Geme JW, Schor NF, Behrman RE, eds. *Nelson Textbook of Pediatrics.* 19th ed. Philadelphia: Elsevier; 2011:1998.

2. Volpe JJ. Intracranial hemorrhage: subdural, primary subarachnoid, intracerebellar, intraventricular (term infant), and miscellaneous. In: *Neurology of the Newborn.* 5th ed. Philadelphia: Saunders; 2008:373.

3. Brett EM, Harding BN. Intracranial and spinal cord tumours. In: Brett EM, ed. *Paediatric Neurology.* 3rd ed. New York: Churchill Livingstone; 1997:537.

4. Curless RG. Subdural empyema in infant meningitis: diagnosis, therapy, and prognosis. *Childs Nerv Syst.* 1985;1:211.

5. Hobbs C, Childs A-M, Wynne J, et al. Subdural hematoma and effusion in infancy: an epidemiological study. *Arch Dis Child.* 2005;90:952.

6. Ney JP, Joseph KR, Mitchell MH. Late subdural hygromas from birth trauma. *Neurology.* 2005;65:517.

7. Whitby EH, Griffiths PD, Rutter S, et al. Frequency and natural history of subdural haemorrhages in babies and relation to obstetric factors. *Lancet.* 2004;363:846.

8. Barone MA. Pediatric procedures. In: McMillan JA, Feigin RD, DeAngelis CD, et al., eds. *Oski's Pediatrics: Principles and Practice.* 4th ed. Philadelphia: Lippincott Williams & Wilkins; 2006:2671.

9. Ferriero D, Buescher ES. Central nervous system. In: Taeusch HW, Christiansen RO, Buescher ES, eds. *Pediatric and Neonatal Tests and Procedures.* Philadelphia: Saunders; 1996:409.

10. Anand KJ, Johnston CC, Oberlander TF, et al. Analgesia and local anesthesia during invasive procedures in the neonate. *Clin Ther.* 2005;27:844.

11. O'Brien L, Taddio A, Lyszkiewicz DA, et al. A critical review of the topical local anesthetic amethocaine (Ametop) for pediatric pain. *Paediatr Drugs.* 2005;7:41.

12. Kaur G, Gupta P, Kumar A. A randomized trial of eutectic mixture of local anesthetics during lumbar puncture in newborns. *Arch Pediatr Adolesc Med.* 2003;157:1065.

13. Taddio A, Ohlsson A, Einarson TR, et al. A systematic review of lidocaine–prilocaine (EMLA) in the treatment of acute pain in neonates. *Pediatrics.* 1998;101:e1.

14. Katona F, Balazs M, Berenyi M, et al. Subdural effusion in the first six months of life. *Acta Paediatr Acad Sci Hung.* 1982;23:219.

15. Gutierrez FA, Raimondi AJ. Acute subdural hematoma in infancy and childhood. *Childs Brain.* 1975;1:269.

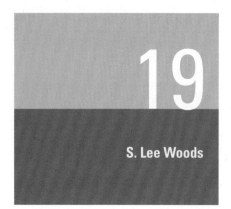

Suprapubic Bladder Aspiration

S. Lee Woods

A. Indications (1–8)

1. To obtain urine for culture

   Suprapubic bladder aspiration is considered the most reliable method of obtaining urine for culture in infants and children <2 years old. In this age group, the distended bladder is located intra-abdominally. Any number of bacteria in urine obtained by this method is considered significant and likely to be indicative of urinary tract infection. Contamination with skin flora can occur but should be avoidable with careful skin preparation. Although bladder catheterization has a higher success rate, it also has a much higher false-positive rate than suprapubic aspiration (3–5,9,10). Reported success rates for suprapubic aspiration vary widely, from 25% to 100% (11). With careful attention to performing the procedure when the infant has a full bladder, success is generally 89% to 95%, even in very low-birthweight infants (7,12). The use of portable ultrasound (11,13–16) or transillumination (17) to determine bladder size can greatly increase the chance of success.

B. Contraindications (1,2,12,18)

1. Empty bladder as a result of recent void or dehydration
   A full bladder is essential for success of the procedure and avoidance of complications.
2. Skin infection over the puncture site
3. Distention or enlargement of abdominal viscera (e.g., dilated loops of bowel, massive hepatomegaly)
4. Genitourinary anomaly or enlargement of pelvic structures (e.g., ovarian cyst, distention of vagina or uterus)
5. Uncorrected thrombocytopenia or bleeding diathesis

C. Equipment

All equipment must be sterile, except transillumination light or ultrasound equipment.

1. Gloves
2. Gauze sponges and cup with iodophor antiseptic solution or

3. Prepared antiseptic-impregnated swabs
4. 3-mL syringe
5. 21- or 22-gauge × 1.5-inch needle
6. Transillumination light or portable ultrasound (optional)

D. Precautions

1. Use strict aseptic technique (see Chapter 5).
2. Delay the procedure if the infant has urinated in the last hour.
   If the infant is systemically ill, do not delay antibiotic therapy to wait for further urine production.
3. Correct bleeding diathesis before the procedure. Consider catheterization as an alternative.
4. Be certain of landmarks. Do not insert the needle over the pubic bone or off the midline.
5. Aspirate urine using only gentle suction. The use of too much suction can draw the bladder mucosa to the needle, obstructing the collection of urine and increasing the risk of injury to the bladder.

E. Technique (1,7,12,18)

1. Have an assistant restrain the infant in the supine, frog-leg position.
2. To avoid reflex urination, ask assistant to
   a. Place the tip of a finger in the anus and apply pressure anteriorly in a female infant, or
   b. Pinch the base of the penis gently in a male infant.
3. Determine the presence of urine in the bladder.
   a. Verify that the diaper has been dry for at least 1 hour.
   b. Palpate or percuss the bladder.
   c. Optionally, use transillumination light (17), or portable ultrasound guidance (11,13–16).
4. *Locate landmarks.* Palpate the top of the pubic bone. The site for needle insertion is 1 to 2 cm above the symphysis pubis in the midline (Fig. 19.1).
5. Wash hands thoroughly and put on gloves.
6. Clean the suprapubic area (including the area over pubic bone) three times with antiseptic solution. Blot dry with sterile gauze.

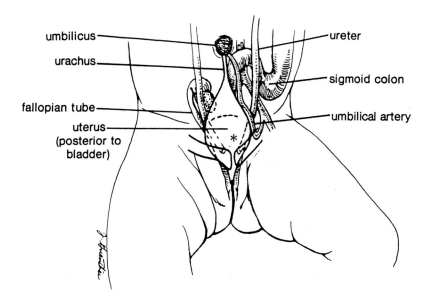

FIG. 19.1. The bladder in the neonate, with immediate anatomical relations. An asterisk indicates approximate site for needle insertion.

Generally, anesthesia is not required, but local injection of lidocaine at this time or application of topical anesthetic cream prior to cleaning the area can be used for local anesthesia at the puncture site and may increase procedure success (19–22).

7. Palpate the symphysis pubis, and insert the needle (with syringe attached) 1 to 2 cm above the pubic symphysis in the midline (Fig. 19.2).
   a. Maintain the needle perpendicular to table or directed slightly caudad.

   b. Advance the needle 2 to 3 cm. A slight decrease in resistance may be felt when the bladder is penetrated.
8. Aspirate gently, as the needle is slowly advanced, until urine enters the syringe. Do not advance the needle more than 3 cms.
   a. Withdraw the needle if no urine is obtained.
   b. Do not probe with the needle or attempt to redirect it to obtain urine.
   c. Wait at least 1 hour before attempting to repeat the procedure.

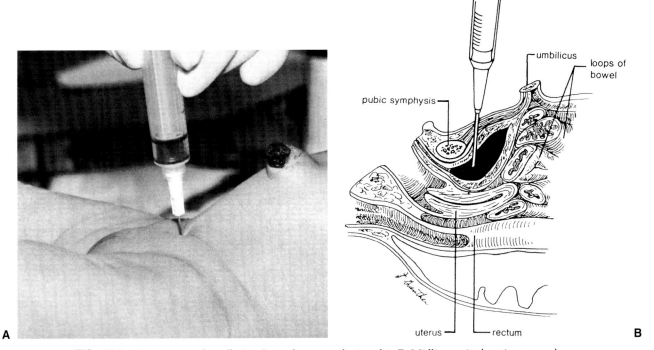

A   **B**

FIG. 19.2. **A:** Insertion of needle 1 to 2 cm above symphysis pubis. **B:** Midline sagittal section to emphasize the intra-abdominal position of the full bladder in the neonate and its posterior anatomic relations.

9. Withdraw the needle after urine is obtained. Apply gentle pressure over the puncture site with sterile gauze to stop any bleeding.

10. Remove the needle and place a sterile cap on the syringe or transfer urine to a sterile container to send for culture.

F. Complications

Minor transient hematuria is the most commonly reported complication, occurring in <1% to 10% of cases (7). Serious complications are very rare, occurring in ≤0.2% of cases (12).

1. Bleeding
   a. Transient macroscopic hematuria (blood-tinged urine) (7)
   b. Gross hematuria (7,23–25)
   c. Abdominal wall hematoma (26)
   d. Bladder wall hematoma (7,27)
   e. Pelvic hematoma (28)
2. Infection
   a. Abdominal wall abscess (29,30)
   b. Sepsis (31,32)
   c. Osteomyelitis of pubic bone (33,34)
3. Perforation
   a. Bowel (30,32,35,36)
   b. Pelvic organ (35)

References

1. Sigman LJ. Procedures. In: Tschudy MM, Arcara KM, eds. *The Harriet Lane Handbook.* 19th ed. Philadelphia: Elsevier; 2012:57.
2. Long SS, Klein JO. Bacterial infections of the urinary tract. In: Remington JS, Klein JO, Wilson CB, et al., eds. *Infectious Diseases of the Fetus and Newborn.* 7th ed. Philadelphia: Elsevier; 2011:310.
3. Karacan C, Erkek N, Senet S, et al. Evaluation of urine collection methods for the diagnosis of urinary tract infection in children. *Med Princ Pract.* 2010;19:188.
4. Phillips B. Towards evidence based medicine for paediatricians. Urethral catheter or suprapubic aspiration to reduce contamination of urine samples in young children? *Arch Dis Child.* 2009;94:736.
5. Jodal U. Suprapubic aspiration of urine in the diagnosis of urinary tract infection in infants. *Acta Paediatr.* 2002;91:497.
6. Ozkan B, Kava O, Akdag R, et al. Suprapubic bladder aspiration with or without ultrasound guidance. *Clin Pediatr.* 2000;39:625.
7. Buescher ES. Immunology and infectious diseases procedures and tests. In: Taeusch HW, Christiansen RO, Buescher ES, eds. *Pediatric and Neonatal Tests and Procedures.* Philadelphia: Saunders; 1996:625.
8. Pollack CV, Pollack ES, Andrew ME. Suprapubic bladder aspiration versus urethral catheterization in ill infants: success, efficiency and complication rates. *Ann Emerg Med.* 1994;23:225.
9. Austin BJ, Bollard C, Gunn TR. Is urethral catheterization a successful alternative to suprapubic aspiration in neonates? *J Paediatr Child Health.* 1999;35:34.
10. Tobiansky R, Evans N. A randomized controlled trial of two methods for collection of sterile urine in neonates. *J Paediatr Child Health.* 1998;43:460.
11. Gochman RF, Karasic RB, Heller MB. Use of the portable ultrasound to assist urine collection by suprapubic aspiration. *Ann Emerg Med.* 1991;20:6.
12. Barkemeyer BM. Suprapubic aspiration of urine in very low birth weight infants. *Pediatrics.* 1993;92:457.
13. Chu RW, Wong YC, Luk SH, et al. Comparing suprapubic urine aspiration under real time ultrasound guidance with conventional blind aspiration. *Acta Paediatr.* 2002;91:512.
14. Munir V, Barnett P, South M. Does the use of volumetric bladder ultrasound improve the success rate of suprapubic aspiration of urine? *Pediatr Emerg Care.* 2002;18:346.
15. Ozkan B, Kaya O, Akdag R, et al. Suprapubic bladder aspiration with or without ultrasound guidance. *Clin Pediatr (Phila.).* 2000; 39:625.
16. Garcia-Neito VG, Navarro JF, Sanchez-Almeida ES, et al. Standards for ultrasound guidance of suprapubic bladder aspiration. *Pediatr Nephrol.* 1997;11:607.
17. Buck JR, Weintraub WH, Coran AG, et al. Fiberoptic transillumination: a new tool for the pediatric surgeon. *J Pediatr Surg.* 1977; 12:451.
18. Barone MA. Pediatric procedures. In: McMillan JA, Feigin RD, DeAngelis CD, et al., eds. *Oski's Pediatrics: Principles and Practice.* 4th ed. Philadelphia: Lippincott Williams & Wilkins; 2006:2671.
19. El-Naggar W, Yiu A, Mohamed A, et al. Comparison of pain during two methods of urine collection in preterm infants. *Pediatrics.* 2010;125:1224.
20. Nahum Y, Tenenbaum A, Isaiah W, et al. Effect of eutectic mixture of local anesthetics (EMLA) for pain relief during suprapubic aspiration in young infants: a randomized, controlled trial. *Clin J Pain.* 2007;23:756.
21. Kozer E, Rosenbloom E, Goldman D, et al. Pain in infants who are younger than 2 months during suprapubic aspiration and transurethral bladder catheterization: a randomized, controlled trial. *Pediatrics.* 2006;118:e51.
22. Anand KJ, Johnston CC, Oberlander TF, et al. Analgesia and local anesthesia during invasive procedures in the neonate. *Clin Ther.* 2005;27:844.
23. Carlson KP, Pullon DHH. Bladder hemorrhage following transcutaneous bladder aspiration. *Pediatrics.* 1977;60:765.
24. Lanier B, Daeschner CW. Serious complication of suprapubic aspiration of the urinary bladder. *J Pediatr.* 1971;79:711.
25. Rockoff AS. Hemorrhage after suprapubic bladder aspiration. *J Pediatr.* 1976;89:327.
26. Kunz HH, Sieberth HG, Freiberg J, et al. Zur Bedeutung der Blasenpunktion fur den sicheren Nachweis einer Bakteriurie. *Dtsch Med Wochenschr.* 1975;100:2252.
27. Morell RE, Duritz G, Oltorf C. Suprapubic aspiration associated with hematoma. *Pediatrics.* 1982;69:455.
28. Mandell J, Stevens P. Supravesical hematoma following suprapubic urine aspiration. *J Urol.* 1978;119:286.
29. Uhari M, Remes M. Suprapubic abscess—a complication of suprapubic bladder aspiration. *Arch Dis Child.* 1977;52:985.
30. Polnay, L, Fraser AM, Lewis JM. Complication of suprapubic bladder aspiration. *Arch Dis Child.* 1975;50:80.
31. Mustonen A, Uhari M. Is there bacteremia after suprapubic aspiration in children with urinary tract infection? *J Urol.* 1978;119: 822.
32. Pass RF, Waldo FB. Anaerobic bacteremia following suprapubic bladder aspiration. *J Pediatr.* 1979;94:748.
33. Wald ER. Risk factors for osteomyelitis. *Am J Med.* 1985;78:206.
34. Kalager T, Digranes A. Unusual complication after suprapubic bladder puncture. *Br Med J.* 1979;1:91.
35. Weathers WT, Wenzel JE. Suprapubic aspiration: perforation of a viscus other than the bladder. *Am J Dis Child.* 1969;117:590.
36. Schreiner RL, Skafish P. Complications of suprapubic bladder aspiration. *Am J Dis Child.* 1978;132:98.

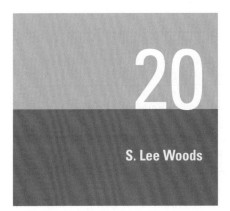

20 Bladder Catheterization

S. Lee Woods

A. Indications (1–7)

1. To obtain urine for culture, particularly when suprapubic collection is contraindicated and when clean-catch specimen is unsatisfactory

   Although suprapubic bladder aspiration is considered the most reliable method of obtaining urine for culture in infants and young children (see Chapter 19), bladder catheterization is an acceptable alternative method. Bladder catheterization has a higher success rate than suprapubic aspiration, especially if the practitioner is inexperienced in bladder aspiration. However, urine samples collected by catheterization have a higher false-positive rate than suprapubic aspiration (3–7,9–11), and catheterization can introduce bacteria colonizing the distal urethra into the bladder, causing a urinary tract infection (see F). The diagnosis of urinary tract infection cannot be made reliably by culturing urine collected in a bag (4,12).
2. To monitor precisely the urinary output of a critically ill patient
3. To quantify bladder residual
4. To relieve urinary retention (e.g., in neurogenic bladder) (13,14)
5. To instill contrast agent to perform cystourethrography (15)

B. Contraindications (1)

Contraindications include pelvic fracture, urethral trauma, and blood at the meatus. In the presence of uncorrected bleeding diathesis, potential risks and benefits must be considered.

C. Equipment

All equipment must be sterile. Commercial prepackaged urinary drainage kits, with or without collection burettes for closed drainage, are available.

1. Gloves
2. Gauze sponges and cup with iodophor antiseptic solution (not containing alcohol), or

3. Prepared antiseptic-impregnated swabs
4. Towels for draping
5. Surgical lubricant
6. Cotton-tipped applicators
7. Urinary catheter

   Silicone urinary drainage catheters are available in 3.5, 5, 6.5, and 8 French (Fr) sizes. A 5-Fr infant feeding tube or a 3.5- or 5-Fr umbilical catheter may be substituted for a urinary catheter.
8. Sterile container for specimen collection or collection burette for continuous closed drainage

D. Precautions

1. Use strict aseptic technique.
2. Use adequate lighting.
3. Try to time the procedure for when the infant has not recently voided (1 to 2 hours after the last wet diaper). Portable ultrasound can be helpful in determining when there is sufficient urine present in the bladder, reducing the chance of an unsuccessful attempt (16,17).
4. Avoid vigorous irrigation of the perineum in preparation for catheterization. This may increase the risk of introducing bacteria into the urinary tract.
5. Avoid separating the labia minora too widely, to prevent tearing of the fourchette.
6. Use the smallest-diameter catheter to avoid traumatic complications. A 3.5-Fr catheter is recommended for infants weighing <1,000 g and a 5-Fr catheter is recommended for larger infants.
7. If the catheter does not pass easily, do not use force. Suspect obstruction and abandon the procedure.
8. To avoid coiling and knotting, insert the catheter only as far as necessary to obtain urine.
9. If urine is not obtained in a female infant, recheck the location of the catheter by visual inspection or by radiographic examination. It may have passed through the introitus into the vagina.
10. Remove the catheter as soon as possible, to avoid infectious complications.
11. If the catheter cannot be removed easily, do not use force. Consult urology, as it may be knotted.

E. Technique

Male Infant (1,8,18–20)

1. Set up equipment and squeeze a small amount of lubricant onto a sterile field.
2. Restrain the infant supine in the frog-leg position.
3. Wash hands thoroughly and put on gloves.
4. Stabilize the shaft of the penis with the nondominant hand. This hand is now considered contaminated.
5. If the infant is uncircumcised, gently retract the foreskin just enough to expose the meatus. Do not attempt to lyse adhesions. The young male infant has physiologic phimosis, and the foreskin cannot be fully retracted (19). If the foreskin is tightly adherent, attempt to line up the preputial ring and the meatus.
6. Apply gentle pressure at the base of the penis to avoid reflex urination.
7. Using the free hand for the rest of the procedure, clean the glans three times with antiseptic solution. Begin at the meatus and work outward and down the shaft of the penis. Blot dry with sterile gauze.
8. Drape sterile towels across the lower abdomen and across the infant's legs.
9. Place the wide end of the catheter or feeding tube into the specimen container.
10. Lubricate the tip of the catheter copiously.
11. Move the specimen container and catheter onto the sterile drape between the infant's legs.
12. Gently insert the catheter through the meatus just until urine is seen in the tube (Fig. 20.1).
    a. During insertion, apply gentle upward traction on the penile shaft to prevent kinking of the urethra (Fig. 20.1).
    b. If the meatus cannot be visualized, insert the catheter through the preputial ring in a slightly inferior direction. If there is any question about catheter position, abandon the procedure.
    c. If resistance is met at the external sphincter, hold the catheter in place, applying minimal pressure.

Generally, spasm will relax after a brief period, allowing easy passage of catheter. If not, suspect obstruction and abandon the procedure.
    d. Do not move the catheter in and out. This will increase the risk of urethral trauma.
    e. Do not insert extra tubing length in an attempt to stabilize a catheter to be left indwelling. This will increase the risk of trauma and knotting.
13. Collect specimen for culture.
14. If the catheter is to remain indwelling, connect the catheter immediately to a closed sterile system for urine collection. Tape the tube securely to the inner thigh.
15. If the catheter is to be removed, gently withdraw it when urine flow ceases.

Female Infant (1,18–21)

1. Follow steps 1 through 3 of technique for male infant.
2. Retract the labia minora.
    a. Use sterile gauze sponges with nondominant hand, or
    b. Have an assistant retract the labia with two cotton-tipped applicators (Fig. 20.2).
3. Using the free hand for the rest of the procedure, cleanse the area between the labia minora three times with antiseptic solution.
    a. Swab in an anterior-to-posterior direction to avoid drawing fecal material into the field.
    b. Blot dry with sterile gauze.
4. Follow steps 8 through 11 of the technique for the male infant.
5. Visualize the meatus (Fig. 20.2).
    a. The most prominent structure is the vaginal introitus. The urethral meatus lies immediately anterior (between the clitoris and the introitus).
    b. The meatus may be obscured by the introital fold. Gently push the fold down with a cotton-tipped applicator.
    c. If the meatus is not visible, the infant may have female hypospadias (the meatus is on the roof of the vagina, just inside the introitus). The urethra

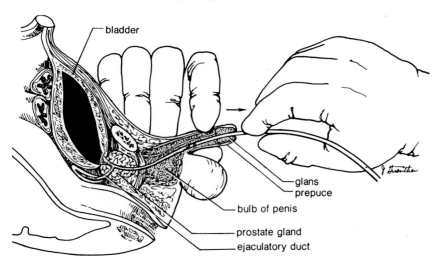

FIG. 20.1. Anatomic drawing demonstrating bladder catheterization in the male.

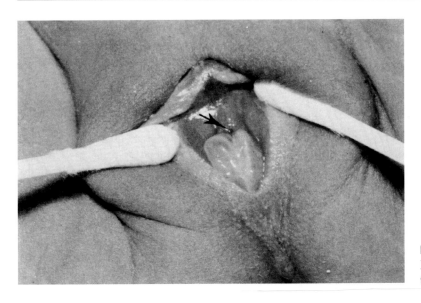

FIG. 20.2. External genitalia in the female. Retraction of labia majora and minora with cotton-tipped applicators. An *arrow* indicates urethral meatus.

must then be catheterized blindly, which may require a curved-tip catheter or urologic assistance.

6. Gently insert the catheter only until urine appears in the tube. Do not insert extra tubing.
7. Follow steps 13 through 15 of technique for the male infant.

Female Infant in Prone Position (22)

This technique is useful in an infant who cannot be placed supine (e.g., one with a large meningomyelocele)

1. Position the infant prone on folded blankets so that the head and trunk are elevated about 3 inches above the knees and lower legs. The hips should be flexed with knees abducted (Fig. 20.3A).
2. Place a gauze pad over the anus and secure with tape across the buttocks, to avoid contamination of the perineum from reflex bowel evacuation (Fig. 20.3B).
3. Place sterile drapes as shown in Fig. 20.3C. Follow the procedure for female catheterization above.

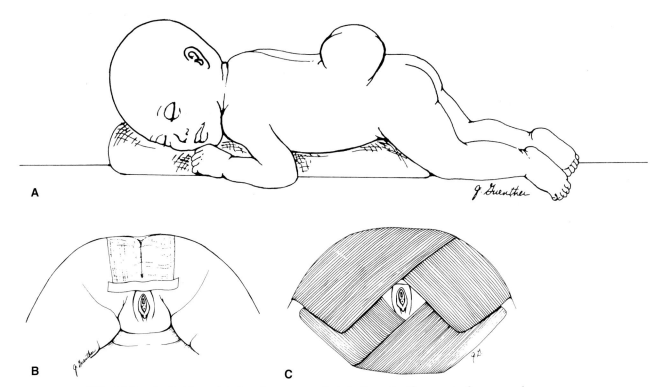

FIG. 20.3.   **A:** Position of infant for prone catheterization. **B:** Placement of gauze pad over anus. **C:** Placement of drapes. (Adapted from Campbell J. Catheterizing prone female infants: how can you see what you're doing? *Am J Matern Child Nurs.* 1979;4:376, based on drawing by N. L. Gahan, with permission.)

F. Complications

1. Infection (23–26)
   a. Urethritis
   b. Epididymitis
   c. Cystitis
   d. Pyelonephritis
   e. Sepsis

   The most common complication of bladder catheterization is the introduction of bacteria into the urinary tract and potentially into the bloodstream. Catheterization is the leading cause of nosocomial urinary tract infection and gram-negative sepsis in adult patients (24). The risk of bacteriuria from straight ("in-and-out") catheterization is 1% to 5% in this population (23,24). The risk of infection is related directly to the duration of catheterization. In infants and children, approximately 50% to 75% of hospital-acquired urinary tract infections occur in catheterized patients, the highest rate being in neonates (25,26). Urinary tract infection developed in 10.8% of catheterized pediatric patients (25), and secondary bacteremia in 2.9% (26). Risk of infection is decreased by adhering to strict aseptic technique during catheter placement, maintaining a closed sterile collection system, and removing the catheter as soon as possible.

2. Trauma
   a. Hematuria
   b. Urethral erosion or tear (27)
   c. Urethral false passage (27,28)
   d. Perforation of the urethra or bladder (Fig. 20.4) (27,29,30)
   e. Tear of the fourchette (27)
   f. Meatal stenosis (20)
   g. Urethral stricture (31)
   h. Urinary retention secondary to urethral edema (27)

3. The risk of trauma is reduced by using the smallest-diameter catheter with ample lubrication, advancing the catheter only as far as necessary to obtain urine, and never forcing a catheter through an obstruction. Erosion and perforation are associated with long-indwelling catheters. This risk is reduced by removing the catheter as soon as possible.

4. Mechanical
   a. Catheter malposition (27)
   b. Catheter knot (32–36)

   The risk of knotting is reduced by using the minimal length of catheter insertion. Standard insertion lengths of 6 cm for male and 5 cm for female term newborns have been suggested (36). Shorter lengths would be appropriate for preterm infants. A more general standard is to insert the catheter only as far as needed to obtain urine. Using a feeding tube as a urinary catheter may also increase the risk of knotting, because these tubes are softer and more likely to coil.

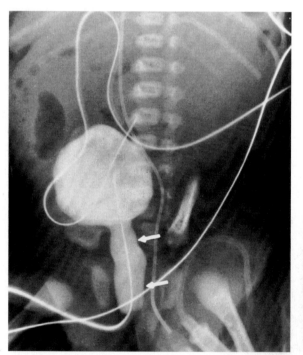 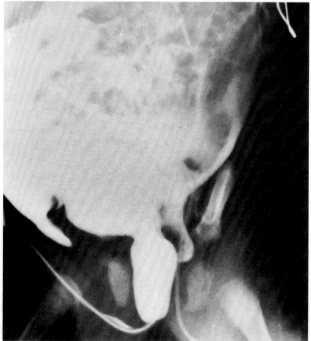

A   B

FIG. 20.4. **A:** Cystogram shows dilated posterior urethra (*arrows*) secondary to posterior urethral valves. **B:** Subsequent film shows perforation of the bladder, with free contrast material in the peritoneal cavity.

References

1. Sigman LJ. Procedures. In: Tschudy MM, Arcara KM, eds. *The Harriet Lane Handbook.* 19th ed. Philadelphia: Elsevier; 2012:57.
2. Long SS, Klein JO. Bacterial infections of the urinary tract. In: Remington JS, Klein JO, Wilson CB, Nizet V, Maldonado YA, eds. *Infectious Diseases of the Fetus and Newborn.* 7th ed. Philadelphia: Elsevier; 2011:310.
3. Wingerter S, Bachur R. Risk factors for contamination of catheterized urine specimens in febrile children. *Pediatr Emerg Care.* 2011;27:1.
4. Karacan C, Erkek N, Senet S, et al. Evaluation of urine collection methods for the diagnosis of urinary tract infection in children. *Med Princ Pract.* 2010;19:188.
5. Phillips B. Towards evidence based medicine for paediatricians. Urethral catheter or suprapubic aspiration to reduce contamination of urine samples in young children? *Arch Dis Child.* 2009;94:736.
6. Cheng YW, Wong, SN. Diagnosing symptomatic urinary tract infections in infants by catheter urine culture. *J Paeditr Child Health.* 2005;41:437.
7. Ma JF, Diariki Shortliffe LM. Urinary tract infection in children: etiology and epidemiology. *Urol Clin NA.* 2004;31:517.
8. Carter HB. Basic instrumentation and cystoscopy. In: Walsh PC, Retik AB, Vaughan ED, et al., eds. *Campbell's Urology.* 8th ed. Philadelphia: Saunders; 2002:11.
9. Austin BJ, Bollard C, Gunn TR. Is urethral catheterization a successful alternative to suprapubic aspiration in neonates? *J Paeditr Child Health.* 1999;35:34.
10. Tobiansky R, Evans N. A randomized controlled trial of two methods for collection of sterile urine in neonates. *J Paediatr Child Health.* 1998;43:460.
11. Pollack CV, Pollack ES, Andrew ME. Suprapubic bladder aspiration versus urethral catheterization in ill infants: success, efficiency and complication rates. *Ann Emerg Med.* 1994;23:225.
12. Al-Orifi F, McGillivray D, Tange S, et al. Urine culture from bag specimens in young children: are the risks too high? *J Pediatr.* 2000; 137:221.
13. Ewalt DH, Bauer SB. Pediatric neurourology. *Urol Clin North Am.* 1996;23:501.
14. Baskin LS, Kogan BA, Benard F. Treatment of infants with neurogenic bladder dysfunction using anticholinergic drugs and intermittent catheterisation. *Br J Urol.* 1990;66:532.
15. Shalaby-Rana E, Lowe LH, Blask AN, et al. Imaging in pediatric urology. *Pediatr Clin North Am.* 1997;44:1065.
16. Milling TJ, Van Amerongen R, Melville L, et al. Use of ultrasonography to identify infants in whom urinary catheterization will be unsuccessful because of insufficient urine volume: validation of the urinary bladder index. *Ann Emerg Med.* 2005;45:510.
17. Chen L, Hsiao AL, Moore L, et al. Utility of bedside bladder ultrasound before urethral catheterization in young children. *Pediatrics.* 2005;115:108.
18. Barone MA. Pediatric procedures. In: McMillan JA, Feigin RD, DeAngelis CD, et al., eds. *Oski's Pediatrics: Principles and Practice.* 4th ed. Philadelphia: Lippincott Williams & Wilkins; 2006:2671.
19. Robson WL, Leung AK, Thomason MA. Catheterization of the bladder in infants and children. *Clin Pediatr.* 2006;45:795.
20. Brown MR, Cartwright PC, Snow BW. Common office problems in pediatric urology and gynecology. *Pediatr Clin North Am.* 1997; 44:1091.
21. Redman JF. Techniques of genital examination and bladder catheterization in female children. *Urol Clin North Am.* 1990;17:1.
22. Campbell J. Catheterizing prone female infants: how can you see what you're doing? *Am J Matern Child Nurs.* 1979;4:376.
23. Nadler BB, Bushman W, Wyker AW. Standard diagnostic considerations. In: Gillenwater JY, Grayhack JT, Howard SS, et al., eds. *Adult and Pediatric Urology.* Philadelphia: Lippincott,Williams & Wilkins; 2002:47.
24. Sedor J, Mulholland SG. Hospital-acquired urinary tract infections associated with the indwelling catheter. *Urol Clin North Am.* 1999;26:821.
25. Lohr JA, Downs SM, Dudley S, et al. Hospital-acquired urinary tract infections in the pediatric patient: a prospective study. *Pediatr Infect Dis J.* 1994;13:8.
26. Dele Davies H, Ford Jones EL, Sheng RY, et al. Nosocomial urinary tract infections at a pediatric hospital. *Pediatr Infect Dis J.* 1992; 11:349.
27. McAlister WH, Cacciarelli A, Shackelford GD. Complications associated with cystography in children. *Radiology.* 1974;111:167.
28. Koleilat N, Sidi AA, Gonzalez R. Urethral false passage as a complication of intermittent catheterization. *J Urol.* 1989;142:1216.
29. Basha M, Subhani M, Mersal A, et al. Urinary bladder perforation in a premature infant with Down syndrome. *Pediatr Nephrol.* 2003;18:1189.
30. Salama H, Al Ju Fairi M, Rejjal A, et al. Urinary bladder perforation in a very low birth weight infant. *J Perinat Med.* 2002;30: 440.
31. Edwards LE, Lock R, Powell C, et al. Post-catheterisation urethral strictures. A clinical and experimental study. *Br J Urol.* 1983;55:53.
32. Anatol T, Nunez J. Intravesical tube knot in a neonate. *J Trop Pediatr.* 2005;51:314.
33. Lodha A, Ly L, Brindle M, et al. Intraurethral knot in a very-low-birth-weight infant: radiological recognition, surgical management and prevention. *Pediatr Radiol.* 2005;35:713.
34. Anbu AT, Palmer K. Urethral catheter knotting in preterm neonates. *Indian Pediatr.* 2004;41:631.
35. Mayer E, Ankem MK, Hartanto VH, et al. Management of urethral catheter knot in a neonate. *Can J Urol.* 2002;9:1649.
36. Carlson D, Mowery BD. Standards to prevent complications of urinary catheterization in children: should and should-knots. *J Soc Pediatr Nurs.* 1997;2:37.

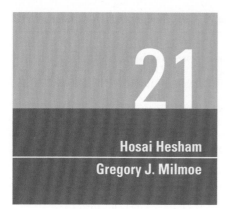

Tympanocentesis

Hosai Hesham
Gregory J. Milmoe

A. Indications

Diagnostic tympanocentesis is indicated in neonatal acute otitis media (AOM) to target antibiotic therapy (1,2). Tympanocentesis may be used for both diagnostic and drainage purposes (3). The specific indications include

1. AOM not responding to antibiotics after 72 hours
2. AOM in severely immunocompromised infant
3. AOM in infant already on antibiotics
4. AOM with suppurative complications (e.g., mastoiditis, facial paralysis, sepsis)
5. To confirm the diagnosis when the clinical exam is not clear
6. To relieve severe otalgia

B. Contraindications

1. Difficulty in confirming ossicular landmarks. One must be able to identify the malleus and the annulus of the tympanic membrane (TM) (Fig. 21.1).
2. Suggestion of abnormal anatomy. This is more likely in patients with congenital malformation syndromes.
3. Suggestion of alternate pathology (e.g., cholesteatoma or neoplasm)

C. Equipment

All Sterile

1. Surgical gloves
2. Otoscope with open operating head and good light
3. Largest speculum that will fit the canal (2, 3, or 4 mm)
4. 18-gauge 3-inch spinal needle with 1-mL or 3-mL syringe
5. Blunt ear curette
6. 70% isopropyl alcohol in 3-mL syringe for cleaning and antisepsis of ear canal
7. Suction setup with 5-Fr Frazier ear suction
8. Culturettes with transport media

D. Precautions

1. Patient safety and comfort require proper restraint, adequate light, and appropriate instruments.
2. The kindest way is to be quick, and this means having the child immobile.
3. Conscious sedation is feasible only if the child is stable and has no issues with airway obstruction. It is not needed past the point of puncturing the TM; usually no medication is used.
4. Good visualization is paramount. Sufficient cleaning must be done so that the malleus and the anterior aspect of the annulus are clearly visible.
5. Avoid the posterior aspect of the tympanic membrane. This is where the round window, stapes, and incus are located.

E. Technique (4,5)

1. Restrain infant (see Chapter 4).
2. Position infant with the head turned so that the involved ear is up. The assistant must keep the head still.
3. Rinse ear canal with alcohol solution from a 3-mL syringe. This will provide antisepsis and initiate cleaning.
4. Let fluid run out or use suction.
5. Use otoscope to visualize canal and remove debris with curette or suction.
6. Align speculum to get best view of TM landmarks. Pulling superiorly and laterally on the pinna will improve visibility (Fig. 21.2).
7. Attach spinal needle to syringe, after bending it 45 to 60 degrees at the hub. This keeps the syringe out of the line of sight.
8. Hold needle at the hub and introduce it through the otoscope. Puncture the drum anterior to the malleus at or below the umbo level (Figs. 21.2 and 21.3).
9. Hold needle securely and have assistant draw back on the syringe to obtain sample.
10. Place sample in appropriate transport medium.

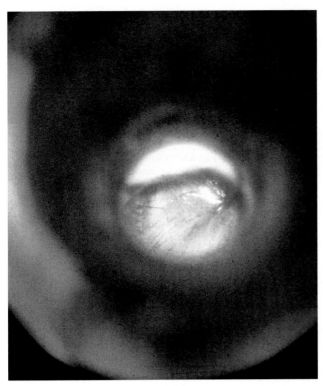

FIG. 21.1. Normal newborn eardrum. View through speculum.

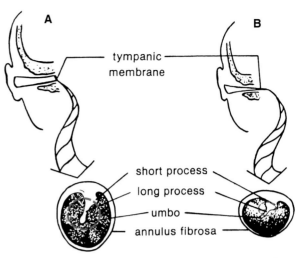

FIG. 21.2. Tympanic membrane in the adult (**A**) and infant (**B**). The portion of the tympanic membrane that may be visualized through the speculum at one time is within the *dotted line*.

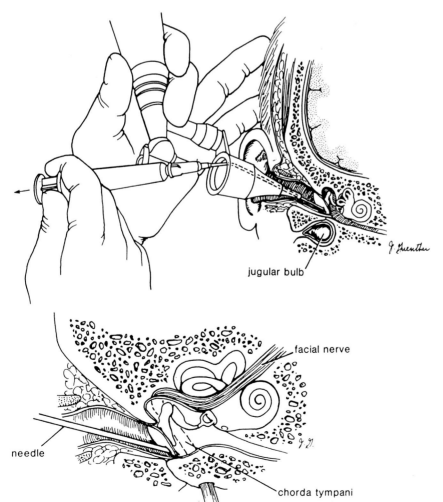

FIG. 21.3. Tympanocentesis. Aspirating the middle ear using a 3-mL syringe. Needle is penetrating eardrum inferiorly.

11. If more drainage is required, a myringotomy blade can be used to widen the opening. This will close in 48 to 72 hours.

F. Complications

1. Most common is bleeding from canal wall. This usually will stop spontaneously, but is preferably avoided.
2. TM perforation that persists. Initially, this is may be helpful for drainage and ventilation of the middle ear space.
3. Disruption of the ossicles from malpositioned needle (see B1 and D5)
4. Major bleeding from dehiscent jugular bulb or carotid artery (6); rare.

References

1. Turner D, Leibovitz E, Aran A, et al. Acute otitis media in infants younger than two months of age: microbiology, clinical presentation and therapeutic approach. *Pediatr Infect Dis J*. 2002;21(7):669.
2. Sakran W, Makary H, Colodner R, et al. Acute otitis media in infants less than three months of age: clinical presentation, etiology and concomitant diseases. *Int J Pediatr Otorhinolaryngol*. 2006;70(4):613.
3. Nomura Y, Mimata H, Yamasaki M, et al. Effect of myringotomy on prognosis in pediatric acute otitis media. *Int J Pediatr Otorhinolaryngol*. 2005;69:61.
4. Guarisco JL, Grundfast KM. A simple device for tympanocentesis in infants and children. *Laryngoscope*. 1988;98:244.
5. Bluestone CD, Klein JO. Otologic surgical procedures. In: Bluestone CD, Stool SE, Kenna M, eds. *Pediatric Otolaryngology*. Philadelphia: Saunders; 1996:28.
6. Hasebe S, Sando I, Orita Y. Proximity of carotid canal wall to tympanic membrane: a human temporal bone study. *Laryngoscope*. 2003;113:802.

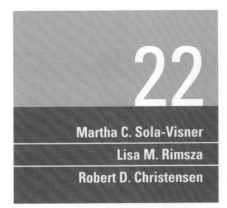

22 Tibial Bone Marrow Biopsy

Martha C. Sola-Visner

Lisa M. Rimsza

Robert D. Christensen

A. Purpose

To obtain a bone marrow clot sample for histologic evaluation of the following[1]
1. Bone marrow cellularity
2. Relative abundance of myeloid, erythroid, lymphoid, and megakaryocytic lineages, using specific immunohistochemical stains on multiple cuts if necessary
3. Maturation and morphology of cells of all lineages
4. Presence of infiltrative nonmalignant diseases
5. Presence of infiltrative malignant diseases (hematologic and nonhematologic)
6. Presence of granulomas or infectious organisms

B. Indications

1. Evaluation of primary hematologic disorders (1–6)
   a. Suspected neonatal aplastic anemia (pancytopenia)
   b. Suspected leukemia, when blood studies are insufficient to confirm the diagnosis
   c. Neutropenia of unclear etiology, which is severe (absolute neutrophil count <500/mL) and persistent.
   d. Thrombocytopenia of unclear etiology, which is severe (platelets <50,000/mL) and persistent
2. Evaluation of suspected metabolic storage disease (e.g., Niemann–Pick disease) (2)
3. Evaluation of suspected hemophagocytic syndrome or familial hemophagocytic lymphohistiocytosis (7,8)
4. Detection of infiltrating tumor cells (9–12) or of congenital systemic Langerhans' cell histiocytosis (13)
5. Certain cultures (e.g., in disseminated tuberculosis or fungal disease) (14)
6. Cytogenetic studies, for chromosomal analysis (even after transfusion of donor blood) within 3 to 4 hours (15). Note: This requires an aspirate rather than a clot.
7. Staging of solid tumors (16,17)

[1]The information listed below (except for maturation and morphology of the cells of all lineages) can be obtained more reliably from biopsies or clot sections than from traditional aspirates (24).

C. Contraindications

1. Sampling from the sternum is not recommended in any neonate because of danger of damage to intrathoracic and mediastinal organs (2,18).
2. Sampling from the anterior iliac crest is not recommended, particularly in the smallest preterm infants, owing to the proximity to intra-abdominal organs.
3. Risks/benefits should be considered carefully in the presence of coagulopathy or when administering anticoagulants or thrombolytics.
4. Risks/benefits should be carefully considered in preterm infants with severe osteopenia of prematurity (19).

D. Limitations

In small preterm infants, the tibial bone marrow biopsy technique sometimes yields no marrow or a very hemodilute sample, mostly because of the small size of the marrow compartment within the tibia.

E. Equipment

Sterile

1. Surgical gloves
2. Cup with antiseptic solution
3. Gauze squares
4. Sterile drapes
5. 1% lidocaine without epinephrine in 1-mL syringe, with 27-gauge needle
6. 19-gauge, 0.5-inch Osgood bone marrow needle (Popper and Sons, New Hyde Park, New York) (Fig. 22.1)
7. 3-mL syringe without Luer-Lok

Nonsterile

1. Cup containing 10% neutral buffered formalin or other appropriate fixative
2. 1- to 2-inch needle to aid in removal of clot from the syringe

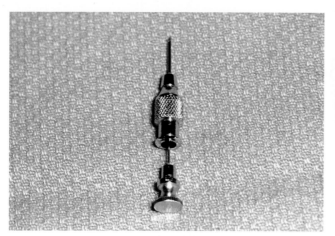

FIG. 22.1.   View of the 19-gauge, 0.5-inch Osgood bone marrow needle. The trocar must be completely inserted in the Osgood needle prior to the procedure.

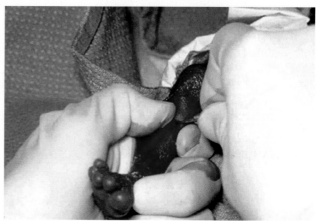

FIG. 22.2.   The Osgood needle is introduced into the tibial marrow cavity with a slow, twisting motion. Notice that the leg is firmly stabilized in the operator's nondominant hand.

F. Precautions

1. Correct coagulopathy as far as possible prior to procedure.
2. Use a total of 0.2 to 0.4 mL of lidocaine. Aspirate before injection to avoid intravascular injection.
3. Stabilize the leg in your hand, between your thumb and forefinger. To avoid bone fracture, be sure to apply counterpressure with your palm directly opposite the site of penetration.
4. Be aware that less pressure is required to insert the bone marrow needle in neonates (particularly in very low-birthweight infants) than in older children.
5. Be careful to enter the bone 1 to 2 cm below the tibial tuberosity, to minimize the risk of injuring the growth plate.
6. After the procedure, apply adequate pressure to control bleeding.

G. Special Circumstances

In cases of suspected osteopetrosis, obtaining a posterior iliac crest bone/bone marrow biopsy is preferable, because it allows quantification of osteoclasts and evaluation of marrow and bony changes consistent with osteopetrosis. In these cases, the tibial bone marrow biopsy technique usually yields only blood or no sample.

H. Technique

1. Place the infant in the supine position.
2. Use the triangular area at the proximal end of the medial (flat) surface of the tibia, approximately 1 to 2 cm distal to the tibial tuberosity (20).
3. Prepare and drape as for a major procedure (see Chapter 5).

4. Infiltrate subcutaneous tissue with lidocaine as the needle is slowly advanced. Inject further small volume when the needle reaches the bone, making sure that the tip of the needle is inserted into the bone for subperiosteal injection.
5. Remove the needle and wait 2 to 3 minutes.
6. Use your nondominant hand to firmly stabilize the leg, providing support with your palm *directly opposite* the site of marrow puncture. This hand cannot be reintroduced into the sterile field.
7. Make sure that the trocar is completely inserted in the Osgood needle.
8. Hold the needle between the thumb and forefinger of your dominant hand.
9. Introduce the needle at a 90-degree angle, and advance it into the marrow cavity with a slow, twisting motion (Fig. 22.2).
10. Continue to advance the needle until it is firmly fixed in bone (does not move when touched) (Fig. 22.3).

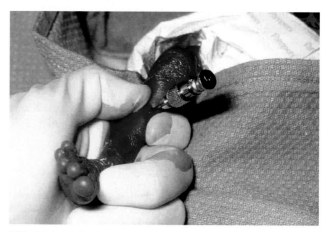

FIG. 22.3.   The Osgood needle is firmly fixed in the bone.

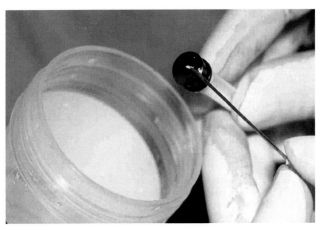

FIG. 22.4. A small amount of bone marrow has been obtained in a 3-mL syringe and allowed to clot at the bottom of the syringe. The plunger has been removed, and the clot is now being gently dislodged from the plunger (with the use of a 1- or 2-inch needle) and placed into the fixative solution.

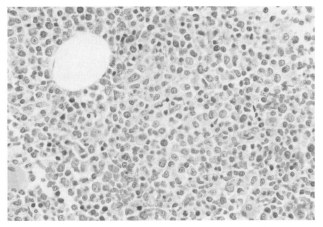

FIG. 22.5. Photomicrograph of a bone marrow clot section obtained from a neutropenic neonate. The cellularity is near 100%. Myeloid precursors, scattered erythroid cells, lymphocytes, and several megakaryocytes are clearly identified. Hematoxylin and eosin; original magnification × 200.

11. Remove the trocar from the needle and advance the hollow needle an additional 2 to 3 mm into the marrow space (this trephinates marrow spicules into the needle).
12. Attach a 3-mL syringe (without a Luer-Lok) firmly to the needle.
13. Withdraw the plunger forcefully until a small drop of marrow (~0.1 mL) appears in the syringe hub. Suction should be stopped as soon as the smallest amount of marrow is obtained, because excessive suction will dilute the sample with peripheral blood.
14. If no marrow is obtained initially, rotate, advance, or retract the needle and try again.
15. Remove the syringe as soon as bone marrow is obtained and withdraw the plunger (with marrow attached) to the bottom of the syringe. Allow the marrow to clot there.
16. Remove the needle and apply pressure over the site to achieve hemostasis.

Preparation of the Bone Marrow Clot

1. After the marrow specimen has clotted, dislodge the clot gently with the use of a 1- or 2-inch needle and place it into the fixative solution (Fig. 22.4).
2. Process the bone marrow clot in a manner identical to a typical bone marrow biopsy, except that decalcification is not required (Fig. 22.5).

I. Complications[2]

1. Subperiosteal bleeding (21)
2. Cellulitis or osteomyelitis (22)

3. Limb fracture (23)
4. Injury to blood vessels (21)
5. Bone changes on x-ray film (24,25)
   a. Lytic lesions
   b. Exostoses
   c. Subperiosteal calcification (secondary to hematoma)

J. Advantages of the Tibial Site

1. It is a safe site, particularly in very small preterm infants, because it avoids any proximity to vital organs.
2. The tibia can be easily positioned without disturbing even the sickest infants (usually maintained in the supine position while on mechanical ventilation).
3. It can be adequately stabilized and supported by the non-dominant hand of the person performing the procedure.

Acknowledgments

This work was partially supported by National Institutes of Health grant HL69990.

References

1. Calhoun DA, Christensen RD, Edstrom CS, et al. Consistent approaches to procedures and practices in neonatal hematology. *Clin Perinatol.* 2000;27:733.
2. Downing V. Bone marrow examination in children. *Pediatr Clin North Am.* 1955;2:243.
3. Garcia L, Valcarcel M, Santiago-Borrero PJ. Chemotherapy during pregnancy and its effects on the fetus—neonatal myelosuppression: two case reports. *J Perinatol.* 1999;19:230.
4. Juul SE, Calhoun DA, Christensen RD. "Idiopathic neutropenia" in very-low birthweight infants. *Acta Paediatr.* 1998;87:963.
5. Calhoun DA, Kirk JF, Christensen RD. Incidence, significance, and kinetic mechanism responsible for leukemoid reactions in patients in the neonatal intensive care unit: a prospective evaluation. *J Pediatr.* 1996;129:403.

---

[2]These complications refer to the bone marrow biopsy procedure in general, not to the tibial site in particular.

6. Mizutani K, Azuma E, Komada Y, et al. An infantile case of cyto-megalovirus induced idiopathic thrombocytopenic purpura with predominant proliferation of CD10 positive lymphoblasts in bone marrow. *Acta Paediatr Jpn.* 1995;37:71.

7. Aygun C, Tekinalp G, Gurgey A. Infection-associated hemo-phagocytic syndrome due to *Pseudomonas aeruginosa* in preterm infants. *J Pediatr Hematol Oncol.* 2003;25:665.

8. Rugolotto S, Marradi PL, Balter R, et al. Familial haemophago-cytic lymphohistiocytosis: survival of a premature twin with immuno-chemotherapy and bone marrow transplantation from an HLA-identical unrelated donor. *Acta Paediatr.* 2005;94:971.

9. Karcioglu ZA, Al-Mesfer SA, Abboud E, et al. Workup for meta-static retinoblastoma. A review of 261 patients. *Ophthalmology.* 1997;104:307.

10. Moscinski LC, Pendergrass TW, Weiss A, et al. Recommendations for the use of routine bone marrow aspirations and lumbar punc-tures in the follow up of patients with retinoblastoma. *J Pediatr Hematol Oncol.* 1996;18:130.

11. Osmanagaoglu K, Lippens M, Benoit Y, et al. A comparison of iodine-123 meta-iodobenzylguanidine scintigraphy and single bone marrow aspiration biopsy in the diagnosis and follow-up of 26 children with neuroblastoma. *Eur J Nucl Med.* 1993;20:1154.

12. Penchansky L. Bone marrow biopsy in the metastatic work-up of solid tumors in children. *Cancer.* 1984;54:1447.

13. Mosterd K, van Marion A, van Steensel MA. Neonatal Langerhans' cell histiocytosis: a rare and potentially life-threaten-ing disease. *Int J Dermatol.* 2008;47(Suppl 1):10.

14. Machin GA, Honore LH, Fanning EA, et al. Perinatally acquired neonatal tuberculosis: report of two cases. *Pediatr Pathol.* 1992;12:707.

15. Page BM, Coulter JB. Bone marrow aspiration for chromosome analysis in newborn. *Br Med J.* 1978;1:1455.

16. Lee ST, Suh YL, Ko YH, et al. Measurement of tyrosine hydroxy-lase transcripts in bone marrow using biopsied tissue instead of aspirates for neuroblastoma. *Pediatr Blood Cancer.* 2010;55:273.

17. Park SJ, Park CJ, Kim S. Detection of bone marrow metastases of neuroblastoma with immunohistochemical staining of CD56, chromogranin A, and synaptophysin. *Appl Immunohistochem Mol Morphol.* 2010;18:348.

18. Bakir F. Fatal sternal puncture. *Dis Chest.* 1963;44:435.

19. Dabezies EJ, Warren PD. Fractures in very low birth weight infants with rickets. *Clin Orthop Relat Res.* 1997;335:233.

20. Sola MC, Rimsza LM, Christensen RD. A bone marrow biopsy technique suitable for use in neonates. *Br J Haematol.* 1999;107:458.

21. McNutt DR, Fudenberg HH. Bone-marrow biopsy and osteopo-rosis. *N Engl J Med.* 1972;1:46.

22. Shah M, Watanakunakorn C. *Staphylococcus aureus* sternal osteomyelitis complicating bone marrow aspiration. *South Med J.* 1978;71:348.

23. Miller D. Normal values and examination of the blood: perinatal period, infancy, childhood, and adolescence. In: Miller D, Pearson H, Bachner R, et al., eds. *Smith's Blood Diseases of Infancy and Childhood.* St. Louis: Mosby; 1978:20.

24. Gilsanz V, Grunebaum M. Radiographic appearance of iliac mar-row biopsy sites. *AJR.* 1977;128:597.

25. Murphy WA. Exostosis after iliac bone marrow biopsy. *AJR.* 1977;129:1114.

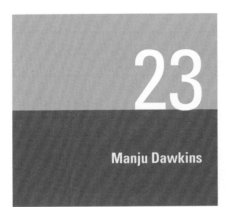

23

Manju Dawkins

Punch Skin Biopsy

A. Definition

1. A small, full-thickness biopsy utilizing a cylindrical instrument

B. Indications

1. Diagnosis of skin lesions (1–8)
2. Electron and light microscopic identification of certain hereditary and metabolic disorders (9–15)
3. Genetic, enzymatic, or morphologic studies on established fibroblast strains (16)
4. Treatment of small skin lesions

C. Types of Skin Biopsy (6,10,17)

1. Punch skin biopsy is appropriate when epidermis, dermis, and, sometimes, subcutaneous fat is required.
   Allows for pathologic evaluation and rapid diagnosis of certain conditions
2. Shave biopsies are performed to obtain epidermis and superficial dermis.
3. Incisional biopsies are used predominantly for disorders of deep subcutaneous fat or fascia (e.g., erythema nodosum).
4. Excision of larger lesions by a trained dermatologist or surgeon is preferable when planning to remove an entire large lesion.

D. Contraindications

There are no absolute contraindications to skin biopsy.

1. Consider whether risk outweighs benefit if a bleeding disorder is present.
2. Caution should be exercised in certain anatomic locations where nerves and arteries are more superficial.
3. Many cephalic and midline lesions may require radiologic examination prior to biopsy to rule out connection to the intracranial or intraspinal space (18,19).

E. Equipment

Sterile

1. Gloves
2. Towel or tray to form sterile area
3. 70% alcohol or other suitable antiseptic agent
4. 4- × 4-in gauze squares
5. Lidocaine HCl 1% with or without epinephrine in 1-mL tuberculin syringe with 27- or 30-gauge needle
6. Blunt tissue forceps
7. Fine, curved scissors or no. 15 scalpel blade
8. Sharp 2- to 6-mm punch (Fig. 23.1). Disposable punches ranging from 2 to 8 mm are available
   Specimens obtained with a 2-mm punch are very small and may not yield enough tissue for an accurate diagnosis. One recent study showed that accurate diagnoses were achieved in 79 out of 84 cases, when comparing 2-mm punch biopsies to excisional specimens (20). In most cases, a 3- to 4-mm punch is appropriate.
   Skin biopsy has been performed on the fetus (11,21,22) and may be done postmortem on stillborn or recently deceased infants to produce fibroblast cultures for karyotype (see Chapter 25). Under the latter circumstances, punch or excisional biopsy from the freshest-appearing, least-macerated skin area(s) is appropriate.
9. 5-0 or 6-0 nylon suture with small curved needle on needle holder, Dermabond (Ethicon, Somerville, New Jersey)

Nonsterile

1. Adhesive bandage with petrolatum jelly
2. Appropriate transport medium affixed with patient's information (Table 23.1)
3. Razor if necessary

F. Precautions

1. Avoid sites, if possible, where a small scar would potentially be cosmetically disfiguring.
   a. Tip, bridge, and columella of nose
   b. Eyelids

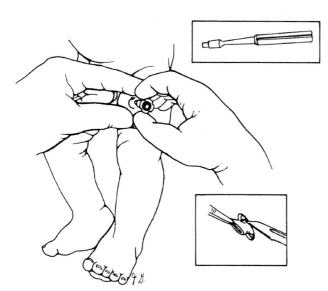

FIG. 23.1. Punch skin biopsy. **Top (inset):** Disposable biopsy punch. **Bottom (inset):** Cutting the dermal pedicle.

c. Lip margins
d. Nipples
e. Fingers or toes
f. Areas overlying joints
g. Lower leg below the knee

2. Avoid a very small punch (2 mm or less), because this may limit the ability to interpret pathologic findings.
3. Avoid multiple procedures at one site.
4. Be gentle, to avoid separating epidermis from dermis.
5. Check biopsy site for signs of infection until healing occurs.
6. Avoid freezing tissue for electron microscopy because cellular detail will then be destroyed (Table 23.1).
7. For specimens undergoing routine microscopic examination, avoid placing biopsy specimen in or on saline because artifactual hydropic degeneration of basal cells and subepidermal bullous formation may occur.

TABLE 23.1	Punch Biopsy Preservatives and Transport Media

Transport Medium	Indications
Formalin 10%	Routine microscopic evaluation
Michel's Medium or Saline-soaked gauze	Blistering or autoimmune disorders (immunofluorence)
	Electron microscopy
	Immunoperoxidase

G. Technique (6,8,17,23,24)

See Fig. 23.1.

1. Restrain and position patient.
2. Choose site for biopsy.
   a. For suspected malignant lesions, choose more atypical areas if unable to excise completely.
   b. For large or chronic lesions, obtain specimen from periphery, including some normal skin.
   c. For most dermatoses, choose site of early or fully developed, but not end-stage, lesion.
   d. For acute eruptions and bullous disease, choose an early lesion, including some normal skin.
   e. For discrete small lesions, try to leave 1- to 2-mm margins of normal skin around the lesions.
   f. Avoid excoriated, crusted, or traumatized lesions.
3. Shave hairs, if necessary.
4. Prepare as for minor procedure (see Chapter 5).
5. Inject 0.25 to 0.5 mL of lidocaine (with/without epinephrine) intradermally beneath the lesion. Some techniques used to minimize pain include: use of a small-bore (30-gauge) needle, buffering anesthetic with sodium bicarbonate, pinching of the site during injection, and applying ice (25–27).
6. Wait 5 minutes for maximal anesthesia. If using lidocaine with epinephrine, maximal vasoconstriction occurs at 15 minutes.
7. Stretch skin surrounding lesion taut, perpendicular to relaxed skin tension lines.
8. Carefully place punch over the lesion and twist in rotary back-and-forth cutting motion until subcutaneous fat is obtained. Biopsy should include epidermis, full thickness of dermis, and some subcutaneous fat.
9. Remove punch.
10. Use blunt forceps in one hand to grasp the lateral edge of the biopsy specimen and elevate it, utilizing care to avoid crush artifact.
11. Use scalpel blade or scissors in the other hand to cut the punch specimen at its base, as deep into the subcutaneous fat tissue as possible.
12. Place specimen in container with appropriate preservative or transport medium.
13. Label container with patient name, date, and exact site of biopsy.
14. Control bleeding at site of biopsy with gentle pressure using sterile 4- × 4-inch gauze square.
15. Approximate wound margins and apply Dermabond. No further care is required.
16. If suture or Steri-Strips are placed, leave on for 5 days on face and for 12 days on trunk, limbs, or scalp.
17. Although not recommended by the author, some practitioners allow the wound to heal by secondary intention. If no suture is placed, expect healing by primary epithelialization in 7 to 14 days, with a residual white

area a few millimeters in diameter if the biopsy extended to the dermis–subcutaneous fat interface.

H. Complications (6)

1. Infection
2. Unsightly scarring or keloid formation (rare)
3. Excessive bleeding (rare, except in patient with coagulation defect)
4. Pathologic uncertainty

References

1. Fretzin D. Biopsy in vesiculobullous disorders. *Cutis*. 1977;20:639.
2. Graham J, Barr R. Papulosquamous eruptions: usefulness of biopsy in establishing diagnosis. *Cutis*. 1977;20:629.
3. Hazelrigg D, Jarratt M. Diagnosis of scabies. *South Med J*. 1975;68:549.
4. Montes L. How useful is a biopsy in a case of suspected fungal infection? *Cutis*. 1977;20:665.
5. Roses D, Ackerman A, Harris M, et al. Assessment of biopsy technique and histopathologic interpretations of primary cutaneous malignant melanoma. *Ann Surg*. 1979;189:294.
6. Solomon L, Esterly N. Diagnostic procedures. In: Solomon L, Esterly N, eds. *Neonatal Dermatology*. Philadelphia: Saunders; 1973:29.
7. Soltani K, Pacernick L, Lorincz A. Lupus erythematosus-like lesions in newborn infants. *Arch Dermatol*. 1974;110:435.
8. Thompson J, Temple W, Lafreniere R, et al. Punch biopsy for diagnosis of pigmented skin lesions. *Am Fam Physician*. 1988;37:123.
9. Carpenter S, Karpati G, Andermann F. Specific involvement of muscle, nerve and skin in late infantile and juvenile amaurotic idiocy. *Neurology*. 1972;22:170.
10. Farrell D, Sumi S. Skin punch biopsy in the diagnosis of juvenile neuronal ceroid-lipofuscinosis. *Arch Neurol*. 1977;34:39.
11. Fleisher L, Longhi R, Tallan H, et al. Homocystinuria: investigations of cystathionine synthase in cultured fetal cells and the prenatal determination of genetic status. *J Pediatr*. 1974;89:677.
12. Martin J, Ceuterick C. Morphological study of skin biopsy specimens: a contribution to the diagnosis of metabolic disorders with involvement of the nervous system. *J Neurol Neurosurg Psychiatry*. 1978;41:232.
13. Martin J, Jacobs K. Skin biopsy as a contribution to diagnosis in late infantile amaurotic idiocy with curvilinear bodies. *Eur Neurol*. 1973;10:281.
14. O'Brien J, Bernet J, Veath M, et al. Lysosomal storage disorders: diagnosis by ultrastructural examination of skin biopsy specimens. *Arch Neurol*. 1975;32:592.
15. Spicer S, Garvin A, Wohltmann H, et al. The ultrastructure of the skin in patients with mucopolysaccharidoses. *Lab Invest*. 1974;31:488.
16. Cooper JT, Goldstein S. Skin biopsy and successful fibroblast culture. *Lancet*. 1973;2:673.
17. Arndt KA. Operative procedures. In: Arndt KA, ed. *Manual of Dermatologic Therapeutics*. Boston: Little, Brown; 1978:223.
18. Kennard CD, Rasmussen JE. Congenital midline nasal masses: diagnosis and management. *J Dermatol Surg Oncol*. 1990;16;1025.
19. Baldwin HE, Berck CM, Lynfield YL. Subcutaneous nodules of the scalp: preoperative management. *J Am Acad Dermatol*. 1991;25;819.
20. Todd P, Garioch JJ, Humphreys S, et al. Evaluation of the 2-mm punch biopsy in dermatological diagnosis. *Clin Exp Dermatol*. 1996;21;11
21. Golbus M, Sagebiel R, Filly R, et al. Prenatal diagnosis of ichthyosiform erythroderma (epidermolytic hyperkeratosis) by fetal skin biopsy. *N Engl J Med*. 1980;302:93.
22. Luu M, Cantatore-Francis JL, Glick SA. Prenatal diagnoses of genodermatoses: current scope and future capabilities. *Int J Dermatol*. 2010;49:353.
23. Ackerman AB. Biopsy: why, where, when, how? *J Dermatol Surg*. 1975;1:21.
24. Ruiz-Maldonado R, Parish LC, Beare JM. Therapeutic aspects of pediatric dermatology. In: Ruiz-Maldonado R, Parish LC, Beare JM, eds. *Textbook of Pediatric Dermatology*. Philadelphia: Grune & Stratton; 1989:50.
25. Arndt KA, Burton C, Noe JM. Minimizing the pain of local anesthesia. *Plast Reconstr Surg*. 1983;72:676.
26. Stewart JH, Cole GW, Klein JA: Neutralized lidocaine with epinephrine for local anesthesia. *J Dermatol Surg Oncol*. 1989;15;1081.
27. Kuwahara RT, Skinner RB. EMLA versus ice as a topical anesthetic. *Dermatol Surg*. 2001;27;495.

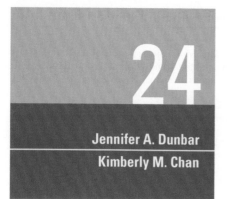

24 Ophthalmic Specimen Collection

Jennifer A. Dunbar
Kimberly M. Chan

Neonatal conjunctivitis is considered an ocular emergency (1,2). Conjunctivitis may be the presenting sign of coexisting life-threatening systemic infection. Signs include diffuse conjunctival injection with mucoid, purulent, or watery ophthalmic discharge. Both bacterial and viral pathogens cause corneal ulceration and opacity, which may lead to blindness. *Neisseria gonorrhea* or *Pseudomonas* species may rapidly perforate the globe.

A. Indications

To obtain specimen for testing to determine the cause of conjunctivitis (Table 24.1)

1. The most common cause of neonatal conjunctivitis is chemical conjunctivitis, which presents in the first 24 hours of life as a reaction to prophylaxis and usually resolves within 48 hours.
2. Infectious neonatal conjunctivitis may be bacterial or viral, and it is often associated with exposure in the birth canal or through spontaneous rupture of membranes. The causes include *Chlamydia*, *Streptococcus* spp., *Staphylococcus* spp., *Escherichia coli*, *Haemophilus* spp., *Neisseria gonorrhea*, and herpes simplex (3).
3. In addition to the classic causes of neonatal conjunctivitis above, methicillin-resistant *Staphylococcus aureus*, group B *Streptococcus* and *Neisseria meningitides* have been described in neonates (4,5).
4. Hospital-acquired conjunctivitis affects 6% to 18% of infants in neonatal intensive care units (NICUs) and may occur in epidemics (6–8).
   a. The eye may be contaminated by respiratory secretions, with coagulase-negative *Staphylococcus*, *S. aureus*, and *Klebsiella* sp. reported as the most common pathogens.
   b. Epidemics of conjunctivitis have been associated with routine ophthalmic screening in the NICU. *Serratia marcescens*, *Klebsiella* sp., *Acinetobacter baumannii*, and adenovirus epidemics have been described (8–11).

B. Relative Contraindications

Corneal epithelial defect

If fluorescein staining of the cornea reveals an epithelial staining defect, then corneal ulceration may be present. This requires referral to an ophthalmologist.

C. Special Considerations for Ophthalmic Specimen Management

1. Conjunctival scrapings are the specimen of choice because many pathogens are intraepithelial (1).
2. The ocular specimen size is small; therefore, special care is given to specimen handling.
3. Direct placement of the conjunctival scrapings on slides for staining and direct plating onto culture medium at the bedside will maximize the yield.
4. Communication with laboratory personnel regarding specimen handling improves culture results (12).

D. Materials

1. Equipment for staining the cornea to rule out epithelial defect
   a. Fluorescein dye or strips
   b. Wood lamp or other blue light source
2. Equipment for obtaining specimen
   a. Choose topical anesthetic (optional):
      (1) 0.5% preservative-free tetracaine in unit-dose containers (Alcon Laboratories, Fort Worth, Texas)
      (2) Preservative-free lidocaine (Elkins-Sinn, Cherry Hill, New Jersey)
      (3) Cocaine 4% preserved with 0.5% sodium benzoate (Schein Pharmaceuticals, Melville, New York) diluted to 1% to 2% with sterile water. A 222C DEA form must be completed to be able to order.

      Many topical ophthalmic anesthetics contain preservatives that may inhibit bacterial growth in culture. For this reason, some physicians choose to perform the procedure without anesthetic. Nevertheless, this may be quite painful for the

TABLE 24.1	Analysis of Conjunctival Scrapings	
Test	**Organisms Identified**	**Finding**
Stain		
Gram stain	*Neisseria gonorrhea*	Gram-negative diplococci
Giemsa stain	*Chlamydia trachomatis*	Intraepithelial intracytoplasmic inclusions
Papanicolaou stain	Herpes simplex virus	Multinucleate giant cells and inclusion-bearing cells
Direct antigen detection techniques		
Immunofluorescent indicator system	*Chlamydia trachomatis*	
Immunosorbent assay (ELISA)	*Chlamydia trachomatis* Herpes simplex virus	
Fluorescein-labeled monoclonal antibodies (MicroTrack)	*Chlamydia trachomatis*	
Indirect fluorescence	Herpes simplex virus	
Culture		
Thayer–Martin	*Neisseria gonorrhea*	
Aerobic	Gram-positive and gram-negative bacteria	
Anaerobic	Anaerobic bacteria	
Viral transport	Herpes simplex virus	
Chlamydia culture (McCoy culture)	*Chlamydia trachomatis*	

ELISA, enzyme-linked immunosorbent assay.

infant. The above-mentioned anesthetics are preservative-free or have been shown to minimally inhibit bacterial growth (13,14).

b. Sterile cotton swabs may be used to evert the eyelids but are not recommended for specimen collection (Fig. 24.1).

c. Choose instrument to obtain cultures.
(1) Calcium alginate swabs
(2) Sterile Dacron polyester-tipped applicator (Harwood Products Company, Guilford, Maine)
 Calcium alginate swabs have been shown to yield equal or better organism retrieval in cultures than spatulas or Dacron swabs (15,16). Moistening the swab with trypticase soy (Becton Dickenson and Company, Franklin Lakes, New Jersey) broth or other culture medium enhances results. However, spatulas have been shown to provide better samples in smear than swabs. Spatulas preserve the conjunctival epithelial cells better, thus providing better opportunity for diagnosing pathogens with intracellular organisms or inclusions (17). Calcium alginate swabs may interfere with immunoassays.

d. Choose instrument for scraping the conjunctiva.
(1) Kimura Platinum spatula E1091 (Storz Ophthalmics, Division of Bausch & Lomb, Rochester, New York) (Fig. 24.2)
(2) Nasopharyngeal swab with metal handle bent for scraping
(3) Calcium alginate swabs
 If spatulas are not available, then swabs should be used vigorously on the tarsal conjunctival surface so as to débride epithelial cells.

e. Equipment for obtaining microscope slides
(1) Frosted, etched glass slides
(2) Microslide holders
(3) Pencil or marker for labeling

E. Equipment for Identifying *Chlamydia* and Viral Agents

1. Equipment for nonculture chlamydial studies
a. The McCoy culture was considered the "gold standard" for identification of *Chlamydia*. However, cultures take several days to provide results, and specimens collected in the first few days of life may have less yield on culture because elementary bodies often take several days to form in neonates (18,19).
b. Nonculture tests listed below, such as direct immunofluorescence, enzyme-linked immunosorbent assay, and polymerase chain reaction (PCR), all perform well for ocular specimens and provide a result more rapidly. (20–24). PCR is the most sensitive nonculture test for *Chlamydia*, with the advantage of increased detection in mild disease (20–24). If PCR is not readily available, direct immunoflourescent monoclonal antibody stain antibody may be the most sensitive and rapid option (25).
(1) *For chlamydial direct fluorescence antibody stain:* MicroTrak *Chlamydia trachomatis* specimen collection kit (Trinity Biotech, Bray, County Wicklow, Ireland)
(2) *For chlamydial enzyme-linked immunosorbent assay:* Place specimen in media advised by the laboratory performing the study.

(3) *For chlamydial PCR:* Place specimen in transport medium appropriate for the assay used. An example is M4 medium for the transport of viruses and *Chlamydia* (Remel, Lenexa, Kansas).

2. Media for culture

Specimens should be plated onto culture medium at the bedside. Each laboratory will have specific media available for a particular type of organism. The following list is a suggestion of classic media used for each type of organism.

a. Bacterial culture media

(1) Trypticase soy broth

(2) Blood agar plate

(3) Chocolate agar plate for *Haemophilus influenzae, Neisseria gonorrhea*

(4) Thayer-Martin medium if gonorrhea suspected

b. Virus-holding medium (i.e., M4 medium for the transport of viruses and *Chlamydia*) (Remel, Lenexa, Kansas)

c. *Chlamydia* culture transport medium (i.e., M4 medium for the transport of viruses and *Chlamydia*) (Remel, Lenexa, Kansas)

d. Sabouraud's agar if fungal conjunctivitis suspected

F. Technique

1. Method for staining the cornea for epithelial defect

a. Instill a very small amount of fluorescein in the lower conjunctival fornix by lightly touching the tear film with a fluorescein strip. Flooding the eye with fluorescein may obscure a small corneal epithelial defect.

b. Evaluate the cornea for staining with a Wood lamp or other blue light source.

c. If a corneal epithelial defect is present, the cornea may be infected and an ophthalmologist should be consulted.

d. Herpes virus may present in the neonate as a geographic-shaped epithelial defect rather than a dendrite.

2. Method for everting eyelids

a. Upper lid (Fig. 24.1)

(1) Grasp lashes and border of lid between thumb and index finger of nondominant hand.

(2) Draw lid downward and away from eyeball.

(3) Indent upper lid, with handle of cotton-tipped applicator held in dominant hand and pull lid back and upward over applicator.

(4) Remove applicator and hold lid in place with nondominant hand by gently pressing border of lid against superior orbital margin.

b. Lower lid (Fig. 24.2)

(1) Place index finger of nondominant hand on margin of lower lid.

(2) Pull downward.

3. Method for obtaining cultures

Obtain cultures prior to conjunctival scraping. Take separate cultures from each eye with a separate sterile swab for each type of medium desired. Culture and

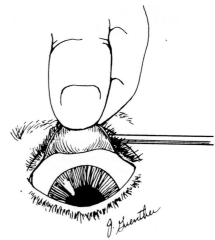

FIG. 24.1.   Everting the upper eyelid.

label each eye separately, even if only one eye is symptomatic. The uninfected eye can serve as a control for indigenous flora (9).

a. Moisten calcium alginate swabs with trypticase soy broth or other liquid culture medium.

b. Evert eyelid.

c. Apply swab to bulbar and palpebral conjunctiva of upper and lower fornices of eye.

d. Apply swab directly to culture medium plates at the bedside with a single row of C-shaped inoculation streaks. Monitoring the growth of organisms along the shape of the inoculation streaks may help the laboratory in the diagnosis of the cultured pathogen.

e. Use a separate sterile swab for each culture plate or culture vial.

f. Label cultures meticulously with eye cultured (right or left) and part of eye cultured (conjunctiva, lid margin, etc.).

g. Incubate cultures immediately.

4. Method for obtaining conjunctival scrapings for smear and nonculture *Chlamydia* tests

a. Evert eyelid as described above.

b. Instill topical anesthetic into conjunctival fornix, if desired.

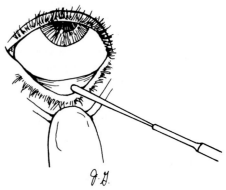

FIG. 24.2.   Using Kimura platinum spatula to take scraping from lower eyelid.

c. Swab off excess discharge.

d. Take scraping 2 mm from eye margin. (Normal keratinized epithelium from the lid margin may confound results of smear.)

e. Pass spatula two to three times in the same direction, avoiding bleeding.

f. Spread specimen from spatula gently into a monolayer on a clean glass slide and label.

g. Fix smears as required for proposed smears and non-culture *Chlamydia* tests.

h. Repeat with separate sterile spatula on second eye.

G. Interpretation of Conjunctival Cytology

1. Cellular reaction
   a. Polymorphonuclear reaction
      (1) Bacterial infections
      (2) Chlamydial infection
      (3) Very severe viral infection
   b. *Mononuclear reactions:* Viral infection
   c. *Eosinophilia and basophilia:* Allergic states
   d. *Plasma cells:* Chlamydial infection
2. Intraepithelial cell inclusions
   a. Chlamydial infection
      (1) Acidophilic inclusions in cytoplasm, capping epithelial cell nuclei
      (2) Basophilic "initial bodies" in cytoplasm
   b. Viral infection
      Giant, multinucleated epithelial cells may be seen (e.g., herpetic keratoconjunctivitis).

H. Complications of Scraping

1. Conjunctival bleeding
   a. Mild conjunctival bleeding, usually self-limiting, frequently occurs.
   b. Instill erythromycin ophthalmic ointment.
2. Corneal injury
   a. Keep the spatula blade flat against the tarsal conjunctiva at all times to avoid trauma to the cornea.
   b. Corneal injury is confirmed by a staining defect on fluorescein staining.
   c. If corneal injury occurs, instill erythromycin ophthalmic ointment and contact an ophthalmologist.
3. Transfer of infection from infected to noninfected eye
   This complication is avoided by using separate sterile instruments when taking samples from each eye.
4. Ocular irritation, pain, photophobia, lacrimation, swelling, and hyperemia
   These problems are usually mild and self-limited.

References

1. Richards A, Guzman-Cottrill JA. Conjunctivitis. *Pediatr Rev.* 2010;31:196.
2. Teoh DL, Reynolds S. Diagnosis and management of pediatric conjunctivitis. *Pediatr Emerg Care.* 2003;19:48.
3. Wright KW. Pediatric conjunctivitis. In: Wright KW, Spiegel PH, eds. *Pediatric Ophthalmology and Strabismus.* 2nd ed. New York: Springer; 2003:335.
4. Sahu DN, Thomson S, Salam A, et al. Neonatal methicillin-resistant *Staphylococcus aureus* conjunctivitis. *BJO.* 2006;90:794.
5. Pöschl JM, Hellstern G, Ruef P, et al. Ophthalmia neonatorum caused by group B *Streptococcus. Scan J Infect Dis.* 2002;34:921.
6. Haas J, Larson E, Ross B, et al. Epidemiology and diagnosis of hospital acquired conjunctivitis among neonatal intensive care unit patients. *Pediatr Infect Dis J.* 2005;24:586.
7. Brito DV, Brito CS, Resende DS, et al. Nosocomial infections in a Brazilian neonatal intensive care unit: a 4-year surveillance study. *Rev Soc Bras Med Trop.* 2010;43:633.
8. Faden H, Wynn RJ, Campagna L, et al. Outbreak of adenovirus type 30 in the neonatal intensive care unit. *J Pediatr.* 2005;146:523.
9. Casolari C, Pecorari M, Fabio G, et al. A simultaneous outbreak of *Serratia marcescens* and *Klebsiella pneumoniae* in a neonatal intensive care unit. *J Hosp Infect.* 2005;61:312.
10. Ersoy Y, Otlu B, Türkçü lu P, et al. Outbreak of adenovirus serotype 8 conjunctivitis in preterm infants in a neonatal intensive care unit. *J Hosp Infect.* 2012;80:144.
11. McGrath EJ, Chopra T, Abdel-Haq N, et al. An outbreak of carbapenem-resistant *Acinetobacter baumannii* infection in a neonatal intensive care unit: investigation and control. *Infect Control Hosp Epidemiol.* 2011;32:34.
12. Miller JM, ed. *A Guide to Specimen Management in Clinical Microbiology.* 2nd ed. Washington, DC: American Society for Microbiology Press; 1999.
13. Mullin GS, Rubinfeld RS. The antibacterial activity of topical anesthetics. *Cornea.* 1997;16:662.
14. Pelosini L, Treffene S, Hollick EJ. Antibacterial activity of preservative-free topical anesthetic drops in current use in ophthalmology departments. *Cornea.* 2009;28:58.
15. Benson WH, Lanier JD. Comparison of techniques for culturing corneal ulcers. *Ophthalmology.* 1992;99:800.
16. Jacob P, Gopinathan U, Sharma S, et al. Calcium alginate swab versus Bard Parker blade in the diagnosis of microbial keratitis. *Cornea.* 1995;14:360.
17. Rapoza PA, Johnson S, Taylor HR. Platinum spatula vs Dacron swab in the preparation of conjunctival smears [Letter]. *Am J Ophthalmol.* 1986;102:400.
18. Talley AR, Garcia-Ferrer F, Laycock KA, et al. Comparative diagnosis of neonatal chlamydial conjunctivitis by polymerase chain reaction and McCoy cell culture. *Am J Ophthalmol.* 1994;117:50.
19. Hammerschlag MR, Roblin PM, Gelling M, et al. Use of polymerase chain reaction for the detection of *Chlamydia trachomatis* in ocular and nasopharyngeal specimens from infants with conjunctivitis. *Pediatr Infect Dis J.* 1997;16:293.
20. Percivalle E, Sarasini A, Torsellini M, et al. A comparison of methods for detecting adenovirus type 8 keratoconjunctivitis during a nosocomial outbreak in a neonatal intensive care unit. *J Clin Virol.* 2003;28:257.
21. Thompson PP, Kowalski RP. A 13-year retrospective review of polymerase chain reaction testing for infectious agents from ocular samples. *Ophthalmology.* 2011;118:1449.
22. Kowalski RP, Thompson PP, Kinchington PR, et al. Evaluation of the Smart Cycler II system for real-time detection of viruses and *Chlamydia* from ocular specimens. *Arch Ophthalmol.* 2006;124:1135.
23. Chichili GR, Athmanathan S, Farhatullah S, et al. Multiplex polymerase chain reaction for the detection of herpes simplex virus, varicella-zoster virus and cytomegalovirus in ocular specimens. *Curr Eye Res.* 2003;27:85.
24. Yip PP, Chan WH, Yip KT, et al. The use of polymerase chain reaction assay versus conventional methods in detecting neonatal chlamydial conjunctivitis. *JPOS.* 2008;45:234.
25. Rapoza PA, Quinn TC, Kiessling LA, et al. Assessment of neonatal conjunctivitis with a direct immunofluorescent monoclonal antibody stain for Chlamydia. *JAMA.* 1986;24:3369.

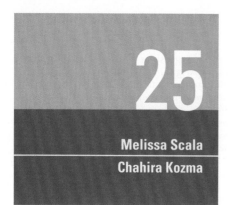

25 Perimortem Sampling

Melissa Scala

Chahira Kozma

A. Background

1. Perimortem sampling may help to establish the diagnosis in infants who die before diagnostic evaluation is completed.
2. Approximately 25% of unexplained infant deaths in the first week of life are due to undiagnosed congenital anomalies. Infectious causes may account for a third of unexplained deaths (1,2).
3. Inborn errors of metabolism are rare individually, but in the general population the incidence may be >1 in 1,000 live births (3).
4. Diagnostic testing for congenital and metabolic disorders can be time-consuming, so some infants may go undiagnosed and even die before the exact cause is elucidated.
5. Autopsy is declining worldwide. Neonatal autopsy rates fell from 80% to 50% by the year 2000 (4).
6. Many parents today question the need for autopsy in an era of sophisticated diagnostic testing. For some families, cultural or religious traditions may be barriers to autopsy consent (5).
7. Even with autopsy, perimortem evaluation may be essential, as some tests have low yield when performed more than a few hours after death (6).
8. Neonatologists and pediatricians should be prepared to independently obtain any necessary samples for diagnosis and to counsel the family regarding options for postmortem evaluation.
9. Information gathered during this period can be very important for current and future generations (7).
10. If time allows, a genetics consult can be very useful in guiding testing. If an inborn error of metabolism or genetic disease is suspected, consultation before or immediately after death is vital.

B. Indications (8,9)

1. Unknown cause of death
2. Suspected genetic disorder
3. Suspected inborn error of metabolism
4. Suspected undiagnosed infection
5. Suspected hypoxic-ischemic encephalopathy (10)

C. Discussion with the Family

1. Families of dying infants are under great strain, particularly if diagnosis is uncertain. An in-depth conversation with the family can answer any questions they may have and create a plan for perimortem sampling and for possible autopsy.
2. Informed consent may be obtained at this time for any planned photographs or procedures.

D. Clinical Information

A detailed history and exam is important, particularly if a geneticist has been unable to see the infant (3,11).

1. History
   a. *Maternal history*: Ethnicity and medical history
   b. *Previous pregnancy history*: Stillbirths or pregnancy losses
   c. History of this pregnancy, including
      (1) Exposure to teratogens
      (2) Amniotic fluid volume
      (3) Results of amniocentesis and ultrasound
      (4) Maternal illness
      (5) Fetal movements
   d. Family history including three-generation pedigree (Table 25.1) (11).
   e. *Infant history*: Report medical course for this infant including diagnoses, treatments, and lab results
2. Physical exam
   a. Should be detailed and performed by specialist in genetic metabolic disorders if possible
   b. Important components include
      (1) Growth parameters
      (2) Hair pattern
      (3) Facial features including eye and ear placement
      (4) Abnormalities of hands and feet
      (5) Genital and rectal exam
      (6) Neurologic findings
      (7) Skin abnormalities

TABLE 25.1	Key Elements of Family History

Gender of each individual using standard pedigree symbols
Male relatives on the maternal side when considering X-linked recessive
 disorder
Consanguinity
Miscarriage and stillbirths
Ethnic origin of family

c. Further resources to guide physical exam are available online from the Wisconsin Stillbirth Service at http://www2.marshfieldclinic.org/wissp/ and from the Perinatal Society of Australia and New Zealand at www.psanz.com.au/special-interest-groups/pnm.aspx.

E. Photographs

1. Digital photographs are the best, but any image is better than none.
2. Use of a blue background allows better definition of findings. Sterile towels or drapes can be used for this purpose.
3. Separate or duplicate copies of photographs should be obtained for diagnostic and bereavement purposes. Full face, body, and profile pictures should be taken (Table 25.2) (12).
4. Every effort should be made to photograph any abnormalities seen on physical examination.

F. Examination of the Placenta

1. Ensure that the placenta is sent for pathology examination for all infants admitted to the neonatal intensive care unit (13).
2. Placental findings are positive in 30% to 60% of neonatal autopsies (14).
3. Evaluation of the placenta may reveal maternal or fetal vascular problems, in utero infections, inflammatory conditions and some inborn errors of metabolism. Cultures for bacteria and fungus as well as viral polymerase chain reactions may be sent as applicable. A discussion with pathology can guide the evaluation (13).

TABLE 25.2	Photographic Format

Whole body
Face: Flat and profile
Right and left ear
Right and left hand: Dorsum and palm
Right and left foot: Dorsum and sole
Palate
Genitalia
Special view of any other abnormality

G. Perimortem Sampling

1. General guidelines
   a. Sterile technique should be used for all procedures, even if they are performed postmortem.
   b. Contact the laboratory to save any unused blood, fluid or tissue samples. (Table 25.3 summarizes sample handling) (1,3,8,11).
   c. If a metabolic disorder is a possibility, tissue samples should be taken within 4 to 6 hours of death.
   d. Resources to guide molecular testing as indicated can be found at http://www.ncbi.nlm.nih.gov/sites/GeneTests/clinic, a voluntary listing of US and international genetics clinics providing genetic evaluation and genetic counseling.
2. Blood
   a. Draw percutaneously or directly from heart (after parental consent) if infant has expired. See Table 25.3 for samples required (1,6).
   b. Be sure newborn screen sample has been sent (15).
   c. Obtain additional dried blood spots on filter paper.
3. Urine
   5 to 10 mL by catheterization or suprapubic tap (8).
4. Cerebrospinal fluid
   Obtain at least 1 mL of cerebrospinal fluid; may be obtained after death by needle insertion through anterior fontanelle (16).
5. Skin sample
   a. Normal skin samples may be sent for fibroblast culture (17).
   b. Any skin lesions should also be biopsied.
   c. Do not use iodine-containing preparations, since cell growth may be impaired.
   d. Best collected within 4 to 12 hours of death. Skin biopsy up to 2 to 3 days postmortem may still provide a viable culture.
   e. Place in viral transport media. If unavailable may use normal saline or saline soaked gauze.
   f. 3- × 2-mm punch or scalpel biopsies can be taken from forearm or anterior thigh (18).
   g. Samples may be kept at room temperature or refrigerated.
   h. Cells can be cultured and archived in liquid nitrogen for many years and still be successfully recovered for analysis.
6. Liver
   a. Obtain if hepatic disease was present or for suspected metabolic disease (19,20).
   b. Collect as soon as possible after death, preferably within 2 to 4 hours.
   c. Tissue may be obtained via open wedge biopsy or percutaneous needle biopsy.
      (1) *Wedge biopsy*: Locate the right costal margin. Make a 2-cm incision just below and incise

TABLE 25.3	Processing of Fluid and Tissue Samples Obtained by Perimortem Sampling			

Tissue Type	Testing	Sample Collection and Handling	Storage
Blood	Inborn errors of metabolism	Newborn screen paper	Room temperature
	Inborn errors of metabolism	Dried spots on filter paper	Room temperature
			No plastic bag
	DNA extraction	5 mL in EDTA tube	Refrigerate at 4°C
			Do not freeze
	Chromosome analysis	5 mL in lithium heparin tube	Keep cool or at room temperature
	Microarray analysis		Do not freeze.
	Quantitative amino acids	5 mL in lithium heparin tube,	Freeze and store at –70°C
	Fatty acids	separate within 20 min	
	Carnitine		
Urine	Organic acids	5–10 mL	Freeze and store at –70°C
	Amino acids		
	Orotic acid		
	Acylglycines		
CSF	Amino acids	1+ mL	Freeze and store at –70°C
Skin	Fibroblast culture	Viral transport media	Keep cool or at room temperature
	• Chromosome analysis		Do not freeze
	• Genetic mutations		
	• Enzyme analysis		
Liver (3 pieces)	Histopathology	5-mm cube each sample	Freeze and store at –80°C
	Enzymology		
	Electron microscopy		
Muscle (3 pieces)	Light microscopy	Wrap in moist saline soaked gauze;	Keep cool (4°C) but do not freeze
		do not immerse in saline	
	Enzyme analysis	Store in available container	Snap freeze in liquid nitrogen and store at –80°C
	Electron microscopy	Place in container with formalin	Room temperature
		or glutaraldehyde	
Other as needed by infant's clinical presentation		Consult geneticist or pathologist	As instructed

EDTA, ethylenediaminetetraacetic acid.

section of right lobe of liver. The sample should be cut into 5-mm cubes.

(2) Percutaneous biopsy (21)

Several needles are available (16 or 18 gauge)

(a) Aspiration or suction needles (Jamshidi, Klatskin, and Menghini)

(b) Cutting type needles (Tru-Cut and Vim-Silverman)

(c) Spring loaded devices

d. Procedure

(i) Make a small (0.25- to 0.5-cm) incision in the right anterior to midaxillary line at the 9th or 10th rib.

(ii) Flush the needle with saline.

(iii) Insert the needle parallel to the bed surface and advance toward the opposite shoulder.

(iv) The needle is advanced 2 to 3 cm into the liver and suction applied, pulling a segment of liver into the needle. Spring-loaded needles do not need suction applied.

7. Muscle

a. Collect if mitochondrial disorder or muscular dystrophy suspected (19,22). Surgeon or neurologist may be more adept at obtaining sample.

b. Collect within 2 to 3 hours of death.

c. Procedure

(1) Make a 2- to 3-cm incision over mid quadriceps.

(2) Muscle clamps are not required but may be used for ease of sample removal.

(3) Excise three 2- by 0.5-cm sections of muscle if possible.

(4) Process the samples as indicated in Table 25.3.

(5) If incisional biopsy is not possible, three cores of quadriceps muscle should be obtained using a percutaneous biopsy needle.

Other tissues may be sampled if specific related diagnoses are being considered. Some metabolic specialists have suggested collecting vitreous fluid for organic acids and bile for acylcarnitines.

Conversation with a genetic or metabolic expert may guide collection of these fluids (6,8,20).

H. Imaging: May be used alone or in conjunction with autopsy

1. X-rays
   a. Important, especially in diagnosing skeletal dysplasia.
   b. Include an anteroposterior and lateral of skull, whole spine, long bones, pelvis, and images of hands and feet (23).
2. MRI
   a. Images of the neonatal brain are very useful and may provide information that is missed on autopsy in some cases (5,23).

I. Autopsy

1. Full autopsy (preferred)
   a. Provides the most complete picture of the infant and has been found to contribute useful information in 40% to 60% cases (2,4,23,24).
   b. Complete inspection of the neonatal brain requires 2 weeks' fixation prior to examination. This may mean that the burial is postponed or that the infant's body is buried without the brain.
2. *Limited examination:* If parents are reluctant to consent to a full autopsy, several choices exist.
   a. *Full autopsy except examination of brain:* This allows the brain to be buried with the body. Postmortem imaging of the brain with MRI may provide useful information on this organ.
   b. *Limited autopsy:* Examination is limited to certain organs or areas of the body. This can also be coupled with imaging for some families.
   c. *Imaging only (MRI and/or x-rays):* A wide range of sensitivities and specificities have been reported. Initial reports were promising, with 90% to 100% sensitivity and specificity in diagnosis with whole-body MRI. Recent studies have shown lower rates of concordance between MRI and autopsy of 30% to 60% (5,25).
   d. Perimortem or postmortem sampling of body tissues and fluids only or in combination with any of the above (26).
3. Consult with pathologist before obtaining consent for limited autopsy so that examination is best directed at questions to be answered.

J. Postmortem Family Conference

1. After results are available from perimortem sampling evaluation and reports generated from autopsy and radiological testing, a conference should be scheduled with the family.
2. The conference has many purposes (6,27)
   a. To give an overview of findings
   b. Explain ramifications for future pregnancies and generations
   c. Allay feelings of guilt parents may have regarding the cause of death
   d. Answer questions regarding decisions made by the medical team
   e. Confirm or dispel allegations of abuse or neglect
   f. Provide emotional support to families
3. The conference should be led by an experienced physician with great sensitivity and communication skills. He or she should be familiar with the case and have a complete understanding of case results and their implications. Nurses, therapists, social workers, and other physicians who are important to the infant's care team may also be present.
4. The meeting should be unhurried, with adequate time available for all the family's questions to be answered.
5. A written report summarizing the results of the meeting and written in language understandable to the family should be provided. A copy of the report should be sent to the family's primary care physician after obtaining appropriate consent from the family.
6. Bereavement photographs of the infant can be given at this time or at an earlier time if possible.

References

1. Christodoulou J, Wilcken B. Perimortem laboratory investigation of genetic metabolic disorders. *Semin Neonatol.* 2004;9:275.
2. Weber M, Ashworth M, Risdon RA. Sudden unexpected neonatal death in the first week of life: Autopsy findings from a specialist center. *J Matern Fetal Neonatal Med.* 2009;22:398.
3. Champion MP. An approach to the diagnosis of inherited metabolic disease. *Arch Dis Child Educ Pract Ed.* 2010;95:40.
4. Laing I. Clinical aspects of neonatal death and autopsy. *Semin Neonatol.* 2004;9:247.
5. Thayyil S. Less invasive autopsy: an evidenced based approach. *Arch Dis Child.* 2011;96:681.
6. Ernst L, Sondheimer N, Deardorff M, et al. The value of the metabolic autopsy in the pediatric hospital setting. *J Pediatr.* 2006;148:779.
7. Cernach M, Patricio F, Galera M, et al. Evaluation of a protocol for postmortem examination of stillbirths and neonatal deaths with congenital anomalies. *Pediatr Dev Pathol.* 2004;7:335.
8. Olpin S. The metabolic investigation of sudden infant death. *Ann Clin Biochem.* 2004;41:282.
9. Chace D, Kalas T, Naylor E. Use of tandem mass spectrometry for multianalyte screening of dried blood specimens from newborns. *Clin Chem.* 2003;49:1797.
10. Enns G. Inborn errors of metabolism masquerading as hypoxic-ischemic encephalopathy. *Neoreviews.* 2005;6:e549.
11. Jorde L, Carey J, Bamshad M. *Medical Genetics.* Philadelphia: Mosby/Elsevier; 2010.
12. Pitt DB, Bankier A, Skoroplas T, et al. The role of photography in syndrome identification. *J Clin Dysmorphol.* 1984;2:2.
13. Roberts DJ, Oliva E. Clinical significance of placental examination in perinatal medicine. *J Matern Fetal Neonatal Med.* 2006;19:255.

14. Wainwright HC. My approach to performing a perinatal or neonatal autopsy. *J Clin Pathol.* 2006;59:673.

15. Kayton A. Newborn screening: a literature review. *Neonatal Netw.* 2007;26:85.

16. Hoffmann GF, Surtees RAH, Wevers RA. Cerebrospinal fluid investigations for neurometabolic disorders. *Neuropediatrics.* 1998;29:59.

17. Lundemose JB, Kolvraa S, Gregerson N, et al. Fatty acid oxidation disorders as primary cause of sudden and unexpected death in infants and young children: an investigation performed on cultured fibroblasts from 79 children who died aged between 0–4 years. *J Clin Pathol: Mol Pathol.* 1997;50:212.

18. Alguire P, Mathes B. Skin biopsy techniques for the internist. *J Gen Intern Med.* 1998;13:46.

19. Wong LC, Scaglia F, Graham BH, et al. Current molecular diagnostic algorithm for mitochondrial disorders. *Mol Genet Metab.* 2010;100:111.

20. Rinaldo P, Yoon HR, Yu C, et al. Sudden and unexpected neonatal death: a protocol for the postmortem diagnosis of fatty acid oxidation disorders. *Semin Perinatol.* 1999;23:204.

21. Al Knawy B, Shiffman M. Percutaneous liver biopsy in clinical practice. *Liver Int.* 2007;27:1166.

22. Kawashima H, Ishii C, Yamanaka G, et al. Myopathy and neurogenic muscular atrophy in unexpected cardiopulmonary arrest. *Pediatr Int.* 2011;53:159.

23. Pinar H. Postmortem findings in term neonates. *Semin Neonatol.* 2004;9:289.

24. Costa S. Diagnosis and cause of death in a neonatal intensive care unit-How important is autopsy? *J Matern Fetal Neonatal Med.* 2011;24:760.

25. Huisman T. Magnetic resonance imaging: an alternative to autopsy in neonatal death? *Semin Neonatol.* 2004;9:347.

26. Putman MA. Perinatal, perimortem and postmortem examination, obligations and considerations for perinatal, neonatal and pediatric clinicians. *Adv Neonatal Care.* 2007;7:281.

27. McHaffie HE. Follow up care of bereaved parents after treatment withdrawal from newborns. *Arch Dis Child Fetal Neonat Ed.* 2001;84:F125.

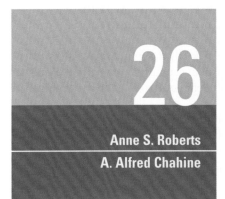

26

Abdominal Paracentesis

Anne S. Roberts

A. Alfred Chahine

A. Indications

1. **Therapeutic:** To reduce intraabdominal pressure in patients with massive ascites causing cardiorespiratory compromise
2. **Diagnostic:** To aid in determining the etiology of neonatal ascites and/or peritonitis
   a. **Necrotizing enterocolitis with suspicion of gangrene or perforation:** Presence of fecal matter or bacteria and white blood cells on a smear (1–3)
   b. **Hepatic ascites:** Comparison of serum and ascitic albumin levels, cell count, and culture in diagnosis of spontaneous bacterial peritonitis (4,5)
   c. **Chylous ascites:** Testing for triglycerides, cholesterol, and lymphocytes on cell count of the fluid (3,5)
   d. **Urinary ascites:** Test for creatinine content (6)
   e. **Meconium peritonitis:** Gross appearance of ascites (7)
   f. **Biliary ascites:** Test for bilirubin level
   g. **Pancreatic ascites:** Test for amylase, lipase levels (8)
   h. **Congenital infections (cytomegalovirus, tuberculosis, toxoplasmosis, syphilis):** Test for inclusion bodies, treponemes (5,9)
   i. **Inborn errors of metabolism (sialic acid storage disorders):** Test for vacuolated lymphocytes and free sialic acid (10)
   j. **Iatrogenic ascites from extravasation of fluid from central venous catheters:** Test for glucose content

B. Contraindications

Coagulopathy is a relative contraindication; the procedure may be performed with concomitant treatment of thrombocytopenia or coagulopathy, though controversy exists over whether administration of blood products is necessary (4,11).

C. Equipment

1. 24- or 25-gauge catheter over a needle (e.g., Angiocath)
2. 5- or 10-mL syringe

3. Skin topical disinfectant (e.g., povidone–iodine, chlorhexidine)
4. Sterile towels
5. Sterile gloves
6. Extension tubing
7. Three-way stopcock
8. Collection tubes and specimen containers for fluid analysis
   Cell count and differential, culture, Gram stain, acid-fast bacillus smear, cytology, total protein, albumin, glucose, lactate dehydrogenase, amylase, bilirubin, creatinine, blood urea nitrogen, electrolytes, specific gravity, pH, cholesterol, triglycerides
9. Tuberculin syringe
10. Lidocaine (1%)
11. Dressing supplies

D. Technique

1. Obtain appropriate informed consent and time out prior to procedure. Patient should be on cardiorespiratory monitor and have appropriate temperature support (Chapter 3).
2. Place a soft support ("bump") is placed under the supine neonate's left flank to allow as much of the fluid to drain into a dependent position and allow the intestines to float away from the right lower quadrant (Fig. 26.1).
3. Prepare the right lower quadrant with the disinfecting solution and drape with sterile towels.
4. Select a point between the umbilicus and the anterior superior iliac spine one third of the way from the anterior superior iliac spine. Avoid the midline to minimize risk to the bladder and a patent umbilical vein, and avoid previous surgical scars to minimize risk of bowel injury. An infraumbilical position avoids the liver and spleen.
5. Infiltrate the skin, muscles, and peritoneum with local anesthetic using the tuberculin syringe.
6. Connect the 10-mL syringe to the 24-gauge catheter and needle.
7. Direct the catheter toward the back at a 45-degree angle (Fig. 26.2). The nondominant hand may be used to

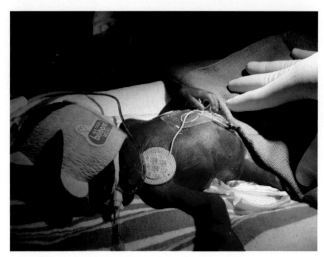

FIG. 26.1. Appropriate position and disinfection of abdomen prior to performing paracentesis in preterm neonate.

retract the skin in a downward direction while advancing the needle to create a Z-track after removal of the needle and catheter.

8. Push the catheter and needle through the skin, muscles, and peritoneal surface while applying gentle suction on the syringe plunger.

9. When a sudden decrease in resistance is felt and peritoneal fluid is aspirated, withdraw the needle and advance the catheter.

10. Connect an extension tube with a three-way stopcock to the syringe and apply gentle, intermittent suction to aspirate as much fluid as possible.

11. If fluid is not free-flowing, the catheter might be inside the intestinal lumen or in the retroperitoneum. Withdraw the catheter, and repeat the maneuver with

the catheter at a slightly different angle. Alternatively, reposition the patient carefully to maintain the catheter site in the dependent position to continue fluid aspiration.

12. When the fluid stops flowing, withdraw the catheter.

13. Distribute the fluid into the various tubes and cups for the appropriate studies.

14. Apply a bandage, holding pressure until leaking has stopped.

E. Complications

1. **Bleeding from the liver or intra-abdominal vessels:** May be severe enough to require a laparotomy

2. **Intestinal perforation:** May lead to abdominal sepsis; however, it is more commonly inconsequential because the catheter and needle are of small diameter. Risk may be reduced with nasogastric or rectal tube decompression if intestinal distension is significant prior to procedure.

3. **Hypotension:** May be due to sudden large fluid shifts during therapeutic paracentesis. Patients should be placed on a monitor during the procedure, and fluid should be withdrawn slowly.

4. **Hematoma:** Take care to avoid the inferior epigastric vessels.

5. **Scrotal or labial edema:** Due to tracking of fluid between layers of the abdominal wall

6. **Persistent ascitic fluid leak:** May require suture closure or bag drainage to prevent skin maceration

References

1. Ricketts RR. The role of paracentesis in the management of infants with necrotizing enterocolitis. *Am Surg.* 1986;52(2):61.

2. Rees CM, Eaton S, Pierro A. National prospective surveillance study of necrotizing enterocolitis in neonatal intensive care units. *J Pediatr Surg.* 2010;45:1391.

3. Sabri M, Saps M, Peters JM. Pathophysiology and management of pediatric ascites. *Curr Gastroenterol Rep.* 2003;5:240.

4. Vieira SMG, Matte U, Kieling CO, et al. Infected and noninfected ascites in pediatric patients. *J Pediatr Gastroentrol Nutr.* 2005;40(3):289.

5. Fitzgerald JF. Ascites. In: Wyllie R, Hyams JS, ed. *Pediatric Gastrointestinal Disease: Pathophysiology, Diagnosis, Management.* 1st ed. Philadelphia: WB Saunders; 1993:1510.

6. Oei J, Garvey PA, Rosenberg AR. The diagnosis and management of neonatal urinary ascites. *J Paediatr Child Health.* 2001;37(5):513.

7. Shyu MK, Shih JC, Lee CN, et al. Correlation of prenatal ultrasound and postnatal outcome in meconium peritonitis. *Fetal Diagn Ther.* 2003;18(4):255.

8. Saps M, Slivka A, Khan S, et al. Pancreatic ascites in an infant: Lack of symptoms and normal amylase. *Dig Dis Sci.* 2003;48(9):1701.

9. Nicol KK, Geisinger KR. Congenital toxoplasmosis: diagnosis by exfoliative cytology. *Diagn Cytopathol.* 1998;18:357.

10. Lemyre E, Russo P, Melancon SB, et al. Clinical spectrum of infantile free sialic acid storage disease. *Am J Med Genet.* 1999;82:385.

11. Grabau CM, Crago SF, Hoff LK, et al. Performance standards for therapeutic abdominal paracentesis. *Hepatology.* 2004;40:484.

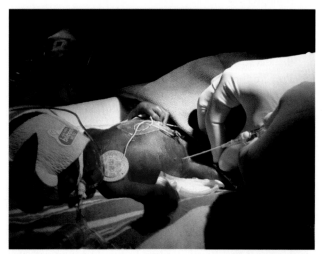

FIG. 26.2. Entry site and direction of needle for abdominal paracentesis in preterm neonate.

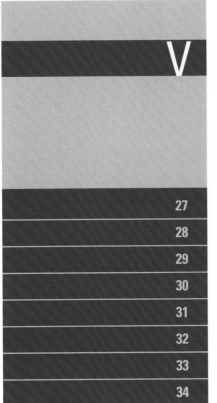

V Vascular Access

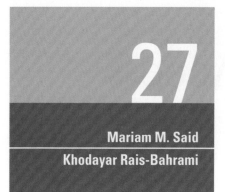

27

Mariam M. Said

Khodayar Rais-Bahrami

Peripheral Intravenous Line Placement

Percutaneous Method

A. Indications

1. Administration of IV medications, fluids, or parenteral nutrition when utilization of the gastrointestinal tract is not possible

B. Equipment

Since the late 1960s, the variety of equipment available for peripheral vascular access has grown from metallic needles of limited size range and stiff polyethylene tubes, to an array of plastic cannulas, single- and multilumen catheters of different sizes and materials, and totally implantable devices (ports). The safest and more effective vascular access is obtained by carefully matching the neonate's size, therapeutic needs, and the duration of required treatment with the most appropriate device and technique. Placement of peripheral IV lines is described in this chapter. Placement of central venous lines (excluding ports, which are not used routinely in neonates) is described in Chapter 32.

Sterile (Fig. 27.1)

1. Povidone–iodine swabs or 70% alcohol swabs (or other antiseptic; see Chapter 5)
2. Appropriate needle (minimum 24 gauge for blood transfusion)
   a. 21- to 24-gauge IV catheter (preferably shielded)
3. Connection for cannula (i.e., T connector)
4. 2- × 2-inch gauze squares
5. Isotonic saline in 3-mL syringe
6. Heparinized flush solution (heparin 0.5 to 1 U/mL normal saline) for heparin lock

Nonsterile

1. Tourniquet
2. Procedure light
3. Materials for restraint (see Chapter 4)
4. Transilluminator (optional, see Chapter 13)
5. Warm compress to warm limb if necessary (heel warmer)
6. Appropriate-sized arm board

7. Cotton balls
8. Scissors
9. Roll of 0.5- to 1-inch porous adhesive tape, transparent tape, or semipermeable transparent dressings (1–5)
   a. If using tape, use the minimum amount necessary on fragile premature skin, and consider using a pectin barrier (DuoDERM, ConvaTec/Bristol-Myers Squibb, Princeton, New Jersey; HolliHesive, Hollister, Libertyville, Illinois).
   b. Transparent tape or dressing will facilitate observation of IV site (Tegaderm, 3M Health Care, St. Paul, Minnesota).
   c. Precut self-adhesive taping devices are available from Veni-Gard Jr. (ConMed IV Site Care Products, Utica, New York).
10. Pacifier, if appropriate. Sucking releases endorphins, which decrease pain. Consider tightly swaddling the baby, leaving the limb needed for IV placement exposed. Swaddling is also a comfort measure (see Chapter 4). In additional, oral sucrose is frequently used as a nonpharmacological intervention for procedural pain relief in neonates (6). Some critically ill infants, such as those with persistent pulmonary hypertension, may require pain medication, sedation, and/or paralysis prior to any invasive procedure, including IV line placement.

C. Precautions

1. Avoid areas adjacent to superficial skin loss or infection.
2. Avoid vessels across joints, because immobilization is more difficult.
3. Take care to differentiate veins from arteries.
   a. Palpate for arterial pulsation.
   b. Note effect of vessel occlusion.
      (1) *Limb vessel:* Arteries collapse, veins fill
      (2) *Scalp vessel:* Arteries fill from below, veins fill from above
   c. Note color of blood obtained (arterial blood is bright red; venous blood is darker).
   d. Look for blanching of skin over vessel when fluid is infused (arterial spasm).

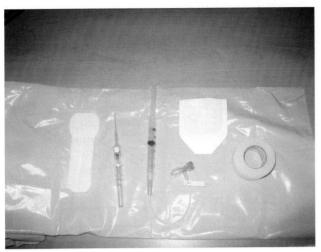

FIG. 27.1. Sterile equipment necessary for peripheral IV line placement.

4. If limb requires warming prior to procedure, use a heel warmer (Warm Gel, Prism Technologies, San Antonio, Texas). "Homemade" compresses such as a diaper soaked in hot water can cause severe thermal injury.

5. Cut scalp hair using small scissors to allow for stabilization of the IV (do not shave the area) (see Chapter 5).

6. Apply tourniquet correctly (see Fig. 14.3).
   a. Minimize time applied.
   b. Avoid use in areas with compromised circulation.
   c. Avoid use for scalp vessels.

7. When using scalp veins, avoid sites outside the hairline.

8. Be alert for signs of phlebitis or infiltration.
   a. Inspect site hourly.
   b. Discontinue IV immediately at any sign of local inflammation or cannula malfunction.
   c. Long plastic catheters are not recommended for use in neonates because their relative rigidity increases the risk of damage to the vascular endothelium, thus increasing the possibility of venous thrombosis (7).

9. Arrange tape dressing at IV site to allow adequate inspection or use transparent sterile dressing over site of skin entry (8).
   Leibovici (9) was unable to show a positive effect of a daily change of the dressing, as compared with a change every 72 hours, on the incidence of infusion phlebitis. Maki and Ringer (3) recommended not removing the transparent dressing until the catheter/needle is removed.

10. Consider using protective skin preparation in small premature infants to prevent skin trauma upon removal of tape or dressing. No Sting Barrier Film (3M Health Care, St. Paul, Minnesota) is a non–alcohol-containing product that is available commercially; however, it, as well as other commercially available skin protectants, has not been tested on neonates.
    a. Forms a tough, protective coating that bonds to skin
    b. Does not require removal when changing dressing

11. The use of tincture of benzoin and other products to increase the adherence of tape should be limited, especially on the premature infant. These products create a tighter bond between the tape and the epidermis than the bond between the epidermis and the underlying dermis. This then causes stripping of the epidermis when the tape is removed. Using a protective skin preparation (e.g., No Sting Barrier Film) prior to the application of these products may decrease damage to the skin when tape is removed (10).

12. Write date, time, and needle/cannula size on piece of tape secured to site.

13. Loop IV tubing and tape onto extremity to take tension off the IV device.

14. Limit to two to three placement attempts per person. Monitor carefully for clinical decompensation, particularly in the very premature infant and in infants with cardiac or respiratory compromise.

D. Technique

Prepare as for minor procedure (see Chapter 5). Ensure that neutral thermal environment is maintained. It is often necessary to transfer small infants to a radiant warmer for peripheral IV placement to avoid cold stress. If the infant has received a recent enteral feeding, consider delaying the procedure until before the next feeding or placing a naso- or orogastric tube to empty the stomach to prevent aspiration.

1. Use transillumination to visualize vessel if needed (see Chapter 13). Other modalities such as ultrasonography (11,12) or bedside near-infrared light devices (13) may also be used for vein identification.

2. Select vessel for cannulation. It is recommended to begin with more distal sites and progress proximally if needed. The following is the suggested order of preference (see Fig. 14.1):
   a. Back of hand—dorsal venous plexus
   b. Foot—dorsal venous plexus
   c. Ankle—small saphenous, great saphenous veins
   d. Forearm—median antebrachial, accessory cephalic veins
   e. Antecubital fossa—basilic or cubital veins
   f. Scalp veins—supratrochlear, superficial temporal, posterior auricular

3. Cut hair with small scissors close to scalp if using scalp vessels.

4. Warm limb with heel warmer for approximately 5 minutes, if necessary.

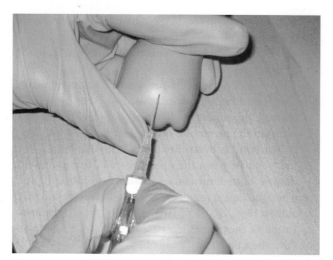

FIG. 27.2. Simulated procedure showing IV needle held in dominant hand, while index finger and thumb of nondominant hand are used to anchor vein and stretch overlying skin.

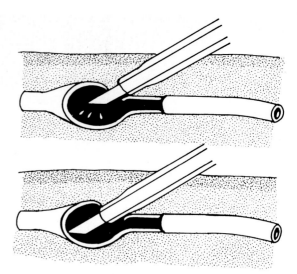

FIG. 27.3. Injecting a small amount of flush solution will distend wall of vein and facilitate cannulation. (Redrawn from Filston HC, Johnson DG. Percutaneous venous cannulation in neonates: a method for catheter insertion without "cutdown." *Pediatrics.* 1971;48:896, with permission of American Academy of Pediatrics.)

5. Apply tourniquet if anatomic site indicates.
   a. Place as close to venipuncture site as possible.
   b. Tighten until peripheral pulsation stops.
   c. Release partially until arterial pulse is fully palpable.
6. Prepare skin area with antiseptic. Allow to dry.

   In the United States, povidone–iodine solution and isopropyl alcohol are the most commonly used skin disinfectant solutions. Povidone–iodine has been shown to have greater efficacy than isopropyl alcohol and, in addition, is less damaging to skin tissue. Povidone–iodine solution should be applied to the proposed insertion site and allowed to dry for at least 30 seconds. It should then be removed with sterile saline or sterile water. The importance of removing the povidone–iodine solution cannot be overstressed, as there have been reports of burns, elevated iodine levels, and hypothyroidism in premature infants caused by prolonged contact and further absorption (10).
7. Select straight segment of vein or confluence of two tributaries.
8. Grasp catheter between thumb and first finger. For winged Angiocaths, grasp plastic wings (Fig. 27.2).
9. Anchor vein with index finger of free hand and stretch skin overlying it. This maneuver may also be used to produce distention of scalp veins.
10. Hold needle parallel to vessel, in direction of blood flow.
11. Introduce needle through skin a few millimeters distal to point of entry into vessel (see Chapter 14).
12. Introduce needle gently into vessel until blood appears in hub of needle or in cannula upon withdrawal of stylet.

    When using a very small vessel or in an infant with poor peripheral circulation, blood may not appear immediately in tubing. Wait. If in doubt, inject a small amount of saline after releasing tourniquet.

13. Remove stylet. Do not advance needle farther, because the back wall of the vessel may be pierced.
14. Advance cannula as far as possible.

    Injecting a small amount of blood or flush solution into the vein prior to advancing the cannula may assist cannulation (Fig. 27.3) (14).
15. Remove tourniquet.
16. Connect T connecter and syringe, and infuse small amount of saline gently to confirm intravascular position.
17. Anchor needle or cannula as shown in Fig. 27.4
18. Attach IV tubing and secure to skin.
19. If an armboard is necessary for securing site, place the affected extremity in an anatomically correct position before taping. Consider placing cotton or a 2- × 2-inch gauze square beneath the hub of T connector to prevent a pressure injury.

E. Complications (15–17)

1. *Hematoma:* The most common but not usually significant complication. Hematomas can often be managed with gentle manual pressure.
2. Phlebitis (18,19)

   Phlebitis remains the most common significant complication associated with the use of peripheral venous catheters. When phlebitis does occur, the risk of local catheter-related infection may be increased (19). The use of heparinized solution to prolong patency of peripheral IV catheters in neonates is controversial (20). The catheter material, catheter size, and tonicity of the infusate also influence the incidence of phlebitis.

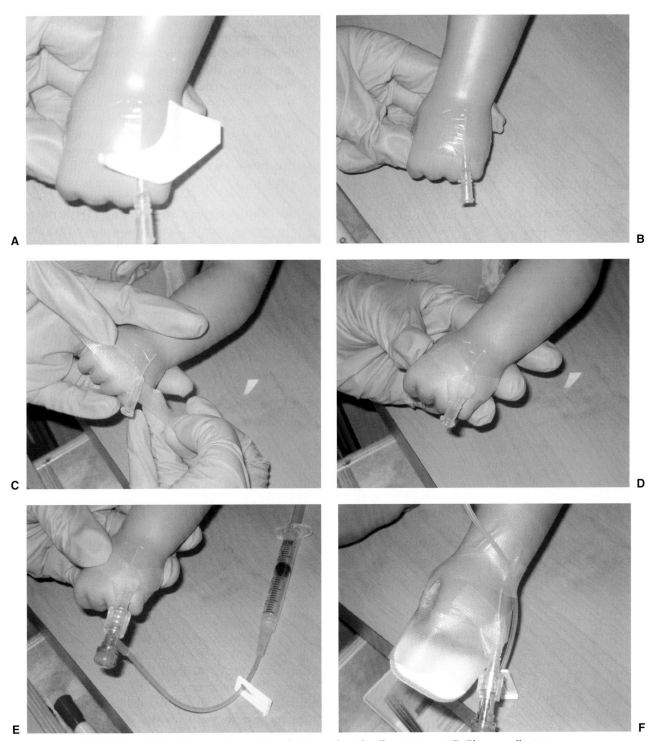

FIG. 27.4. Method for securing peripheral IV cannula with adhesive tape. **A, B:** Place an adhesive transparent tape over the cannula. **C:** Place tape 1 behind cannula as shown, with adhesive side up. **D, E:** Fold tape 1 anteriorly across the catheter–hub junction. **F:** Hold in place with tapes 2 and 3. The area of skin entry can be dressed with semipermeable sterile transparent dressing. Avoid obscuring with opaque dressing.

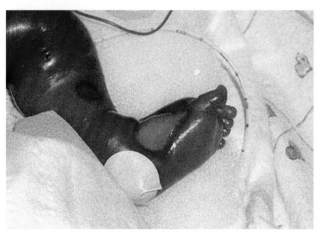

FIG. 27.5.   Result of infusion of lidocaine into subcutaneous tissues of lower limb.

When peripheral lines are used for parenteral nutrition, the coinfusion of a lipid solution with the hyperosmolar total parenteral nutrition solution prolongs the life of the vein (21,22).

3. Infiltration of subcutaneous tissue with IV solution. (For management of this complication, see Chapter 28.) Unfortunately, this is a common complication of peripheral IV infusion. Extreme vigilance and avoidance of hyperosmolar IV solutions will help to reduce the incidence to the minimum possible.
   a. Superficial blistering (Fig. 27.5)
   b. Deep slough, which may require skin graft (Fig. 27.6)
   c. Calcification of subcutaneous tissue due to infiltration of calcium-containing solution
      Note that there may be some extravasation into adjacent tissues even though blood can be aspirated from the needle/cannula.
4. Infection (23–25)

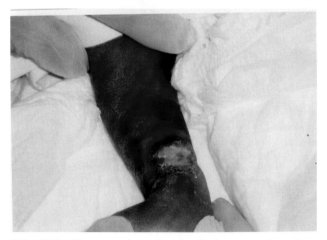

FIG. 27.6.   Extensive deep skin slough that required grafting, caused by IV infiltration.

There is an increase in the incidence of both phlebitis and infection when a needle remains in place longer than 72 hours (8) and is heavily manipulated (25). An increase has also been reported with film-type dressings, but this remains controversial (1–5,19). Catheters made with Teflon or polyurethane appear to be associated with fewer infections in adults than catheters made with polyvinyl chloride or polyethylene (19). Polyurethane catheters appear to have an approximately 30% lower risk of phlebitis than Teflon catheters in adults (19). Batton et al. (18) failed to confirm a difference in the incidence of infection when 25-gauge needles were compared with 24-gauge Teflon cannulas. However, the Teflon cannulas remained functional three times as long as steel needles, with no apparent increase in complications.

5. Embolization of clot with forcible flushing
6. Hypernatremia, fluid overload, or heparinization of the infant due to improper flushing technique or solution; also electrolyte derangements from IV fluid infused at an incorrect rate
7. Accidental injection or infusion into artery, with arteriospasm and possible tissue necrosis (Fig. 27.7)
8. Burn from
   a. Transilluminator (Fig. 27.8; also see Chapter 13)
   b. Compress used to warm limb prior to procedure
   c. Prolonged povidone–iodine or isopropyl alcohol application to very premature skin
9. Air embolus
10. Ischemia or gangrene of lower extremity, complicating infusion into saphenous vein; mechanism unclear (25)

Cutdown Placement of IV Catheter in the Great Saphenous Vein

Modern vascular access catheters and techniques have made the traditional cutdown largely obsolete. However, this means of IV access is occasionally required in emergency situations, particularly shock, when time is of the essence. The saphenous vein at the ankle is the safest, quickest site for the physician with limited surgical experience. Intraosseous vascular access is an alternative method of obtaining IV access in an emergency and is described in Chapter 50. The method described has the advantage of avoiding incision of the vessel prior to introduction of the catheter. This is an important advantage in the very small infant, in whom it is difficult to avoid excessive venotomy and transection of the vein. Even in the most experienced hands, the cutdown procedure may take 10 minutes and last no longer than percutaneous IV access. When other methods cannot be performed, venous cutdowns may provide the only alternative means of emergency venous access.

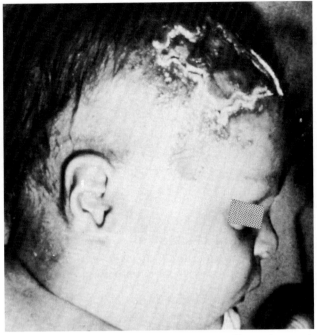

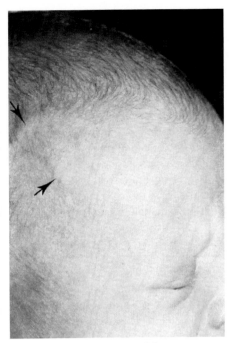

A   **B**

FIG. 27.7.   **A:** Skin slough on scalp caused by inadvertent infusion into the frontal branch of the temporary artery. **B:** This is indicated by arrows.

A. Indications

1. To provide a route for peripheral IV therapy when the percutaneous method is not possible
2. To provide a more stable and reliable IV line in situations where even brief cessation of therapy might compromise the infant
3. To provide emergency IV therapy

B. Contraindications

1. Risks and benefits should be weighed carefully in the presence of bleeding diathesis.
2. Should not be used as routine procedure for starting IV when percutaneous method is technically difficult but not impossible.

C. Equipment

Sterile

1. Gown and gloves
2. Cup with antiseptic solution (e.g., an iodophor)
3. Sterile aperture drape
4. 0.5% lidocaine HCl in 2-mL syringe
5. Two 25-gauge venipuncture needles
6. Two curved mosquito hemostats
7. 22-gauge cannula with needle stylet or a short length of small-diameter (0.6- to 1.2-mm outer diameter) silicone rubber catheter. The small silicone catheters reduce irritation but can slow the process of placing the line.
8. T connector for cannula
9. Heparinized saline (for heparin lock).
10. Half-strength normal saline in a 5-mL syringe
11. Absorbable suture or 5-0 nylon suture on small, curved needle. It is preferable to close the wound with subcuticular absorbable sutures, whenever possible, to avoid inflammation and formation of suture tracts (7).
12. Needle holder
13. No. 11 scalpel blade and handle
14. Semipermeable, sterile transparent dressing

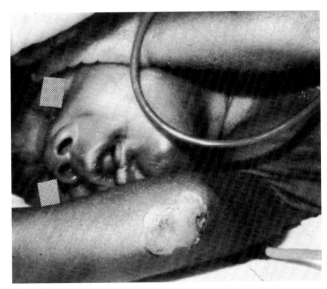

FIG. 27.8.   Burn from transilluminator used to locate vein in antecubital fossa.

Nonsterile

1. Materials for restraint (see Chapter 34)
2. Transilluminator (cover with sterile plastic glove to maintain sterile field; see Chapter 13)
3. Roll of 0.5- to 1-inch porous adhesive tape

D. Precautions

1. Aspirate prior to injection of lidocaine to prevent inadvertent intravascular infusion.
2. To avoid severing underlying vein, take care not to make initial skin incision too deep.
3. Avoid infusing extremely irritating or hypertonic solutions.

E. Technique

Anatomic considerations: The great saphenous vein is constant in its anatomic position, just anterior to the medial malleolus. It is the only structure of importance in this area. The cutdown procedure is facilitated by the fact that the vein lies on tough periosteum and has sufficient elasticity to allow withdrawal through a small incision without the danger of rupture.

1. Restrain foot in equinovalgus position.
2. Palpate medial malleolus, and locate point of incision 1 cm anterior and 1 cm superior to malleolus (Fig. 27.9).
3. Scrub, put on mask, gown, and gloves, and prepare area of incision, as for major procedure (see Chapter 5).
4. Drape area.
5. Indicate line of incision by marking skin with sterile surgical pen prior to infiltration with local anesthetic.
6. Infiltrate skin along line of incision with 0.5 to 1 mL of lidocaine, and then extend infiltration into subcutaneous tissue.
7. Wait 5 minutes for anesthesia to take effect.
8. Make 1-cm transverse incision through skin, down to superficial subcutaneous fat. A vertical, rather than a transverse, incision is optional. The former has the

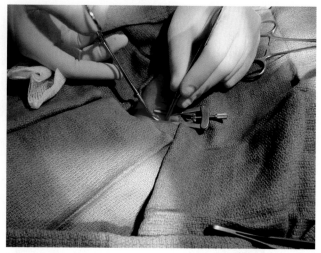

FIG. 27.10. Blades of curved hemostat are spread parallel to vein to dissect the subcutaneous connective tissue down to the periosteum.

advantage that it offers the opportunity to extend the incision cephalad, should the posterior wall of the vein be perforated on the initial attempt at cannulation. However, it has the disadvantage that it may be made too lateral or medial to the vein.

9. Introduce curved hemostat into incision, with tip down. Spread blades of hemostat parallel to vein to dissect tissue down to periosteum. Continue this step until adequate visualization of vein is achieved (Fig. 27.10).
10. Reintroduce curved hemostat into incision, with tip down, and pass down to periosteum. With a "scooping" motion, through approximately 180 degrees, isolate vein and draw into incision (Fig. 27.11).
11. Open hemostat carefully. Spread subcutaneous tissue, leaving the vein surface clean.

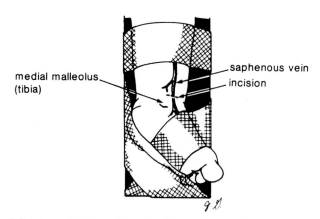

medial malleolus
(tibia)

saphenous vein
incision

FIG. 27.9. Position of restraint for cutdown on the great saphenous vein at the ankle, indicating site of incision.

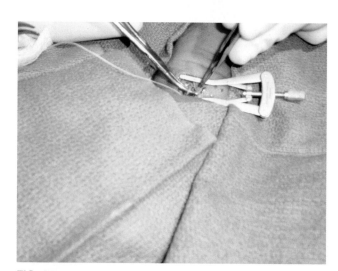

FIG. 27.11. A curved hemostat is used to "scoop" the vein into the incision.

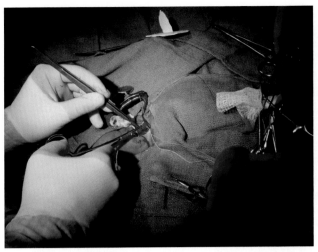

FIG. 27.12. The hemostat has been carefully opened and the subcutaneous connective tissue spread, leaving the vein surface clean. A ligature is placed between the blades of the hemostat.

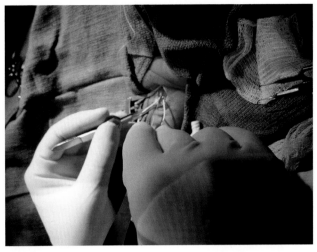

FIG. 27.14. Introducing the cannula into the vein.

12. Place 5-0 silk suture loosely around vein and clamp at end of suture with hemostat to allow for distal control of vessel (Fig. 27.12). (Do not tie ligature.)
13. Place ligature with clamp across extended index finger and inside palm of nondominant hand, retracting it in an upward and caudad direction (Fig. 27.13).
14. Introduce cannula/stylet into vein at a 45-degree angle, with bevel down. Once vein has been entered, angle cannula parallel to vein (Fig. 27.14).
15. Advance cannula into vein while withdrawing inner needle stylet.
16. Advance cannula up to hub, and infuse small volume of saline flush solution to confirm IV position.
17. Remove traction suture and close skin incision with subcuticular absorbable sutures or one or two simple 5-0 nylon sutures.

18. Attach cannula to infusion tubing and regulate IV.
19. Secure cannula to skin, as shown in Fig. 27.4.

F. Complications

1. Same as for percutaneous method
2. Inadvertent infusion of local anesthetic into artery or vein
3. Severance of vein owing to excessively deep initial incision
4. Infiltration of IV infusion into body cavity (Fig. 27.15)
   This is a complication related to placement of very long catheters. When infusion of an extremely irritating or hypertonic solution is required, the catheter is preferably inserted into the central venous system (see Chapter 32).
5. Varicose veins secondary to postinfusion phlebitis (26)

Conversion of Peripheral IV Line to a Saline Lock

A. Technique

1. Wash hands and put on gloves.
2. Clean IV tubing and catheter connection with antiseptic solution.
3. Stop IV infusion and remove IV tubing from hub of IV needle or cannula.
4. Seal hub with a sterile plug or T-connector system (e.g., Argyle intermittent infusion plug [Consolidated Medical Equipment, Utica, New York; Sherwood Medical Co., St. Louis, Missouri] or Burron spin-lock port extension set [Burron Medical, Bethlehem, Pennsylvania] that has been primed with the required

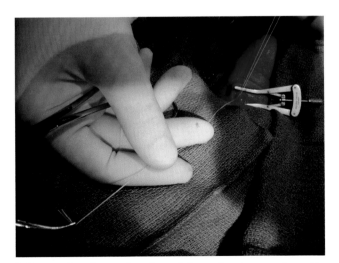

FIG. 27.13. Outward and caudad traction is exerted on the suture.

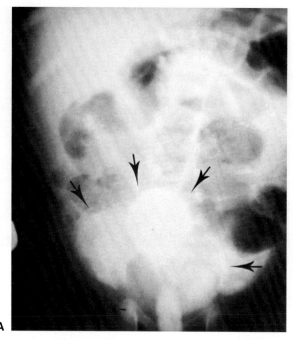
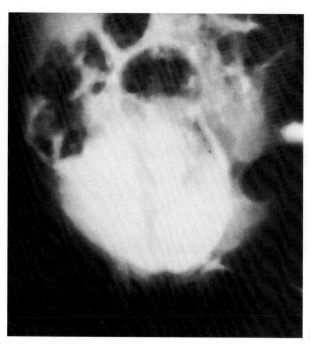

FIG. 27.15.   Cystogram in infant who had not urinated for more than 24 hours despite "adequate" IV fluids. **A:** The bladder appears normal, but there is a "mass effect" displacing the intestines in approximate area indicated by arrows. **B:** Radiographic contrast material, injected through a long catheter introduced into the femoral vein via the great saphenous vein, has extravasated into the abdominal cavity.

quantity of saline). As an improvisation, a stopcock with two dead heads may be used. However, at least 3 mL of flush solution is necessary to flush all parts of a stopcock. This increases the margin for error, with possible fluid overload in very small premature infants.

5. Clean plug with antiseptic, and inject 0.4 to 0.8 mL of saline solution through plug to flush blood from needle or cannula.

6. Clean plug with antiseptic prior to every use.

7. Refill lock with flush solution after every IV infusion. (Flush routinely every 6 to 12 hours, depending on frequency of use.)

References

1. Wille JC, Blussae E, Vanovd Ablas A. A comparison of four film-type dressings by their antimicrobial effect on the flora of the skin. *J Hosp Infect.* 1989;14:153.
2. Vernon HJ, Lane AT, Wischerater LJ, et al. Semipermeable dressing and transepidermal water loss in premature infants. *Pediatrics.* 1990;86:357.
3. Maki DG, Ringer M. Evaluation of dressing regimens for prevention of infection with peripheral intravenous catheters. *JAMA.* 1987;258:3396.
4. Hoffmann KK, Western SA, Kaiser DL, et al. Bacterial colonization and phlebitis-associated risk with transparent polyurethane film for peripheral intravenous site dressings. *Am J Infect Control.* 1988;16:101.
5. Holland KT, Harnby D, Peel B. A comparison of the in vivo antibacterial effects of "Op-Site," "Tegaderm" and "Ensure" dressings. *J Hosp Infect.* 1985;6:299.
6. Stevens B, Yamada J, Ohlsson A. Sucrose for analgesia in newborn infants undergoing painful procedures. *Cochrane Database Syst Rev.* 2010;CD001069.
7. Ganderer MW. Vascular access techniques and devices in the pediatric patient. *Surg Clin North Am.* 1992;72:1267.
8. Downing JW, Charles KK. Intravenous cannula fixing and dressing—comparison between the use of transparent polyurethane dressing and conventional technique. *South Afr Med J.* 1987;721:191.
9. Leibovici C. Daily change of an antiseptic dressing does not prevent infusion phlebitis: a controlled trial. *Am J Infect Control.* 1989;17:23.
10. Lund C, Kuller J, Lane A, et al. Neonatal skin care: the scientific basis for practice. *JOGNN.* 1999;28:241.
11. Stein J, George B, River G, et al. Ultrasonographically guided peripheral intravenous cannulation in emergency department patients with difficult intravenous access: a randomized trial. *Ann Emerg Med.* 2009;54:33.
12. Doniger SJ, Ishimine P, Fox JC, et al. Randomized controlled trial of ultrasound-guided peripheral intravenous catheter placement versus traditional techniques in difficult-access pediatric patients. *Pediatr Emerg Care.* 2009;25:154.
13. Perry AM, Caviness AC, Hsu DC. Efficacy of a near-infrared light device in pediatric intravenous cannulation: a randomized controlled trial. *Pediatr Emerg Care.* 2011;27:5.
14. Filston HC, Johnson DG. Percutaneous venous cannulation in neonates: a method for catheter insertion without "cut-down." *Pediatrics.* 1971;48:896.
15. Johnson RV, Donn SM. Life span of intravenous cannulas in a neonatal intensive care unit. *Am J Dis Child.* 1988;142:968.
16. Duck S. Neonatal intravenous therapy. *J Intravenous Nurs.* 1997;20:121.
17. Wynsma L. Negative outcomes of intravascular therapy in infants and children. *AACN Clin Issues.* 1998;9:49.
18. Batton DG, Maisles JM, Appelbaum JM. Use of intravenous cannulas in preterm infants: a controlled study. *Pediatrics.* 1982;70:487.

19. Pearson ML. Guideline for prevention of intravascular device-related infections. Part I. Intravascular device-related infections: an overview. The Hospital Infection Control Practices Advisory Committee. *Am J Infect Control.* 1996;24:262.

20. Shah PS, Ng E, Sinha AK. Heparin for prolonging peripheral intravenous catheter use in neonates. *Cochrane Database Syst Rev.* 2005;4:CD002774.

21. Pineault M, Chessex P, Pledboeuf B, et al. Beneficial effect of coinfusing a lipid emulsion on venous patency. *J Parenter Enter Nutr.* 1989;13:637.

22. Phelps SJ, Lochrane EB. Effect of the continuous administration of fat emulsion on the infiltration rate of intravenous lines in infants receiving peripheral parenteral nutrition solutions. *J Parenter Enter Nutr.* 1989;13:628.

23. Lloyd-Still JD, Peter G, Lovejoy FH. Infected "scalp-vein" needles. *JAMA.* 1970;213:1496.

24. Lozon MM. Pediatric vascular access and blood sampling techniques. In: Roberts JR, Hedges JR, eds. *Clinical Procedures in Emergency Medicine.* 4th ed. Philadelphia: Saunders; 2004:366.

25. Cronin WA, Germanson TP, Donowitz LG. Intravascular cannula colonization and related blood stream infection in critically ill neonates. *Infect Control Hosp Epidemiol.* 1990;11:301.

26. Shuster S, Laks H. Varicose veins following ankle cut-downs. *J Pediatr Surg.* 1973;8:245.

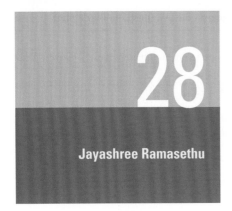

28

Management of Extravasation Injuries

Jayashree Ramasethu

Extravasation or inadvertent infiltration of IV administered solutions into subcutaneous tissue is a common adverse event in intensive care nurseries and may result in partial or complete skin loss, infection, and nerve and tendon damage, with the potential risk of cosmetic and functional impairment (1–3). Parenteral alimentation fluids, calcium, potassium, and sodium bicarbonate solutions, vasopressor agents, and antibiotics such as nafcillin, are often implicated (1,4–6). Early identification and appropriate management are vital to minimize damage (7–9).

A. Assessment (Fig. 28.1; see also Figs. 27.5 and 27.6)

1. Staging of extravasations is recommended for objective evaluation to determine the degree of intervention required. Several staging systems are in use (7–10). Table 28.1 describes one that is commonly used.
2. Detailed descriptions or digital photographs provide better documentation of the extent of the wound and the healing process
3. Fussiness, crying, or withdrawal of the limb when flushing the IV cannula are early warning signs, but these may be absent in an infant who is sedated or critically ill.
4. Blistering and discoloration of skin often portend at least partial skin loss, but visible skin changes do not always indicate the severity of underlying injury, which may evolve over several days (7).

B. Management

The degree of intervention is determined by the stage of extravasation, the nature of the infiltrating solution, and the availability of specific antidotes. There is no consensus on management of stage 3 or 4 lesions. In the absence of randomized controlled trials, some institutions have established management protocols to guide therapy, based on local experience, case series, and anecdotal evidence (1,7–13).

1. In all cases

a. Stop the IV infusion promptly.
b. Remove constricting bands that may act as tourniquets (e.g., armboard restraint).

c. Elevation of the limb may help to reduce edema.
d. The application of warm or cold packs is controversial. Warm packs may, by local vasodilation, help to reabsorb infiltrating solutions. However, warm moist packs have been reported to cause maceration of the skin.

2. Stage 1 or 2 extravasation

a. Remove IV cannula.
b. Consider antidote (see stage 3 or 4 extravasation below).

3. Stage 3 or 4 extravasation

a. Leave the IV cannula in place and, using a 1-mL syringe, aspirate as much fluid as possible from the area. Usually, very little fluid can be aspirated.
b. Remove the cannula unless it is needed for administration of the antidote.
c. Consider use of hyaluronidase or a specific antidote (see below). The use of hyaluronidase may obviate the need for the multiple puncture or saline washout techniques described below.
   i. *Multiple-puncture technique (11):* In infants who develop tense swelling of the site with blanching of the skin owing to infiltration of acidic or hyperosmolar solutions, multiple punctures of the edematous area using a blood-drawing stylet (and strict aseptic technique) has been used to allow free drainage of the infiltrating solution, decrease the swelling, and prevent necrosis. The area is then dressed with saline soaks to aid drainage.
   ii. *Saline flush out:* A technique of saline flushing of the subcutaneous tissue has been advocated by some authors (2,12,14). After cleaning and infiltrating the area with 1% lidocaine, 500 to 1,000 units of hyaluronidase is injected subcutaneously. Four small stab incisions are then made in the tissue plane with a scalpel blade at the periphery of the area. Saline is injected through a blunt cannula inserted subcutaneously through one of the puncture sites and flushed through the other puncture sites, massaging the fluid toward the incisions to facilitate removal of the extravasated material.

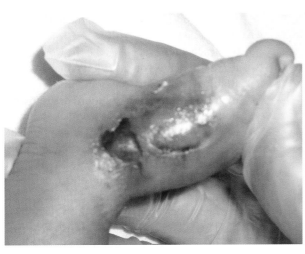 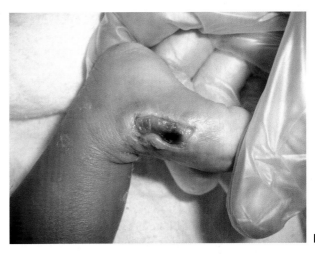

FIG. 28.1. **A:** Stage IV extravasation injury with blistering of skin. **B:** Same area 2 weeks later, with eschar formation.

iii. *Hyaluronidase:* Dispersing agent effective in extravasations involving calcium, parenteral alimentation fluids, antibiotics, sodium bicarbonate, etc. Although standard reference manuals state that hyaluronidase is not recommended for treatment of vasopressor extravasation injury, there have been reports of successful treatment of such extravasations with a combination of hyaluronidase and saline irrigations, as described above (2,12).
Mechanism of action: Breakdown of hyaluronic acid, the ground substance or intercellular cement of tissues; minimizes tissue injury by enhancing dispersion and reabsorption of extravasated fluids

Formulations available:
i. *Animal derived:* Ovine-derived Vitrase (Alliance Medical Products, Irvine, California) or bovine-derived Amphadase (Amphastar Pharmaceuticals, Rancho Cucamonga, California). Amphadase contains small quantities of thimerosal, so it is not recommended in neonates.
ii. *Recombinant human hyaluronidase (rHuPH20) (Hylenex, Baxter Healthcare, Deerfield, Illinois):* This product is reported to have up to 100 times greater enzymatic activity than the animal-derived form, but there is little literature available on its effectiveness in extravasations (15)
Most effective within 1 hour; may be used up to 12 hours
Administration: Use 25- or 26-gauge needles to inject 1 mL (150 USP units/mL of Vitrase) as five separate 0.2-mL injections around the periphery of the extravasation site. If using recombinant human hyaluronidase, a single subcutaneous injection of 150 units using a 25-guage needle may be equally effective (15). Most effective within 1 hour; may be used up to 12 hours after the extraversation.
Adverse effects: None reported in neonates, rare sensitivity reactions to the animal formulations of hyaluronidase reported in adults

d. **Specific antidotes**
Topical nitroglycerine (16,17)
i. Effective in treating injury due to extravasation of dopamine
ii *Mechanism of action:* Vascular smooth muscle relaxant
Application: 2% nitroglycerine ointment, 4 mm/kg body weight, applied over the affected area,

TABLE 28.1	Staging of Extravasation Injury (10)

Stage	Characteristics
1	Pain at site—crying when IV cannula is flushed IV cannula flushes with difficulty No redness or swelling
2	Pain Redness and slight swelling at site Brisk capillary refill
3	Pain Moderate swelling Blanching of area Skin cool to touch Brisk capillary refill below site Good pulse below site
4	Pain Severe swelling around site Blanching of area Skin cool to touch Area of skin necrosis or blistering Prolonged capillary refill time (>4 s) Decreased or absent pulse

may be repeated every 8 hours if perfusion has not improved (17)

Precautions: Absorption through the skin may lead to hypotension.

Phentolamine (6,18)

i. Effective in treating extravasations of vasopressors such as dopamine and epinephrine, which cause tissue damage by intense vasoconstriction and ischemia

ii. *Mechanism of action:* Competitive alpha-adrenergic blockade, leading to smooth muscle relaxation and hyperemia

iii. Effect should be seen almost immediately; most effective within 1 hour but may be used up to 12 hours. The biologic half-life of subcutaneous phentolamine is <20 minutes.

iv. Doses have not been established for newborn infants. The exact dose is dependent on the size of the lesion and the size of the infant.

v. Recommended doses range from 0.01 mg/kg per dose to 5 mL of 1-mg/mL solution.

vi. *Administration:* 0.5 to 1 mg/mL of solution injected subcutaneously into infiltrated area, after removal of IV catheter

vii. *Precautions:* Hypotension, tachycardia, and dysrhythmias may occur; use with extreme caution in preterm infants; consider using repeated small doses.

e. **Wound management**

(1) *Goal:* The goal of wound management in neonates who have partial- or full-thickness skin loss is to achieve primary or secondary healing while avoiding scarring, contractures, and operative intervention. There are several purposes for dressing wounds.

(1) Maintain a moist pH-balanced environment to promote re- epithelialization.

(2) Manage exudates.

(3) Decrease disruption of healing tissue.

(4) Provide an antimicrobial barrier to prevent local and systemic infection.

(5) Decrease pain.

(2) *Wound care:* Wound care regimens differ among experts and institutions (1,3,7,13,19). Consultation with a wound ostomy care nurse is often helpful.

(1) *Evaluate the wound:* Size, depth, edges, wound bed, presence of exudate, necrotic tissue, eschar, undermining of margins, evaluation of skin around the wound for signs of inflammation or for maceration (13).

(2) Evaluate wound healing every day. Time to heal ranges from 7 days to 3 months.

(3) Dressing changes can be painful. Consider using comfort measures, sucrose, and analgesics, as needed.

(4) Irrigate wound with sterile saline to remove exudate and debris.

(5) Topical agents may be used if the wound is colonized, infected, or at risk of being infected. Routine use of antiseptic solutions is not recommended because most solutions destroy granulation tissue.

i. Silver sulfadiazine cream is contraindicated in infants less than 30 days of age because the sulphonamides increase the risk of kernicterus. In addition, the cream can obscure the wound by forming a difficult to remove opaque layer.

ii. Use of povidone–iodine is not recommended because absorption of iodine may suppress thyroid function.

iii. Antibacterial creams and ointments have limited roles.

(6) Wound dressing

i. The selection of dressing material depends on the depth of the wound, the property of the wound bed (presence of granulation tissue, moist, dry, exudative) (19).

ii. Wet wounds require absorptive dressing, whereas dry wounds benefit from hydrating dressings.

iii. Amorphous hydrogels consisting of carboxymethylcellulose polymer, propylene glycol, and water have been shown to keep the wound moist and facilitate wound healing (13,19). They are available in the form of gels or sheets, which may be applied directly to the wound surface and held in place by a secondary dressing. The gel is easily removed with saline and is generally changed every 3 days. More frequent dressing changes may be required if there is excessive exudation.

iv. Silver-impregnated dressings are postulated to decrease wound infection (20).

v. Alginate dressings are fibers derived from brown seaweed and useful for wounds with moderate to heavy exudates (19).

vi. Polyurethane foams are also useful for wounds with exudates.

(7) If the scar involves a flexion crease, passive range-of-motion exercises with each diaper change may help to prevent contractures.

(8) Plastic surgical consultation

a. Recommended for all full-thickness and significant partial-thickness extravasation injuries

b. Enzymatic or surgical débridement or skin grafting may be required (3,21–24).

References

1. Wilkins CE, Emmerson AJB. Extravasation injuries in regional neonatal units. *Arch Dis Child Fetal Neonatal Ed.* 2004;89:F274.
2. Casanova D, Bardot J, Magalon G. Emergency treatment of accidental infusion leakage in the newborn: report of 14 cases. *Br J Plast Surg.* 2001;54:396.
3. Friedman J. Plastic surgical problems in the neonatal intensive care unit. *Clin Plast Surg.* 1998;25:599.
4. McCullen KL, Pieper B. A retrospective chart review of risk factors for extravasation among neonates receiving peripheral intravascular fluids. *J Wound Ostomy Continence Nurs.* 2006;33:133.
5. Zenk KE, Dungy CI, Greene GR. Nafcillin extravasation injury. Use of hyaluronidase as an antidote. *Am J Dis Child.* 1981;135:1113.
6. Subhani M, Sridhar S, DeCristafaro JD. Phentolamine use in a neonate for the prevention of dermal necrosis caused by dopamine: a case report. *J Perinatol.* 2001;21:324.
7. Amjad I, Murphy T, Nylander-Householder L, et al. A new approach to management of intravenous infiltration in pediatric patients. *J Infusion Nurs.* 2011;34:242.
8. Thigpen JL. Peripheral intravenous extravasation: nursing procedure for initial treatment. *Neonatal Netw.* 2007;26:379.
9. Doellman D, Hadaway L, Bowe- Geddes LA, et al. Infiltration and extravasation: update on prevention and management. *J Infusion Nurs.* 2009;32:203.
10. Montgomery LA, Hanrahan K, Kottman K. Guideline for IV infiltrations in pediatric patients. *Pediatr Nurs.* 1999;25:167.
11. Chandavasu O, Garrow D, Valda V, et al. A new method for the prevention of skin sloughs and necrosis secondary to intravenous infiltration. *Am J Perinatol.* 1986;3:4.
12. Harris PA, Bradley S, Moss ALH. Limiting the damage of iatrogenic extravasation injury in neonates. *Plast Reconstruct Surg.* 2001;107:893.
13. Fox MD. Wound care in the neonatal intensive care unit. *Neonatal Netw.* 2011;30:291.
14. Gault DT. Extravasation injuries. *Br J Plast Surg.* 1993;46:91.
15. Kuenstig LL. Treatment of intravenous infiltration in a neonate. *J Pediatr Health Care.* 2010;24:184.
16. Denkler KA, Cohen BE. Reversal of dopamine extravasation injury with topical nitroglycerine ointment. *Plast Reconstruct Surg.* 1989;84:811.
17. Wong AF, McCullough LM, Sola A. Treatment of peripheral tissue ischemia with topical nitroglycerine ointment in neonates. *J Pediatr.* 1992;121:980.
18. Siwy BK, Sadove AM. Acute management of dopamine infiltration injury with Regitine. *Plast Reconstruct Surg.* 1987;80:610.
19. Cisler-Cahill L. A protocol for the use of amorphous hydrogel to support wound healing in neonatal patients: an adjunct to nursing care. *Neonatal Netw.* 2006;25:267.
20. Rustogi R, Mill J, Fraser JF, et al. The use of Acticoat in neonatal burns. *Burns.* 2005;31:878.
21. Falcone PA, Barrall DT, Jeyarajah DR, et al. Nonoperative management of full thickness intravenous extravasation injuries in premature neonates using enzymatic debridement. *Ann Plastic Surg.* 1989;22:146.
22. Tiras U, Erdeve O, Karabulut AA, et al. Debridement via collagenase application in two neonates. *Pediatr Dermatol.* 2005;22:472.
23. Schafer T, Kukies S, Stokes TH, et al. The prepuce as a donor site for reconstruction of an extravasation injury to the foot in a newborn. *Ann Plast Surg.* 2005;54:664.
24. Chen TK, Yang CY, Chen SJ. Calcinosis cutis complicated by compartment syndrome following extravasation of calcium gluconate in a neonate: a case report. *Pediatr Neonatol.* 2010;51:238.

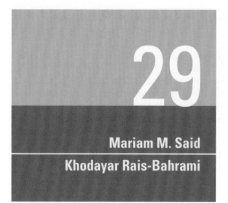

29

Umbilical Artery Catheterization

Mariam M. Said

Khodayar Rais-Bahrami

A. Indications

Catheters should remain in place only as long as primary indications exist, with the exception of secondary indication A3. Because of the risk of complications, catheters should usually not remain in place for more than 2 weeks.

Primary

1. Frequent or continuous (see Chapter 10) measurement of lower aortic blood gases for oxygen tension (PO_2) or oxygen content (percent saturation)
2. Continuous monitoring of arterial blood pressure
3. Angiography
4. Resuscitation (use of umbilical venous line may be first choice)

Secondary

1. Umbilical artery is not usually used for infusion of maintenance glucose/electrolyte solutions or medications. If this line is to be used to provide IV nutrition, the same aseptic techniques used for any central line must be used to prevent line-related sepsis (see Chapter 32).
2. Exchange transfusion
3. To provide vital infusions (1) and a port for frequent blood sampling in the extremely low-birthweight infant

B. Contraindications

1. Evidence of vascular compromise in lower limbs or buttock areas
2. Peritonitis
3. Necrotizing enterocolitis (2)
4. Omphalitis
5. Omphalocele
6. Acute abdomen etiology

C. Equipment

Several standardized graphs for premeasurement of catheter length to be inserted are available (Figs. 29.1–29.3).

Sterile

1. Sterile gown and gloves
2. Cup with antiseptic solution

3. Surgical drape with central aperture (transparent drape recommended)
4. Catheter
   a. Single hole
      (1) Reduces surfaces for potential thrombus formation
      (2) Recorded pressure tracing will change when hole is occluded.
   b. Made of flexible material that does not kink as it follows the curves of vessels
   c. Relatively rigid walls with frequency characteristics suitable for accurate measurement of intravascular pressure
   d. Small capacity (minimum volume of blood to be withdrawn to clear catheter prior to blood sampling)
   e. *Radio-opaque*: The need to visualize the catheter position on x-ray film outweighs the theoretical risk of increased thrombogenicity related to a radio-opaque strip (3).
   f. Smooth, rounded tip (4), nonthrombogenic material (5)
   g. 5-French (Fr) gauge for infants weighing >1,200 g
   h. 3.5-Fr gauge for infants weighing <1,200 g
5. Three-way stopcock with Luer-Lock
6. 10-mL syringe
7. 0.45 to 0.9 normal saline (NS) flush solution (saline with heparin, 1 to 2 U/mL)

In very small premature infants, particularly in the first week of life, hypernatremia may result from receiving excess sodium in flush solutions. We recommend using 0.45 NS rather than more concentrated saline solutions in these infants. The use of hypotonic (0.25 NS) or dextrose solutions has been associated with hemolysis of red blood cells and should be avoided if possible (6). Use of heparinized flush solution is common practice. Rajani et al. and Ankola and Atakent (7,8) have shown that using a heparinized solution containing 1 U/mL heparin for flushing the umbilical arterial line prolonged catheter life by reducing the incidence of fibrin thrombus formation in the catheter lumen. Horgan et al. (9) found that the use of 1 U/mL heparin did not reduce the incidence of umbilical artery catheter (UAC)-related thrombi but did lower the

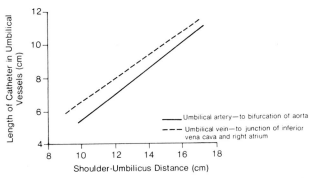

FIG. 29.1. Graph for determination of length of catheter to be inserted for appropriate low aortic or venous placement. Length of catheter is measured from umbilical ring. Length of umbilical stump must be added. The shoulder–umbilicus distance is the perpendicular distance between parallel horizontal lines at the level of the umbilicus and through the distal ends of the clavicles. (Adapted from Dunn P. Localization of the umbilical catheter by postmortem measurement. *Arch Dis Child.* 1966;41:69, with permission.)

incidence of their sequelae. Butt et al. (10) could demonstrate no significant benefit associated with increasing the rate of infusion from 1 to 2 mL/h (heparin 1 U/mL), and Bosque and Weaver (11) showed that continuous infusion of 1 U/mL heparin is more effective than intermittent infusion in maintaining patency of the UAC. More recent data have indicated that heparin decreases the incidence of thrombotic complications (12), and a Cochrane Database Review found that the use of as little as 0.25 U/mL heparin in the infusate decreases the likelihood of line occlusion (13).

8. Tape measure
9. 20-cm narrow umbilical tie
10. No. 11 scalpel blade and holder
11. 4- × 4-inch gauze sponges

12. Two curved mosquito hemostats
13. Toothed iris forceps
14. Two curved, nontoothed iris forceps
15. 2% lidocaine HCl without epinephrine
16. 3-mL syringe and needle to draw up lidocaine
17. Small needle holder
18. 4-0 silk suture on small, curved needle
19. Suture scissors

Nonsterile

1. Cap and mask
2. Wooden tongue depressor

D. Precautions

1. Avoid use of feeding tubes as catheter (associated with higher incidence of thrombosis) (14).
2. Fold drapes so as not to obscure infant's face and upper chest.
3. Take time and care to dilate lumen artery before attempting to insert catheter.
4. Catheter should not be forced past an obstruction.
5. Never advance catheter once placed and secured.
6. Loosen umbilical tie slightly upon completion of procedure and obtain radiographic confirmation of position.
7. Avoid covering the umbilicus with dressing. Dressing may delay recognition of bleeding or catheter displacement.
8. Always obtain radiographic (including a lateral view) or ultrasound (15) confirmation of catheter position. (16,17).
9. Be certain that catheter is secure, and examine frequently when infant is placed in prone position, because hemorrhage may go unrecognized.

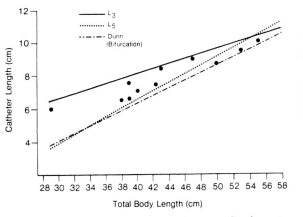

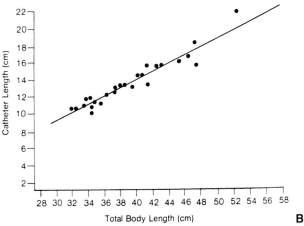

FIG. 29.2. **A:** Graph for distance of catheter insertion from the umbilical ring for L3, L5, and aortic bifurcation. *Large dots* represent catheters positioned at L4. **B:** Graph for catheter insertion to level T8 using total body length. (From Rosenfeld W, Biagtan J, Schaeffer H, et al. Evaluation of graphs for insertion of umbilical artery catheters below the diaphragm. *J Pediatr.* 1981;98:628, with permission.)

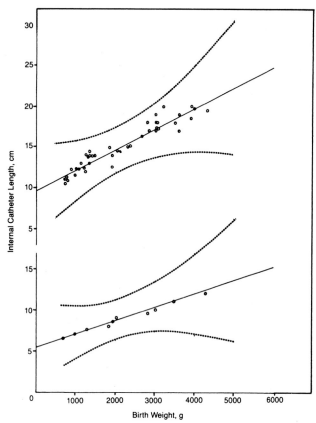

FIG. 29.3. Estimates of insertion length of umbilical catheters (umbilical artery catheter tip inserted between T6 and T10; umbilical vein catheter tip inserted above diaphragm in inferior vena cava near right atrium) based on birthweight (BW) (with 95% confidence intervals). Modified estimating equations utilizing BW are as follows: umbilical artery length = 2.5 BW + 9.7 **(top)** and umbilical vein length = 1.5 BW + 5.6 **(bottom)**, where BW is measured in kilograms and lengths are measured in centimeters. (From Shukla H, Ferrara A. Rapid estimation of insertional length of umbilical catheters in newborns. *Am J Dis Child.* 1986;140:787, with permission.)

10. Take care not to allow air to enter the catheter. Always have catheter fluid filled and attached to closed stopcock prior to insertion. Check for air bubbles in catheter before flushing or starting infusion.
11. When removing catheter, cut suture at skin, not on catheter, to avoid catheter transection.

E. Technique (See also Umbilical Catheterization on the Procedures Website)

Anatomic note: The umbilical arteries are the direct continuation of the internal iliac arteries. Their diameters at their origins are 2 to 3 mm. As they approach the umbilicus, their lumina become small and the walls thicken significantly. In a full-term infant, each artery is approximately 7 cm long (Fig. 29.4). A catheter introduced into the umbilical artery will usually pass into the aorta from the internal iliac artery. Occasionally, it will pass into the femoral artery via the external iliac artery or into one of the gluteal arteries. The latter two sites are unsuitable for sampling, pressure measurement, or infusion.

1. Placement of UAC in high position should be used exclusively. In rare cases if high position is not successful a low position can be used (Fig. 29.5).

    High position is associated with fewer episodes of blanching and cyanosis of the lower extremities (18). High catheters were found to have decreased incidence of clinical vascular complications with a relative risk of 0.53 (95% confidence interval, 0.44 to 0.63) with no statistically significant increase in any adverse sequelae, including the incidence of hypertension, intraventricular hemorrhage, hematuria, necrotizing enterocolitis, or death (19).

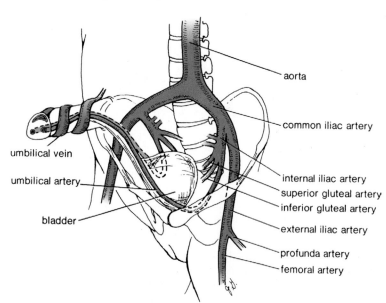

FIG. 29.4. Anatomic relations of the umbilical arteries, showing relationships with major arteries supplying buttocks and lower limb.

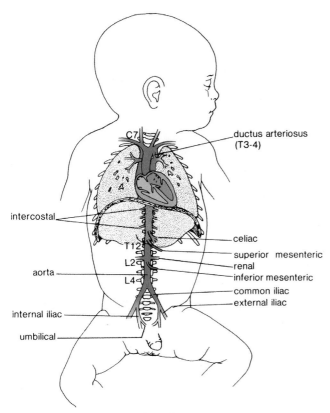

FIG. 29.5. The aorta and branches.

a. *High position (14,19):* Level of thoracic vertebrae T6–T9 (Fig. 29.6); catheter tip above origin of celiac axis
b. *Low position (14,19):* Level of lumbar vertebrae L3–L4 (Fig. 29.7)
   (1) Catheter tip is below major aortic branches such as renal mesenteric arteries.
   (2) In most newborns, this position coincides with the aortic bifurcation at the upper end of the fourth vertebra.
2. Make external measurements as necessary to estimate length of catheter to be inserted (see Figs. 29.1–29.3) (20–23).
3. Prepare as for major procedure (see Chapter 5).
4. Attach stopcock to hub of catheter and fill system with flush solution. Turn stopcock to catheter "off."
5. Place sterile gauze around umbilical stump and elevate out of sterile field or have an ungloved assistant grasp the cord by the cord clamp or forceps and pull the cord vertically out of the sterile field.
6. Prepare cord and surrounding skin with antiseptic solution to radius of approximately 5 cm. The use of chlorhexidine in infants <2 months of age is not recommended (24).
7. Drape area surrounding cord.
8. Place umbilical tie around umbilicus and tie loosely with a single knot.

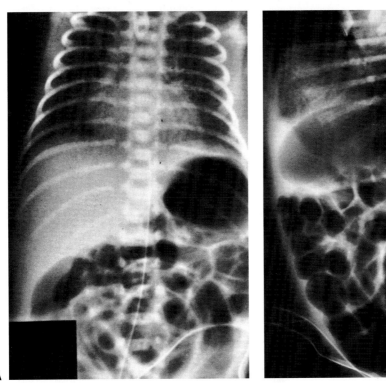

FIG. 29.6. UAC in satisfactory high position at the level of the ninth thoracic vertebral body on anteroposterior (**A**) and lateral (**B**) projections.

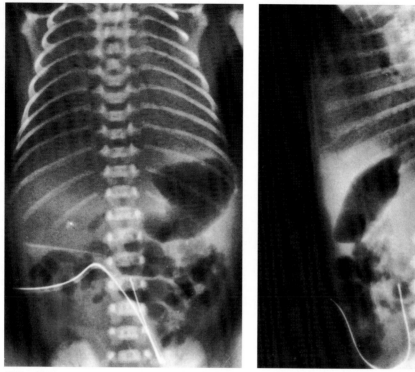

FIG. 29.7. Anteroposterior (**A**) and lateral (**B**) radiographs showing satisfactory low position of a UAC. Catheter tip is at the level of the superior margin of the fourth lumbar vertebral body, which in newborns usually corresponds to the aortic bifurcation.

a. Tighten only enough to prevent bleeding and, if possible, place around Wharton jelly rather than skin.

b. It may be necessary to loosen the tie when inserting the catheter.

9. Cut cord horizontally with scalpel (Fig. 29.8).

a. Approximately 1 to 1.5 cm from skin

b. Avoid tangential slice.

Bloom et al. (25) described an alternative approach to the artery with lateral arteriotomy. To

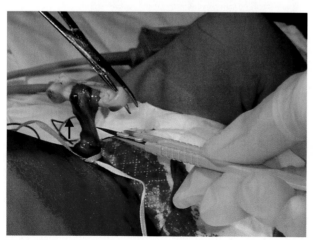

FIG. 29.8. Traction is being placed on cord in direction of the *arrow*. Operator is about to make a horizontal cut across cord.

perform this method, 3 to 4 cm of cord must be preserved because the cord must be rolled over a Kelly clamp 180 degrees (25,26).

(1) Clamp across end of cord with a mosquito hemostat in the nondominant hand and pull firmly toward the infant's head.

(2) Roll cord 180 degrees over hemostat toward abdominal wall.

(3) Identify arteries in superior right and left lateral aspects of cord.

(4) Approximately 1 cm from abdominal wall, incise Wharton jelly down to arterial wall, using a no. 11 scalpel blade.

(5) Incise artery through half of circumference. If necessary, dilate lumen with iris forceps.

(6) Insert catheter into lumen of artery, directed in a caudad direction, for predetermined distance.

10. Control bleeding by gentle tension on umbilical tape.

11. Blot surface of cord stump with gauze swab. Avoid rubbing, as this damages tissue and obscures anatomy.

12. Identify cord vessels (Fig. 29.9).

a. Vein is easiest to identify as large, thin-walled, sometimes gaping vessel. It is most frequently situated at the 12-o'clock position at the base of the umbilical stump.

b. Arteries are smaller, thick-walled, and white and may protrude slightly from cut surface.

c. Omphalomesenteric duct is rarely present.

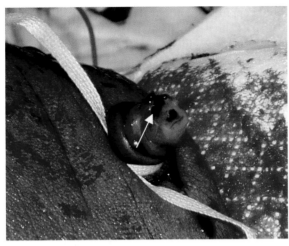

FIG. 29.9. The vessels of the umbilical cord. Thin-walled umbilical vein at 12-O'clock position is indicated by a *white arrow.* One of the two umbilical arteries is to the right and directly below the vein.

13. Grasp cord stump, using toothed forceps, at point close to (but not on) artery to be catheterized. If available, it may be helpful to have an assistant scrub and assist.
    a. Apply two curved mosquito hemostats to Wharton jelly on opposite sides of the cord, away from the vessel to be cannulated.
    b. Apply traction to stabilize cord stump.
14. Introduce one of the points of the curved iris forceps into the lumen of the artery and probe gently to a depth of 0.5 cm.

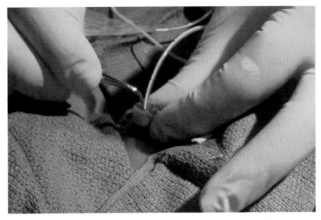

FIG. 29.10. An iris forceps is pointed into the umbilical artery in order to dilate the lumen of the artery.

15. Remove forceps and bring points together before introducing them once more into the lumen.
16. Probe gently to a depth of 1 cm (up to the curved "shoulder" of the forceps), keeping the points together.
17. Allow the points to spring apart, and maintain forceps in this position for 15 to 30 seconds to dilate vessel (Fig. 29.10). Time spent in ensuring dilatation prior to catheter insertion increases the likelihood of success.
18. Release cord and set aside toothed forceps, while keeping curved forceps within artery.
19. Grasp catheter 1 cm from tip, between free thumb and forefinger or with curved iris forceps.

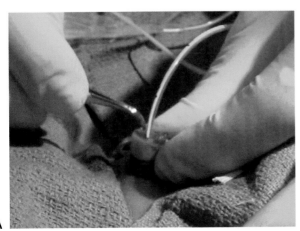

A

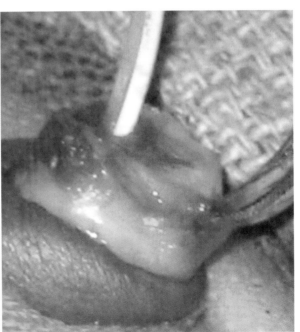

B

FIG. 29.11. **A:** Inserting the catheter into the artery between the prongs of dilating forceps. Note that the umbilical tape has been tied around the skin of the umbilicus; this should be loosened once the catheter is secured in place. **B:** Close-up photo of the umbilical stump with the arterial catheter in place.

20. Insert catheter into lumen of artery, between prongs of dilating forceps (Fig. 29.11).
21. Remove curved forceps, having passed catheter approximately 2 cm into vessel with a firm, steady motion. Grasp cord again with toothed tissue forceps and pull gently toward head of infant. This mild traction will facilitate passage of catheter at an angle between the cord and the abdominal wall.
22. After passing the catheter approximately 5 cm, aspirate to verify intraluminal position. Clear blood by injecting 0.5 mL of flush solution. Advance catheter to calculated appropriate length.
23. Take appropriate action if insertion is complicated (Fig. 29.12).
    a. Resistance before tip reaches abdominal wall (<3 cm from surface of abdominal stump)
        (1) Loosen umbilical tape.
        (2) Redilate artery.

b. "Popping" sensation rather than "relaxation"
    (1) Catheter may have exited lumen and created a false channel.
    (2) Remove and use second artery.
    (3) If unsuccessful, draw 0.5 mL of lidocaine from vial. Reinsert tip of catheter approximately 2 cm into UAC and drip lidocaine into vessel. Apply constant gentle pressure until vessel dilates.
c. Backflow of blood, particularly around vessel
    (1) Tighten umbilical tape.
    (2) Catheter may be in false channel, with extravascular bleeding.
d. Resistance is encountered at anterior abdominal wall or sharp turn in vessel as it angles around bladder toward internal iliac artery (approximately 6 to 8 cm from surface of umbilical stump in 2- to 4-kg neonate).
    (1) Apply gentle but steady pressure for 30 to 60 seconds.

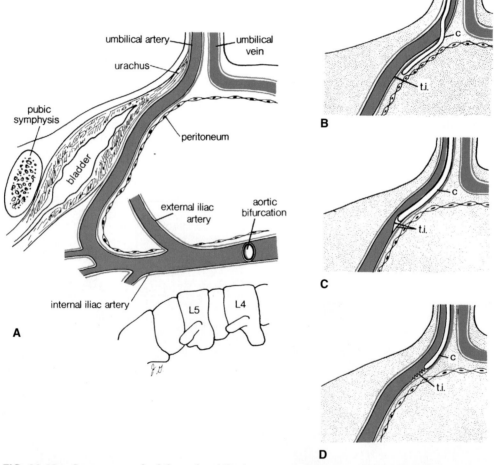

FIG. 29.12.   Some reasons for failure of umbilical artery catheterization. **A:** Sagittal midline section to show normal anatomy of umbilical artery. **B:** Catheter has perforated the umbilical artery within the anulus umbilicalis and is dissecting perivascularly and external to peritoneum. **C:** Catheter has ruptured through the tunica intima (*t.i.*) and dissected into subintimal space. **D:** Catheter invaginating the tunica intima after stripping it from a more distal point. (Adapted from Clark JM, Jung AL. Umbilical artery catheterization by a cut down procedure. *Pediatrics (Neonatol Suppl).* 1977;59:1036, with permission of the American Academy of Pediatrics.)

(2) Position infant on side with same side elevated as artery being catheterized. Flex hip.

(3) Instill lidocaine as for E23b (3). Do not force catheter.

e. Easy insertion, but no blood return

(1) Catheter is outside vessel in false channel.

(2) Remove and observe infant carefully for evidence of complication.

24. Place marker tape on catheter with base of tape flush with surface of cord so that displacement of the catheter may be readily recognized.

25. Remove umbilical tape and place purse-string suture around base of the cord (not through skin or vessels). Three bites into cord (with needle facing away from catheter) are sufficient to include all three vessels within the suture.

If desired, form marker tape into bilateral wings, and sew the tails of the purse-string suture through the wings to anchor the catheter in a symmetrical fashion. This is a useful method in very small premature infants because it avoids sticking tape to the abdominal wall (27). Alternatively, remove needle and wrap ends of suture in opposite direction around catheter for about 3 cm and tie, taking care not to kink catheter.

26. Secure catheter temporarily by looping over upper abdomen and taping.

27. Obtain radiographs or ultrasound to check catheter position.

a. Catheter tip above T6 or between T10 and L2

(1) Measure distance between actual and appropriate position on radiograph.

(2) Withdraw equal length of catheter.

(3) Repeat radiographic study.

(4) Note procedure in chart.

b. Catheter tip below L5

(1) Remove catheter.

(2) Never advance catheter once in situ, because this will introduce a length of contaminated catheter into the vessel.

28. If desired, secure catheter with tape bridge (Fig. 38.14).

29. Continue routine cord care with 70% alcohol swab or other agent of choice.

30. Stabilize catheter, stopcock, and syringe, using tongue depressor (optional).

a. Reduces risk of air embolus if syringe is maintained in vertical position

b. Prevents accidental disconnection of catheter system

F. Alternative Technique: Umbilical Artery Cutdown

This method is usually successful even after failed insertion through the umbilical stump, as there is less tendency for false tracts. The most frequent reason for failed umbilical artery cutdown is mistaking the urachus for a vessel. Because of the time and risks associated with the cutdown procedure, standard insertion should be attempted first.

Indications

1. Failed umbilical artery catheterization through conventional technique described earlier in this chapter

Contraindications

1. Same as for umbilical artery catheterization by conventional technique

2. Bleeding diathesis

Equipment

1. Same as for umbilical artery catheterization by conventional technique.

2. 1% lidocaine HCl without epinephrine in 3-mL syringe with 25- to 27-gauge needle

3. No. 15 surgical blade and holder

4. Curved delicate dressing forceps, two pairs (1/4 or 1/2 curved)

5. Tissue forceps

6. Self-retaining retractor (such as eyelid retractor)

7. Absorbable suture, plain

8. Absorbable suture on small cutting needle

9. Nonabsorbable suture on a small, curved needle

10. Needle holder

11. Suture scissors

12. Skin-closure tapes

Precautions

1. Same as described earlier for conventional technique.

2. If possible, leave catheter from previously attempted standard procedure in place to aid in vessel identification.

3. Ensure that abdominal incision is on abdominal wall and not too close to umbilical stump.

4. Identify landmarks carefully to avoid cutting or catheterizing urachus.

5. When incising mesenchymal sheath, take care to avoid transecting vessel.

6. Secure the catheter with an internal ligature that is just tight enough to prevent accidental removal but loose enough for elective removal or reinsertion, in case the catheter becomes occluded by thrombus or precipitate.

Technique (28)

See Fig. 29.13.

1. Insert an orogastric tube to keep the bowel as decompressed as possible.

2. Prepare infant and drape as for umbilical artery catheterization (see earlier in chapter).

3. If catheter has been left in place after previous attempt, include vessel and catheter in the preparation, leaving the catheter accessible for removal.

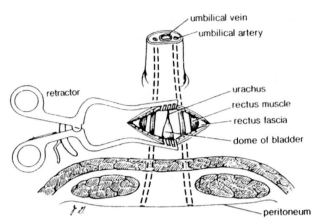

FIG. 29.13. Subumbilical cutdown. Anatomic view through incision. (Redrawn from Sherman NJ. Umbilical artery cutdown. *J Pediatr Surg.* 1977;12:723, with permission.)

4. Anesthetize area of skin immediately below umbilicus, at umbilical stump–abdominal wall junction, with 0.5 mL of lidocaine.
5. Prepare UAC as for standard procedure, leaving catheter filled with flush solution. Estimate length for insertion based on patient size. Subtract 1 to 2 cm from that recommended for standard insertion, as cutdown catheter will enter vessel farther along course.
6. Make a smile-shaped incision from 4 to 8 o'clock through the skin of the abdominal wall at the junction with the umbilical stump.
7. Place self-retaining retractor to maintain exposure.
8. Using blunt dissection through the subcutaneous tissue with mosquito forceps, identify the fascia overlying the urachus and umbilical vessels.

   The mesenchymal sheath is composed of three layers of fascia and is from 1 to 3 mm thick. Although it is barely perceptible in extremely premature infants, in term infants it may be thick enough to require making an incision through the sheath prior to blunt dissection.
9. While elevating the fascia with two forceps, make a small incision between their tips. Enlarge incision with scissors to the same size as skin incision. In very immature infants, simple dissection should suffice.
10. With curved mosquito forceps, dissect in the midline and identify the urachus (Fig. 29.13).

    The urachus is a white, glistening, cordlike structure in the midline. Its position may be confirmed by traction cephalad, pulling the dome of the bladder into view. The umbilical arteries lie posterolaterally on either side but not touching the urachus.
11. Identify the umbilical arteries lying to either side of the urachus.

    The vessels with their surrounding tissues appear larger than expected. When elevated, there will be no caudal bulge, distinguishing them from the urachus. If a previously attempted catheter was left "in place," palpation of the area allows more ready identification of

the vessel. Previously unsuccessful attempts, with failure to pass more than a few centimeters, are usually associated with perivascular hematoma formation from unrecognized perforation and dissection through a false tract. Visualization of a hematoma helps distinguish the vessel from the urachus.

12. Try to avoid entering the peritoneum. In infants with very little subcutaneous tissue, it may be impossible to avoid penetrating the peritoneum. Should this occur, replace any bowel that may protrude and carefully close the peritoneum with absorbable suture, taking extreme care not to include any bowel within the suture. Start antibiotics for peritonitis prophylaxis.
13. Insert the tip of the mosquito forceps under the vessel and pull a doubled strand of plain absorbable suture under the vessel. Position sutures 1 cm apart.
14. While elevating the sutures and with suture scissors directed cephalad, make a V-shaped incision through three fourths of the diameter of the vessel. Take care not to transect the vessel, but cut cleanly into the lumen.

    If the artery is accidentally transected and if the catheter insertion is unsuccessful, tie off the caudal end of the artery to prevent hemorrhage.
15. Use curved tissue forceps or a catheter introducer to dilate the artery.
16. Pass the catheter through the opening for the predetermined distance, checking for blood return after a few centimeters. The catheter should advance without resistance.
17. When the catheter is properly positioned, have an assistant check the perfusion in the lower extremities. If that is satisfactory, secure the catheter by tying the lower ligature firmly around the catheter.
18. Using absorbable suture, close the fascia and approximate the subcutaneous tissues.

    Hashimoto et al. (29) proposed an alternative technique that allows for catheter reinsertion in case of catheter thrombosis or occlusion. They use loose ligation around the artery once the catheter is in proper position. They then fix the artery by using the same sutures that close the fascia, thus creating an arteriocutaneous fistula, making it easy to find the insertion site and use it for reinsertion.
19. Close the skin with nonabsorbable suture or with skin-closure tape after cleaning the area.
20. The catheter may be further secured with a tape bridge (Fig. 38.14).

Removal of Catheter

1. Remove any tape and withdraw catheter slowly, as described earlier in this chapter.
2. If the internal ligature around a catheter is too tight to allow removal with reasonable traction, it may be necessary to dissect and cut the ligature, after sterile skin preparation.

3. Apply pressure for hemostasis.
4. Approximate wound edges with skin-closure tape.

Complications

1. Catheterization of urachus (30)
2. Vesicoumbilical fistula (30)
3. Transection of urachus with urinary ascites (31)
4. Perforation or rupture (32,33) of urinary bladder—although Nagarajan (33) has suggested that the risk of bladder injury is minimal if bladder is emptied prior to procedure.
5. Transection of umbilical artery with hemorrhage
6. Incision of peritoneum (with possible evisceration)
7. Bleeding from incision

G. Care of Dwelling Catheter

For setup and maintenance of arterial pressure transducer, see Chapter 9.

1. Keep catheter free of blood to prevent clot formation.
   a. Flush catheter with 0.5 mL of flush solution, slowly over at least 5 seconds, each time a blood sample is drawn.
   b. Between samples, infuse IV solution continuously through catheter to prevent retrograde flow.
   c. Note amounts of blood removed and IV fluid/flush solution infused, and add to fluid balance record.
2. Watch for indications of clot formation.
   a. Decrease in amplitude of pulse pressure on blood pressure tracing
   b. Difficulty withdrawing blood samples
3. Take appropriate action if clot forms.
   a. Do not attempt to flush clot forcibly.
      Remove catheter. Replace only if critical.
4. Enteral feeding in the presence of UACs remains controversial. Increased risk of mesenteric thromboembolism and its association with the development of necrotizing enterocolitis has been suggested (34). Other studies have shown no increased incidence of feeding problems or complications in infants fed with a UAC in situ (35).

H. Obtaining Blood Samples from Catheter

(With emphasis on aseptic technique and minimizing stress to the vessel)

Equipment

1. Gloves
2. Alcohol swabs
3. Rubber-tipped clamps or disposable IV tubing clamps
4. Syringe of 0.6 mL of flushing solution
5. Syringe for cleaning line
6. Syringe for blood sample
7. Ice, if necessary for sample preservation
8. Appropriate requisition slips and labels

Technique

1. Wash hands and put on sterile gloves.
2. Form sterile field.
3. Clean the connection site of the stopcock/catheter using an alcohol swab.
4. Clamp the umbilical catheter.
5. Connect the 3-mL syringe, release the clamp, and slowly draw back 2 to 3 mL of fluid over 1 minute to clear the line. Reclamp the catheter. Remove syringe and place on sterile field. Data published by Davies et al. (36) indicate that accurate measurements of electrolytes can be obtained after withdrawal of a minimum of 1.6 mL of blood. However, if blood glucose values are desired, a minimum of 3 mL from a 3.5-Fr and 4 mL from a 5-Fr catheter must be withdrawn.
6. Attach sampling syringe. Release clamp and draw back specimen desired. Reclamp the catheter.
7. Reattach the syringe containing the fluid and blood cleared from the line.
   a. Clear the connection of air.
   b. Slowly replace the fluid and blood cleared from the line and remove the syringe.
8. Attach the syringe of flushing solution to the stopcock, clear air from the connection, and slowly flush the line.
9. Clean the stopcock connection with alcohol.
10. Record on infant's daily record sheet all blood removed and volume of flush used.
    A study was carried out that looked at cerebral oxygenation and blood sampling from UAC in high position in preterm infants (median gestational age 30 weeks). Although the clinical significance is unclear, the study showed that blood sampling of 2.3 mL (including flush volumes) through the UAC within 20 seconds resulted in a significantly decreased cerebral oxygenated hemoglobin and tissue oxygenation index. It also caused an increase in deoxygenated hemoglobin. This was not seen when the sampling time was extended to 40 seconds (37).

I. Removal of UAC

Indications

1. No further clinical indication
2. Need for less frequent direct PO_2 measurements
3. Sufficient stabilization of blood pressure to allow intermittent monitoring
4. Hypertension
5. Hematuria not due to other recognizable cause
6. Catheter-related sepsis and/or infections with *Staphylococcus aureus*, gram-negative bacilli, or *Candida* mandate removal of the catheter (38)

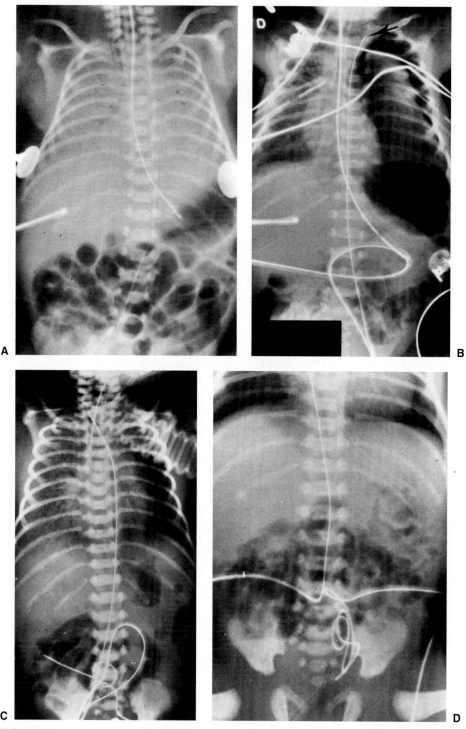

FIG. 29.14.   Various UAC malpositions. **A:** Unacceptable position at L2 because of the proximity of the renal arteries. **B:** UAC in left brachycephalic artery. **C:** UAC in right brachycephalic artery. **D:** UAC in pelvic artery.

7. Catheter-related vascular compromise
8. Onset of platelet consumption coagulopathy
9. Peritonitis
10. Necrotizing enterocolitis
11. Omphalitis

Technique

1. Leave umbilical tie loose around cord stump as precaution against excessive bleeding.

   Reinsertion of purse-string suture through dried Wharton jelly is preferable if

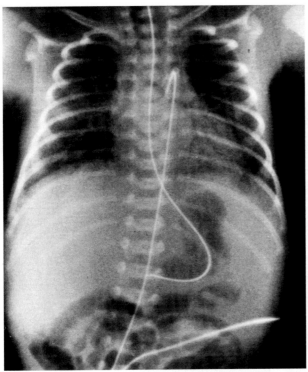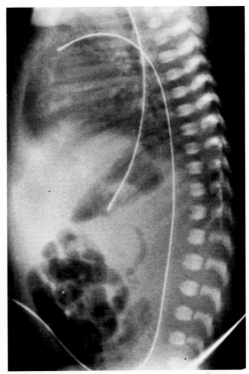

A   B

FIG. 29.15. Anteroposterior (**A**) and lateral (**B**) radiographs demonstrating passage of a UAC into the pulmonary artery via a patent ductus arteriosus.

a. Umbilical tape must be tied on skin rather than Wharton jelly.
b. Catheter has been in situ for longer than 48 hours, because artery may have lost ability to spasm.
2. Withdraw catheter slowly and evenly, until approximately 5 cm remains in vessel, tightening purse-string suture or umbilical tie.
3. Discontinue infusion.
4. Pull remainder of catheter out of the vessel at rate of 1 cm/min (to allow vasospasm). If there is bleeding, apply lateral pressure to the cord by compressing between thumb and first finger.

J. Complications (38–41)

Catheterization of the umbilical artery is probably always associated with some degree of reversible damage to the arterial intima (42,43).

1. Malpositioned catheter (Figs. 29.14–29.16)
   a. Vessel perforation (44)
   b. Refractory hypoglycemia with catheter tip opposite celiac axis (45)
   c. Peritoneal perforation (46)
   d. False aneurysm (47)
   e. Movement of catheter tip position because of changes in abdominal circumference

f. Sciatic nerve palsy (48)
g. Misdirection of catheter into internal or external iliac artery (see Figs. 29.14D and 29.17) (39).
   Schreiber et al. (42) have described a double-arterial catheter technique to correct this problem.
2. Vascular accident
   a. Thrombosis (Fig. 29.18) (49–52)
   b. Embolism/infarction (Fig. 29.17) (17,27) seen days or weeks after line insertion (38)
   c. Vasospasm (17,38,53,54) is seen within minutes to a few hours after insertion.
   d. Loss of extremity (Fig. 29.19) (53)
   e. Hypertension (Fig. 29.20) (18,55)
   f. Paraplegia (56)
   g. Congestive heart failure (aortic thrombosis) (57)
   h. Air embolism (Fig. 29.21)
3. Equipment-related
   a. Breaks in catheter and transection of catheter (58)
   b. Plasticizer in tissues (59,60)
   c. Electrical hazard
      (1) Improper grounding of electronic equipment
      (2) Conduction of current through fluid-filled catheter
   d. Intravascular knot in catheter (61)
4. Other
   a. Hemorrhage (including that related to catheter loss or disconnection and overheparinization) (39,62,63)

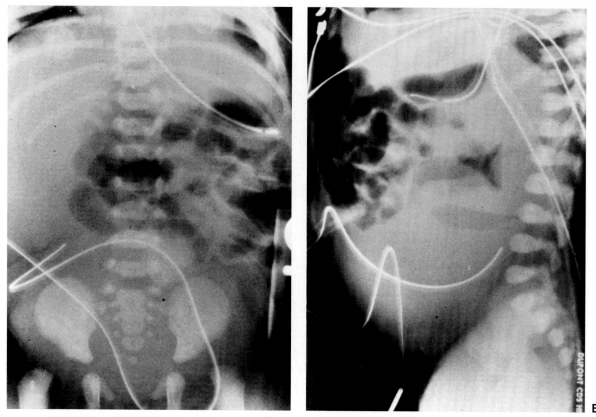

FIG. 29.16.   Effect of abdominal mass stimulating catheter misplacement. Anteroposterior (**A**) and lateral (**B**) films show remarkable displacement of a UAC by a giant hematocolpos in a 1-day-old infant.

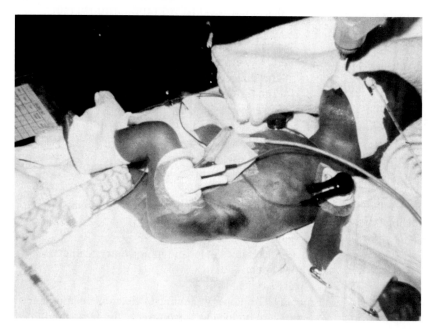

FIG. 29.17.   Vascular compromise in the left buttock and loin owing to a complication of a UAC displaced into the internal iliac artery. For vascular anatomy, see Fig. 29.4.

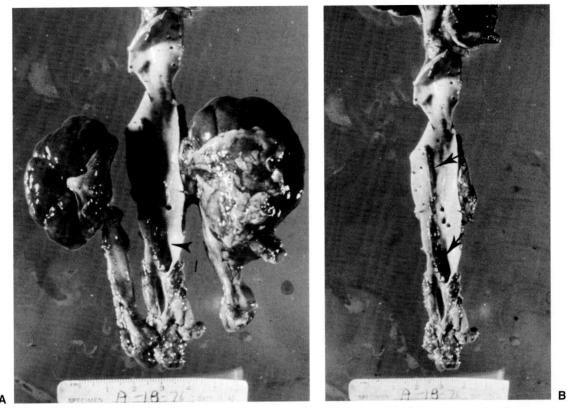

A   B

FIG. 29.18. *Arrows* indicate mural thrombus in the abdominal aorta, which was associated with an umbilical arterial line. Upon further dissection of this autopsy specimen, the left renal artery was found to be occluded by thrombus. The left kidney is showing a degree of atrophy. Both kidneys showed scattered infarction.

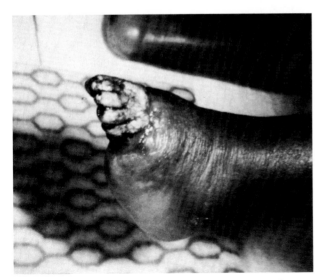

FIG. 29.19.   Autoamputation of forefoot, owing to vascular complication of a UAC.

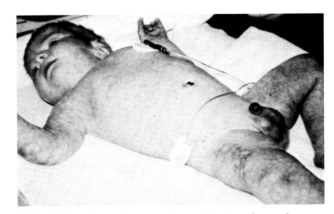

FIG. 29.20.   Generalized mottling of skin in infant with severe hypertension secondary to UAC-associated thrombus in renal artery.

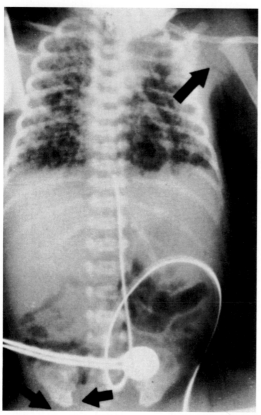

FIG. 29.21. Anteroposterior roentgenogram demonstrating air embolism from a UAC in the left subclavian artery (*upper arrow*) and the femoral arteries (*lower arrows*).

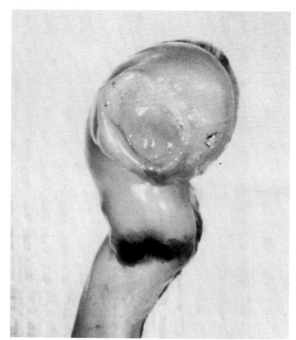

FIG. 29.22. Small omphalocele. This gut-containing hernia was transected during placement of a UAC.

b. Infection (38,64,65)
c. Necrotizing enterocolitis (34,53,54)
d. Intestinal necrosis or perforation (66)
    (1) Vascular accident
    (2) Infusion of hypertonic solution (67)
e. Transection of omphalocele (Fig. 29.22) (68)
f. Herniation of appendix through umbilical ring (69)
g. Cotton fiber embolus (70)
h. Wharton jelly embolus (71)
i. Hypernatremia
    (1) True
    (2) Factitious (60)
j. Factitious hyperkalemia (60)
k. Bladder injury (ascites) (31–33)
l. Curving back of the catheter on itself as a result of it catching in the intima (72)
m. Pseudocoarctation of the aorta (52)
n. Pseudomass in left atrium (73)
o. Displacement by thoracoabdominal abnormality (74)
p. Failure to obtain a lateral x-ray to confirm position of a percutaneous femoral central line. This failure led to the failure to recognize that the line is displaced into a spinal vein; it was interpreted by the radiologist as a correctly placed high umbilical artery line. (Fig. 29.23)(40)

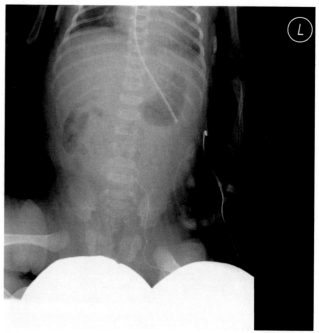

FIG. 29.23. Failure to obtain a lateral radiographic view to confirm the position of this percutaneously placed femoral central venous line led to failure to recognize that the line is displaced into a spinal vein. The line was reported by the radiologist as a correctly positioned high umbilical arterial line.

References

1. Kanarek SK, Kuznicki MB, Blair RC. Infusion of total parenteral nutrition via the umbilical artery. *J Parenter Enter Nutr.* 1991; 15:71.
2. Rand T, Weninger M, Kohlhauser C, et al. Effects of umbilical arterial catheterization on mesenteric hemodynamics. *Pediatr Radiol.* 1996;26:435.
3. Clawson CC, Boros SJ. Surface morphology of polyvinyl chloride and silicone elastomer umbilical artery catheters by scanning electron microscopy. *Pediatrics.* 1978;62:702.
4. Hecker JF. Thrombogenicity of tips of umbilical catheters. *Pediatrics.* 1981;67:467.
5. Boros SJ, Thompson TR, Reynolds JW, et al. Reduced thrombus formation with silicone elastomer (Silastic) umbilical artery catheters. *Pediatrics.* 1975;56:981.
6. Jackson JK, Derleth DP. Effects of various arterial infusion solutions on red blood cells in the newborn. *Arch Dis Child Fetal Neonatal Ed.* 2000;83:F130.
7. Rajani K, Goetzman BW, Wennberg RP, et al. Effects of heparinization of fluids infused through an umbilical artery catheter on catheter patency and frequency of complications. *Pediatrics.* 1979;63:552.
8. Ankola PA, Atakent YS. Effect of adding heparin in very low concentration to the infusate to prolong the patency of umbilical artery catheters. *Am J Perinatol.* 1993;10:229.
9. Horgan MJ, Bartoletti A, Polansky S, et al. Effect of heparin infusates in umbilical arterial catheters on frequency of thrombotic complications. *J Pediatr.* 1987;111:774.
10. Butt W, Shann F, McDonnell G, et al. Effect of heparin concentration and infusion rate on the patency of arterial catheters. *Crit Care Med.* 1987;15:230.
11. Bosque E, Weaver L. Continuous versus intermittent heparin infusion of umbilical artery catheters in the newborn infant. *J Pediatr.* 1986;108:141.
12. Hentschel R, Weislock U, Von Lengerk C, et al. Coagulation-associated complications of indwelling arterial and central venous catheters during heparin prophylaxis: a prospective study. *Eur J Pediatr.* 1999;158:S126.
13. Barrington KJ, Umbilical artery catheters in the newborn: effects of heparin. *Cochrane Database Syst Rev.* 2000;CD000507.
14. Westrom G, Finstrom O, Stenport G. Umbilical artery catheterization in newborns: thrombosis in relation to catheter tip and position. *Acta Paediatr Scand.* 1979;68:575.
15. Fleming SE, Kim JH. Ultrasound-guided umbilical catheter insertion in neonates. *J of Perinatology.* 2011;31:344.
16. Baker DH, Berdon WE, James LS. Proper localization of umbilical arterial and venous catheters by lateral roentgenograms. *Pediatrics.* 1969;43:34.
17. Weber AL, Deluce S, Shannon DL. Normal and abnormal position of umbilical artery and venous catheter on the roentgenogram and review of complications. *AJR.* 1974;20:361.
18. Mokrohisky ST, Levine RL, Blumhagen RD, et al. Low positioning of umbilical artery catheters increases associated complications in newborn infants. *N Engl J Med.* 1978;229:561.
19. Barrington KJ. Umbilical artery catheters in the newborn: effects of position of the catheter tip. *Cochrane Database Syst Rev.* 2000;CD000505.
20. Dunn P. Localization of the umbilical catheter by post-mortem measurement. *Arch Dis Child.* 1966;41:69.
21. Rosenfeld W, Biagtan J, Schaeffer H, et al. A new graph for insertion of umbilical artery catheters. *J Pediatr.* 1980;96:735.
22. Rosenfeld W, Estrada R, Jhaveri R, et al. Evaluation of graphs for insertion of umbilical artery catheters below the diaphragm. *J Pediatr.* 1981;98:627.
23. Shukla H, Ferrara A. Rapid estimation of insertional length of umbilical catheters in newborns. *Am J Dis Child.* 1986;140: 786.
24. Latini G. Potential hazards of exposure to di-(2-ethylhexyl)-phthalate in babies. *Bio Neonate.* 2000;78:269.
25. Bloom BT, Nelson RA, Dirksen HC. A new technique: umbilical arterial catheter placement. *J Perinatol.* 1986;6:174.
26. Squire SJ, Hornung TL, Kirchhoff KT. Comparing two methods of umbilical artery catheter placement. *Am J Perinatol.* 1990;7:8.
27. Stewart DL, Wilkerson S, Fortunate SJ. New technique for stabilizing umbilical artery catheters in very low birth weight infants. *J Perinatol.* 1989;9:458.
28. Sherman NJ. Umbilical artery cutdown. *J Pediatr Surg.* 1977; 12:723.
29. Hashimoto T, Togari H, Yura J. Umbilical artery cutdown: an improved procedure for reinsertion. *Br J Surg.* 1985;72:194.
30. Waffarn F, Devaskar UP, Hodgman JE. Vesico-umbilical fistula: a complication of umbilical artery cutdown. *J Pediatr Surg.* 1980; 15:211.
31. Mata JA, Livne PM, Gibbons MD. Urinary ascites: complication of umbilical artery catheterization. *Urology.* 1987;30:375.
32. Diamond DA, Ford C. Neonatal bladder rupture: a complication of umbilical artery catheterization. *J Urol.* 1989;142:1543.
33. Nagarajan VP. Neonatal bladder injury after umbilical artery catheterization by cutdown. *JAMA.* 1984;252:765.
34. Lehmiller DJ, Kanto WP Jr. Relationships of mesenteric thromboembolism, oral feeding and necrotizing enterocolitis. *J Pediatr.* 1978;92:96.
35. Davey AM, Wagner CL, Cox C, et al. Feeding premature infants while low umbilical artery catheters are in place: a prospective, randomized trial. *J Pediatr.* 1994;124:795.
36. Davies MW, Mehr S, Morley CJ. The effect of draw-up volume on the accuracy of electrolyte measurements from neonatal arterial lines. *J Pediatr Child Health.* 2000;36:122.
37. Schulz G, Keller E, Haensse D, et al. Slow blood sampling from an umbilical artery catheter prevents a decrease in cerebral oxygenation in the preterm newborn. *Pediatrics.* 2003;111:e73.
38. Hermansen MC, Hermansen MG. Intravascular catheter complications in the neonatal intensive care unit. *Clin Perinatol.* 2005;32:141.
39. Miller D, Kirkpatrick BV, Kodroff M, et al. Pelvic exsanguination following umbilical artery catheterization in neonates. *J Pediatr Surg.* 1979;14:264.
40. Ramasethu J. Complications of Vascular Catheters in the Neonatal Intensive Care Unit. *Clin Perinatol.* 2008;35:199.
41. MacDonald MG, Chou MM. Preventing complications from lines and tubes. *Semin Perinatol.* 1986;10:224.
42. Schreiber MD, Perez CA, Kitterman JA. A double-catheter technique for caudally misdirected umbilical arterial catheters. *J Pediatr.* 1984;104:768.
43. Chidi CC, King DR, Bates E. An ultrastructural study of intimal injury induced by an indwelling umbilical artery catheter. *J Pediatr Surg.* 1983;18:109.
44. Clark JM, Jung AL. Umbilical artery catheterization by a cut down procedure. *Pediatrics (Neonatol Suppl).* 1977;59:1036.
45. Carey BE, Zeilinger TC. Hypoglycemia due to high positioning of umbilical artery catheters. *J Perinatol.* 1989;9:407.
46. Van Leeuwen G, Patney M. Complications of umbilical artery catheterization: peritoneal perforation. *Pediatrics.* 1969;44:1028.
47. Wyers MR, McAlister WH. Umbilical artery catheter use complicated by pseudoaneurysm of the aorta. *Pediatr Radiol.* 2002;32:199.
48. Giannakopoulou C, Korakaki E, Hatzidaki E, et al. Peroneal nerve palsy: a complication of umbilical artery catheterization in the full-term newborn of a mother with diabetes. *Pediatrics.* 2002;109:e66.
49. Seibert JJ, Northington FJ, Miers JF, et al. Aortic thrombosis after umbilical artery catheterization in neonates: prevalence of complications on long-term follow-up. *AJR.* 1991;156:567.
50. Martin JE, Moran JF, Cook LS, et al. Neonatal aortic thrombosis complicating umbilical artery catheterization: successful treatment with retroperitoneal aortic thrombectomy. *Surgery.* 1989; 105:793.
51. Greenberg R, Waldman D, Brooks C, et al. Endovascular treatment of renal artery thrombosis caused by umbilical artery catheterization. *J Vasc Surg.* 1998;28:949.

52. Francis JV, Monagle P, Hope S, et al. Occlusive aortic arch thrombus in a preterm neonate. *Pediatr Crit Care Med.* 2010;11:e13.

53. Gupta JM, Roberton NRC, Wigglesworth JS. Umbilical artery catheterization in the newborn. *Arch Dis Child.* 1968;43:382.

54. Lividatis A, Wallgren G, Faxelius G. Necrotizing enterocolitis after catheterization of the umbilical vessels. *Acta Paediatr Scand.* 1970;63:277.

55. Bauer SB, Feldman SM, Gellis SS, et al. Neonatal hypertension: a complication of umbilical artery catheterization. *N Engl J Med.* 1975;293:1032.

56. Muñoz ME, Roche C, Escribá R, et al. Flaccid paraplegia as complication of umbilical artery catheterization. *Pediatr Neurol.* 1993;9:401.

57. Henry CG, Gutierrez F, Joseph I, et al. Aortic thrombosis presenting as congestive heart failure: an umbilical artery catheter complication. *J Pediatr.* 1981;98:820.

58. Murphy KD, Le VA, Encarnacion CE, et al. Transumbilical intravascular retrieval of an umbilical artery catheter. *Pediatr Radiol.* 1995;25:S178.

59. Hillman LS, Goodwin SL, Sherman WR. Identification of plasticizer in neonatal tissues after umbilical catheters and blood products. *N Engl J Med.* 1975;292:381.

60. Gaylord MS, Pittman PA, Bartness J, et al. Release of benzalkonium chloride from a heparin-bonded umbilical catheter with resultant factitious hypernatremia and hyperkalemia. *Pediatrics.* 1991;87:631.

61. Cochrane WD. Umbilical artery catheterization. In: *Iatrogenic Problems in Neonatal Intensive Care. Report of the 69th Ross Conference of Pediatric Research.* Columbus, OH: Ross Laboratories; 1976:28.

62. Johnson JF, Basilio FS, Pettett PG, et al. Hemoperitoneum secondary to umbilical artery catheterization in the newborn. *Radiology.* 1980;134:60.

63. Moncino MD, Kurtzberg J. Accidental heparinization in the newborn: a case report and brief review of the literature. *J Perinatol.* 1990;10:399.

64. Landers S, Moise AA, Fraley JK, et al. Factors associated with umbilical catheter related sepsis in neonates. *Am J Dis Child.* 1991;145:675.

65. Narendran V, Gupta G, Todd DA, et al. Bacterial colonization of indwelling vascular catheters in newborn infants. *J Paediatr Child Health.* 1996;32:391.

66. Hwang H, Murphy JJ, Gow KW, et al. Are localized intestinal perforations distinct from necrotizing enterocolitis? *J Pediatr Surg.* 2003;38:764.

67. Book LS, Herbst JJ. Intraarterial infusions and intestinal necrosis in the rabbit: potential hazards of umbilical artery injections of ampicillin, glucose, and sodium bicarbonate. *Pediatrics.* 1980; 65:114.

68. Simpson JS. Misdiagnosis complicating umbilical vessel catheterization. *Clin Pediatr.* 1977;16:569.

69. Biagtan J, Rosenfeld W, Salazard D, et al. Herniation of the appendix through the umbilical ring following umbilical artery catheterization. *J Pediatr Surg.* 1980;15:672.

70. Bavikatte K, Hillard J, Schreiner RL, et al. Systemic vascular cotton fiber emboli in the neonate. *J Pediatr.* 1979;95:61.

71. Abramowsky CR, Chrenka B, Fanaroff A. Wharton jelly embolism: an unusual complication of umbilical catheterization. *J Pediatr.* 1980;96:739.

72. McGravey VJ, Dabiri C, Bean MS. An unusual twist to umbilical artery catheterization. *Clin Pediatr.* 1983;22:587.

73. Crie JS, Hajar R, Folger G. Umbilical catheter masquerading at echocardiography as a left atrial mass. *Clin Cardiol.* 1989;12:728.

74. Sakurai M, Donnelly LF, Klosterman LA, et al. Congenital diaphragmatic hernia in neonates: variations in umbilical catheter and enteri`c tube position. *Radiology.* 2000;216:112.

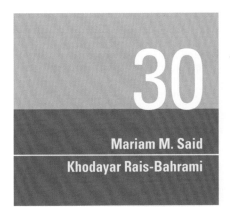

30 Umbilical Vein Catheterization

Mariam M. Said

Khodayar Rais-Bahrami

A. Indications

1. Primary
   a. Emergency vascular access for fluid and medication infusion and for blood drawing
   b. Long-term central venous access in low-birthweight infants. If the line is to be used long-term, particularly if parenteral nutrition is to be infused by this route, the same aseptic techniques must be used to prevent line-related sepsis as are used for any central venous line (see Chapter 32).
   c. Exchange transfusion
2. Secondary
   a. Central venous pressure monitoring (if catheter across ductus venosus)
   b. Diagnosis of total anomalous pulmonary venous drainage below the diaphragm (1)

B. Contraindications

1. Omphalitis
2. Omphalocele
3. Necrotizing enterocolitis
4. Peritonitis

C. Equipment

1. Catheter—same as for umbilical artery catheterization, except:
   a. 3.5-French (Fr) catheter for infants weighing <3.5 kg
   b. 5-Fr catheter for infants weighing >3.5 kg
   c. Double lumen umbilical venous catheters may be used in critically ill neonates to allow administration of inotropes or medications.
   d. Catheters used for exchange transfusion (removed after procedure) should have side holes. This reduces risk of sucking thin wall of inferior vena cava against catheter tip, with possible vascular perforation (2). Avoid double lumen catheters for exchange transfusions.
2. Other equipment as for umbilical artery catheter, but omit 2% lidocaine (see Chapter 29, C)

D. Precautions

1. Keep catheter tip away from origin of hepatic vessels, portal vein, and foramen ovale. Catheter tip should lie ideally at the junction of the inferior vena cava and the right atrium. The tip should at least be well into the ductus venosus to protect the liver from receiving inappropriate infusions (3). Sometimes it will not be possible to advance the catheter through the ductus venosus. Vigorous attempts to advance are to be avoided. In an emergency, vital infusions (avoid very hypertonic solutions) may be given slowly after pulling catheter back into umbilical vein (approximately 2 cm) and checking blood return.
2. Check catheter position prior to exchange transfusion. Avoid performing exchange transfusion with catheter tip in portal system or intrahepatic venous branch (see Fig. 30.1)
3. Once secured, do not advance catheter into vein.
4. Avoid infusion of hypertonic solutions when catheter tip is not in inferior vena cava.
5. Do not leave catheter open to atmosphere (danger of air embolus).
6. Avoid using a central venous pressure monitoring catheter for concomitant infusion of parenteral nutrition (risk of sepsis).
7. Be aware of potential inaccuracies of venous pressure measurements in inferior vena cava (see Chapter 32).

E. Technique (See Procedures Website for Video)

Anatomic note: In the full-term infant, the umbilical vein is 2 to 3 cm in length and 4 to 5 mm in diameter. From the umbilicus, it passes cephalad and slightly to the right, where it joins the portal sinus, a confluence of the umbilical vein with the right and left intrahepatic portal veins. The portal veins have intrahepatic branches that are distributed directly to the liver tissue. The ductus venosus becomes a continuation of the umbilical vein by arising from the left branch of the portal vein, directly opposite where the umbilical vein joins it. The ductus is located in a groove between the right

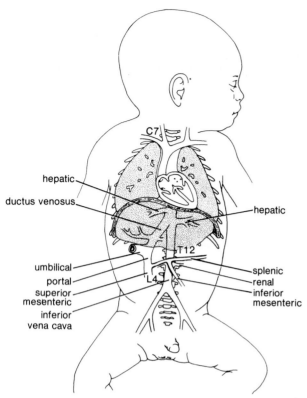

FIG. 30.1.   Anatomy of the umbilical and associated veins, with reference to external landmarks.

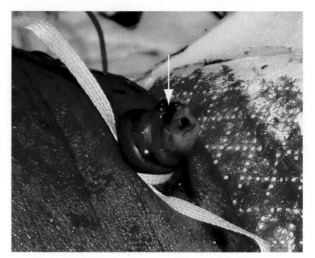

FIG. 30.2.   The umbilical stump. Vein is indicated with an *arrow*.

and left lobes of the liver in the median sagittal plane of the body, at a level between the 9th and 10th thoracic vertebrae; it terminates in the inferior vena cava along with hepatic veins, as shown in Fig. 30.1.

1. Make necessary measurements to determine length of catheter to be inserted, adding length of umbilical stump (Figs. 30.1 and 30.2) (4).
2. Prepare for procedure as with umbilical artery catheter (see Chapter 29, E).
3. Identify thin-walled vein, close to periphery of umbilical stump (Fig. 30.2).
4. Grasp cord stump with toothed forceps.
5. Gently insert tips of iris forceps into lumen of vein and remove any clots.
6. Introduce fluid-filled catheter, attached to the stopcock and syringe, 2 to 3 cm into vein (measuring from anterior abdominal wall).
7. Apply gentle suction to syringe.
   a. If there is not easy blood return, the catheter may have a clot in the tip. Withdraw the catheter while maintaining gentle suction. Remove clot and reinsert catheter.
   b. If there is smooth blood flow, continue to insert catheter for full estimated distance.

8. If catheter meets any obstruction prior to measured distance
   a. It has most commonly
      (1) Entered portal system, or
      (2) Wedged in an intrahepatic branch of portal vein
   b. Withdraw catheter 2 to 3 cm, gently rotate, and reinsert in an attempt to get tip through ductus venosus.
9. If the catheter is in the portal circulation, leave the misdirected catheter in its place. Pass a new 3.5- or 5-Fr catheter into the same vessel. Once the catheter is in a good position, remove the misdirected catheter. This procedure has a 50% success rate (5).
10. Obtain radiographic verification of catheter position. A lateral radiograph will aid in exact localization (Fig. 30.3) (6,7). The desired location is T9 to T10, just above the right diaphragm. The catheter tip position may be estimated clinically by measurement of venous pressure (1) and observation of waveform (Figs. 30.4 and 30.5). The catheter has crossed the foramen ovale if the blood obtained is bright red (arterial in appearance). In this case, pull the catheter back.
    a. As soon as the catheter has been advanced 2 to 3 cm into the vein, have an assistant connect it to a pressure-monitoring system (see Chapter 9).
    b. While continuing to advance the catheter, measure venous pressure and note pressure changes with respiration (Fig. 30.4). The ideal position is with the catheter tip at the junction of the inferior vena cava and the right atrium, although placement in ductus venosus is acceptable for purposes other than measurement of central venous pressure.
11. Other modalities to evaluate catheter placement include ultrasound (8) and echocardiography (9). These techniques may require fewer manipulations during catheter placement and reduce the number of x-rays a patient receives. Additionally, these types of

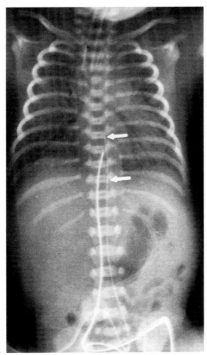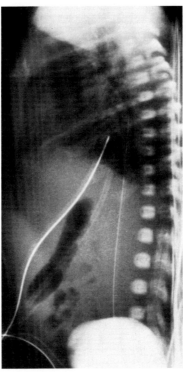

FIG. 30.3. Anteroposterior (**A**) and lateral (**B**) radiographs demonstrating the normal course of an umbilical venous catheter, with an umbilical artery catheter (*arrows*) in position for comparison. Note how the venous catheter swings immediately superior from the umbilicus, slightly to the right as it traverses the ductus venosus into the inferior vena cava (IVC). The distal tip of this line is just superior to the right atrial–IVC junction, and it might optimally be pulled back slightly into the IVC. Note how the thinner umbilical artery catheter (*arrows*) heads inferiorly as it proceeds to the iliac artery and then ascends posteriorly and to the left until it reaches the level of T7.

imaging techniques may provide a more accurate assessment of catheter location.

12. Secure catheter as for umbilical artery catheter (see Chapter 29, E).

There may be more bleeding from the umbilical vein than from the umbilical artery because the vein is not a contractile vessel. Local pressure is usually sufficient to stop oozing. For care of an indwelling catheter, sampling technique, and removal of a catheter, see Chapter 29.

F. Complications

1. Infections (6,10–15)
2. Thromboembolic (10,13,16,17)

Emboli from a venous catheter may be widely distributed. If the catheter tip lies in the portal system and the ductus venosus has closed, emboli will lodge in the liver. If the catheter has passed through ductus venosus, emboli will go to the lungs or, because of right-to-left shunting of blood through foramen ovale or ductus arteriosus in sick newborn infants, emboli may be distributed throughout entire systemic circulation. These emboli may be infected and, therefore, may cause widespread abscesses.

3. Catheter malpositioned in heart and great vessels (Figs. 30.5 and 30.6)
   a. Pericardial effusion/cardiac tamponade (cardiac perforation) (3,18,19)
   b. Cardiac arrhythmias (20)
   c. Thrombotic endocarditis (21)

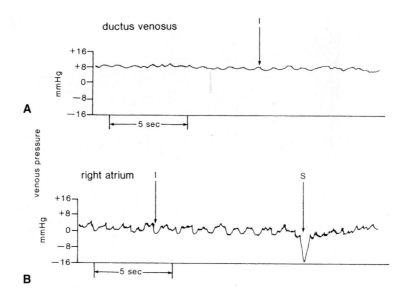

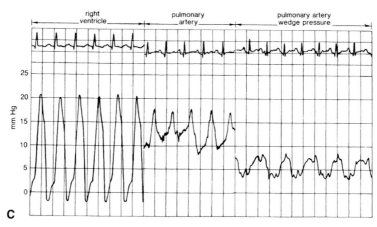

FIG. 30.4. Venous and arterial pressure tracings may be used to facilitate placement and detect misplacement. **A:** The catheter has been pulled back through the ductus venosus, and the tip lies in the portal system. The portal venous pressure is higher than the central venous pressure, there are no venous pressure waves, and there is a small positive deflection during inspiration. **B:** Tip of catheter in the superior vena cava near the right atrium shows a deflection of more than 4 mm Hg during spontaneous inspiration (*I*) and a large negative deflection of more than 15 mm Hg during a sigh (*S*). Atrial tracing shows an AC and a V wave. AC wave occurs with atrial contraction and closure of atrioventricular valve after P wave of ECG. V wave occurs with ventricular contraction near T wave of electrocardiogram. (Based on data from Kitterman JA, Phibbs RH, Tooley WH. Catheterization of umbilical vessels in newborn infants. *Pediatr Clin North Am.* 1970;17:895, with permission.) **C:** Pressure tracing from right ventricle and pulmonary artery. Right ventricular pressure tracing shows a single large rise and fall, beginning just after onset of QRS complex. Pulmonary artery tracing usually shows a dicrotic notch at end of T wave. Diastolic pressure is higher than that in right ventricle. Pulmonary capillary wedge tracing should resemble atrial tracing, inasmuch as it reflects left atrial pressure transmitted to the catheter tip when anterograde pulmonary arterial flow is occluded. *Note:* The marked negative deflection in the right atrial tracing would be more typically seen in infants who are receiving mechanical ventilation and, thus, have a positive airway pressure that exceeds ventricular filling pressures during each inspiration. In a spontaneously breathing neonate, positive airway pressure occurs only during expiration and never exceeds ventricular filling pressures. There are extremely small changes in cardiac pressures (i.e., on inspiration: right atrial [RA] mean pressure ↑, 1 mm Hg; left atrial [LA] mean pressure ↓ 1 mm Hg; on expiration: RA pressure ↓ 1 mm Hg; LA pressure ↑ 1 mm Hg) during the respiratory cycle as a result of changes in venous filling or preload. Right and left atrial pressures remain approximately equal in both inspiration and expiration (36).

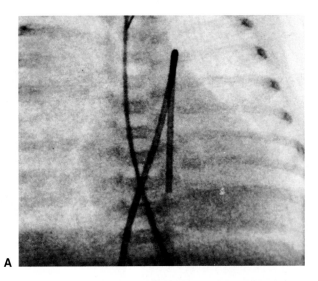

main pulmonary artery   descending aorta

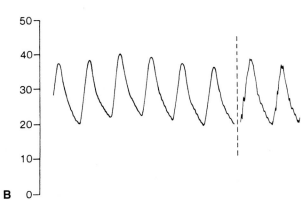

FIG. 30.5. **A:** Radiograph showing venous catheter that has crossed the ductus arteriosus into the thoracic aorta. **B:** In this situation, the arterial pressure markings were not helpful because the presence of pulmonary hypertension in the patient rendered the tracings from the pulmonary artery and descending aorta virtually identical.

d. Hemorrhagic infarction of lung (7)
e. Hydrothorax (catheter lodged in or perforated pulmonary vein) (22)
4. Catheter malpositioned in portal system
  a. Necrotizing enterocolitis (23,24)
  b. Perforation of colon (25)
  c. Hepatic necrosis (thrombosis of hepatic veins or infusion of hypertonic or vasospastic solutions into liver tissues) (Fig. 30.7) (11,12,17,26)
  d. Hepatic cyst (27)
  e. Ascites (secondary to extravasation of fluid through malpositioned catheter) (28)
  f. Hepatic laceration (29)

5. Other
  a. Perforation of peritoneum (30)
  b. Obstruction of pulmonary venous return (in infant with anomalous pulmonary venous drainage) (1)
  c. Plasticizer in tissues (31)
  d. Portal hypertension (16,32)
  e. Electrical hazard (see Chapter 29, J3c) (2)
  f. Fungal mass in right atrium (33)
  g. Pseudomass in left atrium (34)
  h. Digital ischemia (35)
  i. Pneumopericardium (36)

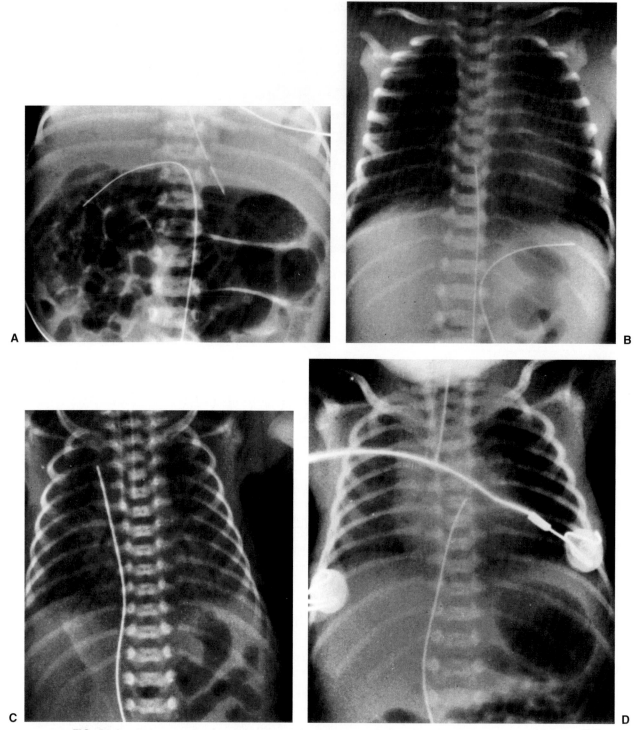

FIG. 30.6.   Spectrum of malpositions of umbilical venous catheters (UVCs) (**A–C**). **A:** UVC in right portal vein with secondary air embolization into portal venous system. **B:** UVC in splenic vein. UAC catheter in good position with its tip at T7. **C:** UVC extending through heart into the superior vena cava. **D, E:** Spectrum of malpositions of UVCs. The anteroposterior film (**D**) shows an indeterminate position of the UVC. The right atrium, the right ventricle, and the left atrium are all possibilities.

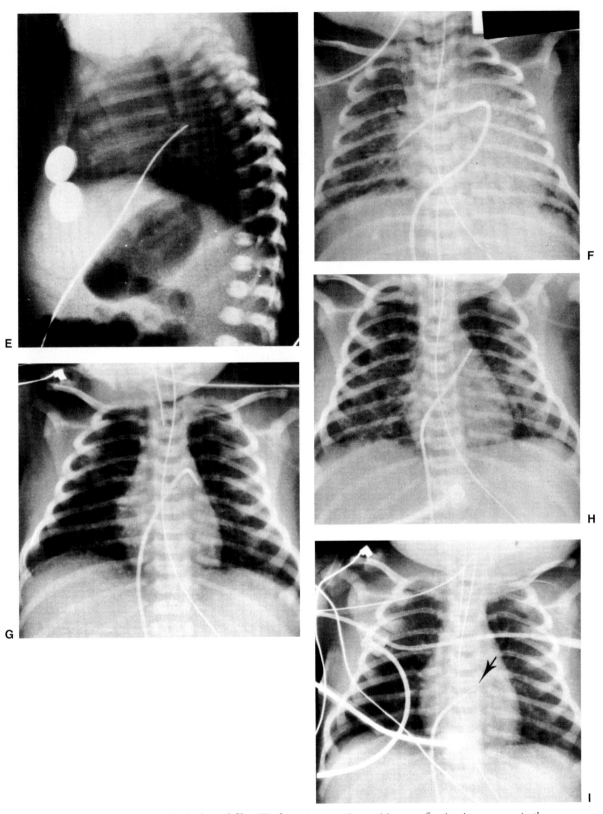

FIG. 30.6. (*Continued*) The lateral film (**E**) shows its posterior position, confirming its presence in the left atrium. The lateral film is particularly important in making this distinction. Measurement of the PO_2 in blood from the catheter will be diagnostic of misplacement, unless the infant has severe persistent pulmonary hypertension or other cause of severe intracardiac shunting. **F–I:** Spectrum of malpositions of UVCs. Series of radiographs demonstrating various malpositions of a venous catheter: right pulmonary artery (**F**), left main pulmonary artery (**G**), main pulmonary artery (**H**), and right ventricle (**I**).

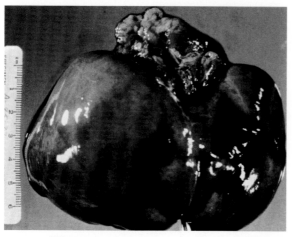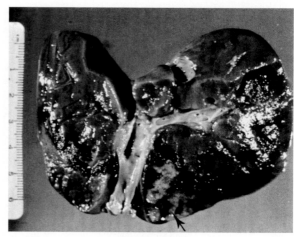

A   **B**

FIG. 30.7. **A:** Hepatic infarction (darkened areas on anterior aspect of liver) related to umbilical vein catheter. **B:** Section through inferior aspect of liver to show internal appearance of infarcted areas (*arrow*).

References

1. Nickerson BG, Sahn DJ, Goldberg SJ, et al. Hazards of inadvertent venous catheterization in a patient with anomalous pulmonary venous drainage: a case report. *Pediatrics.* 1979; 63:929.
2. Kitterman JA, Phibbs RH, Tooley WH. Catheterization of umbilical vessels in newborn infants. *Pediatr Clin North Am.* 1970;17:895.
3. Oestreich AE. Umbilical vein catheterization—appropriate and inappropriate placement. *Pediatr Radiol.* 2010;40:1941.
4. Dunn P. Localization of the umbilical catheter by post-mortem measurement. *Arch Dis Child.* 1966;41:69.
5. Mandel D, Mimouni FB, Littner Y, et al. Double catheter technique for misdirected umbilical vein catheter. *J Pediatr.* 2001;139:5.
6. Baker DH, Berdon WE, James LS. Proper localization of umbilical arterial and venous catheters by lateral roentgenograms. *Pediatrics.* 1969;43:34.
7. Weber AL, Deluce S, Shannan DL. Normal and abnormal position of the umbilical artery and venous catheter on the roentgenogram and review of complications. *AJR.* 1974;20:361.
8. Fleming SE, Kim JH. Ultrasound-guided umbilical catheter insertion in neonates. *J Perinatol.* 2011;31:344.
9. Ades A, Sable C, Cummings S, et al. Echocardiographic evaluation of umbilical venous catheter placement. *J Perinatol.* 2003; 23:24.
10. Anagnostakis D, Kamba A, Petrochilou V, et al. Risk of infection associated with umbilical vein catheterization: a prospective study in 75 newborn infants. *J Pediatr.* 1975;86:759.
11. Brans YW, Ceballos R, Cassady G. Umbilical catheters and hepatic abscesses. *Pediatrics.* 1974;53:264.
12. Centers for Disease Control. Guidelines for prevention of intravascular device-related infections, parts 1 and 2. *Am J Infect Control.* 1996;24:262.
13. Raad II, Luna M, Kaliel S-AM, et al. The relationship between the thrombotic and infectious complications of central venous catheters. *JAMA.* 1994;271:1014.
14. Williams JW, Rittenberry A, Dillard R, et al. Liver abscess in the newborn: complication of umbilical vein catheterization. *Am J Dis Child.* 1973;125:111.
15. Noel GJ, O'Loughlin JE, Edelson PJ. Neonatal staphylococcus epidermitis right sided endocarditis: description of five catheterized infants. *Pediatrics.* 1988;82:234.

16. Oski FA, Allen DM, Diamond LK. Portal hypertension—a complication of umbilical vein catheterization. *Pediatrics.* 1963; 31:297.
17. Sarrut S, Alain J, Allison F. Early complications of umbilical vein perfusion in the premature infant. *Arch Fr Pediatr.* 1969;26:651.
18. Thomson TL, Levine M, Muraskas JK, et al. Pericardial effusion in a preterm infant resulting from umbilical venous catheter placement. *Pediatr Cardiol.* 2010;31:287.
19. Sehgal A, Cook V, Dunn M. Pericardial effusion associated with an appropriately placed umbilical venous catheter. *J Perinatol.* 2007;27:317.
20. Egan EA, Eitzman DV. Umbilical vessel catheterization. *Am J Dis Child.* 1971;121:213.
21. Symchych PS, Krauss AN, Winchester P. Endocarditis following intracardiac placement of umbilical venous catheters in neonates. *J Pediatr.* 1977;90:287.
22. Kulkarni PB, Dorand RD. Hydrothorax: a complication of intracardiac placement of umbilical venous catheters. *J Pediatr.* 1979; 94:813.
23. Livaditis A, Wallgren G, Faxelius G. Necrotizing enterocolitis after catheterization of the umbilical vessels. *Acta Paediatr Scand.* 1974;63:277.
24. Shah KJ, Corkery JJ. Necrotizing enterocolitis following umbilical vein catheterization. *Clin Radiol.* 1978;29:295.
25. Friedman A, Abellera R, Lidsky I, et al. Perforation of the colon after exchange transfusion in the newborn. *N Engl J Med.* 1970;282:796.
26. Venkatavaman PS, Babcock DS, Tsang RC, et al. Hepatic injury: a possible complication of dopamine infusion through an inappropriately placed umbilical vein catheter. *Am J Perinatol.* 1984; 1:351.
27. Levkoff AH, Macpherson RI. Intrahepatic encystment of umbilical vein catheter infusate. *Pediatr Radiol.* 1990;20:360.
28. Nakstad B, Naess PA, Lange C, et al. Complications of umbilical vein catheterization: neonatal total parenteral nutrition ascites after surgical repair of congenital diaphragmatic hernia, *J Pediatr Surg.* 2002;37:1.
29. Yigiter M, Arda IS, Hicsonmez A. Hepatic laceration because of malpositioning of the umbilical vein catheter: case report and literature review. *J Pediatr Surg.* 2008; 43:E39.
30. Kanto WP, Parrish RA. Perforation of the peritoneum and intraabdominal hemorrhage. *Am J Dis Child.* 1977;131:1102.
31. Hillman LS, Goodwin SL, Sherwin WR. Identification and measurement of plasticizer in neonatal tissues after umbilical catheters and blood products. *N Engl J Med.* 1975;292:381.

32. Lauridsen UB, Enk B, Gammeltoft A. Oesophageal varices as a late complication of neonatal umbilical vein catheterization. *Acta Paediatr Scand.* 1978;67:633.

33. Johnson DE, Bass JL, Thomson TR, et al. Candida septicemia and right atrial mass secondary to umbilical vein catheterization. *Am J Dis Child.* 1981;135:275.

34. Crie JS, Hajar R, Folger G. Umbilical catheter masquerading at echocardiography as a left atrial mass. *Clin Cardiol.* 1989;12:728.

35. Welibae MA, Moore JH. Digital ischemia in the neonate following intravenous therapy. *Pediatrics.* 1985;76:99.

36. Long WA. Pneumopericardium. In: Long WA, ed. *Fetal and Neonatal Cardiology* .Philadelphia: WB Saunders; 1990:382.

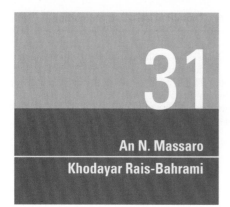

31

An N. Massaro
Khodayar Rais-Bahrami

Peripheral Arterial Cannulation

Arterial access is often needed in the care of the sick neonate for continuous hemodynamic monitoring and blood sampling. For various technical or clinical reasons, catheterization of the umbilical artery is not always possible. Therefore, peripheral arterial cannulation may be required. As a general rule, the most peripheral available artery should be used, to reduce the potential sequelae from any associated vascular compromise or thromboembolic event. The artery chosen should be large enough to measure blood pressure without occlusion, have adequate collateral circulation, be at a site with low infection risk, and be in an area that can be easily monitored and cared for by nursing staff. Common sites for peripheral arterial cannulation include the radial, ulnar, dorsalis pedis, and posterior tibial arteries. Although cannulation of the axillary (1,2) and brachial (3) arteries have been described, these sites are not recommended because of the limited collateral blood flow and high potential for ischemic complications. Cannulation of the temporal artery should likewise be avoided due to potential adverse neurologic sequelae (4,5).

A. Indications

1. Monitoring of arterial blood pressure
2. Frequent monitoring of blood gases or laboratory tests (e.g., sick ventilated neonates or extremely low-birthweight premature infants)
3. When preductal measurement is required (e.g., with persistent pulmonary hypertension) (right upper extremity cannulation)

B. Contraindications

1. Bleeding disorder that cannot be corrected
2. Pre-existing evidence of circulatory insufficiency in limb being used for cannulation
3. Evidence of inadequate collateral flow (i.e., occlusion of the vessel to be catheterized may compromise perfusion of extremity)
4. Local skin infection
5. Malformation of the extremity being used for cannulation
6. Previous surgery in the area (especially cutdown)

C. Equipment

Sterile

1. Gloves
2. Antiseptic solution (e.g., iodophor, chlorhexidine)
3. 4- × 4-inch gauze squares
4. 0.5 to 0.95 normal saline (NS) with 1 to 2 U/mL heparin

    Although hypernatremia has been reported in very small premature infants who received excess sodium in flush solution (6), in our experience 0.5 NS has been used without complications at infusion rates of 0.5 to 1 mL/h. Using heparinized saline has been shown to maintain line patency longer than hypotonic solutions such as heparinized 5% dextrose water (7) or unheparinized NS (8).
5. 3- or 5-mL syringe
6. 20-gauge venipuncture needle (if using larger-sized 22-gauge cannula)
7. Appropriate-sized cannula: 22-gauge × 1-inch (2.5-cm), 24-gauge × 0.75-inch, or 24-gauge × 0.56-inch tapered or nontapered cannula with stylet for larger to smaller neonates, respectively
8. Antiseptic ointment (optional)
9. Arterial pressure transducer and extension tubing (see Chapter 9)
10. 5-0 nylon suture with curved needle (optional)
11. Needle holder (optional)
12. Suture scissors (optional)
13. T connector primed with heparinized flush solution
14. Transparent, semipermeable dressing

Nonsterile

1. Equipment for transillumination (see Chapter 13) or Doppler ultrasound

    Use of Doppler ultrasound for localization of the artery (9,10) and assessment of the adequacy of the palmar circulation has been described (11,12)
2. 0.5-inch, water-resistant adhesive tape
3. Materials for forearm restraint (see Chapter 4) for radial or ulnar cannulation
4. A constant-infusion pump capable of delivering flush solution at rate of 0.5 to 1 mL/h against back pressure

Additional Equipment Required for Cutdown Procedure

All equipment except mask must be sterile.

1. Gown and mask
2. 0.5% lidocaine hydrochloride in labeled 3-mL syringe
3. No. 11 scalpel and holder
4. Two curved mosquito hemostats
5. Nerve hook
6. 5-0 nylon suture

D. Precautions

1. When performing radial artery cannulation, always check ulnar collateral circulation using the Allen test (13–15) prior to undertaking the procedure. This test is recognized to have limitations regarding accuracy and interrater reliability (16), so careful observation for signs of impaired distal perfusion is still required during and after the procedure. Doppler ultrasound (11,12) may also be useful in assessing collateral circulation.

2. When performing dorsalis pedis or posterior tibial cannulation, a modified Allen test can be performed by raising the foot, occluding the dorsalis pedis and posterior tibial arteries, releasing pressure over one, and monitoring for tissue perfusion within 10 seconds, although this technique is less reliable than testing in the hand (17).

3. When performing radial or ulnar cannulation, avoid excessive hyperextension of wrist, because this may result in occlusion of artery and a false-positive Allen test (18) and has been associated with median nerve conduction block (19).

4. Leave all fingertips/toes exposed so that circulatory status may be monitored. Examine limb frequently for changes in perfusion.

5. Never ligate artery.

6. Take care not to introduce air bubbles into cannula while assembling infusion system or taking blood samples.

7. Make sure that a continuous pressure waveform tracing is displayed on a monitor screen at all times.

8. Be aware that the blood pressure measured in the lower extremity may be 5 to 20 mm Hg higher than in the upper extremity, and the reading may be delayed by one tenth of a second (17).

9. Do not administer a rapid bolus injection of fluid via line, because there is a danger of retrograde embolization of clot or air (20). Flush infusion after sampling should be:
   a. Minimal volume (0.3 to 0.5 mL)
   b. Injected slowly

10. To reverse arteriospasm, see Chapter 34.

11. Use cannula for sampling only; no fluids other than heparinized saline flush solution should be administered via cannula.

12. Remove cannula at first indication of clot formation or circulatory compromise (e.g., dampening of waveform on monitor). Do not flush to remove clots.

13. Inspect cannula insertion site at least daily.
   a. If signs of cellulitis are present, remove the cannula and send the cannula tip for culture. Also, send a wound culture if there is inflammation at the cutdown site.
   b. Obtain a blood culture from a peripheral site if signs of sepsis are present.
   c. Inspect the area distal and proximal to the insertion site for blanching, redness, cyanosis, or changes in temperature or capillary refill time.

14. Remove cannula as soon as indications no longer exist.

E. Technique

Standard Technique for Percutaneous Arterial Cannulation

1. Choose a site for cannulation and secure the appropriate limb.
   a. *Radial artery*: This is the most routine site for cannulation (15,21). The infant's forearm and hand can be transilluminated with the wrist in extension 45 to 60 degrees (Fig. 31.1), making sure that fingers are visible to monitor distal perfusion. The artery can be palpated proximal to the transverse crease on the palmar surface of the wrist, medial to the styloid process of the radius, and lateral to the flexor carpi radialis (Fig. 31.2).
   b. *Ulnar artery*: In a small number of infants, the ulnar artery may be easier to locate than the radial artery (22). If an Allen test indicates that the collateral blood supply is adequate, the ulnar artery may be cannulated using the same method as for a radial artery. The ulnar artery runs along the palmar margin of the flexor carpi ulnaris, radial to the pisiform bone.

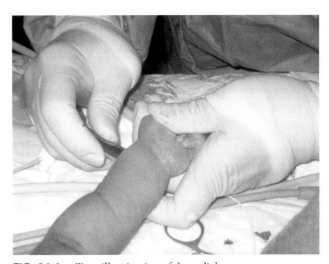

FIG. 31.1. Transillumination of the radial artery.

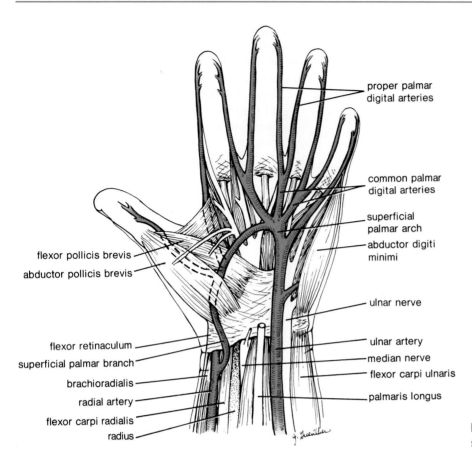

FIG. 31.2. Anatomic relations of the major arteries of the wrist and hand.

Labels (top to bottom, right side):
proper palmar digital arteries
common palmar digital arteries
superficial palmar arch
abductor digiti minimi
ulnar nerve
ulnar artery
median nerve
flexor carpi ulnaris
palmaris longus

Labels (left side):
flexor pollicis brevis
abductor pollicis brevis
flexor retinaculum
superficial palmar branch
brachioradialis
radial artery
flexor carpi radialis
radius

Caution is necessary when cannulating the ulnar artery because it runs next to the ulnar nerve and is smaller in caliber than the radial artery (Fig. 31.2).

   c. *Dorsalis pedis artery:* The dorsalis pedis artery can be found in the dorsal midfoot between the first and second toes with the foot held in plantar flexion (Fig. 31.3). It should be noted that the vascular anatomy of the foot is variable and the dorsalis pedis artery may be absent in some patients (23), whereas it may provide the main blood supply to the toes in others (24).

   d. *Posterior tibial artery:* The posterior tibial artery runs posterior to the medial malleolus with the foot held in dorsiflexion (Fig. 31.4).

2. Identify artery by
   a. Palpation (see anatomic landmarks as described above or individual arterial sites)
   b. Transillumination (see Fig. 13.1 and Chapter 13) (25)
   c. Doppler ultrasound (9–11)
3. Scrub and put on gloves.
4. Prepare skin over site with antiseptic (e.g., an iodophor).
5. Make small skin puncture with venipuncture needle over site (optional; to ease passage of cannula through skin and reduce chances of penetrating the posterior wall of the vessel, especially when using a larger-gauge cannula).
6. Accomplish cannulation of artery (Fig. 31.5).

Method A (Preferred for Small Premature Neonates) (Fig. 31.6)

   a. Puncture artery directly at an angle of 10 to 15 degrees to the skin, with the needle bevel down.
   b. Advance slowly. There will be arteriospasm when the vessel is touched, and blood return may be delayed.
   c. Withdraw needle stylet (blood should appear in the cannula) and advance cannula into artery as far as possible.

Method B (Fig. 31.5B)

   a. Pass needle stylet (with bevel up) and cannula through artery at 30- to 40-degree angle to skin.
   b. Remove stylet and withdraw cannula slowly until arterial flow is established.
   c. Advance cannula into artery.

     The inability to insert the cannula into the lumen usually indicates failure to puncture the artery centrally. This often results in laceration of the lateral wall of the artery with formation of a hematoma, which can be seen on transillumination.

7. Attach cannula firmly to T connector and gently flush with 0.5 mL of heparinized solution, observing for evidence of blanching or cyanosis.
8. Apply iodophor ointment (optional) to puncture site.
9. Suture cannula to skin with 5-0 nylon suture if desired.

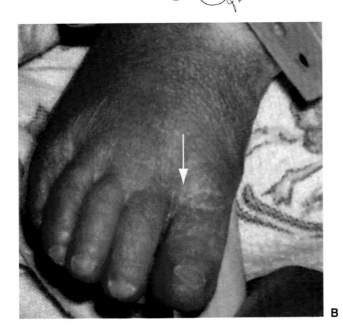

tibialis anterior

inferior extensor retinaculum

lateral malleolus

tendons of extensor digitorum longus

peroneus tertius tendon

dorsalis pedis artery & vein

extensor hallucis brevis

medial tarsal artery & vein

extensor hallucis longus

extensor digitorum brevis

deep peroneal nerve

A

B

FIG. 31.3. **A:** Anatomic relations of dorsalis pedis artery. **B:** *White arrow* shows anatomic location of dorsalis pedis artery.

This step may be omitted as long as cannula is securely taped (Fig. 27.4); use of sutures may produce a more unsightly scar.

10. Secure cannula as done with peripheral IV line, as shown in Fig. 27.4. Transparent semipermeable dressing may be used in place of tape to allow continuous visualization of skin entry site. Guarantee that all digits are visible for frequent inspection.

11. Maintain patency by attaching T connector to extension tubing or arterial pressure line to run 0.5 to 1 mL/h of heparinized flush solution by constant infusion pump.

12. Change IV tubing and flushing solution every 24 hours.

Radial Artery Cutdown

Cutdown technique may be required for the very small neonate, because trauma to the artery causes vasospasm, which makes percutaneous cannulation of a small vessel very difficult.

1. *Technique I:* Cutdown at wrist

The artery is initially exposed by cutdown, and a catheter is inserted under direct vision.

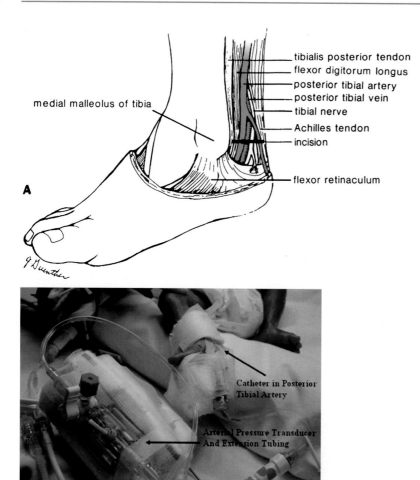

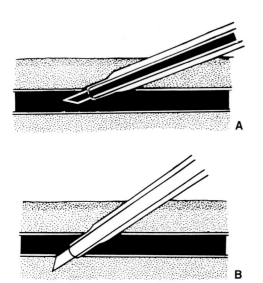

FIG. 31.4. **A:** Anatomic relations of posterior tibial artery, showing site of incision for cutdown. **B:** Cannulation of posterior tibial artery; cannula is attached to a transducer for continuous blood pressure monitoring.

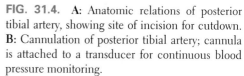

FIG. 31.5. **A:** Cannulation of artery using Method A (see text). **B:** Cannulation of artery using Method B (see text). (Redrawn from Filston HC, Johnson DG. Percutaneous venous cannulation in neonates and infants: a method for catheter insertion without "cutdown." *Pediatrics.* 1971;48:896, with permission of the American Academy of Pediatrics.)

a. Prepare as for percutaneous procedure (Standard Technique, steps 1 to 3).
b. Scrub and prepare as for major procedure (see Chapter 5).
c. Infiltrate site of incision (point of maximum pulsation just proximal to proximal wrist crease) with 0.5 to 1 mL of lidocaine.
d. Wait 5 minutes for anesthesia.
e. Make a 0.5-cm transverse skin incision (Fig. 31.7A).
f. Deepen incision into subcutaneous tissue by blunt longitudinal dissection with curved mosquito hemostat (Fig. 31.7B).
g. Use curved mosquito hemostat to dissect artery free. Be gentle, to avoid arteriospasm.
h. Elevate artery with hemostat or nerve hook (Fig. 31.7C).
i. Loop ligature (5-0 silk) around artery for traction purposes (Fig. 31.7D). Do not tie ligature.
j. Advance cannula stylet into artery with bevel down, until cannula is clearly within vessel lumen (Fig. 31.7E).

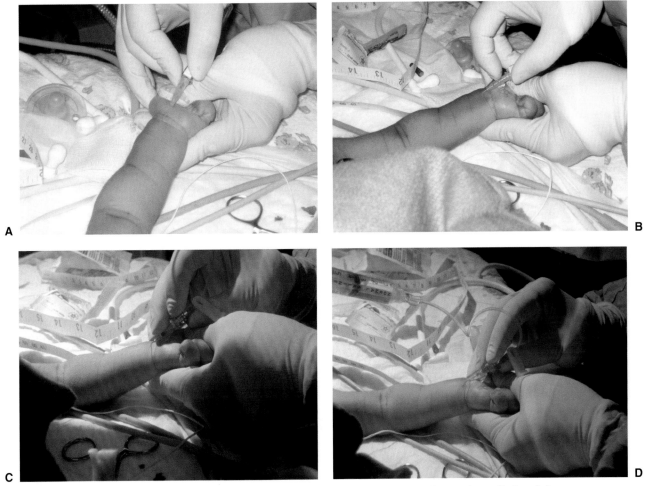

FIG. 31.6. **A:** Puncture artery directly at angle of 10 to 15 degrees to skin, with needle bevel down. **B:** Advance slowly. **C:** Withdraw needle stylet, allow for blood return, and advance cannula into artery. **D:** Attach cannula firmly to T connector.

k. Remove stylet and advance cannula to hub (Fig. 31.7F).

l. Remove ligature.

m. See percutaneous method under E (Standard Technique, steps 7 to 11) for fixation and care of cannula.

   The incision can usually be kept small enough so that the hub of the cannula fills it and no closing suture is needed.

2. Technique II: Cannulation at anatomic snuffbox

   a. Described by Amato et al. (26)

   b. May be used in infants who have undergone previous arterial cutdown at wrist

   c. Should not be a primary approach to radial artery (particularly if cannulation is achieved by cutdown)

      (1) Site is not easy to expose.

      (2) Scar tends to be more disfiguring than at wrist.

   d. The radial artery passes dorsally at the wrist and traverses the anatomic snuffbox, which is bounded medially by the extensor pollicis longus and extensor pollicis brevis muscles (Fig. 31.8A).

   e. The artery becomes superficial immediately after passing the extensor pollicis longus and before passing beneath the first dorsal interosseous muscle.

   f. The point for cannulation is located at the junction of a line drawn along the medial aspect of the extended thumb and another line drawn along the lateral aspect of the extended index finger (Fig. 31.8B).

Posterior tibial Artery Cannulation by a Cutdown Procedure

1. Prepare as for percutaneous method.

2. Put on mask.

3. Tape foot to footboard in equinovarus position (see Chapter 4).

4. Scrub and prepare as for major procedure (see Chapter 5).

5. Infiltrate incision site with 0.5 to 1 mL of 0.5% lidocaine (Fig. 31.4).

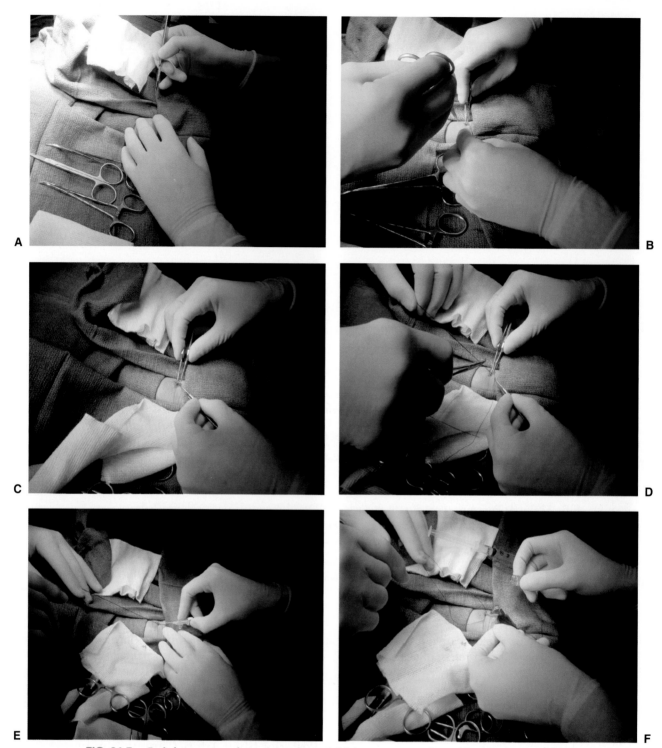

FIG. 31.7.   Radial artery cannulation by cutdown. **A:** Making transverse skin incision. **B:** Blunt dissection with mosquito hemostat. **C:** Elevating artery with artery hook. **D:** Looping ligature around artery. **E:** Introducing cannula into artery while gentle "back traction" is applied to suture. **F:** Cannula advanced to hub.

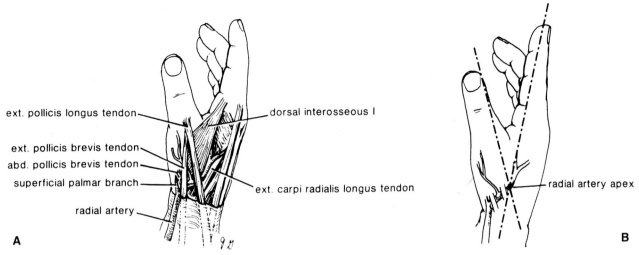

FIG. 31.8. **A:** Anatomic relations of the radial artery on the volar aspect of the wrist. **B:** Point for cannulation of the radial artery is indicated by the junction of the dotted lines. (Redrawn from Amato JJ, Solod E, Cleveland RJ. A "second" radial artery for monitoring the perioperative pediatric cardiac patient. *J Pediatr Surg.* 1977;12:715, with permission.)

6. Wait 5 minutes for anesthesia.
7. Make transverse incision (0.5 cm) posteroinferior to medial malleolus (see Fig. 31.4).

    A vertical, rather than a transverse, incision is optional. The former has the advantage that it offers the opportunity to extend the incision cephalad, should the posterior wall of the vein be perforated on the initial attempt at cannulation. However, it has the disadvantage that it may be made too far lateral or medial to the artery.

8. Identify artery by longitudinal dissection with mosquito hemostat. The artery is usually found just anterior to the Achilles tendon and adjacent to the tibial nerve.
9. Place mosquito hemostat behind artery, and loop 5-0 nylon suture loosely around it.

    Be gentle, to avoid arteriospasm.
10. Elevate artery in wound with suture. Do not ligate artery.
11. While stabilizing artery with suture, insert needle and cannula, with bevel down.
12. Withdraw stylet and advance cannula to hub.
13. Remove nylon suture.
14. Close wound with 5-0 nylon suture (usually requires only one suture).
15. See percutaneous method under E (Standard Technique, steps 7 to 11) for fixation and care of cannula.

F. Obtaining Arterial Samples

Equipment

1. Gloves
2. Alcohol swabs
3. Sterile 2- × 2-inch gauze squares (for three-drop method)
4. 25-gauge straight needle (for three-drop method)
5. Appropriate-sized syringe for sample (heparinized if sample is not processed on site)
6. Syringe with flush (for stopcock method)
7. Ice if necessary for sample preservation
8. Specimen labels and requisition slips

Technique I: Three-Drop Method

1. Wash hands and put on gloves.
2. Clean diaphragm of T connector with antiseptic solution and allow to dry.
3. Clamp T-connector tubing close to hub.
4. Place sterile gauze squares beneath hub.
5. Introduce 25-gauge needle through diaphragm and allow 3 to 4 drops of fluid/blood to drip onto gauze.
6. Attach syringe to needle and withdraw sample.
7. Remove needle from diaphragm.
8. Unclamp T connector and allow residual pump pressure to flush catheter.

Technique II: Stopcock Method (a Three-Way Stopcock Needs to be Interposed between the Patient and the Transducer)

1. Wash hands and put on gloves.
2. Clean hub of stopcock with antiseptic solution.
3. Attach syringe to stopcock.
4. Turn stopcock off to infusion pump.
5. Aspirate waste (volume depends on length of tubing).
6. Using second syringe, withdraw sample.
7. Flush cannula slowly, over 30 to 60 seconds, with 0.5 mL of flush solution.
8. Open stopcock to pump, to allow for continued infusion of heparinized saline.

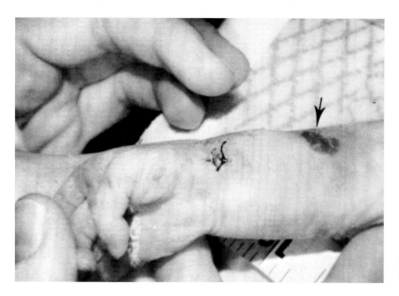

FIG. 31.9. Complication of cannulation of the radial artery. *Arrow* indicates necrotic area on forearm.

G. Removal of the Cannula

Indications

1. Stabilization or resolution of the indications for cannulation of the artery
2. Cannula-related infection
3. Evidence of thrombosis or mechanical occlusion of the artery

Technique

1. Remove tape/dressing and cut stitch (if present) securing cannula to skin.
2. Remove cannula gently.
3. Apply local pressure for 5 to 10 minutes.

H. Complications of Peripheral Arterial Cannulation

1. Thromboembolism/vasospasm/thrombosis
   a. Blanching of hand, gangrene of fingertips, partial loss of digits (14,21,22,27) Topical nitroglycerine has been reported to restore perfusion in some cases. (28,29) Warming of the contralateral limb, to produce reflex vasodilation, can also be used. (30)
   b. Necrosis of forearm and hand (Fig. 31.9) (27,31)
   c. Skin ulcers (31)
   d. Ischemia/necrosis of toes (Fig. 31.10) (32,33)
   e. Cerebral emboli (4,20,34)
   f. Reversible occlusion of artery (14,34)
2. Infiltration of infusate (32)
3. Infection (35)
4. Hematoma (21)
5. Damage to peripheral nerves
   a. Median nerve above medial epicondyle of humerus (Fig. 31.11A) may affect the following
      (1) Pronation of forearm
      (2) Abduction of wrist
      (3) Flexion of wrist and distal phalanges of middle and index fingers
      (4) Opposition, abduction, and flexion of thumb (atrophy of thenar eminence)

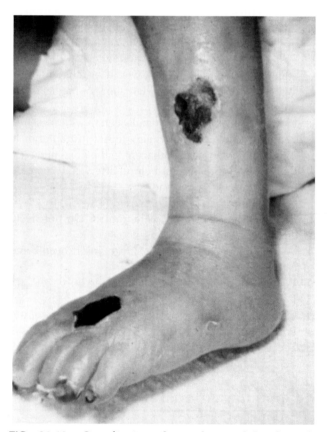

FIG. 31.10. Complication of cannulation of dorsalis pedis artery. Healing areas of sloughed skin are seen at site of skin puncture on dorsum of foot and also on anterior aspect of lower leg. Tips of toes 1, 3, 4, and 5 are necrotic.

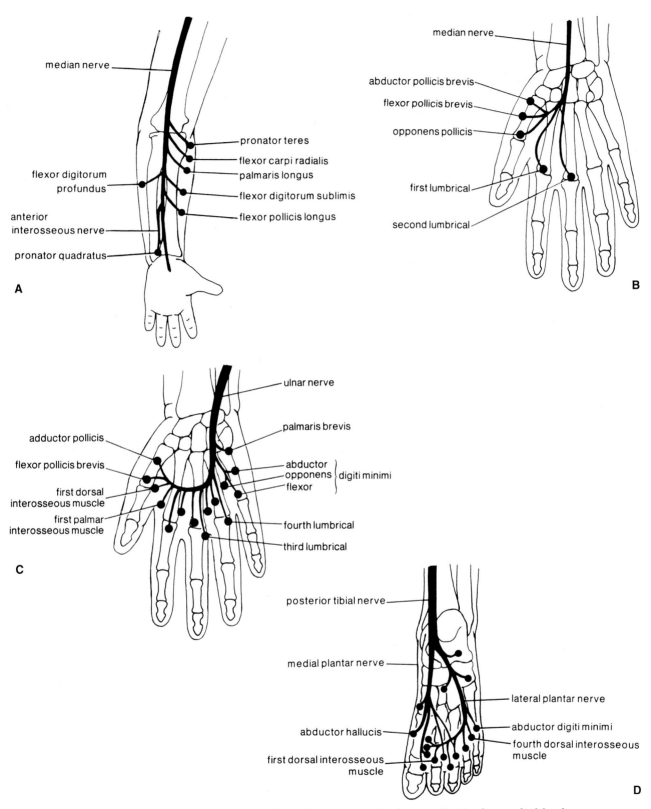

FIG. 31.11. **A:** Muscles supplied by the median nerve in the forearm. **B:** Muscles supplied by the median nerve in the hand. **C:** Muscles supplied by the ulnar nerve in the hand. **D:** Muscles supplied by the posterior tibial nerve in the ankle and foot.

(5) Sensation—maximally over volar aspect index and middle fingers

(6) Vasomotor control in limb

b. Median nerve at wrist (Fig. 31.11B) causes carpal tunnel syndrome (19).

c. Ulnar nerve at wrist causes (Fig. 31.11C)

(1) Atrophy of small hand muscles

(2) Sensory loss over dorsal and palmar surfaces of ring and little fingers and ulnar portion of hand and wrist

d. Peripheral portion of deep peroneal nerve—anesthesia of the lateral aspect of the dorsum of the hand, which results in no significant disability

e. Posterior tibial nerve at medial malleolus (Fig. 31.11D) may affect

(1) Flexor hallucis brevis muscle

(2) Flexor of proximal phalanx of big toe

(3) Muscles of foot that spread and close toes and flex proximal phalanx of toes

(4) Sensation on plantar surface of foot

   Lesions of posterior tibial nerve may be difficult to detect on examination but may lead to significant discomfort in later life owing to loss of plantar arches on weight bearing.

6. False cortical thumbs (36)

7. Burns from transilluminator (37)

8. Hemorrhage (including accidental dislodgement of cannula) (32,34)

9. Hypernatremia caused by heparinized saline infusion through cannula (6)

10. Hypervolemia related to continuous flush device (38)

11. Air embolism (39)

12. Pseudoaneurysm (40)

13. Acquired bone dysplasia (41)

References

1. Greenwald BM, Notterman DA, DeBruin WJ, et al. Percutaneous axillary artery catheterization in critically ill infants and children. *J Pediatr.* 1990;117:442.

2. Piotrowski A, Kawczynski P. Cannulation of the axillary artery in critically ill newborn infants. *Eur J Pediatr.* 1995;154:57.

3. Schindler E, Kowald B, Suess H, et al. Catheterization of the radial or brachial artery in neonates and infants. *Paediatr Anaesth.* 2005;15:677.

4. Prian GW, Wright GB, Rumack CM, et al. Apparent cerebral embolization after temporal artery catheterization. *J Pediatr.* 1978; 93:115.

5. Bull MJ, Schreiner RL, Garg BP, et al. Neurologic complications following temporal artery catheterization. *J Pediatr.* 1980;96:1071.

6. Hayden WR. Hypernatremia due to heparinized saline infusion through a radial artery catheter in a very low-birth-weight infant. *J Pediatr.* 1978;92:1025.

7. Rais-Bahrami K, Karna P, Dolanski EA. Effect of fluids on life span of peripheral arterial lines. *Am J Perinatol.* 1990;7:122.

8. Clifton GD, Branson P, Kelly HJ, et al. Comparison of normal saline and heparin solutions for maintenance of arterial catheter patency. *Heart Lung.* 1991;20:115.

9. Maher JJ, Dougherty JM. Radial artery cannulation guided by Doppler ultrasound. *Am J Emerg Med.* 1989;7:260.

10. Schwemmer U, Arzet HA, Trautner H, et al. Ultrasound-guided arterial cannulation in infants improves success rate. *Eur J Anaesthesiol.* 2006;23:476.

11. Morray JP, Brandford HG, Barnes LF, et al. Doppler-assisted radial artery cannulation in infants and children. *Anesth Analg.* 1984;63:346.

12. Mozersky DJ, Buckley CJ, Hagood CO Jr, et al. Ultrasonic evaluation of the palmar circulation. A useful adjunct to radial artery cannulation. *Am J Surg.* 1973;126:810.

13. Allen EV. Thromboangiitis obliterans: methods of diagnosis of chronic occlusive arterial lesions distal to the wrist with illustrative cases. *Am J Med Sci.* 1929;178:237.

14. Hack WW, Vos A, van der Lei J, et al. Incidence and duration of total occlusion of the radial artery in newborn infants after catheter removal. *Eur J Pediatr.* 1990;149:275.

15. Wallach SG. Cannulation injury of the radial artery: diagnosis and treatment algorithm. *Am J Crit Care.* 2004;13:315.

16. Barone JE, Madlinger RV. Should an Allen test be performed before radial artery cannulation? *J Trauma.* 2006;61:468.

17. Johnstone RE, Greenhow DE. Catheterization of the dorsalis pedis artery. *Anesthesiology.* 1973;39:654.

18. Greenhow DE. Incorrect performance of Allen's test:-ulnar-artery flow erroneously presumed inadequate. *Anesthesiology.* 1972;37:356.

19. Chowet AL, Lopez JR, Brock-Utne JG, et al. Wrist hyperextension leads to median nerve conduction block: implications for intra-arterial catheter placement. *Anesthesiology.* 2004;100:287.

20. Lowenstein E, Little JW 3rd, Lo HH. Prevention of cerebral embolization from flushing radial-artery cannulas. *N Engl J Med.* 1971;285:1414.

21. Adams JM, Rudolph AJ. The use of indwelling radial artery catheters in neonates. *Pediatrics.* 1975;55:261.

22. Kahler AC, Mirza F. Alternative arterial catheterization site using the ulnar artery in critically ill pediatric patients. *Pediatr Crit Care Med.* 2002;3:370.

23. Huber JF. The arterial network supplying the dorsum of the foot. *Anat Rec.* 1941;80:373.

24. Spoerel WE, Deimling P, Aitken R. Direct arterial pressure monitoring from the dorsalis pedis artery. *Can Anaesth Soc J.* 1975;22:91.

25. Pearse RG. Percutaneous catheterisation of the radial artery in newborn babies using transillumination. *Arch Dis Child.* 1978;53:549.

26. Amato JJ, Solod E, Cleveland RJ. A "second" radial artery for monitoring the perioperative pediatric cardiac patient. *J Pediatr Surg.* 1977;12:715.

27. Hack WW, Vos A, Okken A. Incidence of forearm and hand ischaemia related to radial artery cannulation in newborn infants. *Intensive Care Med.* 1990;16:50.

28. Vasquez P, Burd A, Mehta R, et al. Resolution of peripheral artery catheter-induced ischemic injury following prolonged treatment with topical nitroglycerin ointment in a newborn: a case report. *J Perinatol.* 2003;23:348.

29. Baserga MC, Puri A, Sola A. The use of topical nitroglycerin ointment to treat peripheral tissue ischemia secondary to arterial line complications in neonates. *J Perinatol.* 2002;22:416.

30. Detaille T, Pirotte T, Veyckemans F. Vascular access in the neonate. *Best Pract Res Clin Anaesthesiol.* 2010;24:403.

31. Wyatt R, Glaves I, Cooper DJ. Proximal skin necrosis after radial-artery cannulation. *Lancet.* 1974;1:1135.

32. Spahr RC, MacDonald HM, Holzman IR. Catheterization of the posterior tibial artery in the neonate. *Am J Dis Child.* 1979;133:945.

33. Abrahamson EL, Scott RC, Jurges E, et al. Catheterization of posterior tibial artery leading to limb amputation. *Acta Paediatr.* 1993;82:618.

34. Miyasaka K, Edmonds JF, Conn AW. Complications of radial artery lines in the paediatric patient. *Can Anaesth Soc J.* 1976; 23:9.

35. Adams JM, Speer ME, Rudolph AJ. Bacterial colonization of radial artery catheters. *Pediatrics.* 1980;65:94.

36. Skoglund RR, Giles EE. The false cortical thumb. *Am J Dis Child.* 1986;140:375.

37. Uy J, Kuhns LR, Wall PM, et al. Light filtration during transillumination of the neonate: a method to reduce heat buildup in the skin.*Pediatrics.* 1977;60:308.

38. Morray J, Todd S. A hazard of continuous flush systems for vascular pressure monitoring in infants. *Anesthesiology.* 1983;58:187.

39. Chang C, Dughi J, Shitabata P, et al. Air embolism and the radial arterial line. *Crit Care Med.* 1988;6:141.

40. Dzepina I, Unusic J, Mijatovic D, et al. Pseudoaneurysms of the brachial artery following venipuncture in infants. *Pediatr Surg Int.* 2004;20:594.

41. Seibert JJ, McCarthy RE, Alexander JE, et al. Acquired bone dysplasia secondary to catheter-related complications in the neonate. *Pediatr Radiol.* 1986;16:43.

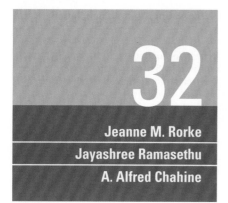

32

Jeanne M. Rorke
Jayashree Ramasethu
A. Alfred Chahine

Central Venous Catheterization

Central venous catheters provide stable IV access to sick or low-birthweight infants who need long-term IV nutrition or medications (1).

A percutaneous central venous catheter, also known as a peripherally inserted central catheter (PICC), is a soft, flexible catheter that is inserted into a peripheral vein and threaded into the central venous system. Central venous lines may be placed by surgical cutdown when percutaneous access is not possible. Totally implantable vascular access devices (ports) are rarely used in neonates and are thus not included in this chapter.

Regardless of the method employed to obtain secure and reliable venous access, the clinician should be familiar with the technique and anatomic considerations unique to the approach. Some form of analgesia and sedation is generally required, with general anesthesia being reserved for more complex access cases. The majority of venous access procedures in the critically ill neonate are performed at the bedside rather than in the operating room.

A. Common Indications

1. Total parenteral nutrition
2. Long-term IV medication administration
3. Administration of hyperosmolar IV fluids or irritating medications that cannot be administered through peripheral IV cannulas.
4. Fluid resuscitation
5. Repetitive blood draws (catheters are not usually inserted primarily for this indication in neonates; only larger-lumen catheters may be used for blood draws without risk of clotting).

B. Relative Contraindications

There are no absolute contraindications, as the clinical situation dictates the need for venous access.

1. Skin infection at insertion site
2. Uncorrected bleeding diathesis (not a contraindication for percutaneous catheters inserted in distal peripheral venous sites)

3. Ongoing bacteremia or fungal infection (which may cause catheter colonization and infection)
4. The patient can be treated adequately with peripheral IV access. Central venous catheters have significant risks of complications and must not be used when peripheral venous access is possible and adequate.

C. General Precautions

1. Central venous catheterization must be performed by trained individuals who are familiar with the venous anatomy of the proposed catheter route.
2. Obtain informed consent prior to performing the procedure.
3. *Plan ahead*: Success with PICC placement is higher if the catheter is inserted electively before peripheral veins are "used up" by frequent cannulations.
4. Infant should be on a cardiorespiratory monitor during the procedure.
5. Follow the manufacturer's instructions for catheter use.
6. Maintain strict aseptic technique for the insertion and care of central catheter. Hand hygiene (with soap and water or with alcohol based hand rub) should be performed before and after palpating catheter insertion sites, as well as before and after inserting, replacing, accessing, repairing or dressing an intravascular catheter (2).
7. Never leave a catheter in a position where it does not easily and repeatedly withdraw blood during the insertion procedure, to ensure that the tip is not lodged against a blood vessel or cardiac wall.
8. Always *confirm* (both AP and lateral radiographs are recommended) the position of the catheter tip by radiography or echocardiography prior to using it.
9. If possible, the line should be inserted and cared for by specifically trained personnel. Central line teams and the use of insertion and maintenance checklists and bundles have been shown to decrease the frequency of catheter-related infections (3).
10. Do not submerge the catheter or catheter site in water.

TABLE 32.1	Vessels Amenable to Central Venous Access	

Blood Vessel	Recommended Technique
Upper extremity: Cephalic, basilic, median cubital, or axillary vein	Percutaneous or surgical
Lower extremity: Saphenous vein or femoral vein	Percutaneous or surgical
Scalp vein	Percutaneous technique, amenable only to PICC lines
External jugular vein	Percutaneous or surgical
Internal jugular vein or common facial vein	Surgical technique

D. Vessels Amenable to Central Venous Access

Table 32.1 lists the sites usually used for central venous catheterization in the newborn.

E. Position of Catheter Tip (Fig. 32.1)

1. The catheter should be placed in as large a vein as possible, ideally outside the heart, and parallel with the long axis of the vein such that the tip does not abut the vein or heart wall. The recommendations for appropriate position of a central venous catheter tip vary, but there is general agreement that the tip should *not* be within the right atrium (4–6). However, one large retrospective audit of 2,186 catheters showed that catheters with their tips in the right atrium *and not coiled* were not associated with pericardial effusions (7).
   a. When inserted from the upper extremity, the catheter tip should be in the superior vena cava (SVC), outside the cardiac reflection, or at the junction of the SVC and right atrium.
   b. When inserted from the lower extremity, the catheter tip should be above the L4–L5 vertebrae or the iliac crest, but not in the heart.

2. Confirmation of catheter tip placement
   a. The tip of the radio-opaque catheter is usually seen on a routine chest radiograph (Fig. 32.1), but there can be significant interobserver variability in assessing the position, even with digital enhancement (8).
   b. Two radiographic views (anteroposterior and lateral) help to confirm that the catheter is in a central vein. This is particularly important for catheters placed in a lower extremity, where the catheter may inadvertently be in an ascending lumbar vein and may appear to be in good position on an anteroposterior view (9).
   c. The use of radio-opaque contrast improves localization of the catheter tip, particularly when the catheter is difficult to see on a standard radiograph. A 0.5-mL aliquot of 0.9% saline is instilled into the catheter to check patency, followed by 0.5 mL of iohexol. The radiograph is taken, and the line is flushed again with 0.5 mL of 0.9% saline. With this technique, there is no need to inject the contrast material while the radiograph is being taken (10).
   d. Ultrasonography may also be useful in localizing the catheter tip (11).
   e. Chest radiographs obtained for any reason should be scrutinized for appropriate catheter position. Routine weekly radiographs taken for this purpose do not appear to reduce the risk of complications (6).

F. Methods of Vascular Access

1. Percutaneous technique
   a. Advantages
      (1) Simpler to perform and relatively rapid procedure
      (2) Vessel is not ligated as in open cutdown methods
      (3) Decreased potential for wound infection/dehiscence complications
   b. Disadvantages
      (1) Beyond the initial insertion into the peripheral vein, further passage of the catheter into its final position is essentially a blind technique, although there is increasing experience with ultrasound imaging (11).
      (2) A smaller-caliber catheter may preclude use for blood transfusions

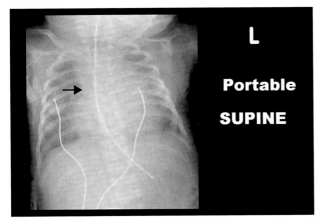

FIG. 32.1. Chest radiograph with PICC tip in appropriate position, just above junction of superior vena cava and right atrium.

2. Cutdown or open surgical technique
   a. Advantages
      (1) Allows for insertion of larger silicone catheter (3 or 4.2 French [Fr])
      (2) The catheters can be tunneled under the skin away from the venotomy site, so they can remain in place longer with a lower risk of infection.
   b. Disadvantages
      (1) Requires general anesthesia or IV sedation
      (2) Requires surgical incision
      (3) Vein is often ligated, so it cannot be reused in the future.
      (4) Potential for injury to adjacent anatomical structures
      (5) Increased potential for wound infection
      (6) An operating room is the ideal setting for the procedure, so risks of transport of critically ill neonates need to be taken into consideration.

G. Types of Central Venous Catheters

1. Catheter materials: See Table 32.2.
2. Types of catheters
   a. Percutaneous (PICC) catheters/introducers
      PICC catheters and kits are available commercially. PICCs are generally made of silicone or polyurethane. Sizes include 1.2, 1.9, 2, and 3 Fr. Larger sizes are generally not used in the neonatal population. Most catheters are single-lumen. Double-lumen catheters can decrease the need for maintaining concurrent IV access when more than one site is required. PICC introducers/needles are available in 20 to 28 gauge. Choice will depend on the size of the vein to be cannulated.
   b. Surgically placed central venous catheters

Surgically placed central venous catheters for neonates are available in sizes 2.5, 2.7, 3, 4.2, and 5 Fr. Catheters are usually silicone or polyurethane, with tissue in-growth cuffs that adhere to the subcutaneous tract, anchoring the catheter. Recently, antimicrobial cuffs have become available. Most catheters are single-lumen, but a few manufacturers make double-lumen catheters.

Percutaneous Central Venous Catheterization (See Procedures Website for video)

A. Insertion Sites (Fig. 14.1)(Table 32.1)

The veins used, in order of preference are

1. *Antecubital veins:* Basilic and cephalic veins
2. *Saphenous veins*
3. *Scalp veins:* Temporal and posterior auricular veins
4. Axillary vein
5. External jugular vein
   Right-sided and basilic veins are preferred because of the shorter and more direct route to the central vein. The cephalic vein may be more difficult to thread to the central position because of narrowing of the vessel as it enters the deltopectoral groove and the acute angle at which it joins the subclavian vein. The axillary and external jugular veins are the last choices because they are close to arteries and nerves.

B. Insertion Variations

1. *Break-away needle (Fig. 32.2):* Needle is inserted into the vein. Next, the catheter is advanced through the needle. The needle is then retracted, split, and

TABLE 32.2	Catheter Materials	
Type of Catheter	**Advantages**	**Disadvantages**
Silicone	Soft, pliable Lower risk of vessel perforation Reported to be thromboresistant	May be more difficult to insert percutaneously Thrombosis reported Fragile material: Less tolerance to pressure Poor tensile strength: Can tear or rupture May be less radio-opaque
Polyurethane	Easier to insert percutaneously Stiffer on insertion but softens within body Some catheters are more radio-opaque Tensile strength: More tolerant to pressure Reported to be thromboresistant	Increased risk of vessel perforation during insertion Thrombosis reported
Polyethylene	Easier to insert Very high tensile strength	High degree of stiffness may increase vessel perforation during insertion or throughout catheter dwell
Polyvinyl chloride (PVC)	Easier to insert percutaneously Stiff on insertion but softens within body	May leach plasticizers into body High incidence of thrombosis

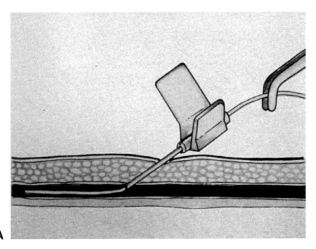

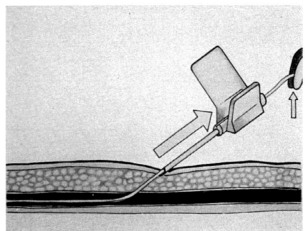

A

B

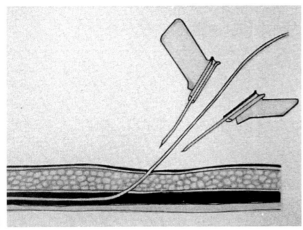

C

FIG. 32.2. PICC using break-away needle technique. (From Gesco International, San Antonio, Texas, with permission.)

removed. Disadvantage: There is a potential for shearing or severing the catheter if it is retracted while the needle is in the vein.

2. *Peel-away introducer (Fig. 32.3):* A needle introducer is used to place a small cannula or sheath into the vein. The needle is then removed and the catheter is threaded through the cannula. The introducer cannula or sheath is then retracted from the vein, split or "peeled" apart, and removed from the catheter.

3. *Intact cannula (Fig. 32.4):* This technique is now rarely used because most commercially available catheters have a hub and introducer needles. A regular IV cannula is used to obtain venous access. The needle is removed. The silicone catheter is threaded through the cannula to its final position. The cannula is then retracted and slipped off the end of the "hubless" catheter. A blunt needle with hub is connected to the end of the catheter. Disadvantage: The blunt needle attachment must be secured well, otherwise leakage can occur.

C. Placement of PICC

1. **Equipment**

All equipment used, except the mask, head cover, and tape measure, must be sterile. Commercial kits contain many of the necessary items. Assemble all supplies before starting procedure.

a. Radio-opaque central venous catheter
b. Break-away or peel-away needle introducer
c. Device for trimming the catheter (based on manufacturer recommendations)
d. Tourniquet (optional)
e. Drapes
f. Smooth iris forceps
g. Gauze pads
h. Skin prep: 10% povidone–iodine or 0.5% chlorhexidine solution (as per institutional policy)
i. Transparent dressing
j. Sterile tape strips
k. Sterile heparinized saline solution (0.5 to 1 U/mL heparin or per institutional policy)
l. 5- to 10-mL syringe with needle
m. Tape measure
n. Sterile surgical gown, sterile gloves, mask, and head cover

2. **Preparation**

a. Although anesthesia is not required, nonpharmacologic comfort measures and pain medication should be provided as needed. A small dose of sedative or narcotic analgesic may be useful.

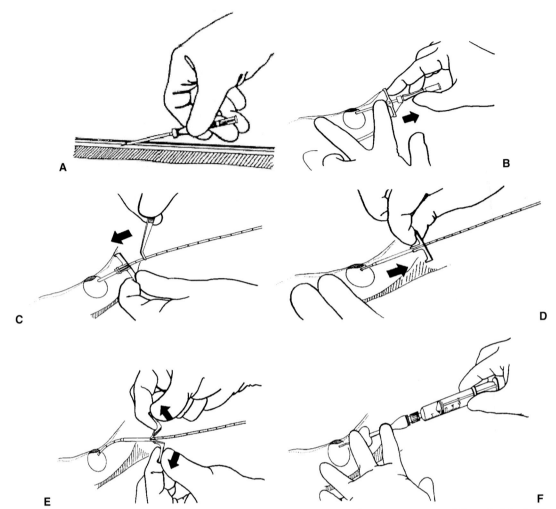

FIG. 32.3. PICC using a peel-away cannula introducer. **A:** Perform venipuncture. When flashback of blood is noted, reduce angle and advance introducer sheath farther to ensure placement in the vein. **B:** Withdraw the introducer needle from the sheath. Note that the introducer sheath is supported to avoid displacement. **C:** Insert the catheter into the introducer sheath using fine nontoothed forceps. **D:** Withdraw the introducer sheath. Note that the catheter is stabilized by applying digital pressure to the vein distal to the introducer sheath. **E:** Remove the introducer sheath by splitting and peeling it away from the catheter. Complete catheter advancement to premeasured length. **F:** Aspirate catheter to check for blood return and flush with heparinized saline to ensure patency. (From Klein C. *NeoPicc: The Neonatal and Pediatric Workshop Manual.* San Antonio, TX: Klein Baker Medical, 1998, with permission.)

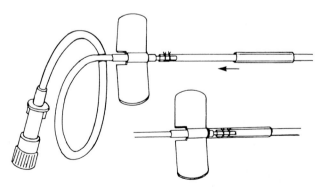

FIG. 32.4. Use of a blunt scalp vein needle to form a hub for a silicone catheter. The plastic needle cover is used to stabilize the needle–catheter junction. A commercially available blunt needle adapter may be inserted and fixed in a similar manner.

b. Gather supplies. Wash hands thoroughly.

c. Identify appropriate vein for insertion (see D).

d. Position infant to facilitate insertion (Table 32.3). Restrain infant; provide comfort measures.

e. Measure approximate distance from the insertion site to the point where the catheter tip will be placed (Table 32.3).

f. Don mask and head cover.

g. Set up/open sterile equipment tray.

h. Perform hand hygiene as for a major procedure and wear sterile surgical gown and gloves.

i. Trim catheter to appropriate size (trimming is based on unit policy and manufacturer recommendations). The catheter is fragile and should be handled with

TABLE 32.3	Patient Position and Measurement for PICC Insertion	
Site of Insertion	**Position of Baby**	**Measurement**
Antecubital veins	Supine, abduct arm 90 degrees from trunk; turn head toward insertion site to prevent catheter from traveling cephalad through ipsilateral jugular vein	From planned insertion site, along venous pathway, to suprasternal notch, to third RICS
Saphenous or popliteal veins	Supine for greater saphenous vein, prone for small saphenous or popliteal; extend leg	From planned insertion site, along venous pathway, to xiphoid process
Scalp veins	Supine, turn head to side; may have to turn head to midline during procedure to assist advancement of catheter	Follow approximate venous pathway from planned insertion site near ear, to jugular vein, right SC joint, to third RICS
External jugular vein	Supine, turn head to side; place roll under neck to cause mild hyperextension	From planned insertion site, to right SC joint, to third RICS
Axillary vein	Supine, externally rotate and abduct arm 120 degrees, flex forearm and place baby's hand behind head; vein is found above artery between medial side of humeral head and small tuberosity of the humerus	From planned insertion site, to right SC joint, to third RICS

PICC, peripherally inserted central catheter; RICS, right intercostal space; SC, sternoclavicular.

care. Do not clamp or suture; stretch or apply tension to catheter.

j. Utilizing sterile technique and a 3- to 5-mL syringe, flush catheter with heparinized saline solution, leaving syringe attached. A small-barreled syringe (such as a 1-mL syringe) may generate too much pressure, resulting in catheter rupture (12).

k. Prepare sterile field: Holding the extremity with sterile gauze prepare a large area at and around the insertion site, working outward in concentric circles. Allow the prep solution to dry. Repeat process with new gauze/prep solution. Place a *large* sterile drape under and above the extremity, leaving only the insertion site exposed. A large drape or multiple sterile towels should be used to cover an area well beyond the extremity to decrease the risk of accidental contamination (2).

3. **Catheter insertion using a break-away needle** (Fig. 32.2) or a peel-away introducer (Figs. 32.3, 32.5)

   a. Apply tourniquet above insertion site on extremity (optional).

   b. Providing slight skin traction, insert needle about 0.5 to 1 cm below the intended vein, at a low angle (approximately 15 to 30 degrees).

   c. When a flashback is obtained, advance the needle about 5 to 6 mm at a lower angle to ensure that the whole bevel of the needle is within the vein. If a peel-away introducer with a needle is used, remove the needle at this time and advance the introducer sheath slightly. If the introducer (needle or sheath) is well within the vein, there will be continued blood flow through it.

   d. Remove the tourniquet.

   e. Using nontoothed iris forceps, gently grasp the catheter about 1 cm from its distal end and thread it

slowly into the introducer, a few millimeters at a time.

Caution: When using a break-away needle, never advance the needle or retract the catheter after inserting it into the needle; the catheter may be severed by this action.

   f. With small, gentle nudges, a few millimeters at a time, advance the catheter through the introducer to a distance of about 6 to 7 cm into the vein.

   g. Once the catheter is successfully advanced to about 6 or 7 cm, withdraw the introducer carefully (an alternative is to insert the catheter to the predetermined distance before withdrawing the introducer).

   h. To withdraw the introducer, stabilize the catheter by applying gentle pressure over the vein proximal to the introducer, and then remove it carefully from the insertion site. Break or peel away the introducer by splitting the wings, and then carefully peel it away from the catheter.

   i. Continue to advance the catheter into the vein to the premeasured length, by nudging it farther, a few millimeters at a time, using the fine forceps.

   j. Difficulties in advancing catheter: Gently massage the vein in the direction of blood flow, proximal to the insertion site, or gently flush the catheter intermittently with 0.5 to 1 mL of heparinized saline; repositioning the extremity or the head may help.

   k. Aspirate to visualize blood return in the catheter, and flush with 0.5 to 1 mL of heparinized saline to clear the catheter.

   l. Verify length of catheter inserted and adjust as necessary.

   m. Attach sterile extension set as per unit protocol.

   n. Apply gentle pressure on insertion site with gauze pad to stop any bleeding.

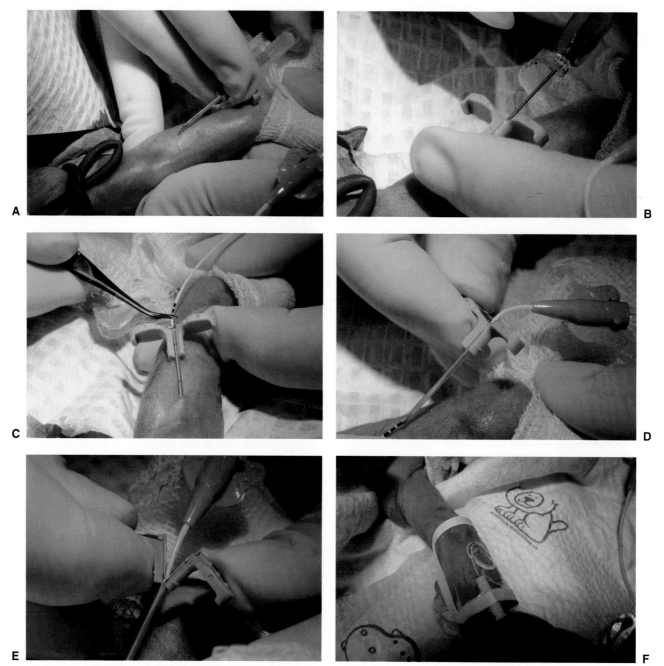

FIG. 32.5.   A: Venipuncture with peel-away cannula introducer. **B:** Withdraw the introducer needle from the sheath. Note that the introducer sheath is supported to avoid displacement. **C:** Insert the catheter into the introducer sheath using fine nontoothed forceps. **D:** Withdraw the introducer sheath. **E:** Remove the introducer sheath by splitting and peeling it away from the catheter. **F:** Transparent dressing on PICC catheter. Note that the excess catheter length has been coiled in place under the dressing.

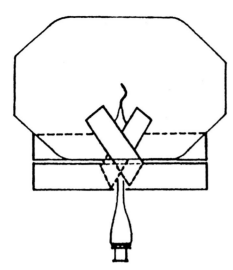

FIG.32.6. PICC dressing with trimmed catheter. No excess catheter is present externally. The silicone heart is anchored with a piece of tape, and a sterile transparent dressing is placed over the insertion site. With use of a "chevron" technique, another piece of tape is placed under the catheter extension, next to the silicone heart, and crossed over on top of the transparent dressing. (From Klein C. *NeoPicc: The Neonatal and Pediatric Workshop Manual.* San Antonio, TX: Klein Baker Medical, 1998, with permission.)

   o. Secure catheter at skin insertion site with a small piece of sterile tape strip (avoid using tape that contains wire) and cover with sterile gauze until radiographic confirmation of position.

D. PICC Dressings (Figs. 32.5, 32.6)

1. Antimicrobial prep solutions should be removed from the skin with sterile water or saline and allowed to dry before dressing is placed. Do not use topical antibiotic ointments or creams on insertion sites (2).

2. To prevent migration of the catheter, secure it to the skin a few millimeters from the insertion site with a small piece of sterile tape (avoid using tape that contains wire).

3. If the catheter has not been trimmed, loosely coil the excess length of catheter close to the insertion site and secure to the skin with more sterile tape. Ensure that there is no kinking or stretching of the catheter under the dressing.

4. Apply a semipermeable transparent dressing over the area surrounding the insertion site.

5. Do not allow tapes or transparent dressing to extend around the extremity. The dressing will form a constricting tourniquet as the infant grows or if there is venous congestion.

6. Place tape under the catheter hub and criss-cross it over the hub (chevron). Do not obscure visualization of the insertion site (Fig. 32.6).

7. To prevent skin breakdown, a skin barrier of hydrocolloid material or soft gauze can be placed under the hub.

E. Dressing Changes

1. Mild oozing of blood from the insertion site may occur for up to 24 hours. If oozing occurs, the initial dressing should be changed when it subsides. If oozing of blood is a problem, a small piece of thrombin foam can be applied over the insertion site and under the dressing for the first 24 hours after insertion.

2. The catheter site dressing should be replaced when it becomes damp, soiled, or loose. Transparent dressings should be changed every 7 days except in those patients in whom the risk of dislodging the catheter outweighs the benefit of changing the dressing (2).

3. Inspect catheter site carefully at each dressing change (Table 32.4).

TABLE 32.4	Examination of the Catheter Site

Assessment	Comments
Catheter: Note external catheter length	Catheter length should be clearly documented. If external length has changed, get radiograph(s) to assess where the catheter tip is located.
	If the catheter is pulled out, cover site with occlusive dressing and measure catheter length to assure that some of the catheter was not retained in the vessel.
Assess for kinks, tension, damage	Kinks and tension can damage catheter. It is recommended that damaged catheters be removed, but some manufacturers provide repair kits.
Insertion site/surrounding skin: Erythema, drainage, bleeding, edema, phlebitis, skin breakdown	Mild erythema and/or phlebitis is common after the catheter is inserted. If condition is severe and/or is persistent, consider removing catheter. Mild oozing of blood should not persist longer than 24 h.
	Edema may be due to venous stasis from lack of extremity movement, constrictive dressings, thrombus, damage to internal structures, localized infection, or infiltration of infusion into soft tissue.
	Avoid skin breakdown by utilizing skin barriers underneath hub, removing dressing adhesives with care, minimizing tape, and removing antiseptics from skin before applying dressing.
Drainage/leaking	Purulent drainage may be due an infectious process. Consider obtaining blood cultures and/or removing the catheter. Clear drainage may be indicative of infusion leakage. This may be due to catheter occlusion, infiltration, or damage to catheter.

4. If the catheter is too far in, as confirmed by radiography or echocardiography, it may be pulled back, prior to replacing dressing. Do not advance the catheter, as the risk of contamination is high.

5. Use sterile technique for dressing changes (mask, cap, and sterile gloves; sterile gown is optional).

6. Prepare sterile field: Place drape under extremity. Utilizing the prep solution, prepare the skin at and around the insertion site, working outward in concentric circles. Allow the prep solution to dry. Repeat process with new gauze/prep solution. Drape prepared area, leaving insertion site exposed.

7. Follow steps D1 through D7 to complete the PICC dressing change.

F. PICC Care and Maintenance

1. Evaluate appearance of the catheter and the tissue around the insertion site frequently.

2. Change IV tubing according to unit policy. Utilize aseptic technique when changing tubing.

3. To prevent contamination of the line, enter the PICC only when absolutely necessary.
   a. Avoid the use of stopcocks in the line.
   b. Always "scrub the hub" with alcohol pad (or similar product) prior to breaking a connection.
   c. If the catheter must be used to infuse medications, arrange the intermittent injection tubing so that it does not come in contact with the parenteral alimentation solution until the terminal infusion site. A dedicated "closed" medication administration system is recommended (13). Gently flush tubing prior to and after medication administration. Ensure that the flush and medication is compatible with the parenteral alimentation.

4. Prime volumes are usually <0.5 mL. Use a 5- to 10-mL syringe when needed to check catheter patency. Do not use force if resistance is encountered. A small-barreled syringe (such as a 1-mL syringe) may generate too much pressure, resulting in catheter rupture (12).

5. Administer a constant infusion of IV fluids at a rate of at least 1 mL/h. Follow the manufacturer's recommendations for maximum flow rates.

6. The addition of heparin in small doses (0.5 units heparin/kg/h or 0.5 units heparin/mL of IV fluids) reduces the risk of occlusion and prolongs catheter patency (14).

7. Do not utilize the PICC for routine blood sampling.

8. Packed red blood cell transfusions should be given through a PICC only if absolutely necessary. Although there is no clinically significant hemolysis, there is a potential for occlusion of the catheter (15).

9. Monitor quality indicators to identify and solve problems. Infection rates, catheter dwell times, patient outcomes, and rates of complications should be monitored (2).

10. Remove catheter as soon as it is no longer medically necessary by slowly withdrawing it from insertion site.

Clean insertion site with prep prior to withdrawing catheter. Hold pressure over site if bleeding is a problem. Remove prep from skin. Place a clean gauze dressing over site. Document length removed.

Placement of Central Venous Catheters by Surgical Cutdown

A. Types of Catheters

Silicone catheters are preferred because they are constructed of relatively inert materials, offer increased pliability, and are associated with lower rates of infection and thrombosis. These catheters are placed in a central vein, and the distal end is tunneled subcutaneously a short distance from the access site to an exit wound. The catheters usually have a single lumen with a Dacron cuff, which adheres to the subcutaneous tract, anchoring the catheter. Polyethylene catheters have a higher rate of infection and thrombolytic complications and are not recommended for long-term IV access.

B. Contraindications

In addition to the relative contraindications delineated earlier, the internal jugular vein should be avoided if the contralateral jugular vein has been catheterized previously, or if there is thrombosis of the jugular venous system on the opposite side.

C. Equipment

Sterile

1. Skin prep: Per institutional policy (e.g., 10% povidone–iodine, or 0.5% chlorhexidine solution)

2. Gown and gloves

3. Cup with antiseptic solution

4. Sterile transparent aperture drape; four sterile towels to ensure a sterile operative field

5. Four 4- × 4-inch gauze squares

6. Local anesthetic: 0.5% lidocaine HCl in labeled 3-mL syringe with 25-gauge venipuncture needle

   Consider sedation and pain medication in addition to local anesthesia. Patients who are intubated may be given a sedative and muscle relaxant in addition to local anesthesia. When patients are taken to the operating room, general anesthesia is preferred.

7. Catheter of choice

8. Heparinized 0.25 N saline flush solution (1 U/mL) in 3-mL syringe

9. 4-0 polyglactin suture (Vicryl; Ethicon, Somerville, New Jersey) and 5-0 nylon suture (black monofilament nylon) on cutting needles (see Appendix B)

10. T connector connected with a sterile 3-mL syringe filled with heparinized saline

11. No. 11 scalpel blade and holder

12. Two small tissue retractors or self-retaining retractor

13. Tissue forceps

14. Fine vascular forceps

15. Two small, curved mosquito hemostats
16. Dissecting scissors
17. 4-0 Vicryl suture on small, curved needle; 6-0 polypropylene on a tapered needle. This is used for a purse-string stitch as an alternative to ligation of the vessels.
18. Needle holder
19. Suture scissors
20. Appropriate materials for occlusive dressing of choice

Nonsterile

1. Cap and mask
2. Roll of 4- × 4-inch gauze
3. Tape measure
4. Adhesive tape

D. Techniques

In the neonate, the cervical veins are preferable to the lower-extremity veins. The cervical veins are easily accessible and are a proportionately larger size. When the lower extremities are used, the greater saphenous vein is often selected in pediatric patients because of its large size and consistent anatomy. It is not established whether femoral or jugular sites have fewer complications in neonates (16,17).

1. **Catheter placement via jugular veins**
   a. Immobilize infant in position similar to that for percutaneous insertion of subclavian venous catheter. Make sure that the patient is in the Trendelenburg position to minimize the risk of an air embolism.
   b. If right side is to be catheterized, turn head to left and extend neck. Care must be taken not to extend the head too much, as this may result in occlusion of the vein.
   c. Estimate length of catheter to be inserted by measuring from a point midway between the nipple and the midpoint of the clavicle to a point over the ster-

nocleidomastoid muscle at the junction of the middle and lower third of the neck (Fig. 32.7).
   d. Put on cap and mask.
   e. Scrub as for major procedure and put on gown and gloves.
   f. Prepare neck and scalp area or right chest wall with antiseptic solution such as iodophor and drape out the sterile field.
   g. Make small, transverse incision (1 to 2 cm) through skin and platysma muscle low in the neck for the external jugular and higher up for the facial vein.
   h. Free external jugular or facial vein by blunt dissection with curved mosquito hemostat. If internal jugular vein is used, sternocleidomastoid muscle must be split to locate vein.
   i. Pass curved mosquito hemostat behind the vein, and place proximal and distal ligatures of 4-0 absorbable suture loosely around vein (Fig. 32.8). Be careful not to twist the vessels as the suture is advanced.
   j. Using a blunt tunneler, create a subcutaneous tract from neck to exit on the chest wall medial to the right nipple. In a baby girl, make sure that the tunnel is far from the breast bud (Figs. 32.9 and 32.10).
   k. Thread the end of the catheter through the opening in the tunneler, and guide the catheter gently through the subcutaneous tract.
   l. Fill the catheter system with heparinized flush solution.

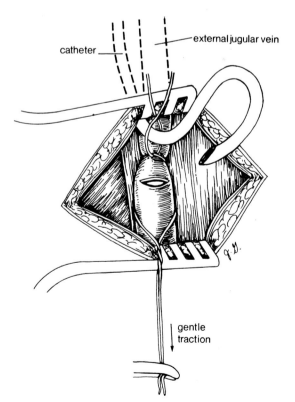

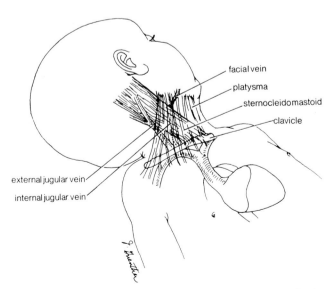

FIG. 32.7. The jugular veins in relation to major anatomic landmarks.

FIG. 32.8. Catheterization of the external jugular vein; venotomy has been performed prior to inserting the catheter.

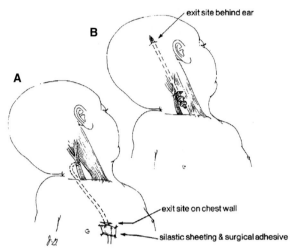

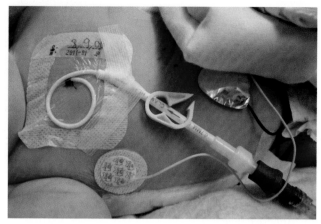

FIG. 32.10.   Broviac catheter with transparent dressing.

FIG. 32.9.   Formation of a subcutaneous tunnel with a Vim-Silverman needle. **A:** Tunnel on the anterior chest wall. **B:** Alternative route under the scalp.

m. Cut the catheter length to the premeasured distance between the neck incision and a point midway between the center of the nipple line and the suprasternal notch.

n. Perform transverse venotomy (Fig. 32.8).

FOR EXTERNAL JUGULAR OR FACIAL VEIN

(1) Tie cephalad-venous ligature, and exert traction on both ligatures in opposite directions with aid of appropriately prepared assistant.

(2) Make short, transverse incision in anterior wall of vein, and enlarge gently by inserting and spreading tips of fine vascular forceps.

FOR INTERNAL JUGULAR VEIN

(3) To avoid ligation of the vessel, use purse-string suture of 6-0 polypropylene, placed in vessel wall around point of catheter entrance.

(4) Make incision in vessel as for external jugular vein.

o. Bevel intravascular end of catheter (optional).

p. Grasp catheter gently with blunt nontoothed tissue forceps, introduce catheter tip, and insert into the vein.

q. Leave loop of catheter in neck wound to dampen effect of head movement (Fig. 32.11).

r. Close wound with subcuticular 5-0 absorbable suture, taking care not to penetrate the catheter.

s. Secure the catheter to the skin with at least one nylon suture to hold it until the cuff has created enough tissue ingrowth.

t. Use selected method for fixation and dressing.

2. **Proximal saphenous vein cutdown**

a. Scrub and prepare as for major procedure.

b. Prepare as for cutdown on jugular vein. Make sure that the patient is in the reverse Trendelenburg position to minimize the risk of an air embolism.

(1) Choose right or left groin area for insertion.

(2) Prepare groin and abdomen on same side.

c. *Make incision 1 cm long:* 1 cm caudad and 1 cm lateral to pubic tubercle (Fig. 32.12).

d. Spread incision into subcutaneous tissues, using curved mosquito hemostat.

(1) Incise superficial fascia.

(2) Identify saphenous vein lying medial and inferior to its junction with femoral vein at foramen ovale (Fig. 32.12).

e. Move 0.5 to 1 cm distally before

(1) Passing curved mosquito hemostat behind vein. This avoids inadvertent damage to femoral vein.

(2) Placing two 4-0 absorbable suture ligatures loosely around vein

f. Create a tunnel, using a small hemostat or tunneling instrument, in subcutaneous plane laterally onto abdomen, just above or lateral to umbilicus or on lateral thigh.

g. Flush catheter with heparinized saline and replace cap.

h. Pull catheter through tunnel into groin wound so that the Dacron cuff is just within the skin incision. Estimate the length of the catheter to be inserted so that the tip will be in inferior vena cava at junction with right atrium.

i. Cut catheter to appropriate length, and bevel intravascular end (optional).

j. Dissect saphenous vein to junction with common femoral vein.

Visualizing the junction prevents inadvertent direction of catheter into lower extremity.

k. Apply traction to vein, using caudad suture. Lateral tension may also be applied by a scrubbed assistant, using fine nontoothed vascular forceps.

l. Make transverse venotomy.

m. Dilate vein, if necessary, with blunt dilatator.

n. Moisten catheter with saline to ease passage into vein.

o. Maintain back-traction on caudad suture to control bleeding.

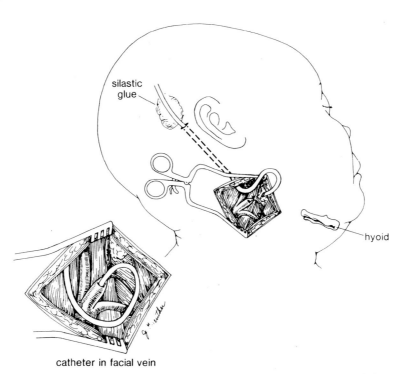

catheter in facial vein

FIG. 32.11.   Insertion of a catheter into the common facial vein. Incision is below the angle of the mandible at the level of the hyoid bone. The facial vein is ligated at the junction of the anterior and posterior tributaries. Alternatively, the subcutaneous tunnel may be made with a catheter exit site on the anterior chest wall. **Inset:** The catheter is looped in the neck wound to "dampen" the effect of head movement. (Reproduced from Zumbro GL Jr, Mullin MJ, Nelson TG. Catheter placement in infants needing total parenteral nutrition utilizing common facial vein. *Arch Surg.* 1971;102:71, with permission of American Medical Association.)

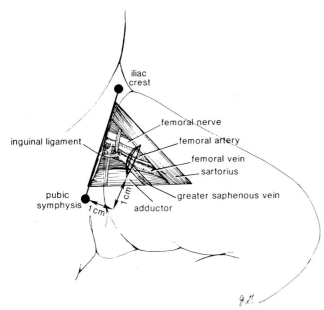

FIG. 32.12.   Anatomic view of the site of incision for proximal saphenous vein cutdown with underlying femoral triangle.

p. Visualize catheter entering common femoral vein to ensure cephalad direction of catheter.

q. Obtain radiograph(s) to confirm position in inferior vena cava, once estimated length is inserted (radiographic contrast material may be required).

r. Ligate vessel with caudad suture, and tie down cephalad suture without occluding catheter.

s. Check for easy backflow of blood in catheter.

t. Flush catheter with 2.5 to 3 mL of heparinized saline. If catheter is capped, while infant is transferred from operating room to intensive care unit, clamp catheter while plunger of heparin syringe is moving forward to ensure positive pressure in line to prevent backflow and clotting of blood.

u. Close groin wound with subcuticular 5-0 absorbable suture, taking care not to penetrate catheter with needle.

v. Secure the catheter to the skin with at least one nylon suture to hold it until the cuff has created enough tissue ingrowth.

w. Cover with dressing of choice.

E. Sterile Dressing for Surgically Placed Central Venous Lines

Routine changing of central venous catheter dressings depends on the type of dressing. Transparent dressings should be changed at least every 7 days, and gauze dressings every 2 days. All dressings should be changed when damp, loose, or soiled (2).

Equipment

Strict sterile technique is used for all central line dressings.

1. Antiseptic skin prep solution: Per institutional policy (e.g., 10% povidone–iodine or 0.5% chlorhexidine solution)
2. Sterile gloves, mask, cap, and sterile gown (optional)
3. Scissors (optional)
4. Cotton-tipped applicator
5. 4- × 4-inch sterile gauze square
6. Dressing of choice
   a. Semipermeable transparent dressing
   b. Sterile 2- × 2-inch gauze squares or presplit 2- × 2-cm gauze dressing
7. Normal saline or sterile water
8. Adhesive tape (if sterile tape not available, use fresh unused roll)

Precautions

1. Procedure should be undertaken by trained personnel.
2. Ensure that all personnel wear masks if within 3 ft radius of sterile area.
3. Use strict aseptic technique.
4. Remove dressing with care, to avoid cutting or dislodging catheter.
5. If it is necessary to clamp the catheter, close the clamp on the catheter according to the manufacturer's directions. If the catheter does not have a clamp, use a rubber-shod clamp. Never place a clamp directly on the catheter.
6. Never advance a dislodged catheter into the patient.
7. Do not place adhesive tape on silicone tubing because this may occlude or damage the catheter.
8. Do not routinely apply prophylactic topical antimicrobial or antiseptic ointment at the insertion site because of the potential for promoting fungal infections and antimicrobial resistance (2).

Technique

When a subcutaneous tunnel is used, occlusive dressing should be applied to both the cutdown site and the catheter exit site. The dressing on the exit site can be removed after 48 hours if there is no oozing.

1. Restrain patient appropriately, utilizing nonpharmacologic comfort measures.
2. Put on head cover and mask.
3. Scrub as for major procedure.
4. Put on gown and gloves.
5. Prepare sterile work area, using "no-touch" technique.
6. Remove old dressing and discard.
7. Inspect catheter site carefully (Table 32.4).
8. Culture site if there is drainage or it appears inflamed.
9. If area around catheter is contaminated with dried blood or drainage, clean with diluted hydrogen peroxide/sterile water solution (1:1).
10. Remove gloves. Don sterile gloves.
11. Cleanse area with antiseptic solution, starting at catheter site and working outward in circular motion for 2 to 4 cm. Repeat twice. Allow area to dry.
12. Remove antiseptic with sterile water or saline gauze and allow to dry.
13. Apply dressing of choice.
    a. Clear, adhesive, hypoallergenic, transparent dressing allows for continuous inspection of catheter insertion site, and is preferred (Fig. 32.10).
       (1) If necessary, cut dressing to desired size.
       (2) Anchor dressing to skin above catheter skin entry site so that the point of skin entry is at the center of the dressing.
       (3) Remove remainder of adhesive backing while applying dressing smoothly over site.
    b. Occlusive gauze dressing
       (1) Cut gauze halfway across, or use presplit gauze. Place around catheter, as shown in Fig. 32.13.
       (2) Cover remainder of external catheter length (not hub) with sterile gauze.
       (3) If sterile tape is not available, discard outer layer of tape on roll.
       (4) Cover gauze with tape.
       (5) Label dressing with initials and date.
       (6) Secure IV tubing with tape to prevent tension on the center (a stress loop can decrease tension on the catheter).

F. Care of the Catheter When Not in Use for Continuous Infusion

Indications

To maintain patency and prevent clotting of the catheter when the line is used intermittently. Only large-bore catheters (2.5 Fr or larger) may be kept patent by this technique. PICC lines that are 2 Fr or smaller tend to clot easily if continuous infusions are interrupted.

Equipment

1. 3 mL of heparin–saline solution (10 unit Heparin /mL) in a 10-mL syringe (follow manufacturer's guidelines for syringe sizes)
2. Alcohol wipes
3. Catheter clamps (must have no teeth or be padded), or use clamp provided on catheter (Fig. 32.10)
4. Clean gloves
5. IV injection cap (needleless is recommended)

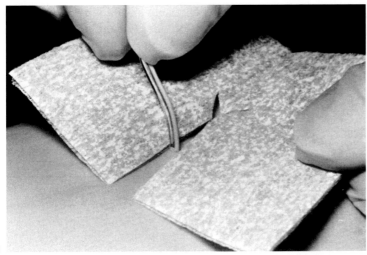

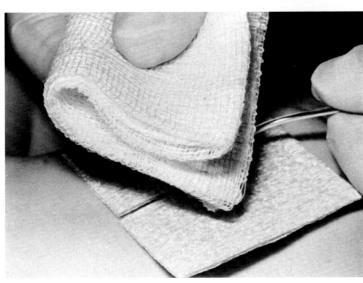

FIG. 32.13. Occlusive dressing for a central venous line using presplit gauze. **A:** Placing split gauze over the skin entry site. **B:** Covering split gauze and the catheter with sterile gauze. Entire dressing is then covered with adhesive tape or clear dressing.

Technique

1. Converting to a heparin lock
   a. Wash hands thoroughly.
   b. Don clean or sterile gloves.
   c. Prepare sterile work area.
   d. Using aseptic technique, open sterile injection cap package and prefill injection cap with heparinized saline.
   e. Clean the outside of the hub–IV tubing connection with an antiseptic such as alcohol wipes. Work outward in both directions. Allow to dry.
   f. Clamp catheter with padded hemostat, or close catheter clamp.
   g. Holding hub with alcohol swab, disconnect catheter hub from IV tubing.
   h. Connect preflushed injection cap into hub of catheter (gently flushing during connecting can prevent air from entering catheter).
   i. Release clamp and flush line with 1 to 3 mL of heparinized saline (depending on size of catheter).
   j. Reclamp catheter while plunger of heparin syringe is depressed to prevent blood from backing into catheter (positive pressure).
   k. Secure catheter and tape to chest or abdomen.
   l. Flush catheter with heparinized solution every 6 to 12 hours (per institution policy).

2. Flushing catheters
   Equipment is same as for heparin lock.
   a. Wash hands thoroughly.
   b. Put on gloves and prepare sterile work area.
   c. Prepare IV injection cap with antiseptic solution. Allow to dry.
   d. If injection cap is part of a needleless system (recommended), connect flush syringe to cap. If the cap is not a needleless device, insert needle into IV catheter plug. Always use a 1-inch or smaller needle. A longer needle can puncture the catheter.
   e. Unclamp catheter and slowly inject 1 to 2 mL of heparinized saline (depending on catheter size). Reclamp catheter while injecting solution to prevent blood

from flowing back into catheter. Positive-pressure injection caps are available to prevent backflow.

f. Changing IV catheter injection cap: Most manufacturers recommend changing injection caps every 3 to 7 days, after blood product administration, or when they appear damaged (see specific manufacturer's instructions).

Catheter Removal

A. Indications

1. Patient's condition no longer necessitates use.
2. Occluded catheter
3. Local infection/phlebitis
4. Sepsis and/or positive blood cultures obtained through the catheter (catheter colonization). There are rare clinical circumstances when a catheter is left in place despite sepsis and antibiotic or antifungal therapy is administered through it in an attempt to clear the infection, but this may be associated with an increased risk of morbidity and mortality (18,19).

B. Technique

Surgically implanted central venous catheters should be removed by a physician or other person specifically trained to remove cuffed and/or tunneled catheters.

1. Remove dressing.
2. Make sure that the patient is in the Trendelenburg position (or reverse Trendelenburg position if the catheter is in the lower extremity) to minimize the risk of an air embolism.
3. Pull catheter from vessel slowly over 2 to 3 minutes. Avoid excessive traction if catheter is tethered, because the catheter may snap (see Complications).
4. Apply continuous pressure to the catheter insertion site for 5 to 10 minutes, until no bleeding is noted.
5. Inspect catheter (without contaminating tip) to ensure that entire length has been removed.
6. The cuff on the tunneled catheter should be dissected out under local anesthesia with IV sedation. If cuffs are retained, they rarely cause more than a persistent small subcutaneous lump, although they can occasionally extrude through the skin.
7. If desired, antibiotic ointment may be placed over site.
8. Dress with small, self-adhesive bandage or gauze pad and inspect daily until healing occurs.

Complications of Central Venous Lines (20)

1. Damage to other vessels and organs during insertion
   a. Possible during both percutaneous and surgical placement of central venous catheters

   b. Complications include bleeding, pneumothorax, pneumomediastinum, hemothorax, arterial puncture, and brachial plexus injury.
2. Phlebitis
   a. Mechanical phlebitis may occur in the first 24 hours after line placement as a normal response of the body to the irritation of the catheter in the vein.
   b. Management of mild phlebitis (mild erythema and/or edema): Apply moist, warm compress, and elevate extremity.
   c. Remove the catheter if symptoms do not improve, if phlebitis is severe (streak formation, palpable venous cord, and/or purulent drainage), or if there are signs of a catheter-related infection.
3. Catheter migration/malposition (Fig. 32.14)
   a. Can occur during insertion or at any point during the dwell time of the catheter (possibly as a consequence of poor catheter fixation at the skin surface and movement of the joints). The catheter can enter a venous tributary during insertion or can reverse direction, causing it to loop back.
   b. Sites of misplacement include the cardiac chambers, internal jugular vein, contralateral subclavian vein, ascending lumbar vein (which communicates with the vertebral venous plexus), superficial abdominal vein, renal vein, and others. Consequences include pericardial effusion or pleural effusion, cardiac arrhythmias, tissue extravasation/infiltration, neurological complications such as seizures or paraplegia, thrombosis, and death.
   c. The decision to remove the catheter or attempt to correct the position is based on the location of the tip. Although PICCs are intended to be placed in central veins (See Section E, page 195), occasionally, the tip is in a noncentral location (e.g., in the subclavian vein). These noncentral PICCs may be used, *provided the fluids administered through them are isotonic*, but the care of the catheters must be as stringent as for centrally placed catheters.
   d. The catheter should be pulled back into an appropriate position if the tip is in the heart, as serious consequences such as cardiac arrhythmia, perforation, or pericardial effusion can occur.
   e. Catheters in the ascending lumbar vein or vertebral venous plexus must be removed, since the infusion of parenteral alimentation fluids in this area may lead to severe CNS damage, manifesting as seizures, paraplegia or death (Figs. 29.3, 32.14D) (20).
   f. Spontaneous correction of malpositioned lines has been demonstrated in some cases (21). If the tip of the catheter is looped into the internal jugular or in the contralateral brachiocephalic vein, the catheter may be used temporarily (using isotonic fluids that are suitable for peripheral venous cannulae) and re-evaluated radiologically in 24 hours. If the catheter

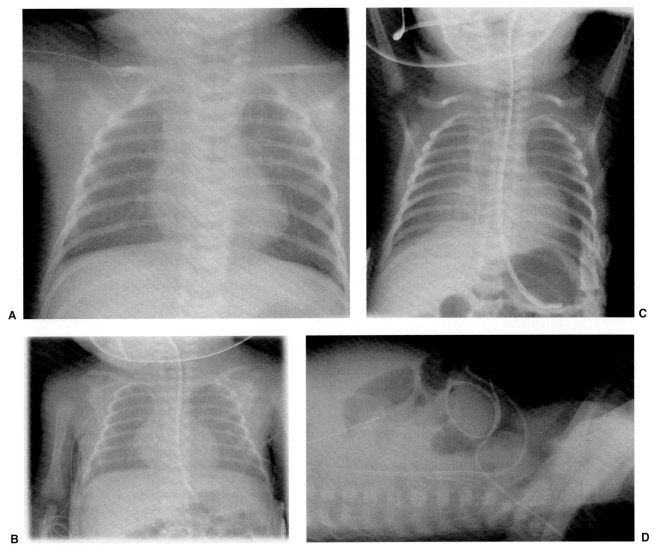

FIG. 32.14. Various venous malpositions of PICCs. **A:** Jugular. **B:** Tip in right atrium **C:** PICC from left arm, through superior vena cava and right atrium, into inferior vena cava. **D:** PICC from saphenous vein in leg entering vertebral venous plexus via ascending lumbar vein.

has not moved spontaneously into the desired location, it should be removed.

4. Infection
   a. Infection is the most common complication of central venous catheters, with the smallest and most immature infants being at greatest risk. Catheter-related sepsis (CRS) rates range from 0% to 29% of lines placed and from 0.4 to 17 per 1,000 catheter days (2,3).
   b. Strict protocols for central line care and a methodology of surveillance with a data feedback mechanism are recommended to decrease CRS (2,3,13).
   c. Management of catheter-related sepsis: Remove central venous line if possible. Prompt removal of the line is recommended for *Staphylococcus aureus*, gram-negative, or *Candida* sepsis. Treatment with appropriate antibiotics without

removal of the line may be attempted in infants with coagulase-negative *Staphylococcus* sepsis, but repeated positive cultures mandate removal of the line (18,19).

5. Catheter dysfunction
   a. Obstruction of the catheter is characterized by increased pump pressures, or inability to infuse fluids or withdraw blood.
   b. Dysfunction may be due to malposition, fibrin thrombosis, precipitates caused by minerals or drugs, or lipid deposits (22).
   c. Management
      (1) Check catheter position on chest radiograph.
      (2) If malposition is ruled out, review history of fluids and drugs administered through the catheter to determine probable cause of occlusion.

(3) Remove the catheter if it is no longer medically critical.

(4) Attempt clot dissolution only if maintenance of catheter is essential.

(5) Equipment required: Face mask, sterile gloves and drape, prep solution, sterile three-way stopcock, a 10-mL syringe, and a 3-mL syringe filled with 0.2 to 0.5 mL of agent for clot dissolution.

(6) Agents for clot dissolution (22)

    (a) Hydrochloric acid 0.1N, for calcium salt precipitates or drugs with pH <7

    (b) Sodium bicarbonate, 8.4%, 1 mEq/mL, for medications with pH >7

    (c) Ethanol, 70% concentration, for lipid deposits

    (d) Recombinant tissue plasminogen activator, 0.5 to 1 mg/mL, for fibrin or blood clot (23,24)

    (e) Recombinant urokinase, 2,000 to 5,000 IU/mL, for fibrin or blood clot (24,25)

(7) Technique (23)

    (a) Use strict aseptic technique.

    (b) Remove IV tubing and cap to maintain sterility. After cleaning with prep, attach a three-way stopcock to catheter hub.

    (c) Attach an empty 10-mL syringe to the side port of the three-way stopcock and a prefilled 3-mL syringe to the other port. Avoid use of 1-mL tuberculin syringe.

    (d) Turn the stopcock off toward the prefilled syringe and open toward the empty syringe.

    (e) Aspirate on the empty syringe, creating negative pressure in the occluded catheter.

    (f) While maintaining the negative pressure, turn the stopcock off to the empty syringe and open to the prefilled syringe. The negative pressure in the catheter will automatically cause the medication in the prefilled syringe to flow into the catheter.

    (g) Allow the medication to dwell in the catheter for 30 minutes to 2 hours.

    (h) Aspirate after the dwell time to check for blood return, discard the aspirate, and flush the catheter with sterile normal saline. Resume catheter use.

    (i) If the procedure is unsuccessful, it may be repeated once, or a different declotting agent may be tried.

    (j) Do not use hydrochloric acid immediately before or after using sodium bicarbonate.

6. Thrombosis, thromboembolism

  a. About 90% of venous thromboembolic events in neonates are associated with central venous catheters (26). They include

    (1) Deep venous thrombosis

    (2) Superior vena cava syndrome

    (3) Intracardiac thrombus

    (4) Pulmonary embolism

    (5) Renal vein thrombosis

  b. The complications of venous thrombosis include loss of venous access, potential danger of injury to affected organ or limb, thrombus propagation, embolization to other areas, and infection.

  c. Management of thromboembolism in neonates is controversial. The severity of thrombosis and the potential risk to organs or limbs dictate the degree of intervention required, including the use of thrombolytic/anticoagulant therapy or surgical intervention (24).

7. Extravascular collection of fluid

  a. Pericardial effusion with or without cardiac tamponade (Fig. 32.15) (4,5,6). This serious complication presents as sudden cardiac collapse or unexplained cardiorespiratory instability. The cardiothoracic ratio is increased, and pulsus paradoxus may be noted (Fig. 39.1). Immediate pericardiocentesis may be life-saving (Chapter 39).

  b. Pleural effusion

  c. Mediastinal extravasation

  d. Hemothorax

  e. Chylothorax

  f. Ascites

8. Catheter breakage

  a. Catheters may be severed by the introducer needle during insertion of a PICC, snap because of excessive tension on the external portion of the catheter, or rupture because of excessive pressure. Other common causes include external clamps, kinking of the catheter, constricting sutures, and poorly secured catheters. The intravascular portion of the broken catheter is at risk for embolization (27).

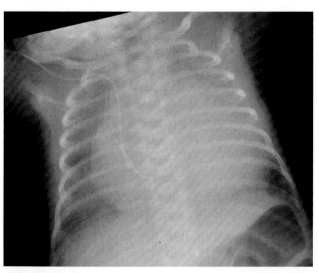

FIG. 32.15. Pericardial effusion in preterm infant with PICC looped in right atrium.

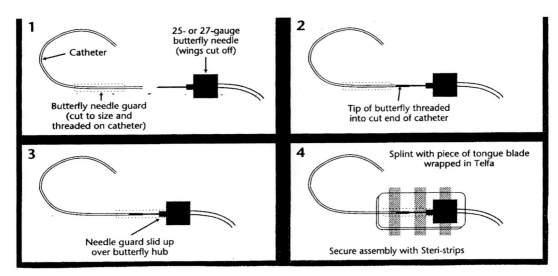

FIG. 32.16. Emergency catheter repair using butterfly needle (46). (From Neonatal Network, Santa Rosa, CA, with permission.)

b. In the event of catheter breakage, immediately grasp and secure the extravascular portion of the broken catheter to prevent migration.

c. If the catheter is not visible outside the baby, apply pressure over the venous tract above the insertion site to prevent the catheter from advancing. Immobilize the infant, and obtain a radiograph immediately to localize the catheter.

d. Surgical and/or cardiothoracic intervention may be required if the catheter is not visible externally (27).

e. Damaged or broken catheters must be removed and replaced. Repaired catheters and catheter replacement over a guidewire place the patient at risk for infection or embolization. If no other options exist owing to limited venous access, the catheter can sometimes be repaired, utilizing meticulous aseptic technique. Repaired PICCs should be considered temporary, and a new catheter should be placed as soon as possible. Some manufacturers offer repair kits and instructions. A butterfly or blunt needle may be used in an emergency (28) (Fig. 32.16).

9. Tethered catheter

a. Difficulty in removing catheter may be due to the formation of a fibrin sheath or secondary to sepsis.

b. Management

(1) Place warm compresses on skin along the vein.

(2) Use gradual, gentle traction on the catheter.

(3) Thrombolytic therapy (29)

(4) Surgical removal through a peripheral incision

References

1. Ainsworth SB, Clerihew L, McGuire W. Percutaneous central venous catheters versus peripheral cannulae for delivery of paren-teral nutrition in newborns. *Cochrane Database Syst Rev.* 2007;CD004219.

2. U.S. Department of Health and Human Services. Centers for Disease Control and Prevention. Guideline for prevention of intravascular catheter related infections; 2011:1. Available at: http://www.cdc.gov/hicpac/BSI/BSI-guidelines-2011.html

3. Schulman J, Stricof R, Stevens TP, et al. Statewide NICU central line associated bloodstream infection rates decline after bundles and checklists. *Pediatrics.* 2011;127:436.

4. Nowlen TT, Rosenthal GL, Johnson GL, et al. Pericardial effu-sion and tamponade in infants with central catheters. *Pediatrics.* 2002;110:137.

5. Beardsall K, White DK, Pinto EM, et al. Pericardial effusion and cardiac tamponade as complications of neonatal long lines: are they really a problem? *Arch Dis Child Fetal Neonatal Ed.* 2003;88:292.

6. Pezzati M, Filippi L, Chiti G, et al. Central venous catheters and cardiac tamponade in preterm infants. *Intensive Care Med.* 2004;30:2253.

7. Cartwright DW. Central venous lines in neonates: a study of 2186 catheters. *Arch Dis Child Fetal Neonatal Ed.* 2004;89:504.

8. Webster NJ, Page B, Kuschel CA, et al. Digital imaging does not improve localization of percutaneously inserted central lines in neonates. *J Paediatr Child Health.* 2005;41:256.

9. Coit AK, Kamitsuka MD. Peripherally inserted central catheter using the saphenous vein: importance of two-view radiographs to determine the tip location. *J Perinatol.* 2005;25:674.

10. Odd DE, Page B, Battin MR, et al. Does radio-opaque contrast improve radiographic localisation of percutaneous central venous lines? *Arch Dis Child Fetal Neonatal Ed.* 2004;89:41.

11. Brissaud O, Harper L, Lamireau D, et al. Sonographaphy guided positioning of intravenous long lines in neonates. *Eur J Radiol.* 2010;74:e18.

12. Primhak RH, Gathercole N, Reiter H. Pressures used to flush venous catheter. *Arch Dis Child Fetal Neonatal Ed.* 1998;78: F234.

13. Aly H, Herson V, Duncan A, et al. Is bloodstream infection pre-ventable among premature infants? A tale of two cities. *Pediatrics.* 2005;115:1513.

14. Shah PS, Shah VS. Continuous heparin infusion to prevent thrombosis and catheter occlusion in neonates with peripherally placed percutaneous central venous catheters. *Cochrane Database Syst Rev.* 2008;16:CD002772.

15. Wong EC, Schreiber S, Criss V, et al. Feasibility of red blood cell transfusions through small bore central venous catheters in neonates. *Pediatr Res.* 2001;49:322A.
16. Vegunta RK, Loethen P, Wallace LJ, et al. Differences in the outcome of surgically placed long-term central venous catheters in neonates: neck vs groin placement. *J Pediatr Surg.* 2005;40:47.
17. Murai DT. Are femoral Broviac catheters effective and safe? A prospective comparison of femoral and jugular venous Broviac catheters in newborn infants. *Chest.* 2002;121:1527.
18. Benjamin DK, Miller W, Garges H, et al. Bacteremia, central catheters, and neonates: when to pull the line. *Pediatrics.* 2001;107:1272.
19. Vasudevan C, McGuire W. Early removal versus expectant management of central venous catheters in neonates with bloodstream infection. *Cochrane Database Syst Rev.* 2011;10:CD008436.
20. Ramasethu J. Complications of vascular catheters in the neonatal intensive care unit. *Clin Perinatol.* 2008;35:199.
21. Rastogi S, Bhutada A, Sahni R, et al. Spontaneous correction of the malpositioned percutaneous central venous line in infants. *Pediatr Radiol.* 1998;28:694.
22. Doellman D. Prevention, assessment and treatment of central venous catheter occlusions in neonatal and young pediatric patients. *J Infus Nurs.* 2011;34:251.
23. Soylu H, Brandao LR, Lee KS. Efficacy of local instillation of recombinant tissue plasminogen activator for restoring occluded central venous catheters in neonates. *J Pediatr.* 2010;156:197.
24. Monagle P, Chalmers E, Chan A, et al. Antithrombotic therapy for neonates and children: American College of Chest Physicians Evidence Based Clinical Practice Guidelines (8th Edition). *Chest.* 2008;133:887S.
25. Svoboda P, Barton RP, Barbarash OL, et al. Recombinant urokinase is safe and effective in restoring patency to occluded central venous access devices: a multiple-center, international trial. *Crit Care Med.* 2004;32:1990.
26. Beardsley DS. Venous thromboembolism in the neonatal period. *Semin Perinatol.* 2007;31:250.
27. Chiang MC, Chou YH, Chiang CC, et al. Successful removal of a ruptured silastic percutaneous central venous catheter in a tiny premature infant. *Chang Gung Med J.* 2006;29:603.
28. Evans M, Lentsch D. Percutaneously inserted polyurethane central catheters in the NICU: one unit's experience. *Neonatal Network.* 1999;18:37.
29. Nguyen ST, Lund CH, Durand DJ. Thrombolytic therapy for adhesions of percutaneous central venous catheters to vein intima associated with Malassezia furfur infection. *J Perinatol.* 2001; 21:331.

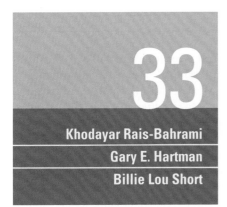

33 Extracorporeal Membrane Oxygenation Cannulation and Decannulation

Khodayar Rais-Bahrami

Gary E. Hartman

Billie Lou Short

Extracorporeal membrane oxygenation (ECMO) is defined as the use of a modified heart–lung machine combined with an oxygenator to provide cardiopulmonary support for patients with reversible pulmonary and/or cardiac insufficiency in whom maximal conventional therapies have failed (1–3). After decades of laboratory and clinical research, ECMO is well accepted as a standard treatment for neonatal respiratory failure refractory to conventional techniques of pulmonary support (4–7). Most causes of neonatal respiratory failure are self-limited, and ECMO allows time for the lung to recover from the underlying disease process and for reversal of pulmonary hypertension, which frequently accompanies respiratory failure in the newborn.

Venoarterial Extracorporeal Membrane Oxygenation — Cannulation

A. Indications

Placement of carotid arterial and internal jugular venous catheters for use in venoarterial (VA) ECMO. VA ECMO should be used in patients with significant cardiovascular instability.

B. Relative Contraindications for ECMO in the Neonatal Period (5,7)

1. Gestational age <34 weeks
2. Birthweight <2,000 g
3. Uncontrolled coagulopathy or bleeding disorders
4. Congenital heart disease without lung disease. Exception: Postoperative cardiac patients, a topic that will not be covered in this chapter.
5. Irreversible lung pathology
6. Intracranial hemorrhage more than grade II
7. Major lethal congenital anomaly
8. Duration of maximum ventilatory support, >10 to 14 days
9. Responding to ventilator management and/or inhaled nitric oxide

C. Precautions

1. Ensure that the patient is paralyzed before placing the venous catheter to prevent air embolus.
2. Recognize that
   a. Internal jugular lines placed for IV access prior to ECMO may cause clot formation, resulting in the need for thrombectomy before placement of the venous ECMO catheter.
   b. Excessive manipulation of the internal jugular vein may cause spasm and inability to place a catheter of appropriate gauge.
   c. A lacerated vessel may result in the need for a sternotomy for vessel retrieval.
      Appropriate instruments should be on the bedside tray or cart.
      A backup unit of blood should be available in the blood bank.
   d. Blood loss sufficient to produce hypotension can occur during a difficult cannulation.
      Emergency blood should be available at the bedside (10 to 20 mL/kg).
   e. The vagus nerve is located next to the neck vessels, and may be injured or manipulated during isolation of the vessels. Manipulation can cause bradycardia or other arrhythmias.
   f. Vital signs and pulse oximetry values must be monitored at all times because clinical observation of the infant is prevented by the surgical drapes.
   g. If the patient has been hand bag–ventilated for stabilization, do not place the Ambu bag on the bedside when surgical drapes are placed. The bag may entrap oxygen, which can result in a fire when electrocautery is used.

D. Personnel, Equipment, and Medications (8)

Personnel

1. Surgical team
   a. A senior surgeon (pediatric, cardiovascular, or thoracic) with assistant
   b. A surgical scrub nurse and a circulating nurse

2. Medical team
   a. A physician trained in management of ECMO patients and cannulation techniques, who will administer anesthetic agents and manage the infant medically during the procedure
   b. A bedside intensive care (neonatal or pediatric intensive care unit) nurse, who will monitor vital signs, record events, and draw up medications as needed by the ECMO physician
   c. A respiratory therapist, who will change ventilator settings as necessary
3. Circuit specialists
   a. A cardiovascular perfusionist, nurse, or respiratory therapist specially trained in this procedure, who will prime the pump
   b. A bedside ECMO specialist (nurse, respiratory therapist, or cardiovascular perfusionist with special training in ECMO management), who will manage the ECMO system after the patient is on ECMO

Equipment (Fig. 33.1)

Sterile

1. Arterial and venous catheters (9)
   a. Arterial
      (1) The size of the arterial catheter determines the resistance of the ECMO circuit because it is the part of the ECMO circuit with the smallest internal diameter and thus the highest resistance.
      (2) This catheter should be as short as possible, with a thin wall and a large internal diameter (resistance is related directly to the length of the catheter and inversely proportional to the diameter). An example of a suitable catheter is the Bio-Medicus Extracorporeal Circulation Cannula, 8 to 10 French (Fr) (Bio-Medicus, Minneapolis, Minnesota).
   b. Venous
      (1) Venous catheter with
         (a) As large an internal diameter as possible, to allow maximal blood flow (the patient's oxygenation is related directly to the rate of blood flow).
         (b) A thin wall/large internal diameter. An example of a suitable catheter is the Bio-Medicus Extracorporeal Circulation Cannula, 8 to 14 Fr. (Bio-Medicus, Minneapolis, Minnesota).
2. Surgical instruments required are listed in Tables 33.1 and 33.2.
3. Gowns and gloves
4. Saline for injection
5. Syringes (1 to 20 mL) and needles (19 to 26 gauge)
6. Povidone–iodine solution
7. Povidone–iodine ointment
8. Semipermeable transparent membrane-type dressing
9. Absorbable gelatin sponge, for example, Gelfoam (Upjohn, Kalamazoo, Michigan)
10. Surgical lubricant, bacteriostatic

Nonsterile

1. Surgical head covers and mask
2. Pulse oximeter
3. Surgical head light
4. Electrocautery
5. Wall suction
6. Shoulder roll, for example, a small blanket, to place under infant's shoulders
7. Tubing clamps

Medications

1. A long-acting paralyzing agent, for example, pancuronium bromide (0.1 mg/kg)
2. Fentanyl citrate (10 to 20 μg/kg)
3. Sodium heparin (75 to 150 U/kg)
4. Topical thrombin/Gelfoam
5. Lidocaine, 0.25%, with epinephrine
6. Lidocaine, 1% (without epinephrine)
7. Cryoprecipitate, thawed, or commercially available fibrin sealant (optional)

E. Technique—Preparation for Cannulation

1. Place infant with head to "foot" of overhead warmer bed.
2. Anesthetize the patient with fentanyl (10 to 20 μg/kg).

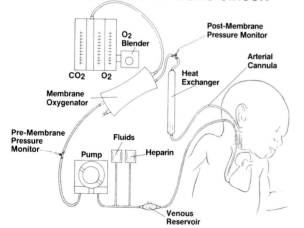

VENOARTERIAL ECMO CIRCUIT

FIG. 33.1. Schematic diagram of VA ECMO circuit, showing the drainage from the right atrium into the bladder of the circuit, with flow through the membrane lung, heat exchanger, and return flow to the arch of the aorta via the carotid artery catheter. (From Polin RA, Fox WC, eds. *Fetal and Neonatal Physiology*, Vol. 1. Philadelphia: WB Saunders; 1992:933, with permission.)

TABLE 33.1	Surgical Instruments for ECMO Cannulation

Number	Item

Place in a 12- × 18-inch mayo tray with a Huck towel on the bottom of the tray.

Number	Item
2	Custard cup (place on inside of other cup with a 3- × 4-inch sponge)
1	Medicine cup (place inside of custard cup with a 3- × 4-inch sponge)
2	Straight bulldog clamps
1	Sauer eye retractor
1	Alm retractor
1	Mastoid Jansen retractor
2	Vein retractors
2	Octagonal forceps
2	7-inch Gerald forceps
2	6-inch DeBakey forceps
1	Adson forceps, plain
2	Adson forceps with teeth
2	No. 3 knife handles
1	Castroviejo needle holder
2	Right-angle retractors
2	Chops retractors
1	Set of Garrett dilators, nine pieces (sizes 1, 1.5, 2, 2.5, 3, 3.5, 4, 4.5, 5)

String the following instruments from left to right on two 9-inch sponge sticks or instrument stringer. Then place on top of a rolled Huck towel.

Number	Item
4	9-inch sponge stick
1	Tonsil clamp (bleeder)
1	6.5-inch Crile
1	5.75-inch Crile
1	Baby right-angle clamp
4	Straight mosquitoes
6	Curved mosquitoes
3	Fine curved mosquitoes
2	Tubing clamp with guard
1	Ryder needle holder
1	Webster needle holder
1	Straight mayo scissor
1	5.75-inch Metzenbaum scissor
1	Curved Steven scissor
1	Straight Iris scissor
4	Small towel clips (nonpenetrating)
1	Baby Satinsky clamp
1	Curved bulldog clamp
1	Straight bulldog clamp
1	Disposable ECMO tray (Table 33.2)

ECMO, extracorporeal membrane oxygenation. For information on suture material, see Appendix B2.

TABLE 33.2	Contents of Disposable ECMO Tray

Number	Item
2	1-mL syringe
1	20-mL syringe
1	6-mL syringe
1	3-mL syringe
1	Needle adapter
3	Single-cavity tray
2	Gauze packages
1	Betadine ointment
1	Surgical blade no. 15 carbon
2	Semipermeable transparent dressings
1	Handle, suction Frazier, 8 Fr
1	Xylocaine insert
1	Mini yellow vessel loops
1	Hand-control cautery
1	Suture, 4-0 Vicryl
1	Suture, 2-0 silk
1	Suture, 6-0 Prolene
4	Forceps, sponge
1	25-gauge needle
1	NaCl, 5-mL amp
1	3-g foil package of Surgilube
1	Surgical blade, no. 11 carbon
2	Steri-Drapes
2	Connectors, straight 0.25 × 0.25 inch
1	Xylocaine 1%
1	Suction tubing, 3/16 inch × 10 ft
1	Package sterile towels (14)

9. At the point of incision, infiltrate the skin with lidocaine (0.25%, with epinephrine) (Fig. 33.2).
10. Wait at least 3 minutes for anesthesia to be effective.
11. Make a 1- to 2-cm vertical incision over the right sternocleidomastoid muscle, starting approximately 1 cm above the right clavicular head, using the electrocautery set on cutting current (Fig. 33.3).

3. Paralyze the patient with pancuronium (0.1 mg/kg).
4. Hyperextend the patient's neck with a shoulder roll, and turn the head to the left (Fig. 33.2). Make sure that the Bovie ground pad is placed at this time.
   Observe closely for hypotension.
5. Monitor vital signs and give additional fentanyl and/or pancuronium as needed (see Chapter 6).
6. Clean a wide area of the right neck, chest, and ear with Betadine solution.
7. Drape the infant and entire bed with sterile towels.
8. Use Steri-Drapes (3M Health Care, St. Paul, Minnesota) to secure the towels to the skin.

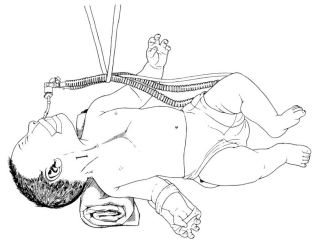

FIG. 33.2. Infant positioned for cannulation with shoulder roll present and head extended to the left. Position of neck incision is indicated.

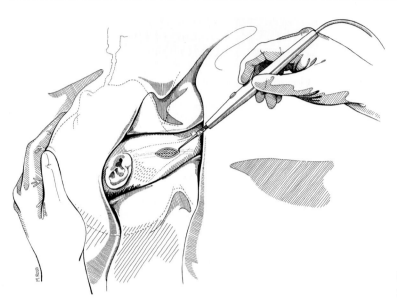

FIG. 33.3. Landmarks over the sternocleidomastoid muscle for making the incision with electrocautery.

12. Continue to use the electrocautery to cut through the subcutaneous tissue.
13. Coagulate all visible bleeding sites.
14. Spread the fibers of the sternocleidomastoid muscle apart with a hemostat and retract using hemostats clamped onto the muscle (Fig. 33.4).
15. Open the carotid sheath, taking care to avoid the vagus nerve.
16. Irrigate both the common carotid artery and internal jugular vein with 1% plain lidocaine to vasodilate the vessels.
17. Encircle the artery with silicone loop, and proximal and distal 2-0 silk ties held with clamps but not tied. Avoid "sawing" the ties on the artery.

18. Avoid excessive handling of the internal jugular vein. Some isolate the vein after cannulation of the carotid artery to avoid spasm.
19. Estimate the length of the cannula to be inserted.
    a. Identify the sternal notch and the xiphoid process.
    b. The arterial catheter is inserted approximately one third of the distance between the sternal notch and the xiphoid process. This is typically between 3 and 4 cm.
    c. The venous catheter is inserted approximately one-half the distance between the sternal notch and the xiphoid process. This is typically between 7 and 7.5 cm.
    d. Mark these distances on the catheters with a 2-0 tie, or note the distance if the cannula is marked.
20. Heparinize the patient with a bolus of 75 to 150 U/kg of heparin, depending on the estimated risk of bleeding, and wait 60 to 90 seconds before proceeding with cannulation.

Arterial Cannulation

1. Tie the distal ligature on the carotid artery, and place a bulldog clamp on the proximal portion of the artery.
     Allow blood to dilate the artery before placing the bulldog clamp.
2. Make an arteriotomy using a no. 11 scalpel blade, and place two traction sutures of 6-0 Prolene (Ethicon, Somerville, New Jersey) on the proximal side of the arteriotomy (Fig. 33.5).
     Always use traction sutures, to prevent intimal tears.
3. If desired, lubricate Garrett dilators with sterile surgical lubricant and dilate the artery to the approximate size of the catheter.
4. Place a sterile tubing clamp on the catheter. Lubricate the catheter and insert the catheter into the vessel as the bulldog clamp is removed.

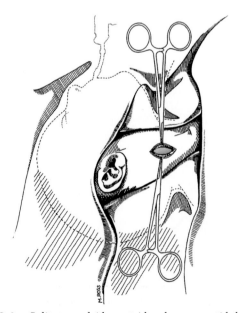

FIG. 33.4. Split sternocleidomastoid and open carotid sheath.

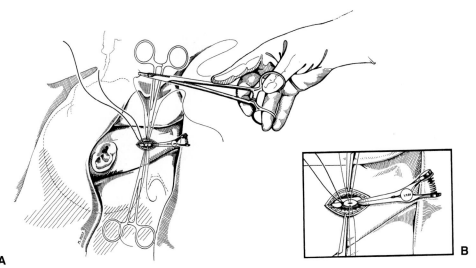

FIG. 33.5. **A:** Carotid artery isolated with vessel clamp in place and with arteriotomy site showing the placement of the 6-0 Prolene traction sutures. **B (inset):** Magnified view of (**A**).

5. Secure the catheter with a 2-0 silk ligature tied over a 0.5- to 1-cm vessel loop ("bootie") (Fig. 33.6).
6. Place a second 2-0 silk ligature. Tie the distal tie around the catheter, and then tie the distal and proximal ties together. Some surgeons place two ties proximally and one distally for added security.
7. Allow blood to back up into the catheter to remove air.

Venous Cannulation

1. Dissect the vein free and isolate with two 2-0 silk ties.
   Do not apply traction to the vein with the ties, to avoid spasm.

2. Place a bulldog clamp on the proximal end of the vein, allowing blood to distend it. Then tie the distal end of the vein with the 2-0 silk ligature.
3. Make a venotomy with a no. 11 scalpel blade, and place two stay sutures of 6-0 Prolene as traction sutures, as for arterial cannulation.
4. Lubricate the venous catheter, place a sterile tubing clamp on the catheter, and dilate the venotomy.
5. Insert the catheter as surgical assistant places traction on the proximal tie, and apply pressure over the liver to increase the backflow of blood out of the catheter (to decrease the risk of an air embolus).

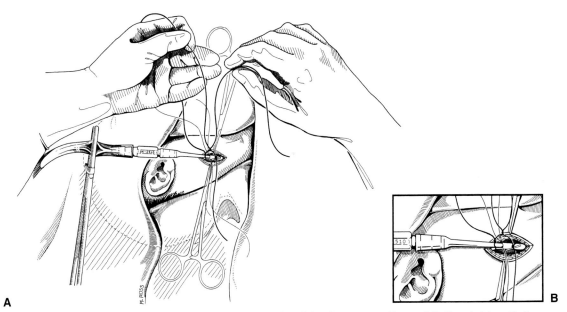

FIG. 33.6. **A:** Securing the catheter with proximal and distal ties onto a "bootie." **B (inset):** Magnified view of (**A**).

There will be slight impedance to catheter advancement at the thoracic inlet—pushing against resistance will tear the vein. Use gentle downward and posterior pressure.

6. Secure, as for the artery, and back blood into the catheter by pressing gently on the liver.

7. If desired, pack the wound with absorbable gelatin sponge soaked in topical thrombin or commercially available topical fibrin sealant, to assist in hemostasis.

Cryoprecipitate and topical thrombin can be used to form a fibrin clot if dropped onto the field from separate syringes in a one-to-one concentration. Note: If they are mixed together in one syringe, they will form a solid clot in the syringe. A similar product is also commercially available as Tisseel-HV Fibrin Sealant (Baxter Hyland Division, Glendale, California).

8. Confirm catheter placement by chest radiography and/ or cardiac echocardiography, if the patient is stable (Fig. 33.7) (10, 11). If the patient is unstable, he or she can be placed on ECMO and the radiograph taken when adequate oxygenation is achieved but prior to closing the surgical wound.

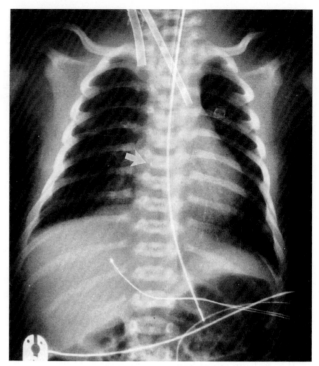

FIG. 33.7. Radiograph at cannulation, showing proper placement of the arterial and venous catheters. Note the radio-opaque dot indicating the end of the Bio-Medicus venous extracorporeal membrane oxygenation catheter (*arrow*).

Venovenous Extracorporeal Membrane Oxygenation—Cannulation

More than 60% of neonatal ECMO patients reported in the ELSO registry have received treatment with VA bypass (12). In neonates with respiratory failure, VA ECMO is gradually being replaced by a venovenous (VV) technique, which uses a single double-lumen catheter (Fig. 33.8). The catheter is placed in the right atrium, where blood is drained and reinfused into the same chamber, thus requiring cannulation of only the right jugular vein, and sparing the carotid artery. Other advantages of VV ECMO include maintenance of normal pulsatile blood flow, and the theoretical advantage that particles entering the ECMO circuit enter by way of the pulmonary rather than the systemic circulation. The design of the original VV catheter resulted in significant recirculation, limiting its use when ECMO flows >350 mL/min were required. Research by Rais-Bahrami et al. (13) resulted in development of a new catheter design that significantly lowers the degree of recirculation. The double-lumen catheter should be placed within the right atrium, directing the oxygenated blood from the return lumen through the tricuspid valve to minimize recirculation. This catheter design in 12-, 15-, and 18-Fr sizes allows the use of VV ECMO in a greater number of infants (14).

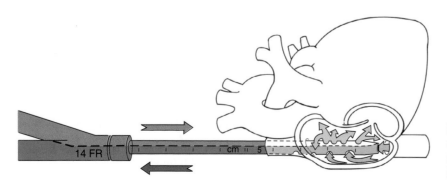

FIG. 33.8. Schematic of the VV ECMO catheter placed in the mid-right atrium. (From Short BL. *CNMC ECMO Training Manual.* 2005, with permission).

A. Double-Lumen VV Catheters

1. Kendall 14-Fr catheter (Kendall Health Care Products, Mansfield, Massachusetts)
2. OriGen 12-, 15-, and 18-Fr catheters (OriGen Biomedical, Austin, Texas)
3. Avalon Elite DLC, 13- to 31-Fr catheter (Avalon Laboratories LLC, Rancho Dominguez, California)

    Note: The Avalon catheter requires insertion under ultrasound or fluoroscopy guidance; refer to company recommendations at www.avalonlabs.com

B. Advantages of VV Bypass

1. Provides excellent pulmonary support
2. Avoids carotid artery ligation
3. Oxygenated blood enters pulmonary circulation.
4. Particles coming from the ECMO circuit enter the venous circulation instead of the arterial circulation.

C. Disadvantages of VV Bypass

1. Lack of cardiac support
2. ECMO support is dependent on the patient's cardiac function.
3. Catheter position and rotation are extremely critical.
4. Amount of recirculation

D. Cannulation Technique

The cannulation technique for VV ECMO is essentially the same procedure as venous cannulation for VA ECMO, with the following exceptions.

1. Both internal jugular vein and carotid arteries are identified and dissected free, although the internal jugular vein is the only vessel cannulated with the double-lumen VV catheter. Both vessels are isolated in case a rapid conversion to VA bypass becomes necessary. A silastic loop may be tied loosely around the artery to facilitate potential conversion to VA flow.
2. The cannula is advanced with the lumen, which will carry oxygenated blood ("arterial side") upward and anterior to the venous side of the double-lumen (Fig. 33.8).

    Caution: Avoid bending the catheter or creating a "crimp" in the catheter.

    Correct positioning of the catheter helps direct the oxygenated blood return toward the tricuspid valve, thus minimizing the recirculation of the oxygenated blood back to the ECMO circuit.
3. The proximal end of the internal jugular vein is also cannulated for cephalad drainage, that is, a jugular bulb catheter. This catheter is connected to the venous tubing of the ECMO circuit via a Luer connector. For this, we use a custom-made Carmeda heparin-coated Bio-Medicus venous catheter, made specifically for use as a cephalad catheter.

    This allows additional venous drainage to the ECMO circuit, prevents venous congestion, and also allows for cephalic venous saturation measurement.
4. If using a jugular bulb catheter to measure cerebral saturations, care should be used when entering the circuit; air will draw into the venous side of the circuit rapidly if a stopcock is loose or is left open.

E. Placing Patient on the Extracorporeal Membrane Oxygenation Circuit

The circuit has been previously primed with packed cells/albumin. The priming procedure and the surgical placement of the ECMO catheters should be timed so that the two are completed at the same time. Priming of the circuit is beyond the scope of this chapter.

1. Fill catheters with sterile saline. Connect them to the ECMO circuit by inserting the 0.25- × 0.25-inch connectors into the tubing as the assistant drips sterile saline into the ends of the circuit tubing and the catheter, to ensure that all residual air is eliminated prior to connection.
    a. Do not squeeze the tubing while attaching; air will enter when the tubing is released.
    b. If air is seen in the tubing, the catheters must be disconnected from the circuit. Prior to reconnection, air is removed, and the catheters are reconnected as described in E1.
2. Remove all sterile tubing clamps from the catheters, and have a nonsterile assistant hold the catheters. Nonsterile tubing clamps remain in place on the arterial and venous sides of the circuit at this juncture.
3. Place the patient on ECMO by removing the arterial clamp, placing a clamp on the bridge (Fig. 33.9A), and removing the venous clamp. This will remove all nonsterile clamps from the circuit.

    Many centers are now using a "bloodless bridge" that has sterile-heparinized saline with stopcock design; thus, a clamp on the bridge is not necessary. The bridge is left closed with the stopcock mechanism during cannulation so that only the clamps on the catheters need to be removed.
4. Increase ECMO flow in 50-mL increments over 20 to 30 minutes, until adequate oxygenation is achieved (usually at 120 mL/kg/min).

    Transfusion may be needed if hypotension occurs at this stage.
5. Decrease the ventilator settings and oxygen concentration gradually as the ECMO flows are increased.

    Typical resting ventilator settings for VA ECMO are at a rate of 10 to 15 breaths/min, a peak pressure

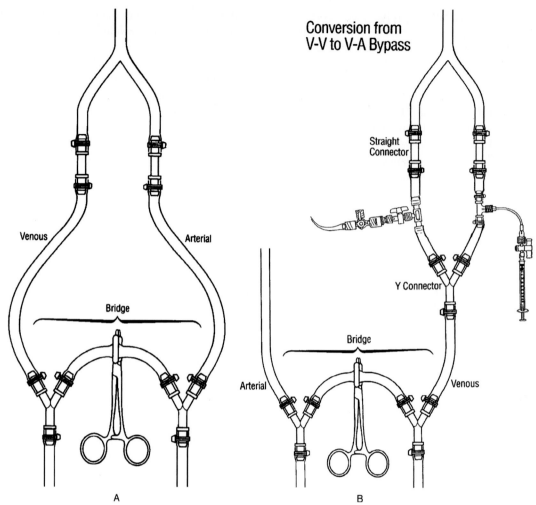

FIG. 33.9.   Schematic view of converting from VA (**A**) to VV (**B**) ECMO. The double-lumen VV catheter is "Y'd" together to make a double-lumen venous drainage catheter.

limit of 15 to 20 cm H_2O, and F_iO_2 of 0.21 to 0.30. For VV ECMO, it is recommended to keep ventilator settings at a rate of 20 to 30 breaths/min, a peak inspiratory pressure of 20 to 25 cm H_2O, and F_iO_2 of 0.30 to 0.35.

F. Closure of the Neck Wound

1. Obtain radiographic confirmation of appropriate catheter position and achievement of an adequate flow rate through the ECMO circuit prior to closure of the neck wound.
2. Cut and remove traction sutures.
3. Approximate the skin with a running 4-0 Vicryl (Ethicon) suture on an atraumatic needle.
4. Tie the Vicryl suture, and use the tails of the suture to secure each catheter.
5. Tie catheters together with another silk tie.

6. Anesthetize the area behind the ear with 0.25% Xylocaine with epinephrine.
7. Use 2-0 silk suture on a noncutting needle to place a stitch behind the ear and tie around the catheter to secure in place. Place a separate stitch for each catheter.
8. Tie catheters together, dress the incision with povidone–iodine ointment, and cover the area with semipermeable membrane dressing.
9. Secure the circuit tubing securely to the bedside to reduce traction on the catheters.

G. Complications

1. Torn vessels, more commonly the vein
   a. This risk is decreased if 6-0 Prolene stay sutures are always used.
   b. Do not attempt to use too large a catheter.

2. Aortic dissection associated with arterial cannulation (15).
3. Blood loss, particularly during the venous cannulation, when side holes in the catheter are outside the vein
4. Venous spasm, resulting in inability to place a large enough venous catheter to meet the required ECMO flow to support the patient adequately

   The rate of blood flow is impeded by the small gauge of the catheter, requiring that a second venous catheter be placed in the femoral vein. The two catheters must be Y-connected together into the ECMO circuit.
5. Arrhythmias and/or bradycardia can occur, owing to stimulation of the vagus nerve
6. Hypotension, due to an increase in the intravascular space when the patient is connected to the ECMO circuit
7. Conversion to VA from VV ECMO. This will occur if
   a. The patient remains hypoxic despite adequate ECMO flow.
   b. The patient remains hypotensive despite vasopressor support.
   c. Cerebral venous saturations remain persistently <60% after adequate flows and ventilator management have been undertaken.

      Converting from VV to VA ECMO requires cannulation of carotid artery with a Bio-Medicus arterial catheter, and the double-lumen VV catheter must be "Y'd" in together to make a double-lumen venous drainage catheter (Fig. 33.9).

Extracorporeal Membrane Oxygenation—Decannulation

A. Indications

1. Removal from ECMO after lung recovery
2. Removal from ECMO because of a complication such as uncontrolled bleeding or failure of lung recovery

B. Contraindications

All intensive support is being withdrawn, and permission for autopsy is obtained. It is usually optimal to remove the catheters during the autopsy.

C. Precautions

1. The patient must be paralyzed during the removal of the venous catheter to avoid an air embolus.
2. The vessels are fragile and may tear. A backup unit of blood should be available at the bedside.
3. Delay removing catheter for 12 to 24 hours after taking the patient off bypass in cases in which there is a high

risk of reoccurrence of pulmonary hypertension and thus need for second ECMO run (e.g., severe congenital diaphragmatic hernia). This procedure places a risk of development of right atrial clots from the venous catheter and, in some patients, has resulted in superior venocaval syndrome. Therefore, the time the catheters are left in place should be limited to no more than 24 hours.

D. Personnel, Equipment, and Medications

Personnel

Same as for cannulation, with the exception that the primer is not required

Equipment

Sterile

1. Surgical tray with towels and suture as for cannulation
2. Semipermeable transparent dressing
3. Povidone–iodine ointment
4. Syringes (1 to 20 mL) and needles (18 to 26 gauge)
5. Unit of blood
6. Absorbable gelatin sponge

Nonsterile

Same as for cannulation

Medications

1. Fentanyl (10 to 20 μg/kg)
2. Vecuronium bromide (0.2 mg/kg)
3. A short-acting paralyzing agent is preferred because of the relatively short duration of the procedure. This allows the infant to breathe spontaneously as soon as possible after decannulation, which facilitates rapid weaning from ventilator support.
4. Lidocaine, 0.25%, with epinephrine
5. Topical thrombin
6. Protamine sulfate (1 mg only)

E. Technique

Postdecannulation vessel reconstruction is beyond the scope of this chapter.

1. Place the neck in an extended position, using the shoulder roll.
2. Give fentanyl for analgesia, prior to giving vecuronium.

   Because of the risk of air embolism during the removal of the venous catheter, the infant must *not* be allowed to breathe during decannulation. If two doses of vecuronium do not produce paralysis, give pancuronium.
3. Increase ventilator setting to a rate of 40 to 50 breaths/min, a peak inspiratory pressure of 20 to 25 cm H_2O

(depending on chest movement), and F_iO_2 of 0.30 to 0.40 after paralytic agent is given.

4. Clean the neck, and drape as for cannulation.
5. Anesthetize with 0.25% lidocaine with epinephrine.
6. Cut and remove the Vicryl suture.
7. Remove absorbable gelatin sponge packing, exposing the catheters and vessels.

   If a jugular bulb catheter is in place, it is usually removed first to allow better visualization for removal of the VV ECMO catheter.

8. The jugular bulb catheter should be clamped off before removal, after the patient is taken off bypass. Be aware that removing the catheter while on bypass without a clamp in place will result in the introduction of air into the circuit.

   In case of VA ECMO, the venous catheter is usually removed first because it is most readily accessible.

9. Separate the catheter from surrounding tissue by blunt dissection.
10. Encircle the vein with a 2-0 silk tie, which is used for traction and hemostatic control.
11. Place a Satinsky clamp around the vein to stabilize the catheter (Fig. 33.10).
12. Place a 2-0 silk tie proximal to the clamp.
13. Cut the silk ties securing the catheter in the vein with a no. 11 scalpel blade. The two proximal ties should be cut where they cross the vessel loop ("bootie").
14. Ask the ECMO specialist to remove the patient from the ECMO circuit.
15. Monitor vital signs and oxygen saturation as an indication that ventilator settings are appropriate. Settings

may have to be increased when the patient is removed from the circuit.

16. Provide an inspiratory "hold" on the ventilator while the surgeon removes the venous catheter. Failure to do this can result in air embolus.
17. Replace any significant blood loss.
18. Cut the 2-0 silk traction suture and tie the suture proximal to the Satinsky clamp. Remove the Satinsky clamp.
19. Isolate the arterial catheter, dissect free, and remove.

   The decannulation procedure is the same as for the venous catheter, with the exception that an inspiratory hold that is not required.

20. Give protamine (1 mg IV) after removal of both catheters.

   Administration of protamine is not mandatory if there is no significant bleeding.

21. Irrigate the wound with sterile saline and cauterize any bleeding sites.
22. If desired, pack the wound with a thrombin-soaked absorbable gelatin sponge and close the neck incision using subcuticular horizontal sutures of 4-0 Vicryl.
23. Remove the sutures holding the cannula behind the right ear.
24. Place povidone–iodine ointment over the incision and cover with semipermeable transparent dressing.

F. Complications

1. Vessel laceration, which may require a sternotomy for correction
2. Excessive blood loss
3. Venous air embolus

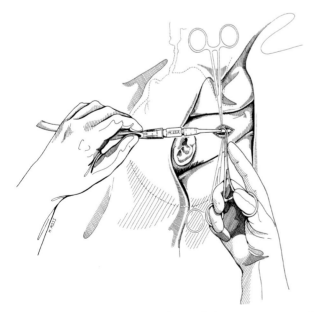

FIG. 33.10. Placement of Satinsky vessel clamp prior to removal of ECMO catheter.

References

1. O'Rourke PP, Crone RK, Vacanti JP, et al. Extracorporeal membrane oxygenation and conventional medical therapy in neonates with persistent pulmonary hypertension of the newborn: a prospective randomized study. *Pediatrics.* 1989;84:957.
2. UK Collaborative ECMO Trial Group. UK Collaborative Randomised Trial of Neonatal Extracorporeal Membrane Oxygenation. *Lancet.* 1996;348:75.
3. Elbourne D, Field D, Mugford M. Extracorporeal membrane oxygenation for severe respiratory failure in newborn infants. *Cochrane Database Syst Rev.* 2002:CD001340.
4. Kanto WP, Shapiro MB. The development of prolonged extracorporeal circulation. In: Zwischenberger JB, Steinhorn RH, Bartlet RH, eds. *Extracorporeal Cardiopulmonary Support in Critical Care.* 2nd ed. Ann Arbor, MI: Extracorporeal Life Support Organization; 2000:27.
5. Rais-Bahrami K, Short BL. The current status of neonatal extracorporeal membrane oxygenation. *Semin Perinatol.* 2000;24:406.
6. Bartlett RH, Roloff DW, Custer JR, et al. Extracorporeal life support: the University of Michigan experience. *JAMA.* 2000;283:904.
7. Rais-Bahrami K, Van Meurs KP. ECMO for neonatal respiratory failure. *Semin Perinatol.* 2005;29:15.
8. Sutton RG, Salatich A, Jegier B, et al. A 2007 survey of extracorporeal life support members: personnel and equipment. *J Extra Corpor Technol.* 2009;41:172.

9. Van Meurs KP, Mikesell GT, Seale WR, et al. Maximum blood flow rates for arterial cannulae used in neonatal ECMO. *ASAIO Trans.* 1990;36:M679.

10. Irish MS, O'Toole SJ, Kapur P, et al. Cervical ECMO cannula placement in infants and children: recommendations for assessment of adequate positioning and function. *J Pediatr Surg.* 1998;33:929.

11. Thomas TH, Price R, Ramaciotti C, et al. Echocardiography, not chest radiography, for evaluation of cannula placement during pediatric extracorporeal membrane oxygenation. *Pediatr Crit Care Med.* 2009;10:56.

12. Neonatal ECMO Registry of the Extracorporeal Life Support Organization (ELSO). Ann Arbor, MI: ELSO; 2011.

13. Rais-Bahrami K, Rivera O, Mikesell GT, et al. Improved oxygenation with reduced recirculation during venovenous extracorporeal membrane oxygenation: evaluation of a test catheter. *Crit Care Med.* 1995;23:1722.

14. Rais-Bahrami K, Waltom DM, Sell JE, et al. Improved oxygenation with reduced recirculation during venovenous ECMO: comparison of two catheters. *Perfusion.* 2002;17:415.

15. Paul JJ, Desai H, Baumgart S, et al. Aortic dissection in a neonate associated with arterial cannulation for extracorporeal life support. *ASAIO.* 1997;43:92.

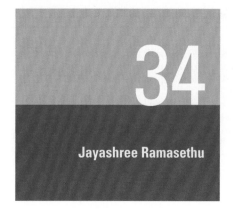

34 Management of Vascular Spasm and Thrombosis

Jayashree Ramasethu

Intravascular arterial and venous catheters are associated with significant risks of vascular thrombosis in newborn infants (1,2). About 90% of neonatal venous thromboses are associated with central venous catheters, although additional risk factors may be present (3).

A. Definitions

1. Vascular spasm is transient, reversible arterial constriction, often triggered by intravascular catheterization or arterial blood sampling.
2. Thrombosis is the complete or partial obstruction of arteries or veins by blood clot(s).

B. Assessment

1. Clinical diagnosis

a. The clinical signs associated with arterial or venous thrombosis are shown in Table 34.1.
b. Vascular spasm of peripheral arteries is characterized by transient pallor, or cyanosis of the involved extremity with diminished pulses and perfusion. The clinical effects of vascular spasm usually last <4 hours from the onset, but the condition may be difficult to differentiate from more serious thromboembolism. The diagnosis of vasospasm of arteries is usually made *retrospectively* after documentation of the transient nature of ischemic changes and complete recovery of circulation (4) (Fig. 34.1 and 34.2).
c. Persistent bacteremia and thrombocytopenia are nonspecific signs associated with vascular thrombosis at any site.
d. Clinical signs may be subtle or absent in many cases of thrombosis, which may be detected incidentally during ultrasonography for other indications.

2. Diagnostic imaging

a. *Contrast angiography:* Gold standard, gives best definition of thrombosis but is difficult to perform in critically ill neonates; requires infusion of radiocontrast material that may be hypertonic or cause undesired increase in vascular volume (3).

b. *Doppler ultrasonography:* Portable, noninvasive, monitors improve over time, but may give both false-positive and false-negative results compared with contrast angiography (5).

3. Additional diagnostic tests

a. Obtain detailed family history in all cases of vascular thrombosis.
b. Laboratory testing for genetic thrombophilic disorder (Table 34.2) has been advocated, but its value is debatable, particularly with catheter-related thrombosis in neonates (6–8). The tests do not influence immediate management, and the volume of blood required (4 to 6 mL) is a limitation. In addition, protein-based assays are affected by age and by the acute thromboembolic event and must be repeated at 3 to 6 months of life before a definitive diagnosis can be made.

C. Management of Arterial Vascular Spasm

1. Warm contralateral extremity (reflex vasodilation).
2. Maintain neutral thermal environment for affected extremity (i.e., keep heat lamps off area).
3. Maintain limb in horizontal position.
4. Correct hypotension or hypovolemia if present.
5. Consider removal of the catheter.

   If mild cyanosis of the fingers or toes is noted after insertion of an arterial catheter but peripheral pulses are still palpable, a trial of reflex vasodilation with close observation is reasonable, as vasospasm may resolve. Continually assess the need for keeping the catheter in place (i.e., the benefits of arterial access vs. the risk of thrombosis and further complications.) A white or "blanched" appearing extremity is an indication for immediate removal of the catheter.
6. Topical nitroglycerine has been demonstrated to reverse peripheral and umbilical artery catheter–induced ischemia in isolated case reports. Maintain good circulatory volume. Monitor for hypotension and be prepared to treat it immediately.

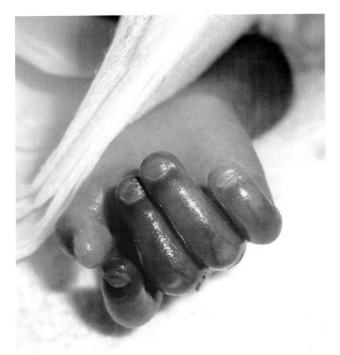

FIG. 34.1. Vasospasm following attempted radial artery catheterization in extremely preterm infant.

Topical application of 2% nitroglycerine ointment at a dose of 4 mm/kg body weight, applied as a thin film over the affected areas; may be repeated after 8 hours (9–11).

D. Management of Catheter-Related Thromboembolism

1. General principles

a. Thrombolysis to restore catheter patency for obstructed central venous catheters is described in Chapter 32.

b. Management of vascular thrombosis may involve one or more of the following: Supportive care with continued close observation, anticoagulation, thrombolytic therapy, or surgical intervention (1,8,12,13).

c. Infant should be managed in an appropriately staffed and equipped neonatal intensive care unit where anticoagulant or thrombolytic therapy can be administered and monitored closely and supportive and surgical care are readily available. Consultation with pediatric hematology is recommended. Plastic or vascular surgical consultation may be required.

d. Treatment of catheter-related thrombosis in neonates is still evolving. Current published guidelines for treatment are based on common clinical practice, case studies, and extrapolation of principles of therapy from adult guidelines (12,13).

e. *Supportive care:* Correct volume depletion, electrolyte abnormalities, anemia, thrombocytopenia, treatment of sepsis.

f. Treatment is *highly individualized* and is determined by the site and extent of thrombosis, and the degree to which diminished perfusion to the affected extremity or organ affects function, and the potential risk of bleeding complications associated with anticoagulant or thrombolytic therapy (8,12,13).

g. Expectant management or "watchful waiting"— close monitoring without anticoagulation or thrombolysis may be appropriate for some infants (1,12).

h. Anticoagulation therapy with unfractionated heparin (UFH) or low-molecular-weight heparin (LMWH) is used for clinically significant clots with the goal of preventing clot extension or embolization.

i. Recombinant tissue plasminogen activator (rTPA) is reserved for thrombolysis of severe life-, organ-, or limb-threatening thrombosis.

j. The International Children's Thrombophilia Network, which is based in Canada, is a free consultative service, maintained 24 hours a day, for

---

| **TABLE 34.1** | **Diagnosis of Vascular Thrombosis** |

Site	Clinical Signs	Diagnostic Imaging
CVL-associated venous thrombosis	Malfunction of CVL, SVC syndrome, chylothorax, swelling and livid discoloration of extremity, dilatation of collateral veins over trunk or abdomen in chronic cases	Contrast angiography Doppler ultrasonography Real-time 2D ultrasonography
Inferior vena cava thrombosis	Lower limbs cool, cyanotic, edematous	
Superior vena cava thrombosis	Swelling of upper limbs and head, chylothorax	
Renal vein thrombosis	Flank mass, hematuria, thrombocytopenia, hypertension	
Aortic or renal arterial thrombosis	Systemic hypertension, hematuria, oliguria	
Peripheral or central (aorta or iliac) arterial thrombosis	Pallor, coldness, weak or absent peripheral pulse(s), discoloration, gangrene	
Right atrial thrombosis	Congestive heart failure	Echocardiography
Pulmonary thromboembolism	Respiratory failure	Lung perfusion scan

CVL, central venous line; SVC, superior vena cava.

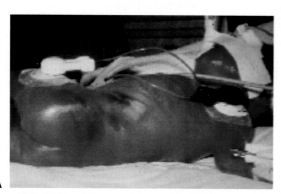
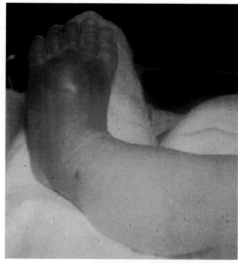

FIG. 34.2.   Skin necrosis associated with an umbilical artery catheter. Such lesions develop after vaso-spasm or embolism. **A:** Spinal injury may be present when ischemia involves this region. **B:** The distal part of an extremity is a common site for embolic arterial loss. The full extent of loss is unpredictable at this stage. (From Fletcher MA. *Physical Diagnosis in Neonatology*. Philadelphia: Lippincott-Raven; 1998:127.)

physicians worldwide who are caring for children with thromboembolic disease. The toll-free number in the North America is 1-800-NO-CLOTS; the number for physicians elsewhere is 1-905-573-4795 (Web site http://www.1800noclots.ca/) The service provides current management protocols as well as links to the network and its services.

2. Management of catheter-related venous thrombosis (12)

a. Either initial anticoagulation or supportive care with radiological monitoring may be appropriate. However, anticoagulation is recommended if extension of the thrombus occurs during supportive care.

b. Remove central venous lines (CVL) or umbilical venous lines associated with confirmed thrombosis, preferably after 3 to 5 days of anticoagulation. This recommendation has been made to reduce

the risk of paradoxical emboli at the time of CVL removal.

c. Intravascular catheters are occasionally left in place if local thrombolysis through the catheter is planned (14).

d. Anticoagulation may be with LMWH or UFH for 3 to 5 days followed by LMWH.

e. Total duration of anticoagulation is between 6 and 12 weeks.

f. Thrombolytic therapy is not recommended for neonatal venous thrombosis unless major vessel occlusion is causing critical compromise of organs or limbs.

3. Management of arterial thrombosis (12)

a. Initiate management as for vasospasm if there are peripheral signs of ischemia.

b. Remove catheter unless catheter-directed thrombolysis is planned (14)

TABLE 34.2 Laboratory Tests for Suspected Prothrombotic Disorders	
Laboratory Test	**Collection Tube**
Antiphospholipid antibody panel, anticardiolipin, lupus anticoagulant (IgG, IgM)	Citrated plasma
Fibrinogen	Citrated plasma
Protein C activity	Citrated plasma
Protein S activity	
Antithrombin (activity assay)	
Factor V Leiden	Ethylenediaminetetraacetic acid
Prothrombin G	
Methylenetetrahydrofolate reductase	
Homocysteine	Citrated plasma
Lipoprotein(a)	

From Saxonhouse MA. Management of neonatal thrombosis. *Clin Perinatol.* 2012;39:191,with permission.

c. Anticoagulation for at least 10 days; UFH or LMWH is recommended for neonates with UAC-related thrombosis.

d. If there are potentially life-, limb-, or organ-threatening signs in neonates with UAC-related thrombosis, thrombolysis with rTPA should be considered.

e. If there are contraindications to thrombolysis, surgical thrombectomy may be indicated.

4. Anticoagulant/thrombolytic therapy

a. **Contraindications**
   (1) Major surgery within the last 10 days
   (2) Active or major bleeding: Intracranial, pulmonary, or gastrointestinal
   (3) Preexisting cerebral ischemic lesions
   (4) Seizures within 48 hours
   (5) Relative contraindications (anticoagulant/thrombolytic therapy may be given after correction of these abnormalities)
      (a) Thrombocytopenia (platelet count $<100 \times 10^9$/L)
      (b) Hypofibrinogenemia (fibrinogen <100 mg/dL)
      (c) Severe coagulation factor deficiency
      (d) Hypertension

b. **Precautions**
   (1) No arterial punctures
   (2) No subcutaneous or intramuscular injections
   (3) No urinary catheterizations
   (4) Avoid aspirin or other antiplatelet drugs.
   (5) Monitor serial head ultrasound scans for intracranial hemorrhage.

c. **Anticoagulants**
   (1) **UFH**
      (a) Anticoagulant, antithrombotic effect limited by low plasma levels of antithrombin in neonates.
      (b) Check complete blood count, platelet count, activated partial thromboplastin time (aPTT), prothrombin time and fibrinogen levels before starting UFH therapy.
      (c) *Dosage:* Is adjusted according to gestational age (12).
         <28 weeks GA: Loading dose 25 U/kg IV over 10 minutes
         Maintenance dose 15 U/kg/h
         28 to 37 weeks GA: Loading dose 50 U/kg IV over 10 minutes
         Maintenance dose 15 U/kg/h
         >37 weeks GA: Loading dose 100 U/kg IV over 10 minutes
         Maintenance dose 28 U/kg/h
      (d) *Monitoring*
         i. **Maintain anti–factor Xa (anti-FXa) level of 0.03 to 0.7 U/mL (aPTT 60 to 85 seconds)**

         ii. **Check anti-FXa level 4 hours after loading dose and 4 hours after every change in the infusion rate.**
         iii. Check platelet counts and fibrinogen levels daily for 2 to 3 days once therapeutic levels are achieved and at least twice weekly thereafter, while on UFH.
         iv. Monitor thrombus closely both during and following treatment.
      (e) *Complications*
         i. *Bleeding:* Discontinue UFH infusion; consider protamine sulphate if anti-FXa level is >0.8 U/mL and there is active bleeding. Dosage: 1 mg/ 100 U heparin received if the time since the last heparin dose is <30 minutes. Use protamine conservatively, starting with a smaller dose than calculated.
         ii. Heparin-induced thrombocytopenia (rare in neonates) (15)
   (2) **LMWH (16,17)**
      (a) LMWHs have specific activity against factor Xa and less activity against thrombin, so therapy is monitored by anti-FXa assay and not by aPTT.
      (b) Different LMWHs preparations (e.g., enoxaparin, dalteparin, reviparin) differ in their molecular weights and dosage regimens. Enoxaparin is the LMWH most commonly used.
      (c) *Advantages:* Subcutaneous administration
      (d) *Dosage:* Administered either by subcutaneous injection or through an indwelling subcutaneous catheter (Insuflon, Unomedical, Birkerod, Denmark)
         Term neonates: 1.7 mg/kg every 12 hours.
         Preterm neonates: 2 mg/kg every 12 hours.
      (e) *Monitoring*
         i. Adjust dose to maintain anti-FXa level between 0.5 and 1 U/mL.
         ii. In neonates, prematurity, rapid growth, and liver and kidney dysfunction make LMWH dosage less predictable. Frequent adjustment of the dose is required to attain target anti-FXa levels.
         iii. Draw blood sample for testing from fresh venipuncture. There must be no contamination from standard heparin (e.g., from an arterial line).
         iv. Check levels 4 hours after subcutaneous administration of LMWH on days 1 and 2 of treatment.
         v. If therapeutic, a weekly check of anti-FXa levels is adequate.
      (f) To discontinue anticoagulation, simply discontinue LMWH therapy. If an invasive

procedure such as lumbar puncture is required, skip two doses of LMWH, and measure anti-FXa level prior to the procedure.

(g) If an immediate antidote is required, protamine may be administered. The dose is usually a 1:1 ratio with LMWH; administration of the dose may be done in 2 to 3 aliquots with monitoring of anti-FXa levels (18).

(3) **Thrombolytic agents**

(a) Thrombolytic agents should be considered in the presence of extensive or severe thrombosis when organ or limb viability is at risk.

(b) The use of streptokinase and urokinase has been superseded by rTPA.

(c) rTPA acts by converting fibrin-bound plasminogen to plasmin, which then proteolytically cleaves fibrin within the clot to fibrin degradation products. rTPA is nonantigenic and has a short half-life. Supplementation with plasminogen in the form of fresh frozen plasma enhances the thrombolytic effect.

(d) Thrombolysis does not inhibit clot propagation, so anticoagulation may be necessary. The administration of heparin, either concomitantly or following thrombolytic therapy, has not been adequately evaluated in neonates.

(e) *Dosage:* A wide variety of dosage protocols have been used (3,12,14,19,20).

   i. *High-dose protocol:* Continuous infusion of rTPA 0.1 to 0.6 mg/kg/h for 6 hours.

   ii. *Low-dose protocol:* Continuous infusion of rTPA 0.01 to 0.06 mg/kg/h over 24 to 48 hours. Simultaneous infusion of UFH at 10 U/kg/h.

   iii. *Catheter-directed thrombolysis:* Infusion of low doses of rTPA through a catheter with the tip adjacent to or within the thrombus. Initial bolus dose ranges from 0 to 0.5 mg/kg, followed by infusion of 0.015 to 0.2 mg/kg/h.

(f) *Monitoring*

   i. Measure thrombin time, fibrinogen and plasminogen levels, and fibrin split products or D-dimers prior to therapy, 3 to 4 hours after initiation of fibrinolytic therapy, and one to three times daily thereafter.

   ii. Imaging studies every 4 to 12 hours during fibrinolytic therapy to allow discontinuation of treatment as soon as clot lysis is achieved.

   iii. Fibrinolytic response is measured by a decrease in fibrinogen concentration and increase in levels of fibrin-degradation products, but the correlation between these hemostatic parameters and efficacy of thrombolysis is poor. Maintain fibrinogen levels of at least 100 mg/dL.

E. Complications of Anticoagulation/ Fibrinolytic Therapy

1. Hemorrhagic complications (1,21,22)

a. *Intracerebral hemorrhage:* Incidence approximately 1% in term neonates, 13% in preterm neonates, increasing to 25% in preterm infants treated in the first week of life. Data in preterm infants is confounded by the risk of "spontaneous" intraventricular hemorrhage (21).

b. *Other major hemorrhage:* Gastrointestinal, pulmonary

c. Bleeding from puncture sites and recent catheterization sites: Bleeding and hematoma at the site of the indwelling catheter for LMWH has been noted (1)

d. Hematuria

2. Embolization

Dislodgement of intracardiac thrombus, causing obstruction of cardiac valves or main vessels, or pulmonary or systemic embolization (23).

F. Surgical Intervention (24,25)

Early consultation is recommended because surgical management may be required concomitantly, particularly for life- or limb-threatening emergencies.

1. Thrombectomy
2. Microvascular reconstruction
3. Decompressive fasciotomy
4. Mechanical disruption of thrombus, using soft wires and balloon angioplasty in conjunction with continuous site-directed thrombolytic infusion into the clot.
5. Amputation

References

1. Van Elteren HA, Veldt HS, te Pas AB, et al. Management and outcome in 32 neonates with thrombotic events. *Int J Pediatr.* 2011; 2011:217564.
2. Brotschi B, Hug MI, Latal B, et al. Incidence and predictors of indwelling arterial catheter related thrombosis in children. *J Thromb Haemost.* 2011;9:1157.
3. Saxonhouse MA, Burchfield DJ. The evaluation and management of postnatal thromboses. *J Perinatol.* 2009;29:467.
4. Haase R, Merkel N. Postnatal femoral artery spasm in a preterm infant. *J Pediatr.* 2008;153:871.

5. Roy M, Turner- Gomes S, Gill G, et al. Accuracy of Doppler ultrasonography for the diagnosis of thrombosis associated with umbilical venous catheters. *J Pediatr.* 2002; 140: 131.

6. Manco- Johnson MJ, Grabowski EF, Hellgreen M, et al. Laboratory testing for thrombophilia in pediatric patients. On behalf of the Subcommittee for Perinatal and Pediatric Thrombosis of the Scientific and Standardization Committee of the International Society of Thrombosis and Haemostasis (ISTH). *Thromb Haemost.* 2002;88:155.

7. Raffini L. Thrombophilia in children: who to test, how, when and why? *Hematology Am Soc Hematol Educ Program.* 2008: 228.

8. Yang JYK, Chan AKC. Neonatal systemic venous thrombosis. *Thrombosis Res.* 2010;126:471.

9. Wong AF, McCulloch LM, Sola A. Treatment of peripheral tissue ischemia with topical nitroglycerine ointment in neonates. *J Pediatr.* 1992;121:980.

10. Vasquez P, Burd A, Mehta R, et al. Resolution of peripheral artery catheter induced ischemic injury following prolonged treatment with topical nitroglycerine ointment in a newborn: a case report. *J Perinatol.* 2003:23:348

11. Baserga MC, Puri A, Sola A. The use of topical nitroglycerine ointment to treat peripheral tissue ischemia secondary to arterial line complications in neonates. *J Perinatol.* 2002;22:416.

12. Monagle P, Chalmers E, Chan A, et al. Antithrombotic therapy in neonates and children: American College of Chest Physicians Evidence Based Clinical Practice Guidelines (8th edition). *Chest.* 2008;133:887S.

13. Saxonhouse MA. Management of neonatal thrombosis. *Clin Perinatol.* 2012;39:191.

14. Albisetti M. Thrombolytic therapy in children. *Thromb Res.* 2006;118:95.

15. Kumar P, Hoppensteadt DA, Prechel MM, et al. Prevalence of heparin- dependent platelet activating antibodies in preterm newborns after exposure to unfractionated heparin. *Clin Appl Thromb Hemost.* 2004;10:335.

16. Streiff W, Goebel G, Chan AKC, et al. Use of low molecular weight heparin (enoxaparin) in newborn infants: a prospective cohort study of 62 patients. *Arch Dis Child Fetal Neonatal Ed.* 2003;88:F365.

17. Malowany JI, Monagle P, Knoppert DC, et al. Enoxaparin for neonatal thrombosis: a call for a higher dose for neonates. *Thromb Res.* 2008;122:826.

18. Wiernikowski JT, Chan A, Lo G. Reversal of anti- thrombin activity using protamine sulphate. Experience in a neonate with a 10 fold overdose of enoxaparin. *Thromb Res.* 2007;120:303.

19. Raffini L. Thrombolysis for intravascular thrombosis in neonates. *Curr Opin Pediatr.* 2009;21:9.

20. Williams MD. Thrombolysis in children. *Br J Haematol.* 2009; 148:26.

21. Zenz W, Arlt F, Sodia S, et al. Intracerebral hemorrhage during fibrinolytic therapy in children. A review of literature of the last thirty years. *Semin Thromb Hemost.* 1997;23:321.

22. Nowak- Gottl U, Auberger K, Halimeh S, et al. Thrombolysis in newborns and infants. *Thromb Haemost.* 1999;82(suppl):112.

23. Yang JY, Williams S, Brando LR, et al. Neonatal and childhood right atrial thrombosis: recognition and a risk-stratified treatment approach. *Blood Coagul Fibrinolysis.* 2020;21:301.

24. Coombs CJ, Richardson PW, Dowling GJ, et al. Brachial artery thrombosis in infants: an algorithm for limb salvage. *Plast Reconstr Surg.* 2006;117:1481.

25. Ade-Ajayi N, Hall NJ, Liesner R, et al. Acute neonatal arterial occlusion: is thrombolysis safe and effective? *J Pediatr Surg.* 2008;43:1827.

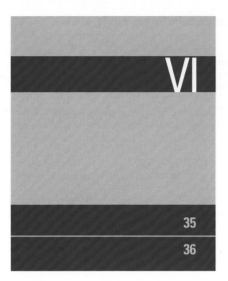

VI Respiratory Care

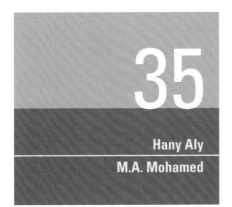

35

Hany Aly

M.A. Mohamed

Bubble Nasal Continuous Positive Airway Pressure

A. Definition

Continuous positive airway pressure (CPAP) is a noninvasive, continuous flow respiratory system that maintains positive pressure in the infant's airway during spontaneous breathing. CPAP was developed by George A. Gregory in the late 1960s (1). Positive pressure was originally applied by placing the neonate's head into a semiairtight "box" (the Gregory box) and, subsequently, by a fitted face mask covering the mouth and nose (2). A major problem with both these methods of application was the fact that it was difficult to feed the baby without discontinuing the CPAP, thus the evolution to the current method of applying CPAP through bilateral nasal prongs (3). "Bubble CPAP" (b-CPAP) is a modern resurgence of the original method of supplying CPAP, wherein pressure is generated in the breathing circuit by immersing the distal end of the expiratory limb of the breathing circuit under a water seal (4–6) (Fig. 35.1).

Bubble CPAP allows provision of CPAP without use of a ventilator, and it is currently primarily used for early treatment of low-birthweight premature infants with or at risk for respiratory distress syndrome and/or with frequent apnea/bradycardia (7). In addition to cost considerations, there is early evidence that b-CPAP may be more effective in small premature babies than ventilator-derived CPAP (8).

CPAP has the Following Physiologic Actions

1. Prevents alveolar collapse and increases functional residual capacity
2. Splints the airway and diaphragm
3. Stimulates the act of breathing and decreases apnea
4. Conserves surfactant via decreased inflammatory responses (9)
5. Stimulates lung growth when applied for extended duration (10)

B. Indications

1. Premature infants with/at high risk for respiratory distress syndrome
2. Premature infants with frequent apnea and bradycardia of prematurity

3. Infants with transient tachypnea of the newborn
4. Infants who have weaned from mechanical ventilation
5. Infants with paralysis of the diaphragm or tracheomalacia

When to Start b-CPAP?

a. Premature infants with a birthweight <1,200 g can be supported with b-CPAP starting in the delivery room, before any alveolar collapse occurs
b. Infants ≥1,200 g may benefit from b-CPAP in the following conditions
   (1) Respiratory rate >60 breaths/min
   (2) Mild to moderate grunting
   (3) Mild to moderate respiratory retraction
   (4) Preductal oxygen saturation <93%
   (5) Frequent apneas

C. Contraindications

1. Choanal atresia
2. Congenital diaphragmatic hernia
3. Conditions where b-CPAP is likely to fail in the delivery room such as
   a. Extremely low gestational age infants (≤24 weeks)
   b. Floppy infants with complete apnea due to maternal anesthesia
4. *Relative contraindication:* Infants with significant apnea of prematurity may require the introduction of nasal intermittent positive pressure ventilation via a variable flow device (11).

D. Equipment

B-CPAP System Consists of Two Components

1. A breathing circuit of light-weight corrugated tubing that has two limbs
   a. Inspiratory limb to provide a continuous flow of heated and humidified gas
   b. Expiratory limb with its terminal end immersed under water seal to create positive pressure
2. A device to safely connect the circuit to patient's nares that includes (Fig. 35.2)

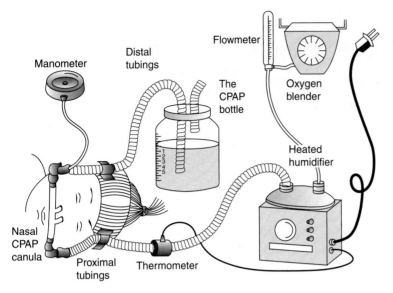

FIG. 35.1. Bubble CPAP circuit. This simplified diagram demonstrates the components of the b-CPAP device that is either assembled at the bedside or commercially manufactured. Gas mixture flows to the infant from the wall source after it is warmed and humidified. The free expiratory limb of the tube is immersed under the surface of sterile water to produce the required CPAP (usually 5 cm H_2O).

a. Short binasal prongs
b. Velcro (to make attachment circles and moustache for upper lip)
c. DuoDERM (to make nasal septum protective layer)
d. CPAP head cap
e. Adhesive tape

E. Technique (See Procedures Website for Video)

1. **Starting b-CPAP**
   Nonventilator-derived b-CPAP apparatus involves making a simple water seal device that can be put together in neonatal units. It consists of a container of water, through which the expiratory gas from the baby is bubbled at a measured level below the surface (e.g., 5 cm below the surface = 5cm H_2O CPAP). The lower the level of the tip of the expiratory tubing below the surface of the water, the higher the CPAP (Fig. 35.1). It is important to fix the water bottle to an IV pole at or below the level of the baby's chest to avoid any accidental displacement or water spills. The recent, commercially available, preassembled circuits rely on the same basic principle.

   a. *Before attaching the device to an infant*
      (1) Position the infant with the head of the bed elevated 30 degrees.
      (2) *Gently* suction the mouth, nose, and pharynx.
          Whenever possible, use size 8-Fr suction catheter. Smaller-sized catheters are not as efficient.
      (3) Place a small roll under the infant's neck/shoulder. Allow slight neck extension to help maintaining the airway open.
      (4) Clean the infant's upper lip with water.

      (5) Place a thin strip of DuoDERM (or Tegaderm) over the upper lip. That should also cover the nasal columella and both sides of nasal apertures (Fig. 35.2).
      (6) Cut a Velcro moustache and fix it over the DuoDERM.
      (7) Cut two strips of soft Velcro (8 mm width) and wrap them around the transverse arm of the device, about 1 cm away, on each side, from the nasal prongs.

   b. *Placing nasal prongs into infant's nostrils (Figs. 35.2 and 35.3)*
      (1) Use appropriate-size CPAP prongs. The correct size nasal prongs should snugly fit the infant's nares without pinching the septum. If prongs are too small, they will increase airway resistance and allow air to leak around them, making it difficult to maintain appropriate pressure. If prongs are too large, they may cause mucosal and septal erosion.
      (2) Curve prongs gently down into the infant's nose.
      (3) Press gently on the prong device until the soft Velcro strips adhere to the moustache.
      (4) Make sure of the following points
          (a) Nasal prongs fit well in the nostrils
          (b) Skin of nares is not stretched (indicated by blanching of the rim of the nostrils)
          (c) Corrugated tubes are not touching the infant's skin
          (d) There is no lateral pressure on the nasal septum
          (e) There is a small space between the nasal septum and the bridge between the prongs
          (f) Prongs are not resting on the philtrum

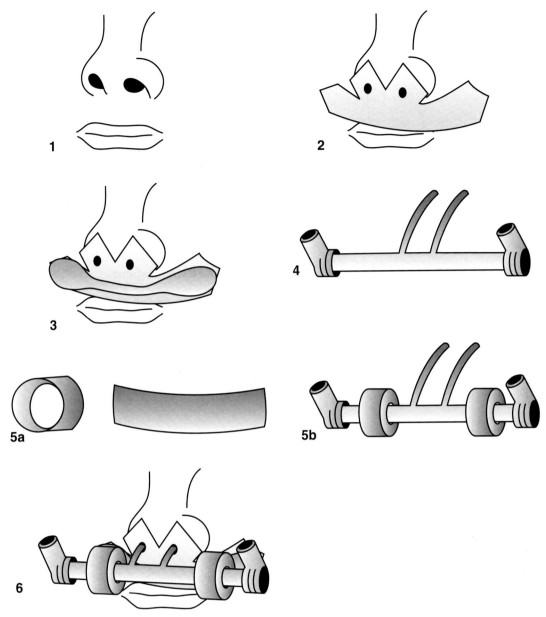

FIG. 35.2. Components of the CPAP attachment device.(1)Infant's nose before applying b-CPAP; (2) protective DuoDERM applied to upper lip and nose; (3) thin Velcro moustache piece: applied to upper lip on top of DuoDERM with sharp edges not touching nose; (4) nasal prongs (prongs are slightly curved to better fit within anatomy of nasal passages); (5a,b) thick Velcro ring pieces: wrapped around both sides of the transverse arm; (6) nasal prongs applied to baby—prongs inserted into nares with thick Velcro rings attached to thin Velcro moustache (allow a space between the transverse arm of the nasal prongs and nose to avoid damage to nasal columella).

c. *Fixing corrugated tubes in place*
 (1) Use appropriate-sized hat and fold rim back 2 to 3 cm.
 (2) Place the hat on the infant's head so that the rim is just over the top of the ears.
 (3) Hold the corrugated tubing to one side of the head.
 (4) Tape the tube to the hat at the side of the head.
 (5) Repeat the same procedure for the tubing on the other side of the head.

d. *Draining excess air from the stomach*
 (1) Pass an orogastric tube and aspirate the stomach contents.
 (2) Fix tube at appropriate position.
 (3) Leave tube open to air to ventilate excess air from stomach.

e. *Maintaining a good seal for CPAP pressure*
 (1) Gently apply a chin strip to minimize air leak from the mouth.

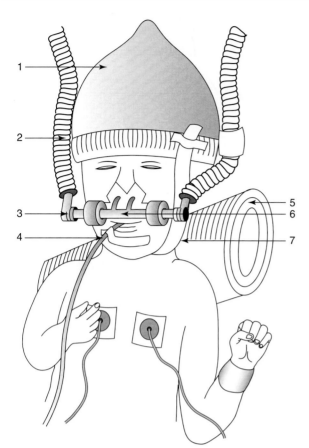

FIG. 35.3. An infant with CPAP properly attached to the head. (1) Head cap (cap fit well on head covering down to eye brows, almost entire ears and back of head); (2) breathing circuit tubes attached to side of hat while avoiding both eyes; (3) three-way elbow on expiratory limb allows the attachment of pressure manometer or could be capped to preserve pressure within circuit; (4) orogastric tube attached to lower lip and chin with Tegaderm; (5) neck roll allowing slight neck extension (sniff position); (6) nasal prongs applied to baby—prongs inserted into nares allowing a space between the transverse arm of the nasal prongs and nose to avoid damage to nasal columella; (7) supporting chin strip.

2. **Maintenance of b-CPAP**
   a. Check the integrity of the entire CPAP system every 3 to 4 hours (Appendix F) (12)
   b. Suction nasal cavities, mouth, pharynx, and stomach every 3 to 4 hours, and as needed.
   c. Keep CPAP prongs off nasal septum at all times.
   d. Change the infant's position every 4 to 6 hours, to allow postural drainage of lung secretions.
3. **Weaning off b-CPAP**
   a. A trial off CPAP should be given when the infant's weight is more than 1,200 g and he or she is breathing comfortably on b-CPAP without supplemental oxygen.
      The nasal prongs should be separated from the corrugated tubing, keeping the tubing in place.

Infant should be assessed during the trial for any tachypnea, retractions, oxygen desaturation, or apnea. If any of these signs are observed, the trial is considered failed. Infant should be restarted immediately on CPAP, for at least 24 hours, before another trial is undertaken.
   b. There is no need to change the level of positive pressure during the weaning process. Infant is either on b-CPAP 5-cm H_2O or off CPAP.
   c. Do not wean the infant off b-CPAP if there is any likelihood of respiratory compromise during the weaning process. It is wise to anticipate and prevent lung collapse, rather than risk having to manage collapsed lungs.
   d. Do not wean infants off b-CPAP if they require supplemental oxygen. (13)
4. **Potential Complications**
   a. *Nasal obstruction:* From secretions or improper positioning of b-CPAP prongs. To avoid obstruction, nares should be suctioned frequently and prongs checked for proper placement. Never use a nasal–pharyngeal tube to supply b-CPAP, because of significant risk of nasal airway obstruction.
   b. *Nasal septal erosion or necrosis:* Due to pressure on the nasal septum. This can be avoided by maintaining a small space (use DuoDERM 2 to 3 mm) between the bridge of the prongs and the septum. Choosing the proper-sized snug-fitting nasal prongs, using a Velcro mustache to secure the prongs in place, and avoiding pinching of the nasal septum, will minimize the risk of septal injury. Significant nasal septal erosion may require consultation with the ENT or Plastic Surgery team.
   c. *Gastric distention:* From swallowing air. Gastric distention is a benign finding and does not predispose the infant to necrotizing enterocolitis or bowel perforation (14). It is important to ensure patency of the indwelling orogastric tube because secretions may block the tube and lead to distention.
   d. *Pneumothorax:* During the first 2 days of life, premature infants usually will require intubation for this complication.
   e. *Unintended increase/decrease in positive end pressure:* The tubing that is placed under water to provide positive end pressure must be firmly fixed in place so that it cannot be displaced to produce unwanted pressure changes.

Acknowledgement

We thank Aser Kandel, MD for drawing the illustrations in this chapter.

References

1. Gregory GA, Kitterman JA, Phibbs RH, et al. Treatment of the idiopathic respiratory distress syndrome with continuous positive airway pressure. *N Engl J Med.*1971;384:133.
2. Gregory GA. Devices for applying continuous positive pressure. In: Thibeault DW, Gregory GA, eds. *Neonatal Pulmonary Care.* Menlo Park, CA: Addison-Wesley; 1979.
3. Katwinkel J, Fleming D, Cha CC, et al. A device for administration of continuous positive pressure by the nasal route. *Pediatrics.* 1973;52:130.
4. Wung JT. Continuous positive airway pressure. In: Wung JT. (ed) *Respiratory care of the newborn: A practical approach.* New York: Columbia University Medical Center; 2009.
5. Aly H. Nasal prongs continuous positive airway pressure: a simple yet powerful tool. *Pediatrics.* 2001;108:759.
6. Aly H, Massaro AN, Patel K, et al. Is it safer to intubate premature infants in the delivery room? *Pediatrics.* 2005;115:1660.
7. Nowadzky T, Pantoja A, Britton JR. Bubble continuous positive pressure, a potentially better practice, reducing the use of mechanical ventilation among very low birth weight infants with respiratory distress syndrome. *Pediatrics.* 2009;123:1534.
8. Courtney SE, Kahn DJ, Singh R, et al. Bubble and ventilator-derived nasal continuous positive pressure in premature infants: work of breathing and gas exchange. *J Perinatol.* 2011; 31:44.
9. Jobe AH, Kramer BW, Moss TJ, et al. Decreased indicators of lung injury with continuous positive expiratory pressure in preterm lambs. *Pediatr Res.* 2002;52:387.
10. Zhang S, Garbutt V, McBride JT. Strain-induced growth of the immature lung. *J Appl Physiol.* 1996;81:1471.
11. Lemyre B, Davis PG, dePaoli AG. Nasal intermittent positive pressure ventilation (NIPPV) versus nasal continuous positive airways pressure (NCPAP) for apnea of prematurity. *Cochrane Database Syst Rev.*2002;1:CD002272.
12. Bonner K.M, Mainous R.O. The nursing care of the infant receiving bubble CPAP therapy. *Adv Neonatal Care.* 2008;8(2):78.
13. Abdel-Hady H, Shouman B, Aly H. Early weaning from CPAP to high flow nasal cannula in preterm infants is associated with prolonged oxygen requirement: a randomized controlled trial. *Early Hum Dev.* 2011;87:205.
14. Aly H, Massaro AN, Hammad TA, et al. Early nasal continuous positive airway pressure and necrotizing enterocolitis in preterm infants. *Pediatrics.* 2009;124:205.

36

Endotracheal Intubation

Mariam M. Said

Khodayar Rais-Bahrami

A. Indications

1. When prolonged positive-pressure ventilation is required
2. To relieve critical upper airway obstruction (Fig. 36.1)
3. To provide a route for selective bronchial ventilation
4. When tracheal suctioning is required to obtain direct tracheal culture
5. To assist in bronchial hygiene when secretions cannot be cleared
6. When diaphragmatic hernia is prenatally diagnosed or suspected

B. Contraindications

There is no absolute contraindication to intubating a neonate who has one of the above-mentioned indications. In older patients, the presence of cervical injuries is a contraindication to intubation with a laryngoscope; however, because the occurrence of cervical injuries/anomalies is infrequent in neonates, we consider that endotracheal intubation is associated with less risk than performance of an emergency tracheotomy.

C. Equipment

The supplies and equipment necessary to perform endotracheal intubation should be kept together on either a resuscitation cart or an intubation tray. Each delivery room, nursery, and emergency room should have a complete set of the following items.

Sterile

1. Gloves
2. 10-French (Fr) suction catheters
3. Endotracheal tube stylet
4. Endotracheal tubes with internal diameters of 2.5, 3, 3.5, and 4 mm
   a. Diameter selected for infant size (Table 36.1)
   b. Length selected for infant's size (1–3)
      In neonates, there is little leeway between a tube that is too high (increased risk for extubation) or too low (increased risk for mainstem intubation or airway trauma). The appropriate length for an endotracheal tube depends on a number of factors, including an infant's size, and it can be quickly and accurately estimated by measuring the nasal–tragus length (NTL) and/or sternal length (STL). The modified prediction formula for insertion by the orotracheal route is NTL or STL + 1. For the nasotracheal route, the formula is NTL or STL + 2 (4).

      It is rarely necessary to insert a tube more than 1 to 2 cm below the vocal cords, regardless of the infant's size. Exceptions include the presence of anatomic defects that necessitate a "bypass" airway, such as a tracheal fistula or subglottic obstruction, and when selective bronchial intubation is intended (5). See Appendix D.

5. Pediatric laryngoscope (with an extra set of batteries and extra bulb)
   a. Miller blade size 1 for full-term infant
   b. Miller blade size 0 for preterm infant (size 00 for extremely low birth weight infant)
      Straight rather than curved blades are preferred for optimal visualization.
   c. Modified blade to allow continuous flow of oxygen at 1 to 2 L/min for better maintenance of oxygenation during procedure. The use of a Viewmax (Rusch, Duluth, Georgia) laryngoscope improves viewing of the larynx but requires a longer time for tracheal intubation (6).
6. Scissors
7. Oxygen tubing
8. Magill forceps (optional)

Nonsterile

9. Humidified oxygen/air source, blender, and analyzer
10. Resuscitation bag and mask
11. Suctioning device
12. Cardiorespiratory monitor
13. Pulse oximetry oxygen saturation monitor
14. Stethoscope
15. *Adhesive tape*: Two 8- to 10-cm lengths of 0.5-inch-wide tape, with half the length split and one 10- to 15-cm length unsplit

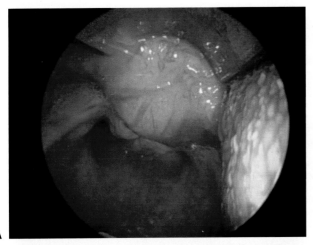

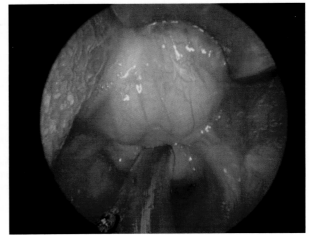

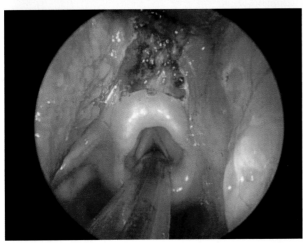

FIG. 36.1. **A:** Vallecula cyst, causing stridor and proximal airway obstruction. **B:** Endotracheal tube passes beneath cyst. **C:** Same patient after laser surgical treatment.

D. Precautions (Table 36.2)

1. Select orotracheal route for all emergency intubations or when a bleeding diathesis is present. Reserve nasotracheal intubation for elective procedures after stabilization with orotracheal tube, unless oral anatomy precludes oral intubation.
2. Prepare all equipment before starting procedure. Keep equipment ready at bedside of patients likely to require intubation.
3. Use appropriate-size tubes (Table 36.1). To minimize upper airway trauma, the tube should not fit tightly between the vocal cords.

TABLE 36.1	Endotracheal Tube Diameter for Patient Weight and Gestational Age	
Tube Size (ID mm)	**Weight (g)**	**Gestational Age (wk)**
2.5	<1,000	<28
3.0	1,000–2,000	28–34
3.5	2,000–3,000	34–38
4.0	>3,000	>38

4. To minimize hypoxia, each intubation attempt should be limited to 20 seconds. Interrupt an unsuccessful attempt to stabilize the infant with bag-and-mask ventilation. In most cases, an infant can be adequately ventilated by bag and mask, so endotracheal intubation can be achieved as a controlled procedure. The one important exception is in a case of prenatally diagnosed or suspected congenital diaphragmatic hernia.
5. Recognize anatomic features of neonatal upper airway (Fig. 36.2).
6. Ensure visualization of larynx. This is the most important step (Fig. 36.3).
   a. Have an assistant maintain proper position of patient.
   b. Avoid hyperextending or rotating neck.
7. Do not use pressure or force that may predispose to trauma.
   a. Avoid using maxilla as fulcrum for laryngoscope blade.
   b. Avoid excessive external tracheal pressure.
   c. Avoid pushing tube against any obstruction.
8. Make certain all attachments are secure.
   a. Avoid obscuring the point of connection of tube and adapter with any fixation device.

TABLE 36.2	Trouble-Shooting Problems with Endotracheal Intubation
Problem	**Suggested Approach for Solution**
Infant's tongue gets in way.	Push tongue aside with finger before inserting blade.
Secretions prevent visualization.	Suction prior to intubation attempt.
Tube seems too big to fit through vocal cords.	Verify correct tube size for patient weight and gestational age.
Vocal cords are closed.	Decrease angle of neck extension. Apply traction to blade. Apply a short puff of air through the tube onto the vocal cords. Select smaller tube size. Evaluate for airway stenosis.
Unsure of appropriate tube length.	Await spontaneous breath. Apply gentle suprasternal pressure.
Difficult to ventilate after intubation.	Insert tube just past vocal cord. Predetermine tube length. Obtain chest radiograph with head in neutral position to confirm tube position relative to carina.
Swelling of neck and anterior chest.	Verify that tube is in trachea. Verify that tube is not in bronchus. Consider tube and/or airway obstruction. **Consider pulmonary air leak into mediastinum/pericardium (Fig. 38.8A, B)**
Blood return from endotracheal tube.	Evaluate for tracheal perforation.
Tube slips into main bronchus.	Avoid neck hyperextension. Secure tape fixation. Maintain correct lip-to-tip distance.
Unplanned extubation.	Regularly verify correct tube distance. Secure tape and replace as necessary. Support neck when moving infant. Avoid neck hyperextension or traction on tube. Secure infant's hands.

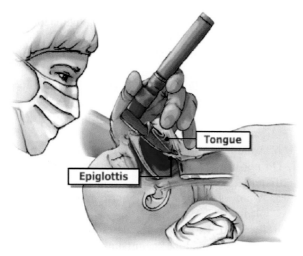

FIG. 36.2.   Anatomic view of neonatal upper airway. The glottis sits very close to the base of the tongue, so visualization is easiest without hyperextending the neck.

b. Secure tube carefully in position to avoid dislodgement, kinking, or movement.
  (1) Vary contact point from side to side to prevent damage to developing palate and palatal ridges (7,8).
  (2) Note relationship of head position to intratracheal depth of tube on radiograph (9).
9. Do not leave endotracheal tube unattached from continuous positive airway pressure; the natural expiratory resistance is lost by bypassing the upper airway.
10. Recognize that in neonates, endotracheal tubes are often pushed in too far because of the short distance from the glottis to the carina. Use a standardized graph or location device (2,5).
11. Recognize the association of a short trachea (fewer than 15 tracheal cartilage rings) with certain syndromes: DiGeorge syndrome, skeletal dysplasias, brevicollis, congenital rubella syndrome, interrupted aortic arch, and other congenital syndromes involving the tracheal area (10).

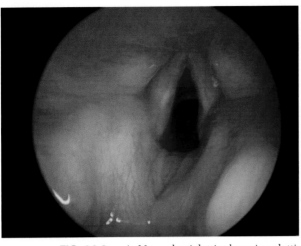
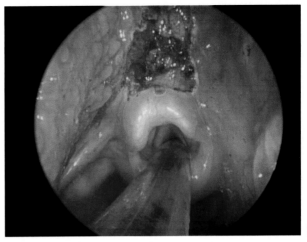

A   B

FIG. 36.3. **A:** Normal epiglottis obscuring glottis. This amount of clear secretions does not require suctioning for visualization. **B:** Same airway as in Figure 36.1 after surgical removal of cyst. Glottic opening is visible just beneath epiglottis. Gentle tracheal, pressure, or decreasing neck extension while lifting tip of laryngoscope blade, will improve visibility.

12. Identify and prevent the factors that are most likely to contribute to spontaneous extubation (11).
    a. Increased secretions
       (1) Necessitating more frequent suctioning
       (2) Loosening of tape
    b. Infant activity
    c. Procedures requiring repositioning infant
    d. Tube slippage

E. Technique (See also Endotracheal Intubation on the Procedures Website, and Appendix D for Techniques of Intubation Specific to Unique Patient Needs) Orotracheal Intubation (Table 36.2)

1. Position infant with the head in midline and the neck slightly extended, pulling chin into a "sniff" position (Fig. 36.4). The head of the infant should be at operator's eye level.

   It may be helpful to place a roll under the baby's shoulders to maintain slight extension of the neck.
2. Put on gloves.
3. Clear oropharynx with gentle suctioning.
4. Empty stomach.
5. Bag-and-mask ventilate and preoxygenate infant as indicated by clinical condition. Follow heart rate and oxygenation.
6. Turn on the laryngoscope light, and hold the laryngoscope in left hand with thumb and first three fingers, with the blade directed toward patient.
   a. Put thumb over flat end of laryngoscope handle.
   b. Stabilize the infant's head with right hand.

The laryngoscope is designed to be held in the left hand, by both right- and left-handed individuals. If held in the right hand, the closed, curved part of the blade may block the view of the glottis, as well as make insertion of the endotracheal tube impossible.

7. Open infant's mouth and depress tongue toward the left with the back of right forefinger (Fig. 36.5).
   a. Continue to steady head with third fourth and fifth fingers of right hand.
   b. Do not use the laryngoscope blade to open mouth.
8. Under direct visualization, insert the laryngoscope blade, sliding over the tongue until the tip of the blade

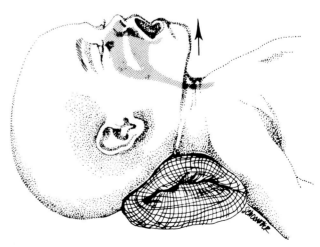

FIG. 36.4. Appropriate sniff position for intubation. Note that the neck is not hyperextended; the roll provides stabilizing support.

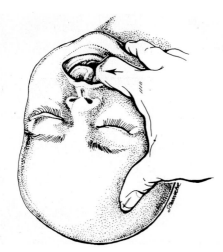

FIG. 36.5.   Open the mouth and push the tongue aside with the forefinger, while stabilizing the head with the thumb and other fingers of the right hand.

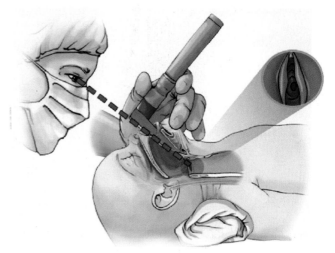

FIG. 36.7.   With the laryngoscope at the proper depth, tilt the blade with the tongue as the fulcrum; at the same time, pull on the laryngoscope handle to move the tongue without extending the infant's neck. Use more traction than leverage.

is resting in the vallecula (the area between the base of the tongue and the epiglottis) (Fig. 36.6).

In general, the blade tip should be placed in the vallecula. However, in extremely premature infants, the vallecula may be too small, in which case it may be necessary to use the blade tip to gently lift the epiglottis.

9. Lift the laryngoscope blade to open mouth further and simultaneously tilt the blade tip slightly to elevate the epiglottis and visualize the glottis (Fig. 36.7).

When lifting the blade, raise the entire blade in the direction that the handle is pointing. Do not lift the tip

of the blade by using the upper gum line as the fulcrum for a rocking motion; this will not produce a clear view of the glottis and will place excessive pressure on the alveolar ridge, potentially impeding future tooth formation.

10. Suction as necessary.
11. Have an assistant apply gentle pressure at the suprasternal notch to open the larynx and to feel the tube pass (12).
12. Hold tube in right hand with concave curve anterior, and pass it down the right side of the mouth, outside the blade, while maintaining direct visualization (Fig. 36.8).
13. Once the vocal cords and trachea are visualized, insert the endotracheal tube through vocal cords, approximately

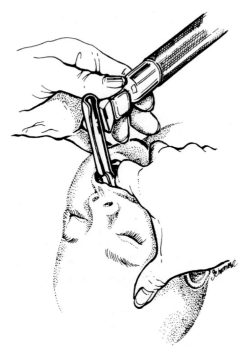

FIG. 36.6.   Pass the laryngoscope carefully along the finger to the back of the oropharynx.

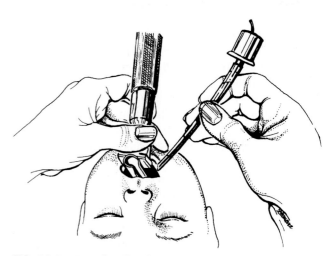

FIG. 36.8.   Visualize the glottis and pass the endotracheal tube into the oropharynx. Keep the tube outside the curve of the laryngoscope blade for better mobility.

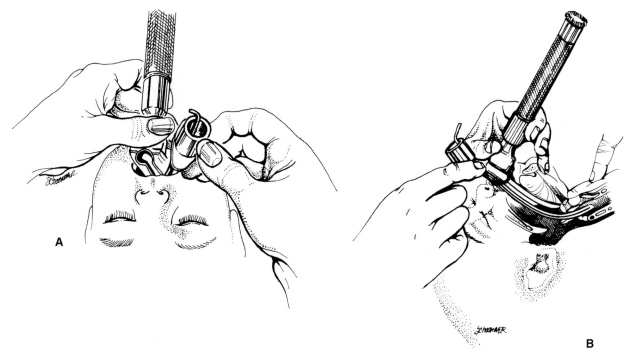

FIG. 36.9. **A:** Pass the endotracheal tube through the glottis to the appropriately predetermined length and remove laryngoscope. **B:** An assistant applies gentle pressure in the suprasternal notch to open the larynx, and to detect when the tube passes into the trachea.

2 cm into trachea or until the tip is felt passing the suprasternal notch by the assistant (Fig. 36.9).
14. If the tube appears too large or does not pass easily, decrease angle of neck extension.
15. Confirm endotracheal tube position within the trachea (13).
   a. We currently use Pedi-Cap (Nellcore, Waukesha, Wisconsin) end-tidal CO_2 detector to verify the position of the endotracheal tube within the trachea. This technique responds quickly to exhaled CO_2 with a simple color change from purple to yellow. It also features an easy-to-see display window that provides constant visual feedback with breath-to-breath response (Fig. 36.10).

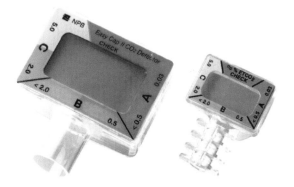

FIG. 36.10. Pedi-Cap CO_2 detector. Pedi-Cap is a trademark of Tyco Healthcare Group LP. (Reprinted by permission from Nellcor Puritan Bennett, Inc).

   b. While gently ventilating with an Ambu bag, auscultate to make sure the breath sounds and chest movement are equal in both sides of the chest.
   c. Observe respiratory wave pattern on oscilloscope to determine that artificial breath is at least as effective as spontaneous breath.
   d. Verify lip-to-tip distance.
16. If the endotracheal tube is correctly placed in the midtracheal region, there should be
   a. Pedi-Cap response to exhaled CO_2 by a reversible color change, purple to yellow
   b. Equal bilateral breath sounds
   c. Slight rise of the chest with each ventilation
   d. No air heard entering stomach
   e. No gastric distention
17. Suction endotracheal tube with sterile catheter, following technique described under F, below.
18. Attach appropriate mechanical ventilatory device.
19. Adjust required F_iO_2.
20. Secure the tube to the infant's face (Figs. 36.11 and 36.12).
      When using adhesive tape, make sure that the face is dried thoroughly to ensure adherence of the tape and to protect the skin. A more permanent fastening can be done later when a radiograph confirms correct placement of the endotracheal tube (14).
21. Obtain chest radiograph with head in neutral position, and note the lip-to-tip distance and direction of bevel (Figs. 36.13 and 36.14).

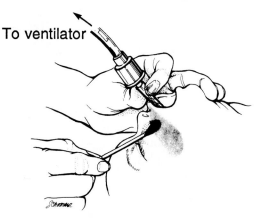

To ventilator

FIG. 36.11. After initially determining that the endotracheal tube is in the correct position, connect the tube to an artificial ventilation source. In the term neonate, begin fixation of the tube by painting the philtrum with tincture of benzoin or Hollister medical adhesive spray and allowing it to dry. Avoid use of tincture of benzoin in low-birthweight infants, as it increases epidermal stripping.

When a correct tube length has been determined for the infant, note the tube marking at the level of the infant's lips.

22. Cut off excess tube length, to leave 4 cm from the infant's lips, and reattach adapter firmly.

If a longer external length is required, before replacing the adapter, slip a short length of a larger endotracheal tube around the narrower tube to prevent kinking, for example, a 6-cm length of 3.5-mm tube over a 2.5-mm tube.

23. Reconfirm tube marking at lip regularly, to avoid unnoticed advancement of the tube into the airway.
24. Retape tube as necessary to maintain stability.

Nasotracheal Intubation

In neonates, orotracheal intubation is preferred because it is easier and faster to perform and there are few proven advantages to nasal intubations in small infants (15). Nasotracheal tubes are preferred in very active infants with copious oral secretions, making it difficult to keep the tube taped in position. When anatomy precludes oral intubation or for oral surgery, nasotracheal intubation may become necessary. There is strong evidence that premedication (sedation and analgesia) allows for a shorter time for intubation and improves physiologic stability (16).

1. Use sterile endotracheal tube. If stylet is used to curve tube, remove it prior to nasal insertion.
2. If desired, premedicate with atropine (20 mcg/kg) and succinylcholine (2 mg/kg) just before inserting tube. Be prepared to provide assisted bag-and-mask ventilation.
3. If orotracheal tube is already in place, release fixation and position at far left of the mouth, to allow continued ventilation during nasotracheal intubation.
4. Directly visualize oropharynx with laryngoscope as described previously, taking particular care not to hyperextend neck.
5. Suction oropharynx while keeping laryngoscope in place.
6. Insert tube through nostril following natural curve of nasopharynx.
7. As tube passes into the pharynx, align the tip with the center of the tracheal orifice, moving infant's head as needed.
8. When the tip of the nasotracheal tube appears to be in direct line with the glottis, have an assistant carefully withdraw the orotracheal tube.
9. Apply gentle pressure over the suprasternal notch and advance tube through cords.

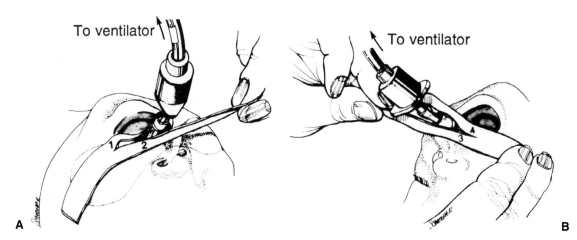

To ventilator

To ventilator

A   **B**

FIG. 36.12. Fixation of tube with half split tape. **A:** Lower half of one split tape (*1*) encircles the tube, and the upper half (*2*) attaches to the upper lip. **B:** Second split tape (*3*) upper half attaches to the upper lip, while the lower half (*4*) encircles the tube.

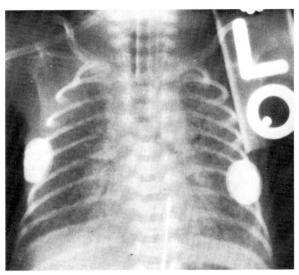
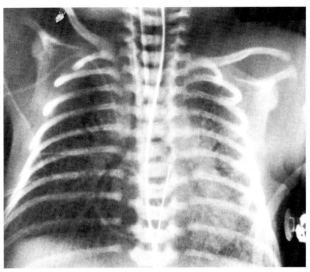

A   B

FIG. 36.13. Although the carina is usually at the level of T4 on the anteroposterior supine chest radiograph, this relationship may be significantly disturbed by a number of factors, including radiographic technique (x-ray tube position, angulation). For this reason, and because the carina is usually easily visualized, as in these cases, one should directly relate the tip of the endotracheal tube to the carina radiographically, knowing the position of the head at the time of film exposure. In both cases, films were taken to verify endotracheal tube position but demonstrated problems with other procedures. A: Appropriate radiographic angle. (Note the oral gastric tube in the esophagus and not reaching the stomach.) B: Slightly lordotic radiographic angle. (Note the central venous line coiled in the heart.)

Use of the Magill forceps is often more cumbersome than helpful in smaller infants. A Magill forceps should always be available, but in a properly positioned infant, a curved tube usually passes directly into the trachea without forceps unless the neck is excessively extended, flexed, or rotated. Secure tube and verify position. The length of a nasotracheal tube for correct positioning of the tip in the trachea is approximately 2 cm longer than the equivalent length of an orotracheal tube.

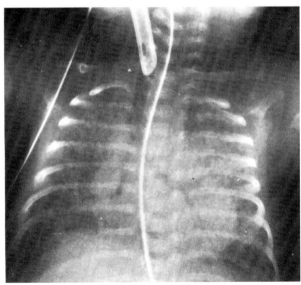
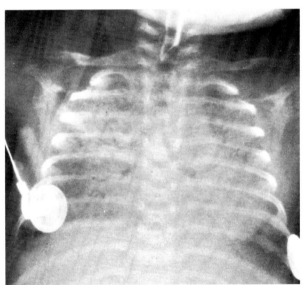

A   B

FIG. 36.14. Sequential radiographs demonstrate the effect of head rotation on bevel direction. A: With the head rotated to the right, the bevel appears to be directed against the tracheal wall. B: The head is rotated to the left, and the bevel is now positioned properly. If the bevel is directed against the posterior tracheal wall in a spontaneously breathing infant, there may be symptoms of tracheal obstruction on expiration. Rather than turning the head to achieve satisfactory position, rotate the endotracheal tube and retape in position.

F. Tracheal Suctioning

Suctioning of the nose, mouth, and pharynx is potentially quite traumatic in neonates. The same equipment, precaution, and complications apply as for tracheal suctioning. Always suction an endotracheal tube before suctioning the mouth; suction the mouth before the nose.

1. Indications

a. To clear tracheobronchial airway of secretions
b. To keep artificial airway patent
c. To obtain material for analysis or culture

2. Relative contraindications

a. Recent surgery in the area
b. Extreme reactive bradycardia
c. Pulmonary hemorrhage
d. Oscillatory ventilation

3. Equipment

Sterile

a. Saline for instillation into airway
b. Saline or water for irrigation of catheter
c. Gloves
d. Suction catheters
   (1) Available safety features
      (a) Markings at measured intervals
      (b) Microscopically smooth surface
      (c) Multiple side holes in different planes
      (d) Large-bore hole for occlusion to initiate vacuum
      (e) No more than half the inside diameter of artificial airway
         (i) *Use 8 Fr for endotracheal tube >3.5 mm.*
         (ii) *Use 5 Fr for endotracheal tube <3.5 mm.*
e. Modified endotracheal tube adapter that allows passage of suction catheter without disconnecting tube from ventilator (Novometrix C/S Suction Adapter; Novometrix Medical Systems, Wallingford, Connecticut) (17)

Nonsterile

a. Adjustable vacuum source and attachments
   (1) Pressure set just high enough to move secretions into suction catheter
   (2) Mechanically controlled pressure source
      Pressure generated by oral suction on mucus extractors can be extremely variable and dangerously high (18).
   (3) Specimen trap, tubing, and pressure gauge
b. Ventilatory device as indicated
   (1) Manometer
   (2) Warmed, humidified oxygen at controlled level
   (3) Bag with positive end-expiratory pressure device

4. Precautions

a. When feasible, use two people when suctioning the airway to minimize the risk of patient compromise and complications and to shorten the procedure time.
b. Determine for each patient if it is better to continue mechanical ventilation during suctioning or to use a sigh with inflation hold after suctioning. Consider the effect of interruption of ventilator therapy and loss of lung volume with each catheter passage.
c. Allow patient to recover between passages of catheter.
d. Stabilize head and airway to prevent tube dislodgement.
e. Assess secretions by auscultation and palpation to determine frequency for suctioning.
   (1) Avoid unnecessary suctioning just to follow a schedule.
   (2) Schedule prophylactic suctioning for tube patency only as often as needed to maintain it.
   (3) Consider increase in monitored airway resistance as indication for suctioning.
f. Readjust humidification as indicated by catheter and volume of secretions.
g. Avoid inadvertent suction during insertion of catheter.
   Use lowest vacuum pressure effective in clearing secretions within a few seconds.
h. Do not insert catheter as far as it will go or until reflex cough occurs. Use prescribed length. Do not suction if catheter is inserted too far; just touching the catheter to the tracheal wall may cause trauma.
i. Limit time of insertion and suctioning to least time required to remove secretions.

5. Technique for intubated patients

a. For artificial airways, use sterile technique with one sterile gloved hand and one free hand.
b. Monitor oxygen saturation continuously during suctioning.
c. Monitor heart rate continuously.
d. It is usually best to remove infant from ventilator and have second person perform assisted ventilation manually, using the following guidelines adjusted to individual needs.
   (1) F_iO_2 set at or up to 10% higher than baseline
      (a) Monitor oxygenation. Adjust F_iO_2 to prevent swings in oxygenation.
      (b) Evaluate effect of procedure.
   (2) Peak inspiratory pressure as on ventilator or up to 10 cm H_2O higher
   (3) Continuous distending airway pressures same as on ventilator
   (4) Respiratory rate 40 to 60 breaths/min, applying an inspiratory hold intermittently
      When there is a high risk of pulmonary air leak as in the presence of significant interstitial emphysema, it may be safer to use a technique of

rapid manual ventilation at lower peak pressure instead of sighing with a prolonged inspiratory pressure. In other cases in which loss of lung volume with suctioning is of greater concern, use sigh with a hold on inflation at a rate similar to ventilator. With suctioning, there is a loss of lung volume with a decrease in compliance. The adverse effect persists for a significant time when mechanical ventilation at the same setting is used during and after the suction procedure.

e. Determine length of endotracheal tube plus adapter and note on suction catheter as limit of depth of insertion.

f. Set vacuum at lowest level to achieve removal of secretions. The level of vacuum required depends on a number of variables, including
   (1) Air tightness of system and fluctuations in generated vacuum pressure
   (2) Accuracy of manometer
   (3) Diameter of catheter (smaller catheter, higher pressure)
   (4) Thickness and tenacity of secretions

g. Holding catheter in one hand, moisten tip with water or saline. Note appropriateness of suction level by rate of liquid uptake. Adjust pressure with free hand.

h. Open artificial airway with free hand.
   (1) Detach from bag; hold oxygen near end of tube, or
   (2) Open suction port of specialized endotracheal tube adapter.

i. With free hand, stabilize airway. Pass catheter down airway to depth limit noted for the patient's endotracheal tube. Do not apply vacuum during insertion (i.e., keep suction control port open).

j. Close proximal suction control port and withdraw catheter.

k. Limit time for insertion and removal to 15 to 20 seconds.

l. Reattach endotracheal tube to bag and ventilate for 10 to 15 breaths or until patient is stable.
   (1) Note oxygenation.
   (2) Note heart rate.
   (3) Note chest excursions.

m. If secretions are thick or tenacious, instill 0.25 mL of saline into endotracheal tube and continue ventilation.

n. Clear catheter with sterile water.

o. Repeat process until airway is clear.

G. Fixation Techniques

Many fixation devices and techniques have been described in the literature. None of them can prevent all accidental extubations or malpositions (11,14,19). Here, we describe a simple and effective method.

1. Prepare two 8- to 10-cm lengths of adhesive tape split half of the length and one 10- to 15-cm length without a split.

2. Paint skin adjacent to the sides of the mouth and above the lips with tincture of benzoin or Hollister medical adhesive spray. Avoid use of tincture of benzoin in low-birthweight infants; it increases epidermal stripping. (Fig. 36.11).

3. Allow to dry while holding the tube in place.

4. Tape the unsplit end of the adhesive to the cheek on one side of the mouth, and wrap the bottom half of the split end clockwise around the endotracheal tube at the lip. Fold the last 2-mm end of tape on itself to leave a tab for easier removal (Fig. 36.12). Secure the other half of the split end above the upper lip.

5. Repeat the procedure from the other side, reversing the direction of the taping and securing half on that side of the upper lip (Fig. 36.12).

6. Secure one end of the long tape to one cheek at the zygoma. Loop the tape around the tube, and secure the other end to a similar point on the opposite cheek.

7. Note the markings on the endotracheal tube at the level of the lips and the tape.

8. Whenever the tape appears loosened by secretions, remove tape and repeat application of benzoin while holding tube at appropriate lip-to-tip depth.

H. Planned Extubation

Various vasoconstrictors and anti-inflammatory medications have been recommended to reduce postextubation stridor and to improve the success of extubation. Systemically administered dexamethasone appears to have very little, if any, effect in reducing acute postextubation stridor in neonates and children (20). Local application of steroids directly to the vocal cords has not been well studied.

1. Perform chest physiotherapy and suction prior to extubation.

2. Release all fixation devices while holding tube in place.

3. Using manual ventilation, provide the infant a sigh breath, and then withdraw tube during exhalation.

4. Avoid suctioning during tube withdrawal, unless specifically utilizing the tube to remove thick foreign material from trachea.

5. Allow recovery time before suctioning oropharynx.

6. Keep the inspired gases well humidified.

I. Complications

1. Acute trauma (21–23)
   a. Tracheal or hypopharyngeal perforation
   b. Pseudodiverticulum
   c. Hemorrhage
   d. Laryngeal edema

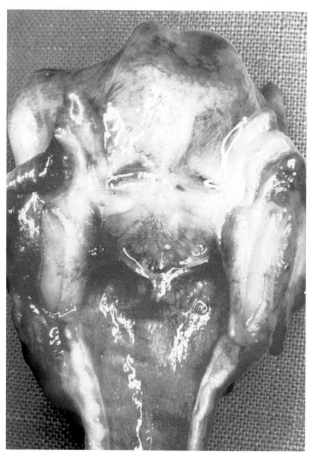

FIG. 36.15.   Subglottic erosion and stenosis after intubation.

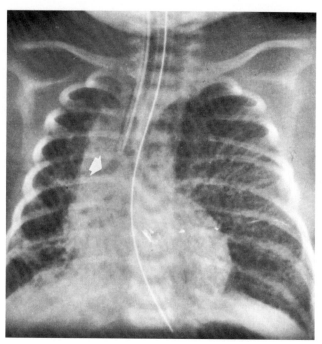

FIG. 36.16.   Radiographic magnification high-kilovoltage film (×2) demonstrating an abrupt cutoff of the right bronchus intermedius (*arrow*) due to an endobronchial granuloma, with secondary volume loss at the right lung base. Although these granulomas may be due to endotracheal tube trauma, in this area they are more likely related to suction tube injury. The endotracheal tube is just entering the right bronchus.

   e. Mucosal necrosis (Fig. 36.15)
   f. Vocal cord injuries
   g. Dislocation of arytenoid
2. Chronic trauma (23–25)
   a. Cricoid ulceration and fibrosis
   b. Glottic and/or subglottic stenosis (Fig. 36.15)
   c. Subglottic granuloma (Figs. 36.16 and 36.17)
   d. Hoarseness, stridor, wheezing
   e. Subglottic cyst
   f. Tracheomegaly
   g. Protrusion of laryngeal ventricle
3. Interference by oral tube with oral development (7,8,26,27)
   a. Alveolar grooving
   b. Palatal grooves (Fig. 36.18)
   c. Acquired oral commissure defect (Fig. 36.19)
   d. Posterior cross-bite
   e. Defective dentition
     (1) Enamel hypoplasia
     (2) Incisor hypoplasia
   f. Poor speech intelligibility
4. Local effects from nasal tube (28–30)
   a. Erosion of nasal septum
   b. Stenosis of nasal vestibule (Fig. 36.20)

   c. Nasal congestion
   d. Midfacial hypoplasia
   e. Otitis media
5. Systemic side effects (31,32)
   a. Infection
   b. Aspiration

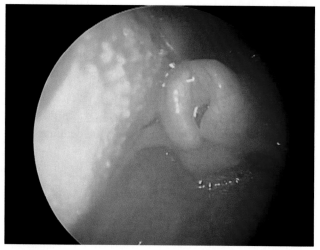

FIG. 36.17.   Glottic granuloma after intubation. Epiglottis is manually retracted to reveal granuloma below cords. Esophageal opening is clearly visible beneath airway.

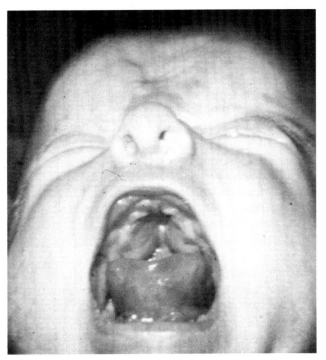

FIG. 36.18. Palatal groove after prolonged oral intubation. Such grooves may be seen after prolonged use of endotracheal or oral gastric tubes when the normal forces of the tongue are prevented from assisting palatal development.

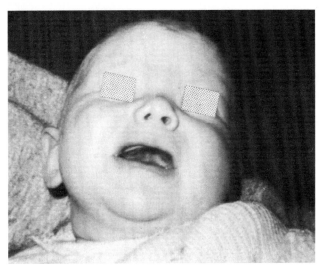

FIG. 36.20. Nasal stenosis due to nasal cartilage necrosis following an indwelling nasotracheal tube.

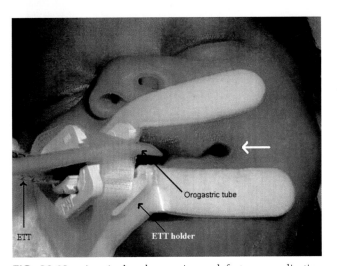

FIG. 36.19. Acquired oral commissure defect: a complication of prolonged endotracheal intubation. (Reprinted by permission from Macmillan Publishers Ltd. *J Perinatol.* 2005;25:612.)

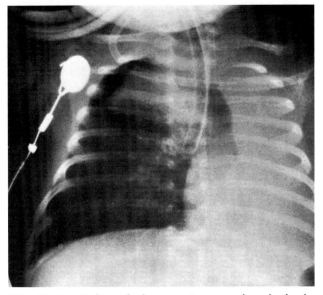

FIG. 36.21. Radiograph demonstrating an endotracheal tube malpositioned in the bronchus intermedius, with resulting atelectasis of the right upper lobe and of the left lung. There is marked overaeration of the right middle and lower lobes but no pneumothorax shown.

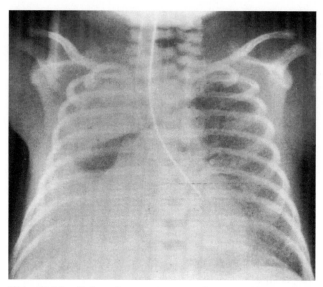

FIG. 36.22. Relatively uncommon malposition of an endotracheal tube in the left bronchus with atelectasis of much of the right lung.

   c. Increased intracranial pressure
   d. Hypoxemia
   e. Hypertension
   f. Apnea
   g. Bradycardia and cardiac arrest
6. Misplacements into esophagus or bronchus (32,33) (Figs. 36.21 through 36.23)
   a. Atelectasis
   b. Pulmonary air leak
   c. Loss of tube into esophagus
   d. Tube crosses tracheoesophageal fistula
7. Displacement; accidental extubation (11,14)
8. Obstruction (34)
9. Kinking, proximally or distally
10. Unrecognized disconnection from adapter or pressure source
11. Rupture of endotracheal tube (35)
12. Foreign body from stylet left unrecognized in airway
13. Swallowed laryngoscope light (36)
14. Postextubation atelectasis (35)
15. Increased airway resistance increasing work of breathing (37)

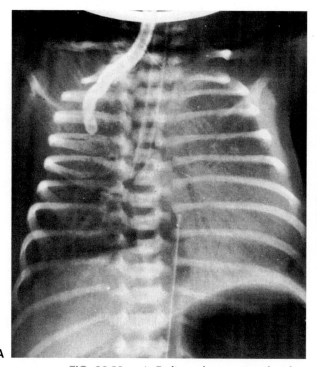

A

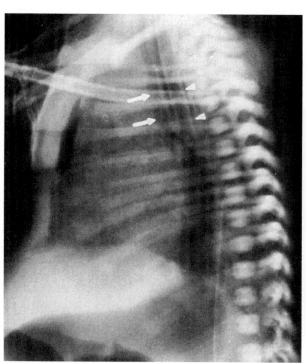

B

FIG. 36.23.   A: Radiograph suggesting that the endotracheal tube is in the right mainstem bronchus. Note the gaseous distension of the stomach. The wavy tube on the right is external. **B:** In the lateral view, the same endotracheal tube is easily seen to be in the esophagus (*arrowheads*) posterior to the trachea (*arrows*).

References

1. Yates AP, Harries AJ, Hatch DJ. Estimation of nasotracheal tube length in infants and children. *Br J Anaesth.* 1987;59:524.

2. De la Sierra Antona M, Lopez-Herce J, Ruperez M, et al. Estimation of the length of nasotracheal tube to be introduced in children. *J Pediatr.* 2002;140:772.

3. Freeman JA, Fredricks BJ, Best CJ. Evaluation of a new method for determining tracheal tube length in children. *Anaesthesia.* 1995;50:1050.

4. Shukla HK, Hendricks-Munoz KD, Atakent Y, et al. Rapid estimation of insertional length of endotracheal intubation in newborn infants. *J Pediatr.* 1997;131:561.

5. Kim KO, Um WS, Kim CS. Comparative evaluation of methods for ensuring the correct position of the tracheal tube in children undergoing open heart surgery. *Anaesthesia.* 2003;58:889.

6. Leung YY, Hung CT, Tan ST. Evaluation of the new Viewmax laryngoscope in a simulated difficult airway. *Acta Anaesthesiol Scand.* 2006;50:562.

7. Erenberg A, Nowak AJ. Palatal groove formation in neonates and infants with orotracheal tubes. *Am J Dis Child.* 1984;138:974.

8. Macey-Dare LV, Moles DR, Evans RD. Long-term effect of neonatal endotracheal intubation on palatal form and symmetry in 8–11 year-old children. *Eur J Orthodont.* 1999;21:703.

9. Lang M, Jonat S, Nikischin W. Detection and correction of endotracheal-tube position in premature neonates. *Pediatr Pulmonol.* 2002;34:455.

10. Wells TR, Wells AL, Galvis DA, et al. Diagnostic aspects and syndromal associations of short trachea with bronchial intubation. *Am J Dis Child.* 1990;144:1369.

11. Lucas da Silva PS, de Carvalho WB. Unplanned extubation in pediatric critically ill patients: a systematic review and best practice recommendations. *Pediatr Crit Care Med.* 2010;11:287.

12. Jain A, Finer NN, Hilton S, et al. A randomized trial of suprasternal palpation to determine endotracheal tube position in neonates. *Resuscitation.* 2004;60:297.

13. Sutherland PD, Quinn M. Nellcor Stat Cap differentiates esophageal from tracheal intubation. *Arch Dis Child Fetal Neonat Ed.* 1995;73:184F.

14. Loughead JL, Brennan RA, DeJuilio P, et al. Reducing accidental extubation in neonates. *Jt Comm J Qual Patient Saf.* 2008;34:164.

15. Spence K, Barr P. Nasal versus oral intubation for mechanical ventilation of newborn infants. *Cochrane Database Syst Rev.* 2000;CD000948.

16. Oei J, Hari R, Butha T, et al. Facilitation of neonatal nasotracheal intubation with premedication: a randomized controlled trial. *J Paediatr Child Health.* 2002;38:146.

17. El Masry A, Williams PF, Chipman DW, et al. The impact of closed endotracheal suctioning systems on mechanical ventilator performance. *Respir Care.* 2005;50:345.

18. Tingay DG, Copnell B, Mills JF, et al. Effects of open endotracheal suction on lung volume in infants receiving HFOV. *Intensive Care Med.* 2007;33:689.

19. Richards S. A method for securing pediatric endotracheal tubes. *Anesth Analg.* 1981;60:224.

20. Khemani RG, Randolph A, Markovitz B. Corticosteroids for the prevention and treatment of post-extubation stridor in neonates, children and adults. *Cochrane Database Syst Rev.* 2009;CD001000.

21. Doherty KM, Tabaee A, Castillo M, et al. Neonatal tracheal rupture complicating endotracheal intubation: a case report and indications for conservative management. *Int J Pediatr Otorhinolaryngol.* 2005;69:111.

22. Mahieu HF, de Bree R, Ekkelkamp S, et al. Tracheal and laryngeal rupture in neonates: complication of delivery or of intubation?. *Ann Otol Rhinol Laryngol.* 2004;113:786.

23. Gomes Cordeiro AM, Fernandes JC, Troster EJ. Possible risk factors associated with moderate or severe airway injuries in children who underwent endotracheal intubation. *Pediatr Crit Care Med.* 2004;5:364.

24. Dankle SK, Schuller DE, McClead RE. Risk factors for neonatal acquired subglottic stenosis. *Ann Otol Rhinol Laryngol.* 1986;95:626.

25. Johnson LB, Rutter MJ, Shott SR, et al. Acquired subglottic cysts in preterm infants. *J Otolaryngol.* 2005;34:75.

26. Angelos GM, Smith DR, Jorgenson R, et al. Oral complications associated with neonatal oral tracheal intubation: a critical review. *Pediatr Dent.* 1989;11:133.

27. Kahn DJ, Spinazzola R. Acquired oral commissure defect: a complication of prolonged endotracheal intubation. *J Perinatol.* 2005;25:612.

28. Gowdar K, Bull M, Schreiner R, et al. Nasal deformities in neonates. Their occurrence in those treated with nasal continuous positive airway pressure and nasal endotracheal tubes. *Am J Dis Child.* 1980;134:954.

29. Rotschild A, Dison PJ, Chitayat D, et al. Midfacial hypoplasia associated with long-term intubation for bronchopulmonary dysplasia. *Am J Dis Child.* 1990;144:1302.

30. Halac E, Indiveri DR, Obergaon RJ, et al. Complication of nasal endotracheal intubation. *J Pediatr.* 1983;103:166.

31. De Dooy J, Leven M, Stevens W, et al. Endotracheal colonization at birth is associated with a pathogen-dependent pro- and antiinflammatory cytokine response in ventilated preterm infants: a prospective cohort study. *Pediatr Res.* 2004;56:547.

32. Marshall TA, Deeder R, Pai S, et al. Physiologic changes associated with endotracheal intubation in preterm infants. *Crit Care Med.* 1984;12:501.

33. Bagshaw O, Gillis J, Schell D. Delayed recognition of esophageal intubation in a neonate: role of radiologic diagnosis. *Crit Care Med.* 1994;22:2020.

34. Rivera R, Tibballs J. Complications of endotracheal intubation and mechanical ventilation in infants and children. *Crit Care Med.* 1992;20:193.

35. Spear RM, Sauder RA, Nichols DG. Endotracheal tube rupture, accidental extubation, and tracheal avulsion: three airway catastrophes associated with significant decrease in peak pressure. *Crit Care Med.* 1989;17:701.

36. Naumovski L, Schaffer K, Fleisher B. Ingestion of a laryngoscope light bulb during delivery room resuscitation. *Pediatrics.* 1991;87:581.

37. Oca MJ, Becker MA, Dechert RE, et al. Relationship of neonatal endotracheal tube size and airway resistance. *Respir Care.* 2002;47:994.

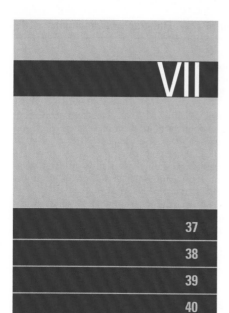

VII Tube Replacement

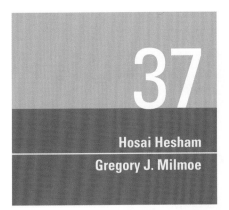

37

Tracheotomy

Hosai Hesham

Gregory J. Milmoe

A. Indications (1–5)

1. Prolonged need for ventilator support — most common
2. Acquired subglottic stenosis after prolonged intubation
3. Craniofacial abnormalities with severe airway obstruction (e.g., Pierre-Robin sequence, Pfeiffer syndrome, Treacher Collins syndrome)
4. Congenital bilateral vocal cord paralysis
5. Laryngeal web, subglottic hemangioma
6. Congenital tracheal stenosis, severe tracheomalacia
7. Congenital neuromuscular disease with insufficient respiratory effort
8. Neurologic disease with aspiration risk, central apnea, or intractable seizures

B. Contraindications

1. Unstable physiology — wait until stabilized
   a. Sepsis
   b. Pneumonia not yet controlled
   c. Pulmonary instability requiring high inspiratory pressures (peak inspiratory pressure >35 to 40 cms H_2O) or need for high-frequency ventilation
   d. Cardiovascular instability (e.g., shunting, arrhythmia, or hypotension)
   e. Evolving renal or neurologic injuries
2. Distal obstruction not relievable by tracheostomy
   a. Congenital stenosis at the carina
   b. External compression from mediastinal mass
3. Congenital anomalies that make the trachea relatively inaccessible
   a. Massive cervical hemangioma — bleeding issues
   b. Massive cervical lymphangioma — severe distortion of neck anatomy
   c. Massive goiter — might be manageable medically
   d. Chest syndromes with severe kyphoscoliosis or tracheal distortion

C. Precautions

1. Patient should be stable (see B); anticipate need for increased pulmonary support temporarily to counter atelectasis and reactive secretions from surgical stimulation.
2. Tracheotomy tubes allow for air leak through the stoma and larynx. In contrast, an endotracheal tube fits more snugly at the cricoid, creating a more closed system for ventilation.
3. Neonates are less able to tolerate bacteremia; use perioperative antibiotic to cover skin flora.
4. If the patient is not currently intubated, have endoscopy equipment available and discuss intubation options with the anesthesiologist.
5. The infant larynx differs from that of the adult and older child (Fig. 37.1).
   a. More pliable and mobile
   b. Relatively higher in neck
   c. Thymus and innominate artery can override trachea in surgical field
6. This procedure should be done only in a facility where there is appropriate support for postoperative management.

D. Equipment

All Sterile

1. Prep tray with brushes, towels, and Betadine
2. Tracheotomy tray
   a. Scalpel with no. 15 blade
   b. Hemostats
   c. Small scissors (iris, tenotomy, small Mayo)
   d. Retractors — Senn or Ragnell
   e. Suction — no. 7 Frazier
   f. Forceps — Adson
3. *Sutures*: 3-0 and 4-0 nonabsorbable on small, curved needles
4. Neonatal tracheotomy tubes
   a. Have several calibers available
   b. Standard tubes are noncuffed, but in special circumstances, a cuff may be needed.

E. Technique

1. Check instruments, sutures, and available tracheotomy tubes.

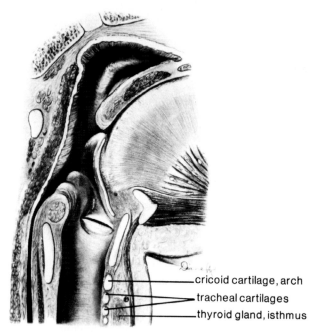

cricoid cartilage, arch

tracheal cartilages

thyroid gland, isthmus

FIG. 37.1. Sagittal section. Larynx lies more cephalad than in adult. Note the proximity of the thyroid isthmus to the tracheal rings. (Drawing contributed by John Bosma, MD)

2. Apply monitors, check IV line, and confirm satisfactory ventilation through endotracheal tube.
3. Have anesthesia team proceed with inhalation agents, oxygen supplementation, and IV agents, as needed for satisfactory level of general anesthesia.
4. Position patient with neck extended, using shoulder roll.
5. Remove nasogastric tube to avoid confusion when palpating trachea. Do *not* place esophageal stethoscope.
6. Inject skin incision and the deeper tissues with local anesthetic (0.5 to 1 mL of 50% lidocaine with 1:200,000 epinephrine).
7. Prep the surgical site from above the chin to below the clavicles. Give IV antibiotic to cover skin flora.
8. Drape the patient with surgical towels, allowing the anesthesiologist access to the endotracheal tube and the securing tape.
9. *Identify the following landmarks:* Suprasternal notch, chin, midline, trachea, and cricoid. In small neonates, the cricoid may be difficult to palpate.
10. Make the skin incision approximately midway between the sternal notch and the cricoid, either vertically or horizontally. Incisions in either plane tend to heal as a circular stoma; however, the horizontal has a slightly better cosmetic effect, whereas the vertical allows more exposure in the midline.
11. Excise excess subcutaneous fat with cautery.
12. Identify the strap muscles and repeatedly palpate the trachea to confirm the midline. Split the raphe to separate the muscles.
13. Grab the fascia of the strap muscles with hemostats to retract them outward and laterally, thereby exposing the thyroid gland, cricoid, and trachea.

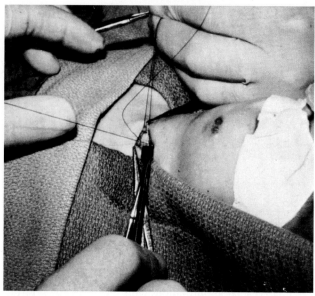

FIG. 37.2. Placement of stay sutures through the tracheal wall.

14. Place Senn retractors on either side of the trachea for optimal visibility.
15. Displace the thyroid gland, using blunt dissection to expose the tracheal rings. If this is not possible, divide the thyroid isthmus, suture, and ligate.
16. Place vertical stay sutures in paramedian position at the level where tracheal entry is planned—usually the third and fourth ring (Fig. 37.2).
17. Incise trachea vertically for two or three rings, depending on the size needed for the tube employed.
18. Have the anesthesiologist loosen the tape and withdraw the endotracheal tube until the tip is just visible (Fig. 37.3).
19. Place the appropriate tracheostomy tube with the flange parallel to the trachea so that the tube more easily enters the trachea and passes posteriorly, then rotate the flange 90 degrees.
20. Have the anesthesiologist confirm placement by checking end-tidal carbon dioxide and oxygen saturation, as well as auscultation of both sides of the chest.

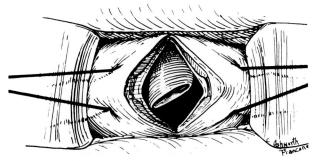

FIG. 37.3. Artistic conception of view through tracheal incision with the tip of the endotracheal tube visible. Stay sutures hold cartilages open.

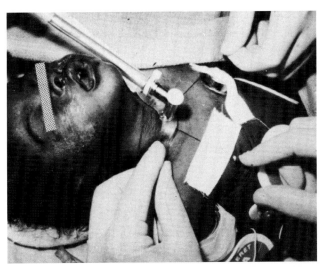

FIG. 37.4. Fixation of stay sutures. As soon as the position of the tracheostomy tube is confirmed and stomal ventilation is started, the tube may be fixed. Equal tension is kept on the stay sutures during taping. Right suture is marked to avoid confusion in future placement.

21. Secure the tracheostomy tube with twill tape tied firmly around the neck. Once tied, only one finger should fit between the tape and the neck when the baby's neck is in neutral position.
22. Secure the stay sutures to the chest with tape labeled as to correct side (Fig. 37.4).
23. Transport the patient back to the intensive care unit with a backup endotracheal tube and laryngoscope.

24. Obtain chest radiograph on arrival in unit, to check tube position and lung status.

F. Postoperative Management

1. Provide intensive nursing (see C).
2. Keep spare tracheostomy tubes at bedside (same size and one smaller).
3. Replace nasogastric tube for nutrition and to avoid aerophagia.
4. Suction secretions as needed to avoid plugging. For first 24 hours, be liberal with saline irrigation.
5. Make sure the ventilator tubing is not pulling on the tracheostomy tube.
6. Be aggressive with wound care so that stoma heals quickly and, thereby, limits granulation. Clean once a shift with half-strength peroxide and cotton swabs, then apply antibiotic ointment.

   The first tracheostomy change is performed by surgical team in 4 to 7 days. Thereafter, weekly changes are sufficient.

G. Early Complications (0 to 7 days)

1. *Bleeding:* Thyroid, venous, arterial
2. Accidental decannulation or displacement in neck— stay sutures are the child's lifeline back to the trachea to allow replacement of the tube.
3. Plugging of tube with secretions (Fig. 37.5)

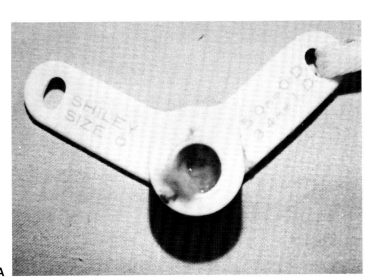

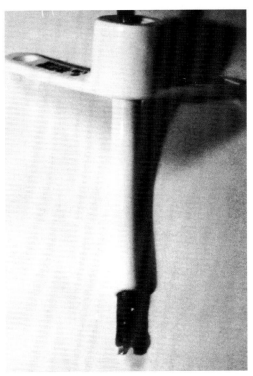

A   **B**

FIG. 37.5. Total obstructions of tracheostomy tubes. **A:** Mucus plug incompletely suctioned. **B:** Dry mucus plug pushed deeper by a suction catheter.

a. Avoid by increasing humidity, saline irrigation, and suctioning.
4. Infection of wound or pneumonia—avoid by local care and by taking care of secretions.
5. Air leaks
    a. Pneumothorax—may need chest tube
    b. Pneumomediastinum—serial films
    c. Subcutaneous emphysema—usually limited (avoid occlusive dressing)
6. Tracheoesophageal fistula—iatrogenic

H. Late Complications (after 1 week)

1. Obstruction and decannulation remain ongoing risks that require vigilant care.
2. Stomal infection and granulation—avoided by careful wound care
3. Proximal tracheal granuloma—commonly occurs at the point where the tube rubs against the superior aspect of the tracheal opening, creating an obstruction between the vocal cords and the tube that can impede routine tracheostomy tube changes. This requires operative removal.
4. Distal tracheal granulation—from overly aggressive suctioning or tube angulation causing rubbing of the tip against the tracheal wall. Hallmark sign is bloody secretions.

5. Stenosis—preventing decannulation later on
    a. Part of original pathology for which tracheotomy was performed
    b. Ongoing obliteration from active inflammatory factors
    c. Consequence of procedure itself; from stomal collapse or distal cicatrix
6. Tracheocutaneous fistula after tube removal—normal physiologic sequela, but needs secondary procedure for closure

References

1. Sisk EA, Kim TB, Schumacher R, et al. Tracheotomy in very low birth weight neonates: indications and outcomes. *Laryngoscope.* 2006;116:928.
2. Wooten CT, French LC, Thomas RG, et al. Tracheotomy in the first year of life: outcomes in term infants, the Vanderbilt experience. *Otolaryngol Head Neck Surg.* 2004;134:365.
3. Kremer B, Botos-Kremer AI, Eckel HE, et al. Indications, complications and surgical techniques for pediatric tracheostomies—an update. *J Pediatr Surg.* 2002;37:1556.
4. Crysdale WS, Feldman RI, Naito K. Tracheostomies: a 10 year experience in 319 children. *Ann Oto Laryngol.* 1988;97:439.
5. Sidman JD, Jaquan A, Couser RJ. Tracheostomy and decannulation rates in a level 3 neonatal intensive care unit: a 12 year study. *Laryngoscope.* 2006;116:136.

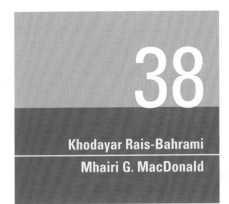

38

Thoracostomy

Khodayar Rais-Bahrami
Mhairi G. MacDonald

Thoracostomy Tubes

Pulmonary air leak is an anticipated risk of mechanical ventilation. Thoracostomy tubes are used in neonatal intensive care units for evacuation of air or fluid from the pleural space. The procedure is often performed because of an emergency. In addition to recognizing pathologic states that necessitate chest tube insertion, intensive care specialists are frequently involved in placement, maintenance, troubleshooting, and discontinuation of chest tubes. As with any surgical procedure, complications may arise. Appropriate training and competence in the procedure may reduce the incidence of complications. This chapter reviews current indications for chest tube placement, insertion techniques, and equipment. Guidelines for chest tube maintenance and discontinuation are also discussed.

A. Indications

1. Evacuation of pneumothorax
   a. Tension
   b. Lung collapse with ventilation/perfusion abnormality
   c. Bronchopleural fistula
2. Evacuation of large pleural fluid collections
   a. Significant pleural effusion
   b. Postoperative hemothorax
   c. Empyema
   d. Chylothorax
   e. Extravasated fluid from a central venous catheter
3. Extrapleural drainage after surgical repair of esophageal atresia and/or tracheoesophageal fistula

B. Relative Contraindications

1. Small air or fluid collection without significant hemodynamic symptoms
2. Spontaneous pneumothorax that, in the absence of lung disease, is likely to resolve without intervention

C. Equipment

Sterile

1. General all-purpose tray with no. 15 surgical blade and curved hemostats (See Appendix B, Table B.1)
2. Gloves
3. Surgical drapes
4. Transparent, sterile bag for tip of transillumination device
5. Thoracostomy tube: Techniques of insertion differ with each type. See original references for description of technique variations (1–3).
   a. Polyvinyl chloride (PVC) chest tube with or without trocar, in sizes 8, 10, and 12 French (Fr)
   b. Pigtail catheter for pleural effusion drainage (Fig. 38.1)
      (1) PVC with pigtail at 90-degree angle to shaft (1)
         (a) 8 to 10 Fr
         (b) Total length 10 cm
         (c) Insertion with or without trocar
      (2) Polyurethane modified vascular catheter with pigtail in same plane as shaft (2)
         (a) 8.5 Fr
         (b) Total length 15 cm
         (c) Insertion guide wire and dilator for insertion by Seldinger technique
      (3) Cook catheter (C-PPD-500/600-MP8561; Cook, Bloomington, Indiana) (3)
         (a) 5 and 6 Fr
         (b) Cutting needle tip joined to a biopsy needle shaft with a collar that prevents the catheter from sliding up the needle during insertion
6. Evacuation device
   a. Infant thoracostomy tube set: Several commercial units are appropriate for infants (Fig. 38.2).
      (1) Evacuation rate (4)
         (a) With single tube, capacity depends on level of water in chamber (cm H_2O).
         (b) With multiple tubes, capacity also depends on applied vacuum.

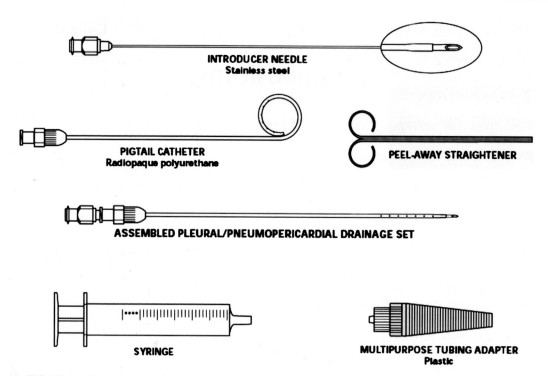

FIG. 38.1. Pigtail catheter for pleural drainage (Fuhrman pleural drainage set). (Illustration provided by Cook Critical Care, Bloomington, Indiana).

(2) Negative pressure of 20 cm H_2O evacuates more than 4 L of air/min in experimental setting (4).

    (a) Appropriate starting point for most infants with lung disease on ventilators is 10 to 15 cm H_2O

    (b) Potentially inadequate in a case of bronchopleural fistula

    (c) Excessive suction pressure may draw tissue into the side holes of the chest tube and could also be potentially harmful by changing intrapulmonary air flow in presence of smaller pleural leak (always start with 10 cm H_2O).

        Measured rates across bronchopleural fistulas in infants have indicated ranges from 30 to 600 mL/min (5). If suction pressure is too high, gas flow to alveoli may be diverted across a fistula. The pressure and flow applied to the endotracheal tube also directly influence flow across a fistula (5). Because there are many interactive factors influencing how much air might have to be evacuated, there can be no single best suction level for all patients; the most effective, least harmful level has to be determined for each situation (6).

7. Nonabsorbable suture on small cutting needle, 4.0
8. Cotton-tipped applicators
9. Semipermeable transparent dressing
10. Antibiotic ointment
11. Petroleum gauze

Nonsterile

1. Tincture of benzoin
2. 0.5-inch adhesive tape
3. Transillumination device
4. Towel roll

D. Factors Influencing Efficiency of Air Evacuation

1. Contiguity of air to chest tube portals; they must be patent
    a. In supine infant, air accumulates in the medial, anterior, or inferior hemithorax, making low anterior location for tip of tube ideal for evacuation (7).
    b. Negative pressure on chest tube may draw tissue into side portals and occlude them.
2. Rate of air accumulation is proportional to
    a. Airway flow and pressure
        Dennis et al. (8) demonstrated in experimental rabbit models that a positive end-expiratory pressure level >6 cm H_2O resulted in greater air leak than peak inspiratory pressures up to 30 cm H_2O.

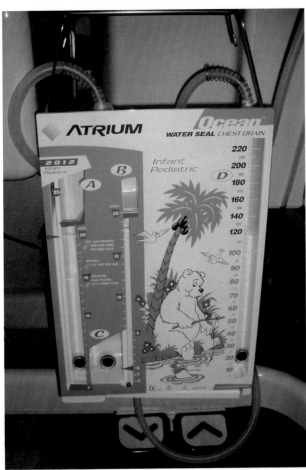

FIG. 38.2. One model of an underwater drainage system, demonstrating the three necessary chambers. Systems now are compact and easy to set up and read. This system is set at 22 cm H₂O, which would be necessary only for a rapid rate of air accumulation.

b. Size of fistula or tear
c. Infant position

The dependent placement of the needle puncture site allows reduction of both the alveolar size and alveolar to pleural pressure difference in the region surrounding the leak, thereby reducing and possibly stopping pneumothorax formation (9).

3. Rate of evacuation
a. Directly proportional to
   (1) Internal radius of chest tube (r^4)
   (2) Pressure gradient across tube (DP)
       (a) Suction pressure applied
           The negative pressure applied may effect intrapleural pressure only in the immediate vicinity of the tip of the tube (4).
       (b) Positive intrathoracic pressure during exhalation and spontaneous or mechanical ventilation

b. Inversely proportional to length of tube and viscosity

Poiseuille's law regarding flow across a tube is $F = DP\pi r^4/8hl$, where F = flow; DP = pressure gradient; r = radius; h = viscosity; and l = length.

E. Precautions

1. Anticipate which infant is at risk of developing pulmonary air leakage and keep equipment for diagnosis and emergency evacuation at bedside (6,10,11).
2. Recognize that transillumination may be misleading (12,13).
   a. True positive
      (1) Follows shape of thoracic cavity (not corona of light source)
      (2) Varies with respiration and position
      (3) Has larger area compared with corona of light
   b. False positive
      (1) Subcutaneous edema
      (2) Subcutaneous air
      (3) Severe pulmonary interstitial emphysema
   c. False negative
      (1) Thick chest wall
      (2) Darkly pigmented skin
      (3) Area over air accumulation obscured by dressing/monitor probe
      (4) Weak light due to fiberoptic deterioration or voltage turned too low
      (5) Room too bright
      (6) Abnormal color vision in observer
3. Distinguish pleural air collections from skin folds, thymus, Mach effect*, artifacts, or other nonpleural intrathoracic air collections on radiograph (Figs. 38.3–38.6) (7,14).
4. Select the appropriate insertion site (Figs. 38.7 and 38.8).

   Allen et al. (15) recommend inserting the thoracostomy tube in the anterosuperior portion of the chest wall, in the first to third intercostal space at the midclavicular line, to ensure anterior placement of the chest tube tip. However, although an anterior insertion may be appropriate for the right-angled pigtail tube used by Allen et al., a properly placed lateral tube will have its tip anterior but, more important, will not leave a (more visible) scar on the anterior chest and completely avoids the nipple (see Fig. 38.9).
   a. Reduces complications
   b. Facilitates insertion of thoracostomy tube into appropriate position
      (1) Anteromedial tip position for air collections
      (2) Posterior tip position for fluid accumulation (Fig. 38.9A, B).

---

*Appearance on x-ray of a dark or light line where there is a convex or concave curve in the body shape of the patient.

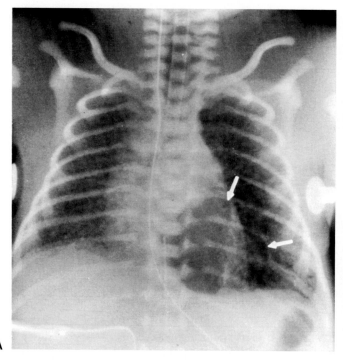

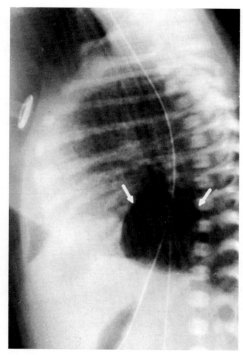

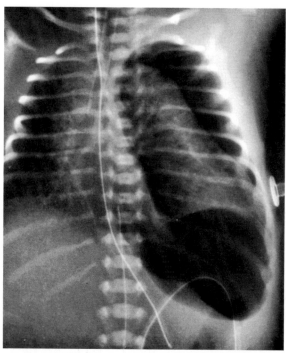

FIG. 38.3. Sequential radiographs. **A:** Anteroposterior radiograph demonstrating a cystic lucency at the left base behind the heart (*arrows*) that resembles the artifact caused by taking a film through the hole in the top of an incubator. Note also the coarse, irregular lucencies of interstitial emphysema (PIE) in the left lung. **B:** Lateral film showing the lucency to be real (*arrows*) and, in this case, a pneumomediastinum located most probably in the left inferior pulmonary ligament. **C:** PIE and air in the pulmonary ligament are often harbingers of impending pneumothorax, in this case, a tension pneumothorax. Note low position of endotracheal tube.

5. While inserting the chest tube, allow some air to remain within pleural space as protective buffer between lung and chest wall (6).
   a. Use emergency pneumothorax evacuation only if patient is critically compromised. If emergency evacuation is used, remove air only until vital signs are stable.
   b. Position infant so that point of entry is the most elevated area of the chest.
      (1) Allows air to rise to provide protective buffer

      (2) Direct tip of the chest tube anteriorly, toward the apex of the thorax.
6. Consider the possibility that a rapid, complete evacuation may cause an abrupt increase in mean arterial blood pressure and cerebral blood velocity to undesirable, supranormal levels (16).
7. To avoid further compromising ventilation, avoid positioning infant in lateral decubitus position with more normal lung dependent for any longer than necessary.

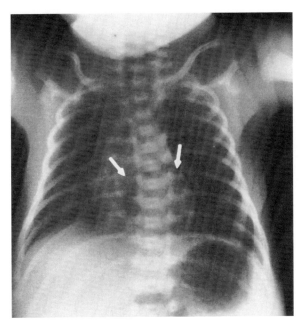

FIG. 38.4. Radiographic artifact of cystic lucency behind the heart (*arrows*) caused by taking film through top of incubator. The lateral film was negative, therefore excluding a cystic pulmonary lesion or air in the pulmonary ligament.

8. To prevent laceration of lung parenchyma, avoid inserting needles beyond parietal pleura for diagnostic or emergency taps. Use a straight clamp perpendicular to the needle shaft to limit depth of penetration (Fig. 38.10).

9. Do not use purse-string suturing of the incision site because resulting scars tend to pucker (6,17) (see Fig. 38.9).

10. Recognize that air leaks are likely to persist after initial evacuation in the presence of continuing lung disease or positive-pressure ventilation. Air leaks resolve in 50% of patients within the first 4 days after chest tube placement, and 83% resolve after 7 days (18).
    a. Continue to watch for patency of the chest tube (Fig. 38.11).
    b. Verify the correct position of the tube.
    c. Modify positive-pressure ventilator patterns to minimize risk of further air leaks (10).
       (1) Decrease inspiratory time.
       (2) Decrease mean airway pressure.

F. Technique (See also Procedures Website)

Insertion of Anterior Tube for Pneumothorax

1. Determine location of air collection.
   a. Physical examination
      Auscultation of the small neonatal chest may be misleading because the breath sounds normally are bronchotubular and may be relatively well transmitted across an air-filled hemithorax. In addition, a shift of the point of maximal cardiac impulse toward the other side is unusual in the presence of noncompliant lungs. Physical findings of acute

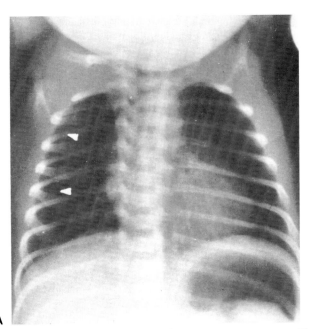

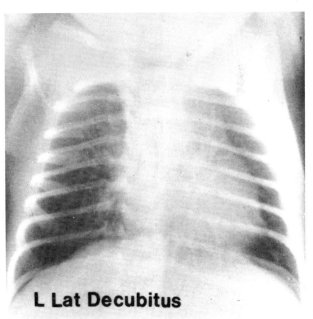

A　　　　　　　　　　　　　　　　　　　　　　　　**B**

FIG. 38.5. **A:** On this anteroposterior supine film, there is a line that parallels the chest wall (*arrowheads*), which suggests the presence of a pneumothorax. **B:** This left decubitus film (right side up) confirms this line to be a skin fold, negative for air. When there is a question of potential adventitial air or of the anatomic location of real adventitial air, a decubitus film with the side in question up is the most important radiographic study.

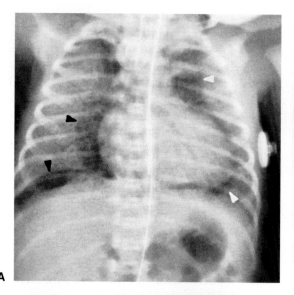

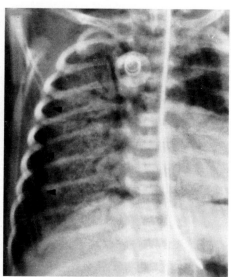

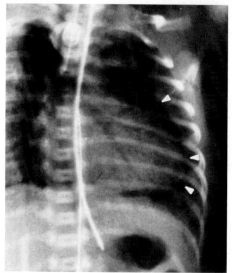

FIG. 38.6. **A:** Anteroposterior radiograph demonstrates ventral air over the hemidiaphragms and around the heart (*arrowheads*). The sometimes difficult question of pneumothorax versus pneumomediastinum is answered by the decubitus films. **B:** The left lateral decubitus radiograph (right side up) shows that the right-sided gas is a pneumothorax (*arrowheads*). **C:** The right decubitus film indicates that the adventitial air fails to come up over the lung and is located in the mediastinum (*arrowheads*). This important distinction is made obvious by the decubitus radiographs.

abdominal distention, irritability, and cyanosis and/or a change in transthoracic impedance suggest an air leak but not its location (19,20). Supplementary diagnostic procedures are usually necessary.

  b. Transillumination (12)
  c. Radiograph (7,21)

2. Provide ventilatory support as needed. Majority of infants with a pneumothorax requiring chest tube also need mechanical ventilatory support.
3. Monitor vital signs. Move any electrodes from the operative site to alternative monitoring areas.
4. Position infant with affected side elevated 60 to 75 degrees off the bed, and support the back with a

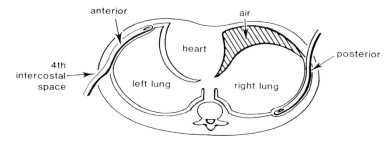

FIG. 38.7. Anterior versus posterior position of the tube for drainage of air or fluid. Because air collects anteromedially in the supine neonate, the posterior tip is less appropriate.

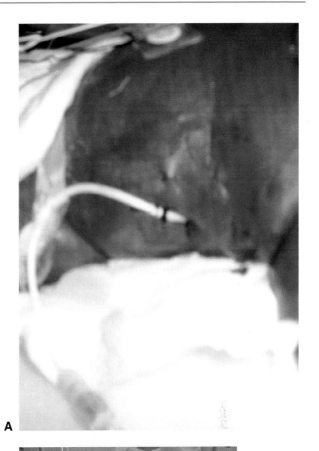

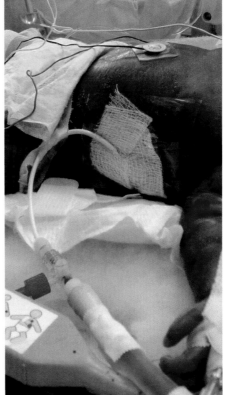

FIG. 38.8. Sequential radiographs in a patient with right pneumothorax. An air collection in supine neonates (**A**) is most effectively treated with an anteromedial chest tube (**B, C**). The medial extension is falsely exaggerated by the slight right posterior oblique rotation of the chest. Pulling this tube back might put the side holes outside the pleural space. There is a pneumomediastinum, most evident on the lateral view, not drained by the pleural tube. Note the nuchal air on all three films.

FIG. 38.9. **A:** Photograph of a pigtail catheter placed posteriorly for pleural fluid drainage. **B:** Serosanguineous pleural fluid collection into the chest tube set.

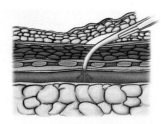

FIG. 38.10.   Chest wall in cross-section. If there is need to use a needle or trocar to enter the pleural space, its depth of penetration should be limited by a perpendicular clamp.

towel roll. Secure arm across the head, with shoulder internally rotated and extended (Fig. 38.12A).

This position is very important because it allows air to rise to the point of tube entry within the thoracic cavity, outlines the latissimus dorsi muscle, and encourages the correct anterior direction of the tube.

5. Prepare the skin with an antiseptic solution over the entire lateral portion of chest to the midclavicular line, and allow skin to dry.
6. Drape surgical area from third to eighth ribs, and from latissimus dorsi muscle to midclavicular line (Fig. 38.12B). Using a transparent drape allows for visualization of landmarks.
7. Locate essential landmarks (Fig. 38.12C).
   a. Nipple and fifth intercostal spaces
   b. Midaxillary line
   c. Skin incision site is at point midway between midaxillary and anterior axillary lines, in the fourth or fifth intercostal space. A horizontal line from the nipple is a good landmark for identifying the fourth intercostal space. Keep well away from breast tissue (22).
8. Remove trocar from tube.

Using a trocar during tube insertion is not recommended because of the greater risk of lung perforation. Dissection to the pleura should be performed, with puncture of the pleura by the tip of the closed forceps, not by a trocar. If a trocar is to be used after dissecting to the pleura, there should be a straight clamp perpendicular to the shaft at 1 to 1.5 cm from the tip to avoid penetrating too deeply (Fig. 38.10).

9. Estimate length of insertion for intrathoracic portion of tube (skin incision site to midclavicle). This should be approximately 2 to 3 cm in a small preterm infant and 3 to 4 cm in a term infant. (These are approximate guidelines only.)
10. Infiltrate skin at incision site with 0.125 to 0.25 mL of 1% lidocaine.
11. Using a no. 15 blade, make incision through skin approximately the same length as chest tube diameter, or no more than 0.5 to 1 cm (Fig. 38.12C).
12. Puncture pleura immediately above the fifth rib by applying pressure on the tip of the closed forceps with index finger (Fig. 38.12D).
    a. Place the forefinger as shown in Fig 38.12D and not further forward on the forceps, to prevent the tip from plunging too deeply into the pleural space.
    b. A definite "give" will be felt as the forceps tip penetrates the pleura; there may also be an audible rush of air.

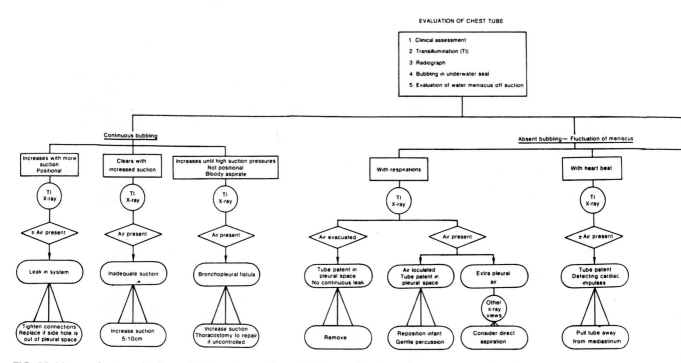

FIG. 38.11.   Evaluation of a chest tube: Flow chart to determine how well a chest tube is evacuating pleural air leak and when the tube should be removed.

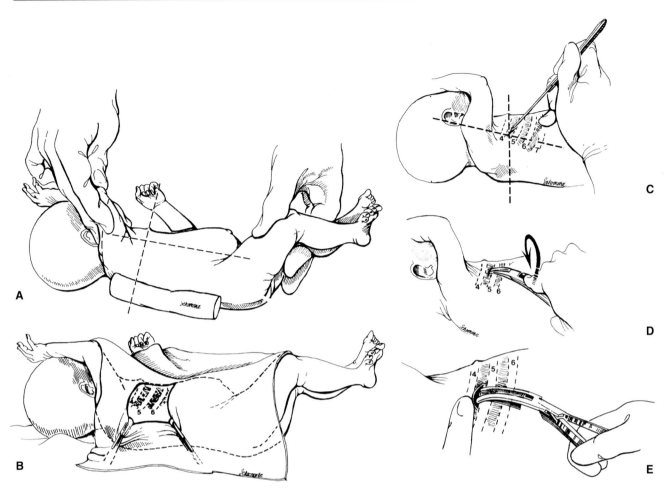

FIG. 38.12. Insertion of a soft chest tube. **A:** Position the infant with back support so the point of tube entry will be highest. Fix arm over the head without externally rotating it. Note the midaxillary (MA) line and the line from the nipple through the fourth intercostal space (ICS). **B:** Drape so head of the infant is visible. **C:** Same landmarks without the drape, showing the incision in the fourth ICS in the MA line with entry into the chest at the intersection of the nipple line and the MA line. **D:** Turning the hemostat to puncture into the pleura in the fourth ICS. **E:** With the index finger marking the fourth ICS puncture site, the tube may now be passed between the hemostat blades, along the tunnel into the pleural space.

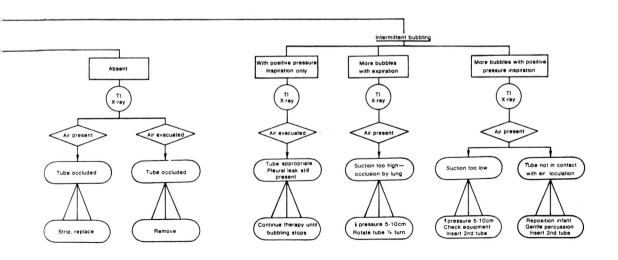

c. After puncturing pleura, open hemostat just wide enough to admit chest tube.

13. Leaving hemostat in place, thread tube between opened tips to the predetermined depth (Fig. 38.12E).

   a. Alternatively, insert closed tips of mosquito hemostat into side port of tube to its end. The disadvantage of this method is that the forceps will have to be withdrawn from the opening in the chest; it is common that the intercostal muscles then render the opening undetectable (22,23).

   b. Direct chest tube cephalad toward apex of the thorax (midclavicle), and advance tip to midclavicular line, ensuring that all side holes are within the pleural space.

   c. Observe for humidity or bubbling in the chest tube, to verify intrapleural location.

14. Connect tube to vacuum drainage system and observe fluctuations of meniscus and pattern of bubbling (Fig. 38.11). Avoid putting tension on tube.

15. Secure chest tube to skin with suture (Fig. 38.13A).

   a. Use one suture to close the end of the skin incision and make an airtight seal with the chest tube. Tie the ends of the suture around the tube in alternating directions, without constricting the tube.

      Using a traditional purse-string suture to secure the tube leaves an unsightly scar and is, therefore, not recommended. Unless the skin incision has been made unnecessarily long, a single suture is usually sufficient.

   b. Apply tincture of benzoin to chest tube near chest wall and to skin several centimeters below incision. When tacky, encircle tube with a 2-inch length of tape, leaving the tab posterior (Fig. 38.13B).

   c. Place suture through skin and tab of tape to stabilize the chest tube in a straight position (Fig. 38.13B).

   d. Alternatively, secure tube with a tape bridge (Fig. 38.14) or clear adhesive dressing (the latter may not be optimal; chest tubes tend to function optimally when allowed to exit from the skin at as close to a 90-degree angle as possible).

16. Apply antibiotic ointment or petroleum gauze around skin incision. Cover with a small semiporous transparent dressing.

   It is important not to cover the wound with a heavy dressing, as this restricts chest wall movement, obscures tube position, and makes transillumination more difficult. If the position of tube is in doubt, secure with a temporary tape bridge before covering with dressing, until the correct position is confirmed.

17. Verify proper position of tube.

   a. Anteroposterior and lateral radiographs (6,24–26)

      Both views are recommended to detect anterior course of tube. See Tables 38.1 and 38.2 for radiographic clues on malpositions. A malpositioned tube tip results in an increased risk of complications and/or poor air evacuation. A chest radiograph should confirm that the side holes are within the chest cavity.

   b. Pattern of bubbling (Fig. 38.11)

18. Strip tube if meniscus stops fluctuating or as air evacuation decreases. Take extreme care not to dislodge tube by holding tube firmly with one hand close to chest wall.

Insertion of Posterior Tube for Fluid Accumulation

The technique is similar to that for an anteriorly positioned tube, with the following differences.

1. Position infant supine, elevating the affected side by 15 to 30 degrees from the table. Secure the arm over the head (Fig. 38.15).

2. Prepare skin over lateral portion of hemithorax from anterior to posterior axillary line.

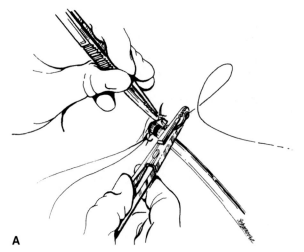
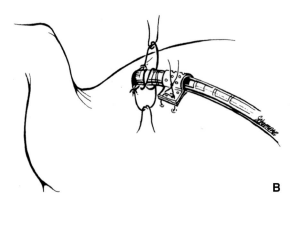

FIG. 38.13.   Securing a chest tube. **A:** Make the incision site airtight with the tube. Do not use a purse-string suture around the incision because it will form a puckered scar. The initial incision should be made small enough to require only a single suture. **B:** After painting the tube and skin with benzoin, encircle the suture around the tube or attach a tape and suture it to the skin.

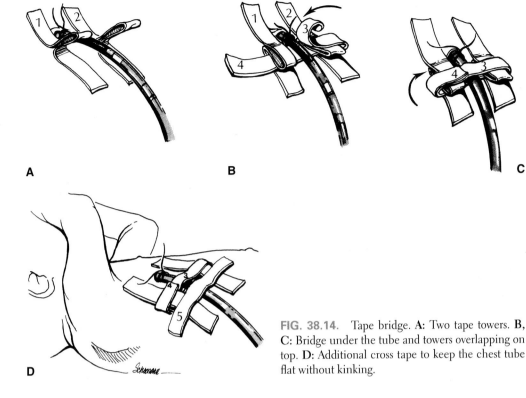

FIG. 38.14. Tape bridge. **A:** Two tape towers. **B, C:** Bridge under the tube and towers overlapping on top. **D:** Additional cross tape to keep the chest tube flat without kinking.

3. Make a skin incision 0.5 to 0.75 cm in length, just behind the anterior axillary line in the fourth to sixth intercostal space and following direction of rib.
   a. Fourth or fifth space for high posterior tube tip
   b. Sixth space for low posterior tube tip
4. Take care to position forceps tip immediately above a rib to avoid the intercostal vessels that run under the inferior surface of the rib. Penetrate the pleura as described for an anterior chest tube.
5. Insert tube only deeply enough to place side holes within pleural space.
6. Collect drainage material for culture, chemical analysis, and volume.
7. Connect to an underwater seal drainage system that includes a specimen trap.
8. Strip tube regularly.
9. Monitor and correct any imbalance caused by loss of fluid, electrolytes, protein, fats, or lymphocytes.

TABLE 38.1 **Clues to Recognize Thoracostomy Tube Perforation of the Lung**

1. Bleeding from endotracheal tube
2. Continuous bubbling in underwater seal
3. Hemothorax
4. Blood return from chest tube
5. Increased density around tip of tube on radiograph
6. Persistent pneumothorax despite satisfactory position on frontal view
7. Tube lying neither anterior nor posterior to lung on lateral view
8. Tube positioned in fissure

Removal of Thoracostomy Tube

1. Ascertain that tube is no longer functioning or needed.
   a. Evaluate as suggested in Fig. 38.11.
   b. Leave chest tube connected to water seal without suction for 4 to 12 hours. Do not clamp tube.
      (1) Transilluminate to detect reaccumulation.
      (2) Obtain radiograph.
   c. Document absence of significant drainage.
2. Assemble equipment.

Sterile

a. Antiseptic solution
b. Gloves
c. Scissors
d. Forceps
e. Petroleum gauze cut and compressed to 2-cm diameter
f. Gauze pads, 2 × 2 inch

TABLE 38.2 **Clues to Thoracostomy Tube Positioned in Fissure**

1. Major interlobar fissure
   a. Frontal view: Upper medial hemithorax
   b. Lateral view: Oblique course posterior and upward
2. Minor fissure (on right)
   a. Horizontal course toward medial side of lung

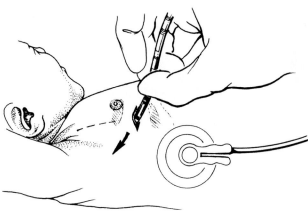

FIG. 38.15. Insertion of a posterior chest tube. With the infant supine, the incision is in or just below the anterior axillary line, with the tube entry into the pleura more posteriorly Take care to enter pleural space over the top of a rib.

Nonsterile

1-inch tape
  3. Cleanse skin in area of chest tube with antiseptic.
  4. Release tape and suture holding tube in place. Leave wound suture intact if skin is not inflamed.
  5. To prevent air from entering chest as tube is withdrawn until petroleum gauze is applied, palpate pleural entry site and hold finger over it. After removing tube, approximate wound edges and place petroleum gauze

over the incision. Keep pressure on the pleural wound until dressing is in place.
  6. Cover petroleum gauze with dry, sterile gauze. Limit taping to as small an area as possible so that transillumination will be possible.
  7. Remove sutures when healing is complete.

G. Complications

  1. Misdiagnosis with inappropriate placement
  2. Burn from transillumination devices (27)
  3. Trauma
      a. Lung laceration or perforation (28) (Fig. 38.16)
      b. Perforation and hemorrhage from a major vessel (axillary, pulmonary, intercostal, internal mammary) (15) (Fig. 38.17)
      c. Puncture of viscus within path of tube (Fig. 38.18)
      d. Residual scarring (17) (Fig. 38.19)
      e. Permanent damage to breast tissue (17)
      f. Chylothorax (29)
  4. Nerve damage
      a. Horner syndrome caused by pressure from tip of right-sided, posterior chest tube near second thoracic ganglion at first thoracic intervertebral space (30)
      b. Diaphragmatic paralysis or eventration from phrenic nerve injury (31)

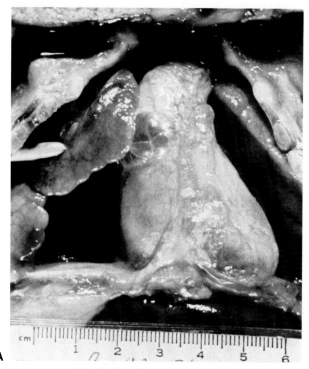

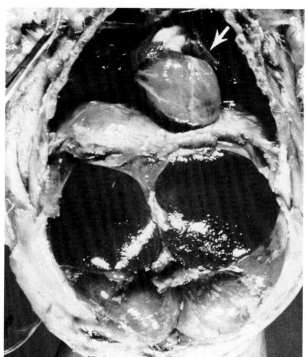

FIG. 38.16. Postmortem examination of infants who died with uncontrolled air leaks. **A:** Perforation of the right superior lobe by a chest tube inserted without a trocar, demonstrating that virtually any tube can penetrate into the lung. **B:** Perforation of the left upper lobe by a chest tube (*arrow*).

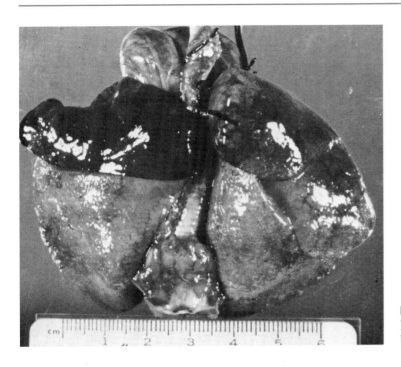

FIG. 38.17. Posterior view of thoracic organs. Traumatic hemorrhage of the left upper lobe was due to perforation by a thoracostomy tube.

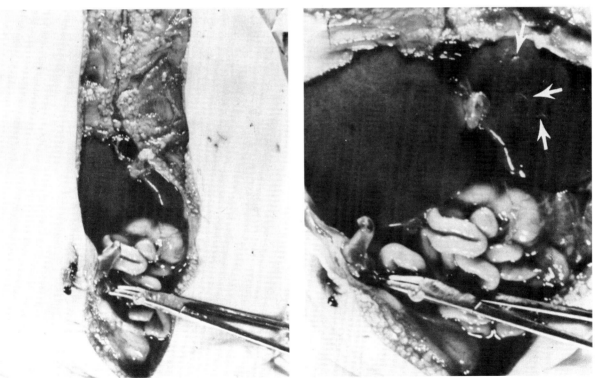

A   B

FIG. 38.18. Postmortem examination of an infant with bilateral pneumothorax, pneumomediastinum, and pneumoperitoneum secondary to pulmonary air leaks. Attempted needle aspirations, as shown by multiple skin puncture sites of the pneumomediastinum and pneumothorax (**A**), resulted in needle punctures of the liver (*arrows*, **B**) with peritoneal hemorrhage.

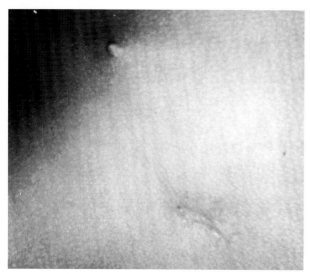

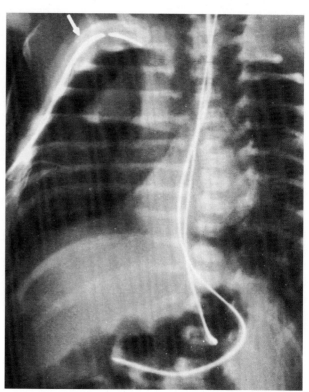

FIG. 38.19.   Scar from thoracostomy insertion, emphasizing the importance of avoiding the breast area. Massaging the healed wound with cocoa butter helps break down adhesions that lead to dimpling at the scar.

FIG. 38.20.   The thoracostomy tube is completely outside the pleural space on this slightly oblique chest film. Note that the long feeding tube is not in an appropriate position for transpyloric feeding. Indwelling tubes may dislodge when other emergency procedures are performed.

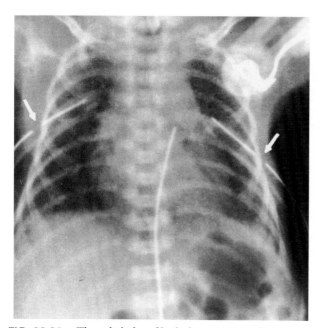

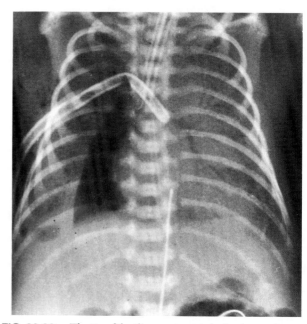

FIG. 38.21.   The side holes of both thoracostomy tubes are outside the pleural space on this radiograph.

FIG. 38.22.   The tip of the thoracostomy tube has been advanced too far medially and is kinked against the mediastinum. Withdrawing the tube 1 or 2 cm would improve drainage at the medial thorax. Note the endotracheal tube tip in the right mainstem bronchus.

5. Misplacement of tube
   a. Tube outside pleural cavity in subcutaneous placement (Fig. 38.20)
   b. Side hole outside pleural space (Fig. 38.21)
   c. Tip across anterior mediastinum (Fig. 38.22)
6. Equipment malfunction
   a. Blockage of tube by proteinaceous or hemorrhagic material
   b. Leak in evacuation system, usually at connection sites
   c. Inappropriate suction pressures (32) (Fig. 38.11)
      (1) Excessive pressure
         (a) Aggravation of leak across bronchopleural fistula
         (b) Interference with gas exchange
         (c) Suction of lung parenchyma against holes of tube
      (2) Inadequate pressure with reaccumulation
7. Infection
   a. Cellulitis
   b. Inoculation of pleura with skin organisms, including *Candida* (33)
8. Subcutaneous emphysema secondary to leak of tension pneumothorax through pleural opening
9. Aortic obstruction with posterior tube (34)
10. Loss of contents of pleural fluid
    a. Water, electrolytes, and protein (effusion)
    b. Lymphocytes and chylomicrons (chylothorax)

Emergency Evacuation of Air Leaks

Life-threatening air accumulations require emergency evacuation. This provides temporary relief to the patient while preparing for thoracostomy tube placement. The following techniques using modified equipment are less traumatic than using straight needles or scalp vein sets. We suggest using an anterior approach for emergency evacuation because position will not interfere with the preparation of the lateral chest site for an indwelling chest tube.

Tubes used for emergency evacuation require suction pressures as high as 30 to 60 cm H_2O to overcome the resistance of their small diameters (35). This requirement and their tendency to occlude make these cannulas unreliable for continuous drainage of a significant air leak.

A. Indications

Temporary evacuation of life-threatening air accumulations while preparing for permanent tube placement

B. Contraindications

1. When patient's vital signs are stable enough to allow placement of permanent thoracostomy tube without prior emergency evacuation
2. When air collection is likely to resolve spontaneously without patient compromise (nontension pneumothorax)

A. Equipment

All sterile

1. Gloves
2. Antiseptic solution
3. 18- to 20-gauge angiocatheter (36)
4. IV extension tubing
5. Three-way stopcock
6. 10- and 20-mL syringes

B. Technique

1. Prepare skin of appropriate hemithorax with antiseptic.
2. Connect a three-way stopcock to an IV extension tubing. Connect syringe to three-way stopcock.
3. Insert angiocatheter at point that is
   a. At a 45-degree angle to skin, directed cephalad
   b. In second, fourth, or fifth intercostal space, just over top of rib, *well above or below the areola of the breast*
   c. In midclavicular line (Fig. 38.23A)
4. As angiocatheter enters pleural space, decrease angle to 15 degrees with the chest wall and slide cannula in while removing stylet (Fig. 38.23A).
5. Attach IV extension tubing to angiocatheter, open stopcock, and evacuate air with syringe (Fig. 38.23B).
6. Continue evacuation as patient's condition warrants, while preparing for permanent tube placement.
7. Cover insertion site with petroleum gauze and small dressing after procedure.

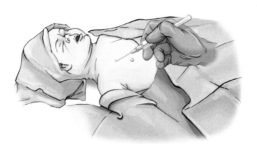

A

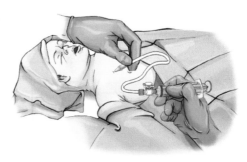

B

FIG. 38.23. Emergency evacuation with a vascular cannula. Puncture the skin and enter the pleura at a 45-degree angle, immediately above a rib.

Diagnostic Tap of Pleural Fluid

Follow the procedure for the insertion of a posterior chest tube, with the following differences.

A. Differences

1. Use a 20-gauge angiocatheter.
2. Position patient without elevating the hemothorax on the side of fluid collection. It will be necessary to lower the affected side only if the quantity of fluid is small.
3. Select insertion site in anterior or midaxillary lines below breast tissue for diffuse pleural collections. Direct catheter tip posteriorly, after penetrating into pleural space.
4. Keep system closed to prevent leakage of air into pleural space.

Anterior Mediastinal Drainage

Most mediastinal air collections cause only mild symptoms and are not under sufficient tension to require drainage. Their presence often precedes tension pneumothorax in the presence of lung disease and positive-pressure ventilation. Posterior mediastinal tube insertion is rarely required (37).

A. Indications

1. Significant air accumulation with physiologic compromise (38)
   a. Increased intracranial pressure (39)
   b. Poor cardiac output because of impeded venous return
   c. Critical interference with artificial ventilation
      (1) Competition with lungs for thoracic volume
      (2) Negative effect on pulmonary compliance
2. Drainage of fluid
   a. Mediastinitis after esophageal perforation
   b. Postoperative

B. Contraindications

No absolute contraindications

C. Equipment

Sterile

1. Antiseptic for skin preparation
2. Gauze pads
3. Aperture drapes
4. Surgical gloves
5. No. 11 surgical blade
6. Local anesthetic, as required
7. Curved mosquito hemostat
8. Drainage tube (see equipment for emergency evacuation of air leaks)
   a. 10-Fr soft thoracostomy tube
   b. IV cannula system
      (1) 14- to 16-gauge angiocatheter
      (2) IV extension tubing
      (3) Three-way stopcock
9. 10- to 20-mL syringe
10. Connecting tubing and underwater suction device for indwelling tube
11. 4-0 nonabsorbable suture on small cutting needle with needle holder
12. Transparent bag to cover tip of transillumination device.

Nonsterile

1. 0.5-inch adhesive tape
2. Transillumination device

D. Precautions and Complications

The problems encountered in evacuating material from the mediastinum are similar to those encountered in placement of chest tubes. In contrast to tension pneumothorax, mediastinal collections tend to accumulate more gradually. For this reason, careful preparation of the patient and use of sterile technique are possible and essential. For precautions and complications, refer to E and G under Thoracostomy Tubes at the beginning of this chapter.

E. Technique

Drainage for longer than 12 hours normally dictates placing a 10- to 12-Fr tube by direct dissection because smaller tubes occlude readily. Select indwelling tubes only in the presence of significant lung disease or mediastinitis, where continued accumulations are anticipated. Remove the tubes as soon as possible to reduce the risk for infection.

Soft Mediastinal Tube Insertion

1. Follow sterile technique throughout.
2. Monitor infant's vital signs and oxygenation.
3. Determine, by transillumination or radiograph, the region of maximal mediastinal air accumulation (Fig. 38.24).
4. Cover tip of transillumination light with sterile, clear plastic bag for use after skin preparation.
5. Cleanse skin with antiseptic.
6. Drape patient with aperture drape, without obscuring infant.
7. Infiltrate insertion site with 0.25 mL of local anesthetic.
8. With a no. 11 blade, make a small stab wound through the skin at the subxiphoid.

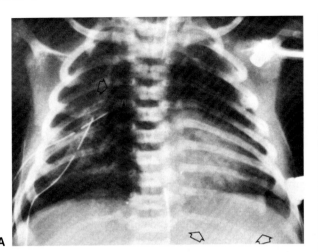

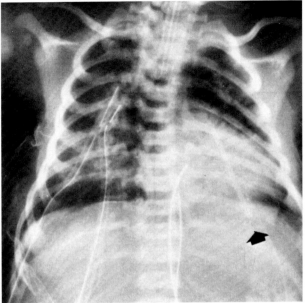

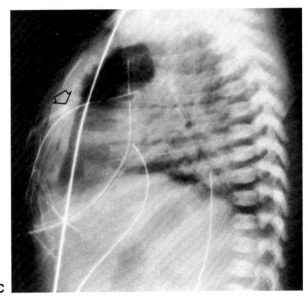

FIG. 38.24. Sequential radiographs. **A:** Tension pneumomediastinum (*arrows*). A mediastinal collection this massive is unusual. **B:** Successful drainage tube (*arrow*). **C:** The apparent slipping of the mediastinal cannula (*arrow*) is an artifact of patient rotation on this lateral view. There is residual mediastinal air superiorly, but there was no patient compromise at this time.

9. Using a curved mosquito hemostat, dissect in the midline at 30-degree angle to chest wall in cephalad direction until entering mediastinal space. The mediastinum under tension should bulge downward.
10. Insert soft chest tube into dissected tunnel, and direct tube cephalad and toward area of maximal transillumination.
11. Observe tube for air rush or condensation while completing insertion. If loculations are evident, break them up using blunt dissection.
12. Connect to closed drainage system at vacuum of 5 cm H_2O, and increase to 10 cm H_2O if necessary.
    Accumulation in mediastinum is usually relatively slow; therefore, lower suction pressures are effective.
    a. Use low pressure to keep tube side holes patent while clearing air collection.
    b. Monitor efficacy by radiograph and transillumination (Fig. 38.24).
13. Secure tube with suture, and tape as for thoracostomy tubes.

14. If drainage stops with significant accumulation still evident on transillumination or radiograph
    a. Verify that accumulation is in mediastinum by lateral decubitus and lateral radiographs.
    b. Verify tube position on radiographs.
    c. Rotate tube.
    d. Aspirate, but do not irrigate, tube; reattach to continuous drainage.
    e. Change position of infant to move air toward tube.

Temporary Mediastinal Drainage with IV Cannula

1. Assemble equipment and prepare patient as for insertion by mediastinal dissection.
2. Make a small stab wound in subxiphoid notch.
    Mediastinal air under tension should be located in this area, pushing the liver and heart away from needle tip.
3. Insert cannula with stylet at 45-degree angle to chest wall in cephalad direction.

4. As soon as cannula passes through skin, lower cannula to a 30-degree angle with skin.

5. Remove stylet, and attach connecting tubing, stopcock, and syringe.

6. Advance cannula into mediastinal space cephalad and medially, but toward area of maximal transillumination. Aspirate while advancing, and monitor cardiac tracing. Stop insertion if there is resistance, blood, or arrhythmia.

7. Secure cannula in effective position, and attach IV extension tubing to underwater drainage system with suction pressure of 10 cm H_2O. The smaller cannula will require higher suction pressures unless the air accumulates slowly. Because air loculates within the mediastinum and the side holes occlude easily, small catheters are rarely effective for anything other than acute relief of tension. Remove cannula as soon as possible.

References

1. Dull KE, Fleisher GR. Pigtail catheters versus large-bore chest tubes for pneumothoraces in children treated in the emergency department. *Pediatr Emerg Care.* 2002;18:265.

2. Lawless S, Orr R, Killian A, et al. New pigtail catheter for pleural drainage in pediatric patients. *Crit Care Med.* 1989;17:173.

3. Wood B, Dubik M. A new device for pleural drainage in newborn infants. *Pediatrics.* 1995;96:955.

4. Rothberg AD, Marks KH, Maisels MJ. Understanding the Pleurevac. *Pediatrics.* 1981;67:482.

5. Gonzalez F, Harris T, Black P, et al. Decreased gas flow through pneumothoraces in neonates receiving high-frequency jet versus conventional ventilation. *J Pediatr.* 1987;110:464.

6. MacDonald MG. Thoracostomy in the neonate: a blunt discussion. *NeoReviews.* 2004;5:c301.

7. Chan L. Medial pneumothorax: a radiographic sign that should not be overlooked on the supine view. *Am J Emerg Med.* 1999;17:431.

8. Dennis J, Eigen H, Ballantine T, et al. The relationship between peak inspiratory pressure and positive end expiratory pressure on the volume of air lost through a bronchopleural fistula. *J Pediatr Surg.* 1980;15:971.

9. Zidulka A. Position may reduce or stop pneumothorax formation in dogs receiving mechanical ventilation. *Clin Invest Med.* 1987;10:290.

10. Stevens TP, Harrington EW, Blennow M, et al. Early surfactant administration with brief ventilation vs. selective surfactant and continued mechanical ventilation for preterm infants with or at risk for respiratory distress syndrome. *Cochrane Database Syst Rev.* 2007;17:CD003063.

11. Ryan CA, Barrington KJ, Phillips HJ, et al. Contralateral pneumothoraces in the newborn: incidence and predisposing factors. *Pediatrics.* 1987;79:417.

12. Kuhns LR, Bednarek FJ, Wyman ML. Diagnosis of pneumothorax or pneumomediastinum in the neonate by transillumination. *Pediatrics.* 1975;56:355.

13. Wyman ML, Kuhns LR. Accuracy of transillumination in the recognition of pneumothorax and pneumomediastinum in the neonate. *Clin Pediatr.* 1977;16:323.

14. Albelda SM, Gefter WB, Kelley MA, et al. Ventilator-induced subpleural air cysts: clinical, radiographic, and pathologic significance. *Am Rev Respir Dis.* 1983;127:360.

15. Allen RW, Jung AL, Lester PD. Effectiveness of chest tube evacuation of pneumothorax in neonates. *J Pediatr.* 1981;99:629.

16. Batton DG, Hellmann J, Nardis EE. Effect of pneumothorax-induced systemic blood pressure alterations on the cerebral circulation in newborn dogs. *Pediatrics.* 1984;74:350.

17. Cartlidge PH, Fox PE, Rutter N. The scars of newborn intensive care. *Early Hum Dev.* 1990;21:1.

18. Bhatia J, Mathew OP. Resolution of pneumothorax in neonates. *Crit Care Med.* 1985;13:417.

19. Merenstein GB, Dougherty K, Lewis A. Early detection of pneumothorax by oscilloscope monitor in the newborn infant. *J Pediatr.* 1972;80:98.

20. Noack G, Freyschuss V. The early detection of pneumothorax with transthoracic impedance in newborn infants. *Acta Paediatr Scand.* 1977;66:677.

21. Grim P 3rd, Keenan WJ. Two uncommon radiographic signs of an anterior neonatal pneumothorax. Correlated with clinical finding. *Clin Pediatr.* 1986;25:440.

22. Genc A, Ozcan C, Erdener A, et al. Management of pneumothorax in children. *J Cardiovasc Surg.* 1998;39:849.

23. Mehrabani D, Kopelman AE. Chest tube insertion: a simplified technique. *Pediatrics.* 1989;83:784.

24. Mauer JR, Friedman PJ, Wing VW. Thoracostomy tube in an interlobar fissure: radiologic recognition of a potential problem. *AJR.* 1981;139:1155.

25. Strife JL, Smith P, Dunbar JS, et al. Chest tube perforation of the lung in premature infants: radiographic recognition. *AJR.* 1983;141:73.

26. Bowen A, Zarabi M. Radiographic clues to chest tube perforation of neonatal lung. *Am J Perinatol.* 1985;2:43.

27. Perman MJ, Kauls LS. Transilluminator burns in the neonatal intensive care unit: a mimicker of more serious disease. *Pediatr Dermatol.* 2007;24:168.

28. Strife JL, Smith P, Dunbar JS, et al. Chest tube perforation of the lung in premature infants: radiographic recognition. *AJR Am J Roentgenol.* 1983;141:73.

29. Kumar SP, Belik J. Chylothorax—a complication of chest tube placement in a neonate. *Crit Care Med.* 1984;12:411.

30. Rosegger H, Fritsch G. Horner's syndrome after treatment of tension pneumothorax with tube thoracostomy in a newborn infant. *Eur J Pediatr.* 1980;133:67.

31. Nahum E, Ben-Ari J, Schonfeld T, et al. Acute diaphragmatic paralysis caused by chest-tube trauma to phrenic nerve. *Pediatr Radiol.* 2001;31:444.

32. Grosfeld JL, Lemons JL, Ballantine TVN, et al. Emergency thoracostomy for acquired bronchopleural fistula in the premature infant with respiratory distress. *J Pediatr Surg.* 1980;15:416.

33. Faix RG, Naglie RA, Barr M. Intrapleural inoculation of *Candida* in an infant with congenital cutaneous candidiasis. *Am J Perinatol.* 1986;3:119.

34. Gooding C, Kerlan R Jr, Brasch R. Partial aortic obstruction produced by a thoracostomy tube. *J Pediatr.* 1981;98:471.

35. Ragosta KG, Fuhrman BP, Howland DF. Flow characteristics of thoracotomy tubes used in infants. *Crit Care Med.* 1990;18:662.

36. Arda IS, Gurakan B, Aliefendioglu D, et al. Treatment of pneumothorax in newborns: use of venous catheter versus chest tube. *Pediatr Int.* 2002;44:78.

37. Purohit DM, Lorenzo RL, Smith CE, et al. Bronchial laceration in a newborn with persistent posterior pneumomediastinum. *J Pediatr Surg.* 1985;20:82.

38. Moore JT, Wayne ER, Hanson J. Malignant pneumomediastinum: successful tube mediastinotomy in the neonate. *Am J Surg.* 1987;154:687.

39. Tyler DC, Redding G, Hall D, et al. Increased intracranial pressure: an indication to decompress a tension pneumomediastinum. *Crit Care Med.* 1984;12:467.

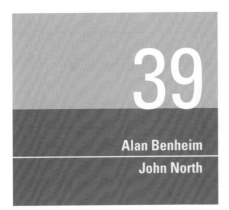

39

Pericardiocentesis

Alan Benheim

John North

A. Definitions

1. Pericardium
   a. A double layer of mesothelial lining surrounding the heart, consisting of the visceral pericardium on the epicardial surface and the parietal pericardium as an outer layer
   b. Between the two layers, there is normally a small amount of pericardial fluid (typically <5 mL for a neonate) that is thought to reduce friction.
2. Pneumopericardium
   a. Collection of air in the pericardial space
3. Pericardial effusion
   a. Accumulation of excess fluid in the pericardial space
4. Pericardiocentesis
   a. A procedure to remove air or excess fluid from the pericardial space, usually through a needle, small cannula, or drainage catheter
5. Pericardial drain
   a. A catheter or other drainage device left in place to allow intermittent or continuous evacuation of air or fluid from the pericardial space
   b. Placed in select situations with recurring accumulation of air or fluid in the pericardial space
6. Tamponade
   a. Clinical condition with limited cardiac output because of external restriction of expansion of the heart, preventing normal cardiac filling, resulting in a decreased stroke volume and impaired cardiac output
   b. May be caused by
      (1) Fluid or air in the pericardial space
      (2) Abnormalities of the pericardium (restrictive or constrictive)
      (3) Increased intrathoracic pressure associated with obstructive airway lung disease or tension pneumothorax
7. Pulsus paradoxus (Fig. 39.1)
   a. Respiratory variation in blood pressure, with a decrease in systolic blood pressure during spontaneous inspiration. (During positive-pressure ventilation, this is reversed, with a rise in systolic pressure during inspiration.)
   b. This finding occurs during tamponade.

B. Purpose

1. To evacuate air to relieve cardiac tamponade
2. To evacuate fluid to relieve cardiac tamponade
3. To obtain fluid for diagnostic studies

C. Background (See also A)

1. The heart lies within a closed space, covered by the pericardium. The pericardial space lies between the two layers of the pericardium. If the pericardial space fills with excess fluid or if air accumulates, the heart has less space available, and the pressure within the pericardium increases. Increased intrapericardial pressure restricts venous return and impairs cardiac filling. The decrease in venous return and cardiac filling results in a reduced cardiac output. This clinical situation is known as cardiac tamponade (1–5).
2. Neonates are at increased risk for cardiac tamponade when there is
   a. Accumulation of air dissecting into the pericardium from the respiratory system (Fig. 39.2) (4–7)
   b. Pericardial fluid accumulation due to perforation or transudate from umbilical or central venous catheter (Figs. 32.15, 39.3) (1,8–12)
   c. Cannulation for extracorporeal membrane oxygenation (13,14)
   d. Cardiac catheterization, either diagnostic or therapeutic (15)
   e. Postoperative pericardial hemorrhage following cardiac surgery (2,16)
   f. Postpericardiotomy syndrome, typically 1 to 3 weeks after cardiac surgery (2,16,17)
   g. Pericardial effusion as part of generalized edema/hydrops (3,16)
   h. Pericardial effusions due to infectious or autoimmune causes. (These are less common in neonates than in older children.)

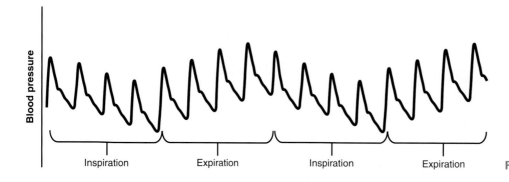

FIG. 39.1.   Pulsus paradoxus.

3. Clinical signs of cardiac tamponade may evolve gradually or rapidly (1,3,18).
4. The primary therapy for cardiac tamponade is to evacuate the pericardial space. Volume expansion and pressor agents may be of transient benefit, but they usually do not result in sustained clinical improvement (1,8,12,16,19).
5. Cardiac tamponade may require urgent treatment with pericardiocentesis in infants with severe hemodynamic compromise (1,16,17).

D. Indications (1,12,15–17)

1. Cardiac tamponade due to pneumopericardium
2. Cardiac tamponade due to pericardial fluid
3. Aspiration of pericardial fluid for diagnostic studies

E. Contraindications

1. There are no absolute contraindications to performing pericardiocentesis in the setting of cardiac tamponade.

2. Relative contraindication for diagnostic pericardiocentesis
   a. Coagulopathy
   b. Active infection. (However, infection may also be an indication for diagnostic pericardiocentesis in some clinical situations.)

F. Precautions

Draining a large volume from the pericardial space can alter cardiac preloading conditions significantly, and some infants may require a supplemental intravascular fluid bolus after the pericardium is drained.

G. Limitations

1. Cannot readily evacuate thrombus
2. Cannot remove mass lesions

H. Equipment

Sterile

1. Antiseptic solution
2. Aperture drape or multiple drapes to be arranged around access site

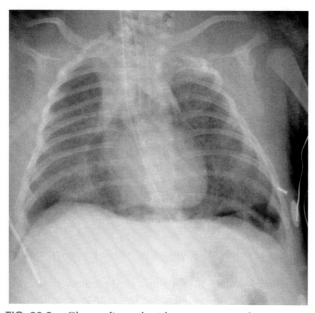

FIG. 39.2.   Chest radiograph with pneumopericardium.

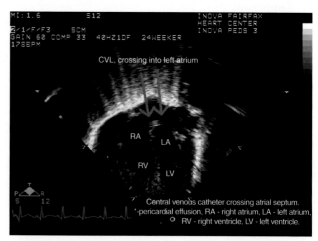

FIG. 39.3.   Echocardiogram image of preterm infant with pericardial effusion and central venous line in left atrium.

3. Swabs or gauze pads
4. Gloves
5. Local anesthetic
6. 16- to 20-gauge IV cannula over 1- to 2-inch needle
7. Indwelling drainage catheter (optional)
8. Three-way stopcock
9. Short IV extension tubing (optional)
10. 10- to 20-mL syringes
11. Preassembled closed drainage system as for emergency evacuation of air leaks, thoracostomy tubes described in Chapter 38 (optional)
12. Connecting tubing and underwater seal for indwelling drain (optional)
13. Specimen containers for laboratory studies, if procedure is diagnostic

Nonsterile (See also I)

1. Transillumination device (optional, for pneumopericardium)
2. Echocardiogram/sonography imaging device (optional in urgent situations)

I. Procedure

1. If ultrasound/echocardiographic imaging is available, and if time permits, imaging can be performed to determine an optimal needle entry site and angle. In addition, the approximate distance required to reach the pericardial space can be estimated (15). Even after a sterile field is created, ultrasound imaging can be performed from a nonsterile area of the chest to monitor the effusion during the procedure. If imaging is done from a part of the sterile field, the transducer can be placed in a sterile sheath (or a sterile glove). Care should be taken to avoid moving a probe with sterile cover back and forth between sterile and nonsterile areas.
2. Similarly, evaluation with transillumination can be performed in cases of pneumopericardium, if time permits.
3. Cleanse skin over xiphoid, precordium, and epigastric area with antiseptic. Allow to dry.
4. Arrange sterile drapes, leaving the subxiphoid area exposed.
5. Administer local anesthesia if the patient is conscious. For example, 0.25 to 1 mL of subcutaneous 1% lidocaine instilled within 1 to 2 cm of the xiphoid process. (See also Chapter 6.)
6. Form a closed system by assembling a syringe, three-way stopcock, and extension tubing so that the stopcock is open to both the syringe and the extension tubing, but closed to the remaining side-port.
7. Using the IV needle/cannula, enter the skin 0.5 to 1 cm below the tip of the xiphoid process, in the midline or slightly (0.5 cm) to the left of the midline. The needle should be at a 30- to 40-degree angle to the skin, and

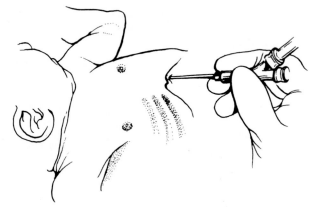

FIG. 39.4. Insertion of needle/cannula attached to three-way stopcock, in the subxiphoid space, directed toward the left shoulder.

the tip should be directed toward the left shoulder (Fig. 39.4). A different approach may be used in certain cases, for example, if an echocardiogram suggests that most of the fluid is right-sided or apical.

8. Advance the needle until air or fluid is obtained.
   a. A rhythmic tug, corresponding to the heart rate, may be felt as the needle enters the pericardium.
   b. If ultrasound imaging is available, needle position can be determined either by visualizing the tip of the needle within the pericardial space or by demonstrating that the amount of pericardial fluid is diminishing as fluid is aspirated (Fig. 39.5). Some authors have described reinfusing a small amount of the aspirated fluid while imaging to observe the location of microcavitation echoes (15,20,21).
9. Fix the needle in position and advance the cannula over the needle into the pericardial space. Remove the needle, and connect the cannula to the closed system syringe for aspiration.
10. Aspirate as much fluid/air as possible. If the syringe fills, use the third port of the stopcock to empty the syringe, or to attach a second syringe, and then aspirate more, repeating as needed. If diagnostic studies are desired, the fluid should be transferred to appropriate specimen containers.
    a. If bloody fluid is aspirated, there could be a serosanguineous or hemorrhagic effusion, or the needle might have entered the heart (usually the right ventricle). There are a few clues that can be helpful in determining whether the needle has entered the heart (see J).
    b. Note that small single-lumen catheters may easily become blocked.
    c. A decision will need to be made whether to leave the cannula in place for any length of time or to remove it once the pericardium has been drained. This decision will vary in individual cases, but factors to consider include the likelihood of reaccumulation and

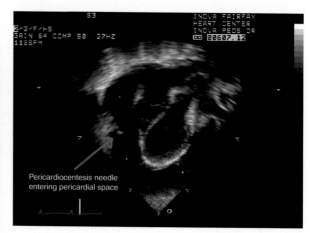

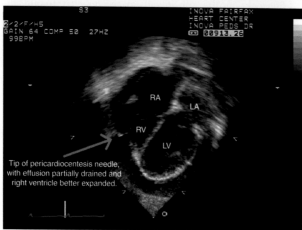

FIG. 39.5. Echocardiogram images of pericardiocentesis. **A:** Echocardiogram image of pericardial effusion. **B:** Tip of needle in pericardial space. **C:** Pericardial effusion partially drained.

the need for repeat drainage versus the risk of infection or entry of free air with an indwelling cannula.

d. In certain cases, the operator may elect to evacuate the pericardial space directly through the needle, rather than placing a cannula.

J. Special Circumstances

1. If ultrasound imaging is available, it may be helpful in planning the needle entry site and angle, as well as anticipating the distance required to reach the pericardial space (2,15,17,20,21).

2. If transillumination is positive for free air before the procedure, it can be used to assess the adequacy of air evacuation after the procedure and to look for evidence of reaccumulation. Because pneumothorax and pneumomediastinum are potential complications, the availability of transillumination may also be helpful after the procedure. Transillumination is not a reliable method to rule out free air or to distinguish between pericardial air and mediastinal air (5,6).

3. On initial aspiration of the pericardium, air, serous fluid, serosanguineous or grossly bloody fluid, or fluid resembling infusate from a central line (including parenteral feeding fluids) (8,11) may be encountered. Bloody fluid raises the concern that the needle may have entered the heart. The following may be helpful in distinguishing between pericardial fluid and intracardiac blood.

a. In an infant with tamponade, aspirating 10 mL of blood from the heart will have minimal effect on the acute hemodynamics, whereas draining as little as 5 to 15 mL from the pericardial space can result in significant hemodynamic improvement within 30 seconds.

b. If ultrasound is being used, the pericardial fluid volume will appear to be decreased if the needle is correctly positioned. In some cases, one can reliably identify the needle in the pericardial space (Fig. 39.5) (15).

c. Placing a few drops on a gauze swab may help distinguish the two sources, because serosanguineous fluid will separate into a central dark red zone and a more serous peripheral zone, but this can take several minutes.

d. Alternatively, a spun hematocrit can be performed rapidly if the unit has a readily available centrifuge; this also takes a few minutes.

4. Draining a large volume from the pericardial space can alter cardiac preloading conditions significantly, and some infants may benefit from intravascular fluid boluses after the pericardium is drained.

5. Pericardiocentesis is often an urgent or emergency procedure. The technique for pericardiocentesis described above applies when there is time for each step. In an infant with significant hemodynamic compromise, the operator may be forced to omit certain steps in the interest of time. This requires a judgment as to the baby's clinical status and the time delay involved for any given step, such as waiting for the ultrasound machine, preparing a larger sterile field, or assembling a three-way stopcock system. In extreme cases, this life-saving procedure might consist of pouring or swabbing Betadine over the subxiphoid area, followed by "blind" aspiration using any available needle and syringe, without anesthetic, and before any other equipment is available at the bedside (15).

K. Complications (15–17,20,21)

1. Pneumopericardium
2. Pneumomediastinum
3. Pneumothorax
4. Cardiac perforation
5. Arrhythmia
6. Hypotension (if a large effusion is drained)

References

1. Nowlen TT, Rosenthal GL, Johnson GL, et al. Pericardial effusion and tamponade in infants with central catheters. *Pediatrics.* 2002;110:137.
2. Tsang TS, Barnes ME, Hayes SN, et al. Clinical and echocardiographic characteristics of significant pericardial effusions following cardiothoracic surgery and outcomes of echo-guided pericardiocentesis for management: Mayo clinic experience. 1979–1998. *Chest.* 1999;116:322.
3. Tamburro RF, Ring JC, Womback K. Detection of pulsus paradoxus associated with large pericardial effusions in pediatric patients by analysis of the pulse-oximetry waveform. *Pediatrics.* 2002;109:673.
4. Heckmann M, Lindner W, Pohlandt F. Tension pneumopericardium in a preterm infant without mechanical ventilation: a rare cause of cardiac arrest. *Acta Paediatr.* 1998;87:346.
5. Hook B, Hack M, Morrison S, et al. Pneumopericardium in very low birthweight infants. *J Perinatol.* 1995;15(1):27.
6. Cabatu EE, Brown EG. Thoracic transillumination: aid in the diagnosis and treatment of pneumopericardium. *Pediatrics.* 1979; 64:958.
7. Bjorklund L, Lindroth M, Malmgren N, et al. Spontaneous pneumopericardium in an otherwise healthy full-term newborn. *Acta Pediatr Scand.* 1990;79:234.
8. Ramasethu J. Complications of vascular catheters in the neonatal intensive care unit. *Clin Perinatol.* 2008;35:199.
9. van Engelenburg KC, Festen C. Cardiac tamponade: a rare but life-threatening complication of central venous catheters in children. *J Pediatr Surg.* 1998;33:1822.
10. Fioravanti J, Buzzard CJ, Harris JP. Pericardial effusion and tamponade as a result of percutaneous silastic catheter use. *Neonatal Netw.* 1998;17:39.
11. van Ditzhuyzen O, Ronayette D. Tamponnade cardiaque après catheterisme veineux central chez un nouveaune. *Arch Pediatr.* 1996;3:463.
12. Pezzati M, Filippi L, Chiti G, et al. Central venous catheters and cardiac tamponade in preterm infants. *Intensive Care Med.* 2004; 30:2253.
13. Kurian MS, Reynolds ER, Humes RA, et al. Cardiac tamponade caused by serous pericardial effusion in patients on extracorporeal membrane oxygenation. *J Pediatr Surg.* 1999;34:1311.
14. Becker JA, Short BL, Martin GR. Cardiovascular complications adversely affect survival during extracorporeal membrane oxygenation. *Crit Care Med.* 1998;26:1582.
15. Tsang TS, Freeman WK, Barnes ME, et al. Rescue echocardiographically guided pericardiocentesis for cardiac perforation complicating catheter-based procedures: The Mayo Clinic experience. *J Am Coll Cardiol.* 1998;32:1345.
16. Tsang TS, Oh JK, Seward JB. Diagnosis and management of cardiac tamponade in the era of echocardiography. *Clin Cardiol.* 1999;22:446.
17. Tsang TS, El-Najdawi EK, Seward JB, et al. Percutaneous echocardiographically guided pericardiocentesis in pediatric patients: evaluation of safety and efficacy. *J Am Soc Echocardiogr.* 1998; 11:1072.
18. Berg RA. Pulsus paradoxus in the diagnosis and management of pneumopericardium in an infant. *Crit Care Med.* 1990;18: 340.
19. Traen M, Schepens E, Laroche S, et al. Cardiac tamponade and pericardial effusion due to venous umbilical catheterization. *Acta Paediatr.* 2005;94:626.
20. Muhler EG, Engelhardt W, von Bernuth G. Pericardial effusions in infants and children: injection of echo contrast medium enhances the safety of echocardiographically-guided pericardiocentesis. *Cardiol Young.* 1998;8:506.
21. Watzinger N, Brussee H, Fruhwald FM, et al. Pericardiocentesis guided by contrast echocardiography. *Echocardiography.* 1998; 15:635.

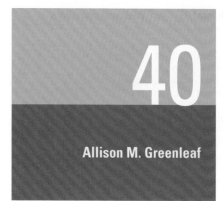

40 Gastric and Transpyloric Tubes

Allison M. Greenleaf

A. Definitions

1. Enteral feeding is defined as providing nutrients distal to the oral cavity.
2. A gastric tube is a tube inserted via the nose or mouth to the stomach.
3. A transpyloric tube is a tube passed via the nose or mouth, through the stomach and pylorus to the duodenum or jejunum.

B. Purpose

1. To provide a route for feeding (1)
2. To administer medications
3. To sample gastric or intestinal contents
4. To decompress and empty the stomach

C. Background

1. Oral feeding may be compromised in neonates due to neurobehavioral immaturity, physiological instability, or respiratory compromise.
2. In preterm infants, enteral feeds stimulate the secretion of gastric hormones, influence development of the gastrointestinal (GI) tract, reduce the risk of sepsis, and decrease length of hospitalization (2).
3. Incorrect placement of gastric and transpyloric tubes is common, with incidence ranging from 21% to 59%, and can lead to substantial morbidity and mortality (3–5).

D. Types of Tubes (6,7)

1. Feeding tubes
   a. Single-lumen tubes are used for gastric or transpyloric feeding via the oral or nasal route, or for temporary gastric decompression of air or gastric contents. They are made of silastic, silicone, polyurethane, or polyvinyl chloride (PVC) and are radio-opaque for location on radiography. They are incrementally marked in centimeters, and usually have two to four side holes at the distal end (Fig. 40.1A).

   (1) Silastic, silicone, and polyurethane tubes are softer and can remain in situ for up to 30 days, or per manufacturer's recommendations, although individual practice guidelines should be followed. Silastic tubes are preferred, especially in preterm infants weighing <750 g (8).
   (2) PVC tubes are stiffer and easier to insert. However, they are not recommended for long-term use because the plasticizers are leached, stiffening the tube and can lead to esophageal perforation (8,9). Manufacturer recommendations for frequency of tube change can range from every 6 hours to every 5 days, so individual practice guidelines should be followed.
   b. Available for neonates in sizes 3.5 to 8 Fr and in a variety of lengths. The smaller diameter tubes will have slower rates of flow. Tube length will vary depending on the depth of placement and whether the tube is to be gastric or transpyloric.
   c. Weighted, stylet-containing tubes are not recommended in the neonatal population due to the risk of perforation.
2. Suction/decompression tubes
   a. Single-lumen feeding tubes maybe used for occasional or intermittent nasogastric aspiration of stomach contents.
   b. Double-lumen (Replogle) tubes are preferable for continuous gastric decompression or for continuous suction to clear secretions from the upper esophageal pouch in infants with esophageal atresia prior to surgery (10–12).
   (1) The wider lumen is attached to the suction device for gastric decompression or esophageal clearing, and the second, smaller lumen is for airflow to prevent adherence of the catheter to the mucosal wall (Fig. 40.1B).
   (2) These catheters are also radio-opaque, marked incrementally and have multiple side holes at the distal end.
   (3) Available in 6, 8, and 10 Fr; vary in length. Manufacturer's recommendations should be followed for frequency of tube change.

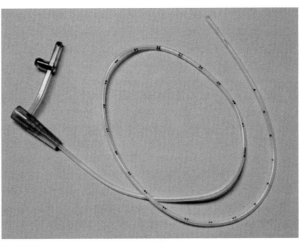 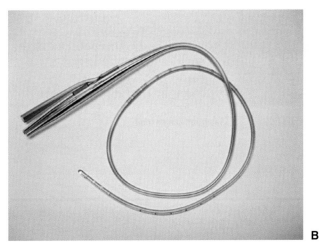

FIG. 40.1. **A:** Silastic gastric feeding tube. **B:** Double-lumen replogle tube.

Oral or Nasal Gastric Tubes

A. Indications (1)

1. Neurologic immaturity or impairment
2. Poor oral skills
3. Respiratory instability
4. Physiologic instability

B. Contraindications

Recent esophageal repair or perforation

C. Limitations

1. Size of nares
2. Type and amount of respiratory support
3. Congenital anomalies of the nasopharynx

D. Equipment

1. Suction equipment
2. Cardiac monitor
3. Infant tube of appropriate size
4. 0.5-inch hypoallergenic tape
5. Sterile water
6. 3- or 5-mL syringes
7. Stethoscope
8. Gloves

E. Precautions

1. When determining oral or nasal placement, individual assessment must be done to weigh the risks of compromising the nasal airway.
2. Measure and note appropriate length for insertion.
3. Have suction apparatus readily available in case there is regurgitation.
4. Do not push against any resistance. Perforation may occur with very little force or sensation of resistance.
5. Do not instill any material before verifying tube placement.
6. Evaluate for possible esophageal perforation if any of the following occur (8,13–15)
   a. Bloody aspirate
   b. Increased oral secretion
   c. Respiratory distress
   d. Pneumothorax
7. Stop the procedure immediately if there is any respiratory compromise.

F. Special Circumstances

1. Feeding with umbilical catheters in situ is controversial and should be done with caution, as there are insufficient data to guide practice (8,16).
2. Tubing should be vented between feedings if continuous positive airway pressure is in place (3).

G. Technique

1. Wash hands and put on gloves, maintaining aseptic technique.
2. Clear infant's nose and oropharynx by gentle suctioning as necessary.
3. Monitor infant's heart rate and observe for arrhythmia or respiratory distress throughout procedure.
4. Position infant on back with head of bed elevated.
5. Measure length for insertion by measuring distance from tip of the nose to ear to halfway between the xiphoid and umbilicus (3,17) (Table 40.1). Mark length on feeding tube with a loop of tape.
6. Moisten end of tube with sterile water or saline.
7. Oral insertion
   a. Depress anterior portion of tongue with forefinger and stabilize head with free fingers.
   b. Insert tube along finger to oropharynx.

TABLE 40.1	Guidelines for Minimum Orogastric Tube Insertion Length to Provide Adequate Intragastric Positioning in Very Low-Birthweight Infants

Weight (g)	Insertion Length (cm)
<750	13
750–999	15
1,000–1,249	16
1,250–1,500	17

Data from Gallaher KJ, Cashwell S, Hall V, et al. Orogastric tube insertion length in very low birth weight infants. *J Perinatol.* 1993;13:128.

8. Nasal insertion (avoid this route in very low-birthweight infants in whom nasal tubes may be associated with periodic breathing and apnea) (1,8).
    a. Stabilize head. Elevate tip of nose to widen nostril.
    b. Insert tip of tube, directing it toward occiput rather than toward vertex (Fig. 40.2).
    c. Advance tube gently to oropharynx.
    d. Monitor for bradycardia.
9. If possible, use pacifier to encourage sucking and swallowing.
10. Tilt head forward slightly.
11. Advance tube to predetermined depth.
    a. Do not push against any resistance.

b. Stop procedure if there is onset of any respiratory distress, cough, struggling, apnea, bradycardia, or cyanosis.
12. Determine location of tip using a combination of several measures. Radiograph of the abdomen to verify placement is the gold standard but is expensive and subjects neonates to additional radiation. Injecting air to verify placement is not a reliable method, as the sound of air in the respiratory tract can be transmitted to the GI tract (5,8,18,19). Measuring the pH of the aspirate as the sole method to verify tip position is not reliable, as stomach acid in infants can be weakly acidic, and the degree of acidity of the aspirate can be affected by the timing of feeding, the exact location in the stomach of the tube tip (distal versus proximal), and timing of medication delivery (18–22).
    a. Aspirate any contents; describe and measure.
        (1) Gastric contents may be clear, milky, tan, pale green, pale yellow, or blood stained.
        (2) Determine acidity by measuring pH. If the pH of the aspirate is <5, one can be reasonably certain the tube is in the stomach. If the pH is ≥5, placement should be confirmed using an additional method, such as radiography or character of secretions (4,18,20,23).
        (3) Assess for any respiratory compromise or instability.
    b. If there is difficulty obtaining aspirate, use a larger-sized syringe, reposition the infant, and instill a small

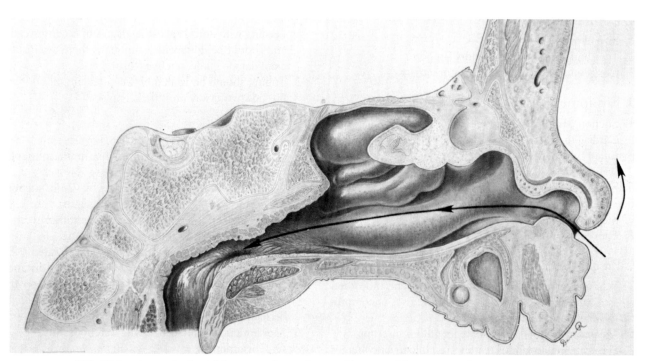

FIG. 40.2. Anatomic view of the neonatal nasopharynx. The natural direction in tube insertion is toward the nasal turbinates, where it might stop and give an impression of obstruction. By pushing the nostril up, one can direct a tube toward the occiput with less trauma.

amount of air into the tube to reposition the nasogastric tube away from the stomach wall. Avoid pushing against any resistance. If no aspirate is obtained, consider verifying placement by radiography (18).

   c. Suspect perforation or misplacement if no air or fluid is returned or if there is onset of respiratory distress, blood in the tube, or difficult insertion.

   d. Verify tube placement on all subsequent radiographs.

13. Secure indwelling tube to face with 0.5-inch tape.

   a. For feedings, attach to syringe.

   b. For gravity drainage, attach specimen trap and position below level of stomach.

   c. For decompression, a dual-lumen tube, connected to low intermittent or continuous suction, is preferred.

14. Pinch or close gastric tube during removal to prevent emptying contents into pharynx.

15. Document patient response, observing any physiologic changes and verifying tube placement. Note the location of the tube at the nares, and document it on the chart. Check this location before each use.

H. Complications

1. Apnea, bradycardia, or desaturation
2. Obstruction of obligatory nasal airway (15)
3. Irritation and necrosis of nasal mucosa (15)
   a. Epistaxis
   b. Ulceration
4. Misplacement on insertion (Fig. 40.3)
   a. Coiled in oropharynx
   b. Trachea leading to aspiration (5,15)
   c. Esophagus
   d. Duodenum
5. Displacement after insertion because of inappropriate length or fixation
   a. Pulling back or coiling into esophagus (24)
   b. Prolapsing into duodenum (5)
6. Coiling and clogging of tube
7. Perforation (Fig. 40.4)
   a. Posterior pharynx, particularly at level of cricopharynx
   b. Esophagus
     (1) Submucosal, remaining within mediastinum
     (2) Complete into thorax
     (3) Symptoms can mimic esophageal atresia or tracheoesophageal fistula (13)
     (4) Chylothorax or pneumothorax (25)
   c. Stomach
   d. Duodenum (26)
8. Grooved palate with long-term use of indwelling tube (8)
9. Increased gastroesophageal reflux
10. Infection (8)
11. Breakage of tube with retention of distal portion in stomach (27).

Transpyloric Feeding Tube

A. Indications

1. Severe gastroesophageal reflux with risk of aspiration
2. Suspected gastroesophageal reflux-associated apnea (28)
3. Gastric distention with continuous positive airway pressure
4. Delayed gastric emptying
5. Gastric motility disorders
6. Sampling of duodenojejunal contents
7. Intolerance to gastric feeds

B. Contraindications

Clinical condition that compromises duodenojejunal integrity: Necrotizing enterocolitis, fulminant sepsis, shock, patent ductus arteriosus, recent small-bowel surgery

C. Limitations

1. Long-term use may be associated with fat malabsorption, although recent studies suggest that there is no significant impact on growth over time (29).
2. There are no data to support routine use in preterm infants (2,29,30)

D. Equipment (see also Oral or Nasal Gastric Tubes, D.)

1. Silastic tube of appropriate size. Silastic tubes are preferred over PVC tubing, as they can remain in place for a longer duration; PVC tubes are not recommended for long-term use (8).
2. Continuous-infusion pump and connecting tubing

E. Precautions

1. When determining oral or nasal placement, individual assessment must be done to weigh the risks of compromising the nasal airway.
2. Avoid pushing against any obstruction or resistance.
3. Most often, if the tube does not cross the pylorus within the first 30 minutes after passage, it is unlikely to pass in the next few hours, and it may be better to restart the procedure.
4. Replace tubes per manufacturer's recommendations. If the tube is stiff on removal, replace next tube sooner.
5. If a tube has become partially dislodged, replace it rather than pushing it in farther.
6. When using feedings that tend to coagulate in tubing, it may be necessary to flush the tube periodically with air or water.
7. Use reliable infusion pumps that control rate and detect obstruction.
8. Limit infusion of hypertonic solutions and do not deliver bolus feedings beyond the pylorus.
9. Consider the effect of continuous feedings on medication absorption.

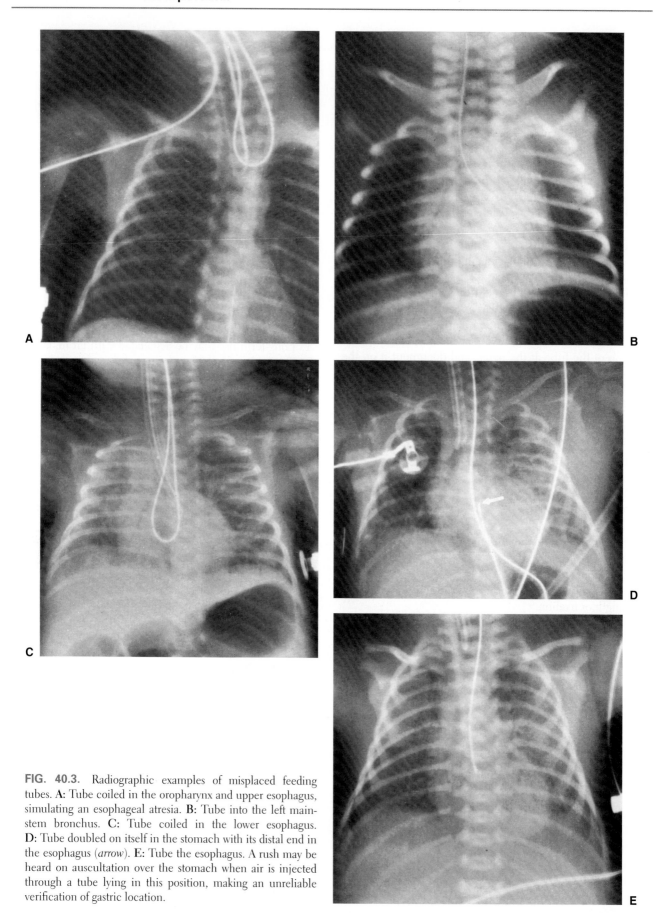

FIG. 40.3. Radiographic examples of misplaced feeding tubes. **A:** Tube coiled in the oropharynx and upper esophagus, simulating an esophageal atresia. **B:** Tube into the left mainstem bronchus. **C:** Tube coiled in the lower esophagus. **D:** Tube doubled on itself in the stomach with its distal end in the esophagus (*arrow*). **E:** Tube the esophagus. A rush may be heard on auscultation over the stomach when air is injected through a tube lying in this position, making an unreliable verification of gastric location.

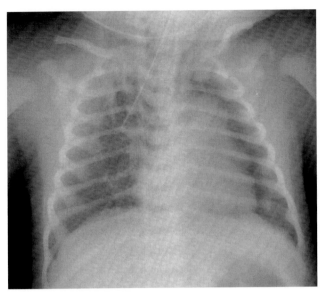

FIG. 40.4. Chest radiograph showing esophageal perforation by an orogastric tube.

F. Special Circumstances

1. See Oral or Nasal Gastric Tubes (F).

G. Technique

1. Follow steps 1 through 4 above under Oral or Nasal Gastric Tubes (G).

2. Measure distance from glabella to heels or from the tip of the nose to the ear to the xiphoid to the right lateral costal margin (19). Mark point with tape on transpyloric tube.

3. Turn patient onto right side and elevate the head of the bed 30 to 45 degrees.

4. Pass transpyloric tube to predetermined depth.

5. After approximately 10 minutes with infant remaining on right side, gently aspirate through transpyloric tube. Tube may be in position within duodenum if aspirate is
   a. Without air
   b. Bilious (gold or yellow in color)
   c. pH >6, although this method alone is not reliable (4,19)

6. Verify placement with radiograph. The tip of the tube should be just beyond the second portion of duodenum (4,19) (Fig. 40.5).

7. Avoid pushing to advance tube after initial placement. If tube is not in far enough, retape to give external slack and to allow peristalsis to carry tip to new position.

8. After verifying correct positioning, close transpyloric tube or start continuous infusion.

9. Document patient response, observing any physiologic changes and verifying tube placement. Note the location of the tube at the nares and document it on the chart. Check this location before each use.

10. Transpyloric tubes may also be placed with fluoroscopic guidance.

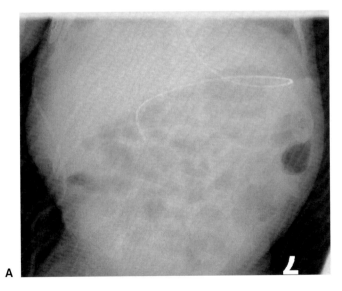

A

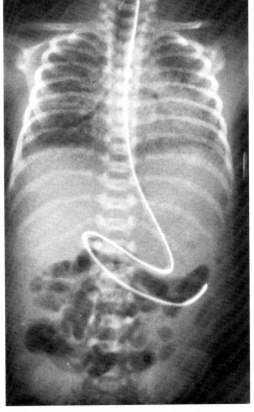

B

FIG. 40.5. **A:** Abdominal radiograph showing appropriate position of transpyloric tube. **B:** Radiographic demonstration of a transpyloric feeding tube that has passed the ligament of Treitz, well below the appropriate level, increasing the risk of perforation or nutritional dumping.

H. Complications (See also Oral or Nasal Gastric Tubes, H.)

1. The risk of aspiration with transpyloric feeding does not appear to be different from the risk with gastric feeding (29).
2. Kinking or knotting of tube
3. Hardening of PVC tube with leaching of bioavailable plasticizers (8)
4. Perforation of esophagus, stomach, duodenum (31)
5. Development of pyloric stenosis (32)
6. Possible interference with absorption of medications
7. Malabsorption and GI disturbance (29,31)
   a. Risk of fat malabsorption with nasojejunal feeds
   b. Dumping syndrome if hypertonic medications or feedings instilled too rapidly
   c. GI disturbance as characterized by abdominal distention, gastric bleeding, and bilious vomiting
8. Intussusception (33)

References

1. Birnbaum R, Limperopoulos C. Nonoral feeding practices for infants in the neonatal intensive care unit *Adv Neonatal Care.* 2009;9(4):180.
2. Hay W. Strategies for feeding the preterm infant. *Neonatology.* 2008;94:245.
3. deBoer J, Smit B. Nasogastric tube position and intragastric air collection in a neonatal intensive care population. *Adv Neonatal Care.* 2009;9(6):293.
4. Westhus N. Methods to test feeding tube placement in children. *MCN Am J Matern Child Nurs.* 2004;29:282.
5. Quandt D, Schraner T, Bucher H, et al. Malposition of feeding tubes in neonates: is it an issue? *J Pediatr Gastroenterol Nutr.* 2009;48:608.
6. Koong Shiao SP, Novotny DL. The features of different gastric tubes used in nurseries. *Neonatal Netw.* 1998;17(4):78.
7. Pedron Giner C, Martinez-Costa C, Navas-Lopez VM, et al. Consensus on Paediatric enteral nutrition access: a document approved by SENPE/SEGHNP/ANECIPN/SECP. *Nutr Hosp.* 2011;26(1):1.
8. Premji SS. Enteral feeding for high-risk neonates: a digest for nurses into putative risk and benefits to ensure safe and comfortable care. *J Perinat Neonat Nurs.* 2005;19:59.
9. Filippi L, Pezzati M, Poggi C. Use of polyvinyl feeding tubes and iatrogenic pharyngo-oesophageal perforation in very-low-birthweight infants. *Acta Paediatr.* 2005;94(12):1825.
10. Replogle RL. Esophageal atresia: plastic sump catheter for drainage of the proximal pouch. *Surgery.* 1963:54:296.
11. Petrosyan M, Estrada J, Hunter C, et al. Esophageal atresia/ tracheoesophageal fistula in very low birth weight neonates: improved outcomes with staged repair. *J Pediatr Surg.* 2009;44: 2278.
12. Berman L, Moss RL. Necrotizing enterocolitis: an update. *Semin Neonatal Med.* 2011;16:145.
13. Schuman T, Jacobs B, Walsh W, et al. Iatrogenic perinatal pharyngoesophageal injury: a disease of prematurity. *Int J Pediatr Otorhinolaryngol.* 2010;74:393.
14. Su B, Lin HY, Chiu H, et al. Esophageal perforation: a complication of nasogastric tube placement in premature infants. *J Pediatr.* 2009;154:460.
15. Metheny N, Meert K, Clouse R. Complications related to feeding tube placement. *Curr Opin Gastroenterol.* 2007;23:178.
16. Tiffany KF, Burke BL, Collins-Odoms C, et al. Current practice regarding the enteral feeding of high-risk newborns with umbilical catheters in situ. *Pediatrics.* 2003;112:20.
17. Cirgin Ellett ML, Cohen MD, Perkins SM, et al. Predicting the insertion length for gastric tube placement in neonates. *JOGNN.* 2011;40:412.
18. Farrington M, Lang S. Nasogastric tube placement verification in pediatric and neonatal patients. *Pediatr Nurs.* 2009;35:17.
19. Ellett MLC. Important facts about intestinal feeding tube placement. *Gastroenterol Nurs.* 2006;29:112.
20. Khilnani P. Errors in placement of enteral tubes in critically ill children: are we foolproof yet? *Pediatr Crit Care Med.* 2007;8(2): 193.
21. Lopez-Alonso M, Moya MJ, Cabo JA, et al. Twenty-four hour esophageal impedance-pH monitoring in healthy preterm neonates: rate and characteristics of acid, weakly acid, and weakly alkaline gastroesophageal reflux. *Pediatrics.* 2006;118(2):e299.
22. Omari TI, Davidson GP. Multipoint measurement of intragastric pH in healthy preterm infants. *Arch Dis Child Fetal Neonatal Ed.* 2003;88(6):F517.
23. Gilbertson HR, Rogers EJ, Ukoumunne OC. Determination of a practical pH cutoff level for reliable confirmation of nasogastric tube placement. *JPEN.* 2011;35(4):540.
24. Crisp CL. Esophageal nasogastric tube misplacement in an infant following laser supraglottoplasty. *J Ped Nurs.* 2006;21(6):454.
25. Kairamkonda VR. A rare cause of chylo-pneumothorax in a preterm neonate. *Indian J Med Sci.* 2007;61:476.
26. Agarwala S, Dave S, Gupta AK, et al. Duodeno-renal fistula due to a nasogastric tube in a neonate. *Pediatr Surg Int.* 1998;14:102.
27. Halbertsma FJ, Andriessen P. A persistent gastric feeding tube. *Acta Paediatrica.* 2010;99:162.
28. Misra S, Macwan K, Albert V. Transpyloric feeding in gastro-esophageal-reflux-associated apnea in premature infants. *Acta Paediatrica.* 2007;96:1426.
29. McGuire W, McEwan P. Transpyloric versus gastric tube feeding for preterm infants. *Cochrane Database Syst Rev.* 2007;(3):CD003487.
30. MacDonald PD, Skeoch CH, Carse H, et al. Randomized trial of continuous nasogastric, bolus nasogastric, and transpyloric feeding in infants of birth weight under 1400 g. *Arch Dis Child.* 1992; 67:429.
31. Flores JC, Lopez-Herce J, Sola I, et al. Duodenal perforation caused by a transpyloric tube in a critically ill infant. *Nutrition.* 2006;22:209.
32. Latchaw LA, Jacir NN, Harris BH. The development of pyloric stenosis during transpyloric feedings. *J Pediatr Surg.* 1989;24:823.
33. Hughes U, Connolly B. Small-bowel intussusceptions occurring around nasojejunal enteral tubes—three cases occurring in children. *Pediatr Radiol.* 2001;31:456.

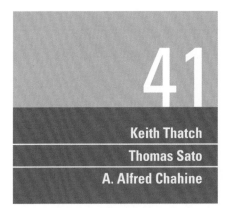

41

Keith Thatch

Thomas Sato

A. Alfred Chahine

Gastrostomy

First performed over 150 years ago, gastrostomy is one of the most commonly performed procedures by pediatric surgeons, in the neonatal and pediatric population (1,2). Although neonatologists do not usually perform gastrostomies, a range of procedures are described to support the principles of good gastrostomy care. Surgical advances, including endoscopy and laparoscopy, have expanded the applications of gastrostomy while making placement faster and safer (3–5).

A. Indications

1. Inability to swallow/dysphagia
   a. Neurologic impairment resulting in uncoordinated swallowing
   b. Complex congenital malformations (e.g., esophageal atresia or Pierre Robin sequence) not undergoing early correction.
2. Failure to thrive/need for supplemental feedings
   a. Anatomic intestinal anomalies (i.e., short gut syndrome)
   b. Functional intestinal dysmotility (i.e., gastrointestinal malabsorption)
   c. Malignancy/tumor
   d. Chronic pulmonary disease (i.e., persistent pulmonary hypertension)
   e. Congenital heart disease
   f. Glycogen storage disease (need for consistent glucose source)
3. Frequent aspiration
   a. Gastroesophageal reflux disease (GERD) leading to pulmonary disease
4. Nonpalatable diet or medications
   a. Renal failure diet
   b. HAART therapy for HIV
   c. Cholestyramine for Alagille syndrome
5. Gastric decompression
   a. Severe respiratory compromise necessitating long-term gastric decompression
   b. Esophageal atresia with distal tracheoesophageal fistula with acute decompensation requiring emergency gastric decompression.

B. Contraindications

1. Treatable medical conditions that increase operative risks (i.e., active infection or coagulopathy).
   Treat aggressively prior to elective gastrostomy placement.
2. Pure esophageal atresia
   Small stomach volumes (microgastria), making gastrostomy placement more difficult and potentially contraindicated secondary to possible need for gastric transposition to repair long-gap esophageal atresia.

C. Preoperative Workup

Prior to operative planning, it is important to make sure that the patient meets the proper anatomical and physiologic indications for gastrostomy. For example, identifying neonates in need of concomitant procedures such as antireflux surgeries requires more extensive preoperative workup.

1. Antireflux procedure workup (6–8)
   a. Upper gastrointestinal (UGI) study (primary study)
      Anatomic anomalies (e.g., malrotation, delayed gastric emptying) alter operative planning.
   b. 24-hour pH probe, especially in severely neurologically impaired neonates (9)
      (1) Gold standard in establishing GERD diagnosis.
      (2) DeMeester score—composite of
         (a) Frequency and duration of episodes of pH ≤4
         (b) Number of episodes lasting >5 minutes
         (c) Duration of longest episodes
         (d) Total percentage of time of GERD
      (3) DeMeester score >14.7 correlates with pathologic GERD and need for antireflux surgery.
   c. Gastric emptying study
      If emptying is delayed, the use of a gastrojejunostomy tube to allow for gastric drainage and jejunal feeds might be considered.
   d. Endoscopy (rarely utilized in neonatal population)

D. Stamm Gastrostomy (Open)

Neonatal gastrostomy placement often necessitates general anesthesia. Classically, the open, or Stamm, gastrostomy, described by Dr. Martin Stamm in 1894, was frequently used in premature infants and neonates (2). The Stamm technique, however, is now being used with less frequency secondary to its invasive approach. Current indications include altered gastric anatomy, multiple previous abdominal surgeries, concurrent laparotomy for other procedures, and unstable patients.

1. Sterile preparation of the skin, and delivery of IV antibiotics (first-generation cephalosporin) within the hour prior to the skin incision.
2. Transverse abdominal or supraumbilical midline incision (Fig. 41.1).
3. Identify the stomach and elevate the greater curvature of the stomach through the wound.
   Choose a dependent portion of the anterior wall of the stomach.
4. Place two concentric, seromuscular purse-string sutures on the greater curvature of the stomach (Fig. 41.2).
   a. The inner purse-string suture allows for hemostasis.
   b. The outer purse-string suture inverts the gastric mucosa while fixating the stomach to abdominal wall.
   c. Take care to avoid injury to the gastroepiploic vessels.
5. Make a stab incision through the stomach wall (gastrostomy) in the center of the purse-string absorbable sutures.
   a. With a stylet inside the catheter, gently direct the catheter through the gastrostomy.
   b. Verify position of the tube inside the stomach.
   c. Inflate the balloon if present.

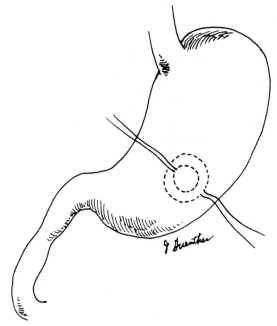

FIG. 41.2. Site for concentric sutures for Stamm procedure. Entrance into stomach is on greater curvature midway between esophagus and pylorus.

6. Tie sutures.
   a. The inner suture secures the stomach around the catheter while providing hemostasis.
   b. The outer suture allows for mucosal inversion and a watertight abdominal wall to stomach wall seal.
7. At a separate and previously identified exit site, make a stab wound through the abdominal wall.
8. Insert a curved hemostat through the abdominal wall exit site and into the intraperitoneal cavity.
9. Secure the stomach and abdominal wall to each other with three to four absorbable sutures in a seromuscular fashion.
10. With the hemostat, pull the gastrostomy tube through the abdominal wall stab wound until the stomach is snug against the abdominal wall.
11. Tie the previously placed inner and outer sutures while placing gentle traction on the gastrostomy tube.
12. Secure the gastrostomy tube to the skin with a suture to prevent inadvertent removal (Fig. 41.3).
    Document the length of the gastrostomy tube outside the abdomen.
13. Close the abdominal incision in standard surgical fashion.
14. Anatomically, this will allow the gastrostomy tube to lie in the center of a triangle formed by the left costal margin, umbilicus, and xiphoid (Fig. 41.1).
15. Tubes utilized in a Stamm gastrostomy include balloon- and mushroom-tip catheters, and/or low-profile buttons (e.g., Mic-Key buttons, Kimberly-Clark Worldwide, Inc., Neenah, Wisconsin).

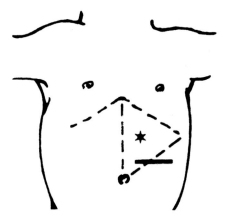

FIG. 41.1. Landmarks for gastrostomy. The primary horizontal incision is left supraumbilical. The gastrostomy tube will pass through the abdomen at a separate site in the center of a triangle formed by the xiphoid, umbilicus, and left costal margin.

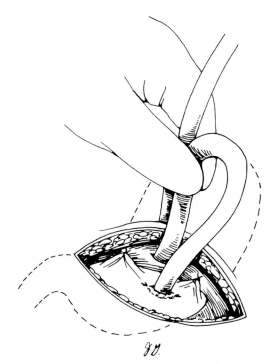

FIG. 41.3. After the tube is secured inside the stomach and passed through a stab wound in the abdominal wall, the anterior wall of the stomach is sutured to the inner wall of the abdomen.

E. Percutaneous Endoscopic Gastrostomy (PEG)

Developed in 1980 by Drs. Gauderer and Ponsky, percutaneous endoscopic gastrostomy (PEG) has become the primary method of gastrostomy in children (1,4,10). Infants and children require general anesthesia for PEG placement.

1. The gastrostomy site preparation and antibiotic prophylaxis are similar to the open technique.
   Standard PEG kits include a drape for the abdomen.
2. A flexible endoscope is inserted through the oropharynx and guided down to the stomach.
3. The stomach is insufflated to approximate the stomach to the abdominal wall.
4. An introducer needle is placed percutaneously into the insufflated stomach under direct endoscopic visualization.
   a. Transillumination of the stomach along the greater curvature through the abdominal wall with the endoscope can aid in introducer placement.
   b. Proper gastrostomy site is about 2 cm inferior to the left costal margin along the paramedian plane, which can also be palpated and visualized by the endoscope.
   c. A looped guidewire is inserted through the introducer into the stomach and the proximal end is captured with an endoscopic snare. The snared

guidewire is then pulled through the mouth with the endoscope, with the distal end remaining externally on the abdomen.
5. A gastrostomy tube is attached to the proximal end of the guidewire.
   Simultaneously, a small nick (~8 mm) is made with a scalpel at the site of the introducer to allow for the gastrostomy placement.
6. The guidewire is gently pulled back from the abdominal end, guiding the gastrostomy tube through the oropharynx, esophagus, and into the stomach.
7. The tapered end of the gastrostomy is pulled through the abdominal wall until the intragastric mushroom-type flange fits snugly up against the abdominal wall (1).
8. An external bolster/immobilizing ring is slid over the tube down to the abdominal wall to secure the gastrostomy in place.
9. The gastrostomy tube is cut to the desired external length and a feeding adaptor is placed on the end of the tube.

F. Laparoscopic Gastrostomy

Laparoscopic placement of gastrostomy tubes, one of the most popular methods, has been described as safe and efficacious (11). Some believe that the laparoscopic gastrostomy technique has a lower complication rate than the PEG technique in neonates and small children (12).

1. The gastrostomy site preparation and antibiotic prophylaxis are similar to the open technique.
   a. Mark the costal margin and proposed gastrostomy site.
   b. Oro- or nasogastric tube decompression of the stomach.
2. A 3- to 5-mm 30-degree laparoscope is inserted through an umbilical incision.
   The abdomen is insufflated to 8 to 10 torr with carbon dioxide.
3. A small subcostal incision is made at the aforementioned proposed site.
   A 5-mm trocar and then a laparoscopic grasper are inserted.
4. Under direct visualization, the stomach is grasped along the greater curvature and pulled toward the abdominal wall.
   The abdomen is desufflated, the trocar is removed, and the stomach is pulled through the abdominal wall.
5. A traction suture is placed and the stomach is secured to the abdominal fascia in four quadrants.
   Inner purse-string is placed.
6. A gastrostomy is created by stab incision or with cautery and a gastrostomy tube is inserted. The gastrostomy tube can either be a Pezzer-type tube, or more

frequently, a balloon retention tube (MIC-Key® or AMT® button gastrostomy tube).

The purse-string is tied down to secure the gastrostomy tube in place.

7. The abdomen is reinsufflated and the laparoscope is reinserted to confirm placement.

G. Laparoscopic Percutaneous Endoscopic Gastrostomy

Laparoscopic gastrostomy may be difficult to place in neonates or children with thick abdominal walls. Some surgeons recommend the use of laparoscopic PEG. Other indications for laparoscopic PEG include failed PEG attempts, altered anatomy secondary to previous operations, and when combined with another laparoscopic procedure (11,13). It is basically a hybrid of the laparoscopic and percutaneous techniques to prevent hollow viscus and solid organ injury and confirm accurate placement.

1. A laparoscope is inserted through a supra-umbilical incision and the abdomen is moderately insufflated to 8 to 10 torr.
2. A standard PEG procedure as previously described is completed under direct intra-abdominal visualization.
3. Additionally, in order to secure the stomach to the abdominal wall, 2 to 4 T fasteners may be placed percutaneously through the gastric wall with laparoscopic visualization.

H. Image-guided Percutaneous Gastrostomy

A recent advance in minimally invasive gastrostomy placement utilizes fluoroscopy to guide percutaneous gastrostomy placement. Interventional radiologists typically perform this technique (14,15).

1. Insufflation of the stomach with an oro- or nasogastric tube.
2. A needle is advanced into the distended stomach under fluoroscopic visualization.

Contrast injection confirms intragastric positioning.

3. T fasteners (2 to 4) are advanced into the stomach to secure it to the abdominal wall.
4. A second needle is then inserted in the center of the T fasteners and again is confirmed by contrast injection.
5. A wire is advanced through the second needle and the tract is dilated over the wire.
6. A balloon-type gastrostomy tube is inserted into the stomach over the wire and positioning is confirmed with contrast injection.
7. The T fasteners are tied externally over abdominal bolsters.

I. Emergent Percutaneous Gastric Decompression

The ability to decompress the stomach urgently is a life-saving measure that may be required in neonates who have severe respiratory compromise or a high probability of gastric rupture secondary to the presence of extreme gastric distention.

1. Primary indication
   a. Respiratory failure secondary to massive abdominal distention that cannot be decompressed by either an oro- or nasogastric tube. For example, premature neonates with esophageal atresia and a tracheo-esophageal fistula (prerepair) with massive gastric distention from preferential ventilation of the compliant stomach rather than the stiff premature lungs.
2. Procedure
   a. Prepare the abdomen with Betadine or chlorhexidine and then drape the skin in the upper left abdomen.
   b. If possible, utilize a light to transilluminate the abdomen to locate and verify the position of the distended stomach away from liver.
   c. Make a small skin weal with 1% lidocaine to provide local anesthesia.
   d. Using a 20- or 22-gauge catheter with needle stylet, puncture the abdominal wall at the junction of the left anterior rib cage and the lateral border of the rectus abdominus muscle.
   e. Advance the needle through the wall into the stomach.
   f. Remove the needle and advance the catheter into the stomach.
   g. Attach a short IV extension tubing, three-way stopcock, and syringe.
      (1) Aspirate only enough air to relieve tamponade effect and improve ventilation.
      (2) Avoid completely emptying stomach.
   h. Secure the catheter and keep in place until surgical evaluation is possible.
   i. Secure with tape or suture if necessary.

J. Postoperative and Maintenance Gastrostomy Care

Postoperative gastrostomy care begins immediately with meticulous attention to wound care to prevent infection and skin irritation. Initiation of feeds through the new gastrostomy tube may begin within 12 to 24 hours postplacement. Certain complications, however, such as a postoperative ileus, as seen in more complicated operations, may require further bowel rest prior to gastrostomy feeding.

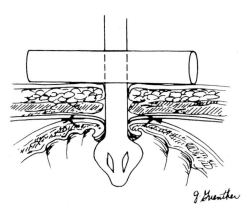

FIG. 41.4. Latex bridge at gastronomy exit stabilizes tube perpendicular to skin, keeping stoma narrow to avoid leakage. Rotating the bridge around the tube allows change in contact points with the skin. Note how the flared end of the mushroom catheter is pulled to keep the stomach apposed to the abdominal wall.

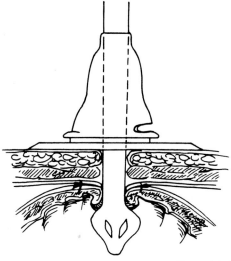

FIG. 41.5. Modified feeding nipple. The elliptical hole at the base allows air circulation and regular cleaning of the skin as important factors in avoiding maceration of the site. (From Kappell DA, Leape LL. A method of gastrostomy fixation. *J Pediatr Surg.* 1975;10:523, with permission.)

Tube feeds should be started slowly and advanced to the goal rate over the next few days.

1. Maintain fixation of gastrostomy between stomach and abdomen.
   a. Prevent gastric distention.
   b. Keep the gastrostomy balloon or flange pulled snugly against the stomach wall by maintaining the external bolster snug against the skin (take time to recognize and record the gastrostomy level mark at the skin) (Fig. 41.4).
   c. *Avoid pressure necrosis of the abdominal wall*: the external bolster should be snug enough to be gently twisted around but not too tight.
   d. Avoid inadvertent dislodgement of the gastrostomy (i.e., patient restraints, minimize tension on the gastrostomy tube by providing secondary fixation points on the skin or keeping the tube secure within the diaper). Nursing staff and parents should be informed of the type of gastrostomy tube inserted, how much fluid has been placed in the retention balloon, and anticipated time of first gastrostomy tube exchange.
2. Maintain gastrostomy immobility at the insertion site to minimize the formation of granulation tissue.
   a. Use careful fixation to maintain the perpendicular position.
      (1) This will decrease the amount of soft tissue stretching at the stoma site.
   b. Keep some slack in the tube when it is suspended.
      This prevents stoma tension and widening, thereby decreasing the risk of stoma leak.
3. Prevent migration of gastrostomy
   a. Proper fixation (Fig. 41.5)

If not fixed on the outside with a bolster or tape, the gastrostomy tube may migrate through the pylorus or up into the esophagus.
   b. Compare the length of external tube with the postoperative length (again checking and monitoring the level at the skin).
   c. Observe for signs of obstruction.
      (1) Gastric distention
      (2) Feeding intolerance, nausea/vomiting
      (3) Increased drainage from oral gastric or gastrostomy tube
      (4) Bilious drainage
      (5) New-onset or increased gastroesophageal reflux
4. Minimize leak rate from the gastrostomy site
   a. Maintain adequate fit of tube in stoma.
      Long-term gastrostomy tubes may need to be upsized if the stoma site increases in diameter.
   b. Avoid local infection—continue meticulous wound care.
      Daily cleansing with soap and water starting 48 hours after placement.
5. Close follow-up after placement to screen for and reduce risk of tube-related complications (see below).

K. Replacing Gastrostomy Tubes

Healing of gastrostomy sites requires 4 to 6 weeks for fibrosis to occur and create a well-epithelialized tract attaching the stomach to the anterior abdominal wall and. This process may take several months with PEG tubes, as there is generally no suture or fastener deployed to form a seal between the stomach and the abdominal wall. During the initial postoperative period (2 to 4 weeks postgastrostomy placement), loss of the tube can be treacherous in that the stomach can separate from the abdominal wall; therefore, the surgical team should always be notified. Loss of the tube can result spontaneous stoma closure if not reintroduced promptly.

1. Steps to reintroduce a gastrostomy tube
   a. Replace within 4 to 6 hours to avoid stoma closure.
   b. In the initial postoperative period prior to the formation of a well-epithelialized tract, replace with a balloon-type catheter (a button or a Foley-type catheter). For well-epithelialized tracts, mushroom catheter tubes or balloon-type gastrostomy tubes may be used for placement
   c. Lubricate the catheter generously with water-soluble lubricant, and insert gently.

      If resistance is felt and/or the catheter does not pass easily, stop and reassess.
      (a) Attempt passing a flexible guidewire through the tract.
      (b) A catheter is inserted over the wire or the stoma may be dilated by sequential dilators.
      (c) Fluoroscopy can confirm gastric position.
      (1) Inflate the balloon with 2 to 4 mL of water, then pull firmly against the stomach wall.
      (2) Secure with a fixation/external bolster device.
      (3) Mark outside length of catheter to help detect internal or external migration of the balloon.
      (4) Prior to feeding, confirm placement of gastrostomy with water-soluble contrast study if replacement is difficult or uncertain or if performed within 4 to 6 weeks of surgical placement.
2. Confirm intragastric position
   a. For recent gastrostomy (initial postoperative period)
      Instill 15 to 30 mL of water-soluble contrast through the gastrostomy under fluoroscopic guidance to confirm accurate positioning.
   b. For epithelialized gastrostomy tracts
      (1) Aspirate for gastric contents and observe for fluctuation of the gastric fluids in the tube with respiration. Fluids should flow back to stomach with gravity.
      (2) If there is any doubt, obtain contrast study prior to initiating feeding.

L. Discontinuation of Gastrostomy (16)

1. General principles
   a. Remove gastrostomy tube and apply gauze dressing.
      (1) Spontaneous closure usually occurs in 4 to 7 days.
      (2) May also approximate the skin edges with surgical tape.
2. Persistent gastrocutaneous fistula
   a. Granulation and epithelialization of gastrocutaneous tract (well-established tract).
      (1) Remove gastrostomy tube.
      (2) Cauterize the stoma granulation tissue and/or epithelium with silver nitrate.
      (3) Seal orifice with Stomahesive.
      (4) Approximate the edges with surgical tape.
   b. Persistent gastrocutaneous fistula (>4 to 6 weeks)
      (1) Requires surgical closure
      (2) If the skin is becoming macerated, replace the gastrostomy and use protective skin ointment prior to surgical closure.

M. Complications (1,15,17–19)

Gastrostomy placement can have serious complications. Early recognition of such complications allows for prompt intervention and prevention of devastating sequelae. The complications associated with neonatal gastrostomy placement may be characterized as intraoperative, early, or remote (late).

1. Intraoperative complications
   a. Pneumoperitoneum
      Some pneumoperitoneum is expected after the laparoscopic and open placement but is most common with PEG placement.
   b. Liver or splenic injury
   c. Colonic placement
   d. Hollow viscus injury
   e. Injury to posterior wall of stomach on initial insertion or upon reinsertion (gastrostomy replacement)
   f. Bleeding
2. Early complications (within the first 4 postoperative weeks)
   a. Most early complications are technical or mechanical in nature.
   b. *Presentation may be subtle*: recognition requires a high index of suspicion.
   c. Symptoms range from early feeding intolerance to worsening abdominal pain/peritonitis and signs of systemic infection.
   d. Common early complications
      (1) Wound infection, dehiscence
      (2) Prolonged ileus, gastric atony leading to feeding intolerance
      (3) Gastric separation from anterior abdominal wall
      (4) Intraperitoneal spillage/gastric leak leading to peritonitis
      (5) Early tube dislodgement
      (6) Early tube occlusion
      (7) Gastric outlet obstruction
3. Remote (late) complications
   a. Common remote complications
      (1) Dislodgement
         (a) Inadvertent removal
         (b) Internal or external gastrostomy migration (20)
      (2) Catheter deterioration
         (a) Tube erosion/fracture
         (b) Balloon rupture

(3) Tube occlusion

(4) Granulation tissue formation

(5) Persistent leak

  (a) Wound breakdown

    i. Granulation tissue and skin irritation

    ii. Infection

    iii. Enlargement of tract leading to loose gastrostomy with leakage

    iv. Skin ulceration

  (b) Electrolyte imbalance

  (c) Malnutrition

(6) New-onset or worsening GERD (21).

(7) Persistent gastrocutaneous fistula (post removal)

(8) Prolapse of gastric mucosa

  (a) Bleeding

  (b) Excessive leakage.

(9) Gastric torsion around catheter

  b. Prevention

  (1) Requires meticulous hygiene and appropriate perpendicular positioning to avoid trauma to the skin and subcutaneous tissues

  (2) Parental education is essential to long-term care and prevention of complications.

4. Treatment of Common Complications

  a. Gastrostomy leak—treat early

  (1) Remove tube for up to 24 hours to allow partial tract closure.

  (2) Replace mushroom catheter with a balloon-type catheter.

    Secure tube by pulling the balloon (inflated with 2 to 5 mL of water) against the abdominal wall.

  (3) Apply Stomahesive around catheter.

    (a) Decrease excoriation.

    (b) Encourage epithelialization.

    (c) Change Stomahesive every 3 to 4 days to maintain seal.

  (4) Maintain perpendicular positioning of gastrostomy tube.

  (5) Do not clamp the gastrostomy tube.

  (6) Maintain skin and stoma hygiene

5. Cleanse daily with soap and water.

  Consider half-strength hydrogen peroxide for areas of fibrinous exudate.

6. Frequent dressing changes to maintain a dry site.

  a. Granulation tissue at gastrostomy site

  (1) Silver nitrate

    (a) Apply daily for up to 3 to 5 days.

    (b) Avoid spilling the liquefied silver nitrate onto normal adjacent skin since this will cause a chemical burn.

  (2) 0.5% Triamcinolone ointment

    Apply three times a day for 5 to 7 days.

(3) Cautery

  May require local or general anesthesia.

References

1. Gauderer MW, Stellato TA. Gastrostomies: evolution, techniques, indications, and complications. *Curr Probl Surg.* 1986;23:657.
2. Stamm M. Gastrostomy by a new method. *Med News (NY).* 1894;65:324.
3. Jones VS, La Heir ER, Shun A. Laparoscopic gastrostomy: the preferred method of gastrostomy in children. *Pediatr Surg Int.* 2007;23:1085.
4. Gauderer MW. Percutaneous endoscopic gastrostomy-20 years later: a historical perspective. *J Pediatr Surg.* 2001;36:217.
5. Charlesworth P, Hallows M, Van der Avoirt A. Single-center experience of laparoscopically assisted percutaneous endoscopic gastrostomy placement. *J Laparoendosc Adv Surg Tech A.* 2010; 20:73.
6. Valusek PA, St. Peter SD, Keckler SJ, et al. Does an upper gastrointestinal study change operative management for gastroesophageal reflux? *J Pediatr Surg.* 2010;45:1169.
7. Wheatley MJ, Wesley JR, Tkach DM, et al. Long-term follow-up of brain-damaged children requiring feeding gastrostomy: should an anti-reflux procedure always be performed? *J Pediatr Surg.* 1991;26:301.
8. Cuenca AG, Reddy SV, Dickie B, et al. The usefulness of the upper gastrointestinal series in the pediatric patient before anti-reflux procedure or gastrostomy tube placement. *J Surg Res.* 2011; 170:247.
9. Soares RV, Forsythe A, Hogarth K, et al. Interstitial lung disease and gastroesophageal reflux disease: key role of esophageal function tests in the diagnosis and treatment. *Arq Gastroenterol.* 2001;48:91.
10. Gauderer MW, Ponsky JL, Izant Jr. RJ. Gastrostomy without laparotomy: a percutaneous endoscopic technique. *J Pediatr Surg.* 1980;15:872.
11. Zamakhshary M, Jamal M, Blair GK, et al. Laparoscopic vs. percutaneous endoscopic gastrostomy tube insertion: a new pediatric gold standard?. *J Pediatr Surg.* 2005;40:859.
12. Akay B, Capizzani TR, Lee AM, et al. Gastrostomy tube placement in infants and children: is there a preferred technique? *J Pediatr Surg.* 2010;45:1147.
13. Lantz M, Larsson MH, Arnbjornsson E. Literature review comparing laparoscopic and percutaneous endoscopic gastrostomies in a pediatric population. *Int J Pediatr.* 2010;507:616.
14. Nah SA, Narayanaswamy B, Eaton S, et al. Gastrostomy insertion in children: percutaneous endoscopic vs. percutaneous image-guided?. *J Pediatr Surg.* 2010;45:1153.
15. Fortunato JE, Cuffari C. Outcomes of percutaneous endoscopic gastrostomy in children. *Curr Gastroenterol Rep.* 2011;13:293.
16. Ducharme JC, Youseff S, Tilkin R. Gastrostomy closure: a quick, easy and safe method. *J Pediatr Surg.* 1977;12:729.
17. Gallagher MW, Tyson KRT, Ashcraft KW. Gastrostomy in pediatric patients: an analysis of complications and techniques. *Surg.* 1973;536:74.
18. Gauderer MW. Percutaneous endoscopic gastrostomy: a 10-year experience with 220 children. *J Pediatr Surg.* 1991;26:288.
19. Gordon JM, Langer JC. Gastrocutaneous fistula in children after removal of gastrostomy tube: incidence and predictive factors. *J Pediatr Surg.* 1999;34:1345.
20. Curriano G, Votteler T. Prolapse of the gastrostomy catheter in children. *AJR Radium Ther Nucl Med.* 1975;123:737.
21. Jolley SG, Tunnel WB, Hoelzer DJ, et al. Lower esophageal pressure changes with tube gastrostomy: a causative factor of gastroesophageal reflux in children?. *J Pediatr Surg.* 1986;21:624.

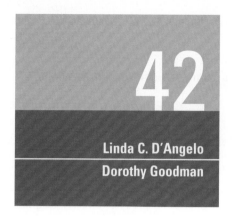

42

Linda C. D'Angelo
Dorothy Goodman

Neonatal Ostomy and Gastrostomy Care

An ostomy is the construction of a permanent or temporary opening in the intestine (enterostomy) or urinary tract (urostomy) through the abdominal wall to provide fecal or urinary diversion, decompression, or evacuation (1). Gastrostomies (G tubes) are stomas that allow direct access into the stomach and are used for feeding, medication administration, and decompression. This chapter discusses care of simple and complex ileostomies, colostomies, urostomies, and gastrostomies (see also Chapter 41). Tracheostomy care is discussed in Chapter 37.

Enterostomies and Urostomies

A. Indications

Ostomies may be indicated in the neonate for a variety of congenital or acquired conditions (Table 40.1). The stoma is usually temporary, and reanastomosis of the bowel or urinary tract with closure of the stoma is performed during infancy or early childhood (2, 3).

B. Types of Ostomies

1. There are several types of intestinal stoma. The patient's condition, the segment of bowel affected, and the size of the patient's abdomen often determine the type of stoma and its external location. Figure 42.1 depicts the most common types of neonatal stoma (1).
2. Urostomies are urinary diversions constructed to bypass a dysfunctional portion of the urinary tract. Ileal conduits and ureterostomies are rarely performed in the neonatal period.
3. A vesicostomy is an opening directly from the bladder through the abdominal wall and is a more common urinary diversion in the neonate. Urine flows freely through the stoma from the bladder.

C. Ostomy Assessment

The neonate with a stoma needs careful observation and assessment for a variety of potential complications (4). Monitoring the infant for function of the ostomy is vital in

the initial postoperative period. Possible surgical complications are paralytic ileus, intestinal obstruction, anastomotic leak, and stomal necrosis. The factors to be considered during evaluation of the stoma are listed below.

1. *Type of stoma:* The segment of bowel from which the stoma is made.
2. *Viability:* A healthy stoma should be bright pink to beefy red and moist, indicating adequate perfusion and hydration (Fig. 42.2). The stoma is formed from the intestine, which is very vascular and therefore may bleed slightly when touched or manipulated, but the bleeding usually resolves quickly. The stoma is not sensitive to touch because it does not have somatic afferent nerve endings (4).
   a. A purple or dark brown to black stoma with loss of tissue turgor and dryness of the mucous membrane may indicate ischemia and possible stomal necrosis.
   b. A pale pink stoma is indicative of anemia.
3. *Size:* The stoma shape (round, oval, mushroom, or irregular) and diameter (length and width) in inches or millimeters is noted. In the early postoperative period, the stoma will be edematous. After the first 48 to 72 hours, the edema should resolve and result in a reduction in size of the stoma, which should, however, still remain everted from the skin surface. Stomas generally continue to decrease in size over 6 to 8 weeks postoperatively. It is not uncommon for the stoma to become edematous when exposed to air while changing the pouch; this edema generally resolves quickly when the pouch is replaced.
4. *Stomal height:* The degree of protrusion of stoma from the skin. Ideally, the surgeon will evert the stoma prior to suturing it to the skin to produce an elevation, which will promote a better seal with the ostomy wafer. With the stoma elevated above the surface of the skin, the effluent will be more likely to go into the pouch instead of staying in contact with the skin (2). Eversion of the stoma, referred to as maturing the stoma, is not always possible in neonates, in whom blood supply may be

TABLE 42.1	Conditions Necessitating Ostomy in the Neonate

Disease/Congenital Anomaly	Most Common Location of Stoma
Intestinal atresia	Duodenum, ileum, or jejunum
Meconium ileus	Ileum
Necrotizing enterocolitis	Ileum or jejunum
Hirschsprung disease	Sigmoid colon
Imperforate anus/anorectal malformations	Colon
Volvulus	Ileum or jejunum
Bladder exstrophy	Bladder

tenuous, and in situations in which the bowel is markedly edematous (1,5).

5. *Stomal construction:* The ostomy may be an end, loop, or double barrel (Figs. 42.1 and 42.3).

6. **Abdominal location**

7. *Peristomal skin:* Ideally the peristomal skin should be intact, nonerythematous, and free from rashes. However, frequently the stoma(s) is not separate from the surgical incision (Fig. 42.4). There is often not enough space on the baby's abdomen for the surgeon to create separate incisions. In addition, stomas are often in close proximity to the umbilicus, ribs, or groin, which may interfere with pouch selection and adherence (6).

8. **Stomal complications**
   a. *Bleeding*
      (1) Hemorrhage during the immediate postoperative period is caused by inadequate hemostasis (4).
      (2) Trauma to stoma caused by improper fitting pouch. A wafer cut too close to the stoma can injure the delicate tissue. Stomal lacerations can occur as a result of the edge of the wafer rubbing back and forth against the side of the stoma (4).
   b. *Necrosis:* Caused by ischemia and may be superficial or deep. Necrosis extending below the facial level may lead to perforation and peritonitis, requiring additional surgical intervention (4).
   c. *Mucocutaneous separation:* This condition is caused by a breakdown of the suture line securing the stoma to the surrounding skin, leaving an open wound next to the stoma.
   d. *Prolapse:* Telescoping of the bowel out through the stoma. In infants, this condition is frequently related to poorly developed fascial support or excessive intra-abdominal pressure caused by crying.
   e. *Retraction:* The stoma is flush or recessed below the skin surface. This condition may result from insufficient mobilization of the mesentery or excessive tension on the suture line at the fascial layer, excessive

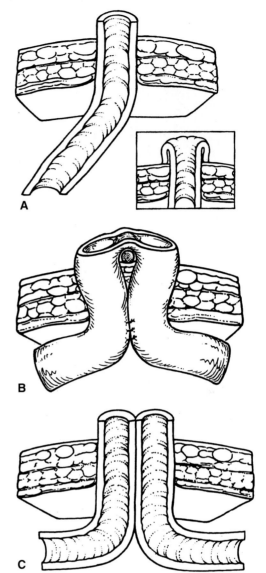

FIG. 42.1.   A: End stoma. The end of the bowel is everted at the skin surface. **B:** Loop stoma. Entire loop of bowel is brought to the skin surface and opened to create a proximal, or functioning, end and a distal, or nonfunctioning, end. The distal side is called a mucus fistula because of the normal mucus secretions it produces. **C:** Double-barrel stoma. Similar to a loop stoma, except the bowel is divided into two stomas, a proximal and a distal stoma. The distal stoma functions as a mucus fistula. (Adapted from Gauderer MWL. Stomas of the small and large intestine. In: O'Neil JA, Rowe MI, Grosfeld JL, et al., eds. *Pediatric Surgery.* 5th ed. St. Louis: Mosby; 1998:1349, with permission.)

scar formation, or premature removal of a support device (4).
   f. *Stenosis:* The lumen of the ostomy narrows at either the cutaneous level or the fascial level. Sudden decrease in output may indicate stenosis.

9. **Peristomal complications**
   a. *Dermatitis*
      (1) Allergic dermatitis

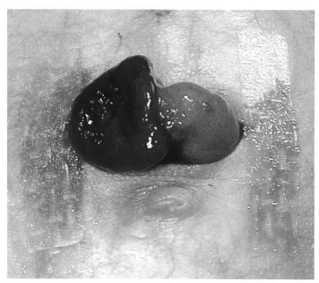

FIG. 42.2. Immediately postoperative loop ileostomy. Segment of bowel on left is the exteriorized perforation from necrotizing enterocolitis.

  (2) *Contact dermatitis:* Most common type of peristomal skin complication seen, generally from the leakage of fecal effluent on the skin.
 b. *Infection*
  (1) Bacterial
  (2) Candidal
 c. *Mechanical trauma:* Epidermal stripping, abrasive cleansing techniques, or friction due to ill-fitting equipment are the most common causes of mechanical injury to the perist-omal skin.
 d. *Hernia:* A peristomal hernia appears as a bulge around the stoma that occurs when loops of the bowel protrude through a facial defect around the stoma into the subcutaneous tissue (4).

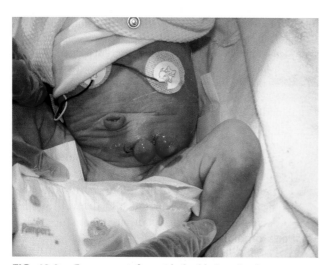

FIG. 42.3. Premature infant with double-barrel colostomy.

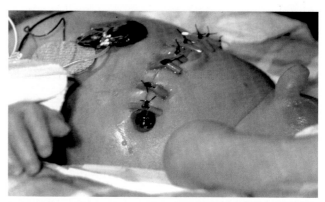

FIG. 42.4. End ileostomy and wound closure with retention sutures posing a challenge for placing a pouch.

D. Ostomy Care

1. **Immediate postoperative care**
 a. Assess stoma for adequate perfusion.
 b. Until there is output from the stoma, it is not necessary to apply an ostomy pouch
  Keep stoma protected and moist with petrolatum gauze. When an enterostomy begins to produce, it is preferable to pouch. The pouch will protect the stoma, the peristomal skin, the suture line, and any central lines in that area. Pouching allows for qualifying and quantifying output. Before applying pouch, make sure to gently remove any residue of petrolatum gauze, which will interfere with the pouch adhesion.
 c. Cover the mucus fistula with a moisture-retentive dressing to keep it from drying out. When securing a dressing on a neonate, use low-tack adhesives. There is increased risk of skin tears in neonates, especially when they are premature with delayed epidermal barrier development. Avoid placing petrolatum gauze over the pouching surface for the stoma, as it can impede adherence.

2. **Subsequent care**
 a. Regular assessment of the stoma
 b. Protect peristomal skin from the effects of the effluent by pouching (Fig. 42.5). The effluent from a small bowel stoma contains proteolytic enzymes that can rapidly cause skin erosion. Ideally the pouch should remain in place for at least 24 hours. In some low-birthweight neonates, the pouch may only last 12 hours. The average wear time is 1 to 3 days.
 c. The pouch *must* be changed if there is any evidence of leaking effluent under the skin barrier wafer. Frequent pouch changes, however, can result in denuded skin, especially in the premature infant (2,4,7). In situations with frequent leaking and pouch changes, expert help (certified wound ostomy continence nurse) may be required to preserve the

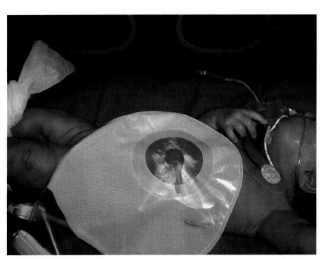

FIG. 42.5. One-piece ostomy appliance on small newborn dwarfs this infant but provides longer wear time and holds larger volume of output than the preemie pouches previously used.

skin and obtain acceptable wear time. In the rare instance when a pouch cannot be maintained, it may be necessary to leave the pouch off and protect the peristomal skin with a protective barrier oint-

ment that will adhere to denuded skin to allow the skin to heal. The barrier ointment can be covered with petrolatum-impregnated gauze; fluff gauze can then be placed on top to absorb the effluent and changed as needed. In some cases of severe skin damage, some neonatal centers stop enteral feedings briefly to limit stool production and allow the skin to heal (2). The more damaged the skin, the more difficult it is to maintain a seal. It is best to heal the skin, get a good seal, and then resume the feeding.

   d. Protect stoma from trauma. Measures include accurate sizing of the pouch opening to clear the stoma as the size changes. If the infant's movements cause the inner edge of the barrier to rub against the stoma, a moldable barrier between the stoma and the wafer can be used to protect the stoma.

E. Equipment

A variety of pouches and ostomy care supplies are available (Tables 42.2). One-piece pouches come with a barrier and pouch attached as a single unit. Two-piece appliances have a barrier and pouch separate, with a mechanism for attaching the pouch to the wafer. The type of pouch used for a

TABLE 42.2	Ostomy Accessory Products
Product	**Indications and Precautions**
Barrier powder	This product is used to dry moist and/or weepy skin. It can add extra adhesiveness to the skin. It must be sealed by padding with a moistened finger and allowed to dry. In cases of severely moist weeping skin, it may be necessary to apply powder and seal two or three times to attain a dry peristomal skin surface. It adds an additional barrier over the skin to protect from drainage. Apply in limited amounts and wipe off excess. Protect infant from inhalation of aerosolized powder by using minimal amounts and wiping away gently; do not blow powder away.
Paste	Barrier product that is semiliquid because of addition of alcohol. Best if applied to barrier and allowed to air for 1 to 2 minutes to allow the alcohol to evaporate (Fig. 42.6). Not recommended for use on premature infants or term infants <2 weeks old.
Skin sealants	Sealants use plasticizing agents to form a barrier on the skin that can protect from effluent and also improve adherence of some adhesives. Most skin sealants contain alcohol and are, therefore, contraindicated for use in preemies or term neonates <2 weeks old. One skin sealant that does not contain alcohol is Cavilon No Sting Barrier Film (3M, St. Paul, Minnesota).
Moldable barrier	Barriers that are adhesive and can be shaped to fill in uneven spaces; generally hold up very well to corrosive effluent. Common types are Eakins Seals (ConvaTec, Princeton, New Jersey), Barrier No. 54 (Nu-Hope Laboratories, Pacoima, California), and Adapt Rings (Hollister, Libertyville, Illinois)
Caulking strips	Similar to moldable barriers but come in narrow strips; they can be used to provide an extra barrier between the edge of the stoma and the barrier. May come in contact with stoma; soft enough that it does not injure the mucosa. Examples are Ostomy Strip Paste (Coloplast, Marietta, Georgia), Skin Barrier Caulking Strips (Nu-Hope Laboratories, Pacoima, California), and Adapt Strips (Hollister, Libertyville, Illinois)
Belt	Elastic belt with tabs that fit to ostomy pouch of some two-piece appliances. Belt can help maintain the appliance in place by holding it firmly to abdomen. Generally used as a last resort when unable to obtain acceptable wear time.

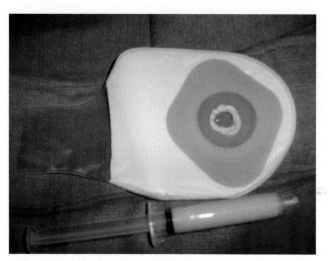

FIG. 42.6.   Barrier paste applied to wafer.

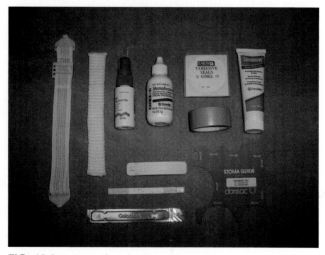

FIG. 42.8.   Examples of ostomy accessories.

neonate is generally either an open-end pouch that allows the passage of thick or formed effluent or a urostomy pouch with a spout designed for drainage of urine or liquid effluent. The type of pouch and the need for accessory products varies depending on the size of the child, the condition of the peristomal skin, abdominal size and contours, and institutional preference. In general, it is best to keep the procedure simple and to use as few products as possible (2). Special consideration needs to be given to the premature infant whose skin is immature and fragile. Several companies manufacture pouches for neonates and premature infants (Fig. 42.7). Neonatal units should have several varieties to choose from in order to meet each patient's individual needs.

Supplies

1. Clean gloves
2. Warm sterile water or normal saline
3. Clean, soft cloth

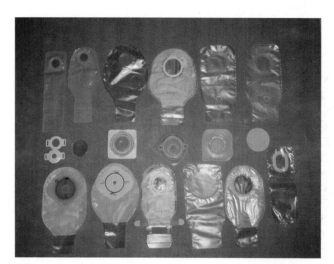

FIG. 42.7.   Examples of appliances for pouching a neonate.

4. 2 × 2-inch gauze
5. Appropriate-size pouch with closure device
6. Protective skin barrier and pouch
7. Other ostomy accessories as appropriate (Table 42.2 and Fig. 42.8).
8. Scissors or seam ripper
9. Stoma-measuring device

F. Applying the Pouch: Routine/Simple Ostomies (2,6,8)

1. Remove old pouch by gently lifting up the edges and using water to loosen while pressing down gently on the skin close to the edge to reduce traction on the epidermis. Adhesive remover should not be used on a neonate <2 weeks of age. Limited use of adhesive remover, followed by thorough cleansing of the area to remove any chemical residue, is recommended only when the adhesive bond of the barrier to the skin is so strong that the skin might be injured during removal (2).
2. Use damp soft gauze or paper washcloth to gently cleanse the stoma to remove adherent stool or mucus. It is common to have a little bleeding of the stoma when it is cleansed.
3. Wash peristomal skin with water; pat dry. Soap is not recommended because it may leave a chemical residue that could cause dermatitis; furthermore, many soaps contain moisturizers that can adversely affect the adherence of the barrier to the skin. It is also not advisable to use commercial infant wipes, because most are lanolin-based and contain alcohol (2).
4. Measure stoma(s) using stoma measuring device (Fig. 42.9). The opening generally is cut 2 to 3 mm larger than the stoma, to limit the skin exposed to effluent. In tiny infants, in whom the mucus fistula may be immediately adjacent to the functional stoma, one pouch may be sized to fit over both the stoma and the mucus

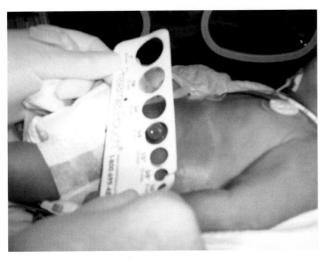

FIG. 42.9. Measuring the stoma.

fistula. Further discussion about pouching mucous fistula below in F8.

5. Trace hole size onto wafer. Cut hole(s) using small scissors or a seam ripper (Fig. 42.10). After cutting and before removing the paper backing, check the fit around the stoma and trim more if needed. Run a finger along the inside of the opening to make sure there are no sharp edges; these can be cut or smoothed by rubbing with the finger. It may be necessary to trim the wafer to avoid umbilicus, groin, and so on. Cutting small slits along the edges of the wafer may help the barrier conform to the contour of the stomach.

6. Warm wafer in hands to promote flexibility and enhance bonding to the skin. Avoid using a radiant heater to heat the wafer because the amount of heat absorbed cannot be controlled and may burn immature skin (2).

7. Press wafer to skin and hold for 1 to 2 minutes. Secure the edges of the wafer down to the skin to improve wear time. Avoid the use of high-tack adhesives. Pink

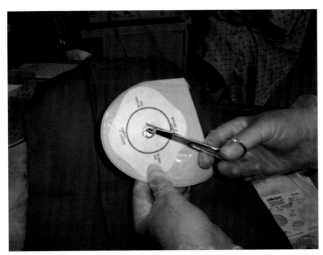

FIG. 42.10. Cutting a hole in the wafer.

tape is a waterproof tape that contains zinc oxide; it is very gentle and generally can be used safely. Other low-tack alternatives are silicon tape or clear film dressing.

8. Change dressing to mucus fistula using a folded 2- × 2-inch gauze piece and low-tack adhesive or secure with diaper or tubular elastic dressing. If the drainage from the mucus fistula is more than can be contained in the gauze and is interfering with the pouch adhering or the drainage may potentially contaminate wounds or central line sites, then the mucus fistula can be pouched. It is always preferable to pouch the mucus fistula separately from the active stoma to keep the stool from contaminating the bowel anastomosis or draining into the vagina or bladder in the case of a patient with high imperforate anus defect with fistula. It is advisable to discuss with the surgeon before placing both stomas in one pouch.

G. Emptying the Pouch

1. Supplies
   a. Clean gloves
   b. Diaper or syringe for withdrawing stool/effluent
   c. 30- to 60-mL syringe for irrigating/washing the bag
   d. Tap water

2. The pouch should be emptied when it is one-third to one-half full. Gas must also be released or vented to prevent pulling the adhesive wafer away from skin. Neonates generally produce large amounts of gas, related to increased intake with sucking and crying (2). Effluent can be drained directly into a diaper or withdrawn from the bag with a syringe. Use of two or three cotton balls placed in an open-end pouch can improve wear time by wicking the effluent away from the barrier and also may facilitate easy drainage of the pouch. It is generally not necessary to wash the pouch, but it may be necessary to add fluid to help loosen up thick or pasty stool. For the hospitalized neonate, measurement of ostomy output is usually indicated.

3. Close the pouch with an integrated closure device or rubber band.

H. Complicated Stomas and Peristomal Skin Problems (5,9)

Table 42.3 lists complications and interventions for treating complex stomas and common stoma problems. Note that many of items used are not generally recommended for use on premature neonates or neonates <2 weeks of age, but in situations of deterioration of the peristomal skin, they are sometimes used cautiously to prevent further deterioration and maintain an effective seal.

I. Vesicostomy Care

A vesicostomy does not require pouching; urine drains directly into the diaper. Care is similar to general perineal

TABLE 42.3	Complications and Complex Ostomies

Complication	Interventions
Multiple stomas	Customize pouch to fit around or accommodate stomas in bag; mucous fistulas may be in or out of pouch.
Open incision or wound	Two-piece pouches without starter hole may allow for easier customization. Keep wound as clean as possible. Use hydrocolloid wound dressing (e.g., DuoDERM, ConvaTec, Skillman, New Jersey; Replicare, Smith and Nephew, London, UK; Memphis, TN) or calcium alginate in wound bed covered with a piece of clear film dressing to protect wound from stool. Paste and powders may also be used to protect peristomal skin. In some cases it may not be possible to apply a pouch; however, the skin must be protected from caustic effluent, using a barrier such as Sensi-Care Protective Barrier (ConvaTec, Skillman, New Jersey), or Calmoseptine Ointment (Calmoseptine Inc., Huntington Beach, California).
Flush/retracted stoma	Apply paste or moldable barrier around hole in wafer. Use convex insert/convex pouch and belt to push skin back and allow stoma to protrude.
Prolapsed stoma	Notify surgeon if evidence of circulatory compromise. Protect the stoma from injury. When using two-piece pouch with plastic flange, the stoma could be pinched in the flange that secures the pouch to the wafer when closed. Adjust size of hole accordingly; cover exposed skin with moldable barrier or paste.
Peristomal hernia	Use a flexible wafer and pouching system to adjust to contour of the skin.
Mushroom-shaped stoma	Modify opening to accommodate size of "crown"; protect skin around base with moldable barrier or paste.
Irritant dermatitis	Ensure that hole is cut to fit properly. Use paste/moldable barrier to protect from leakage. Apply powder to open, weepy skin. Assess for sensitivity to products. Apply topical steroids if needed to decrease inflammation, pain, and itching.
Peristomal *Candida albicans*	Appears as red, shiny, macular, papular rash that is pruritic. Apply topical antifungal powder (e.g., nystatin) to skin. The powder should be mixed with a small amount of water, painted smoothly on the skin with a cotton swab, and allowed to dry before placing the appliance. Continue to use with each pouch change until rash resolves. Dry skin completely when changing pouch. Resize pouch so that no skin is exposed.
Dehydration, metabolic acidosis, electrolyte imbalance	Monitor intake and output carefully, especially for infants with ileostomy and/or high output. Assess lab values regularly. Infants can develop electrolyte imbalance rapidly.

Data from Borokowski S. Pediatric stomas, tubes, and appliances. *Pediatr Clin North Am.* 1998;45:1419; Craven DP, Fowler JS, Foster ME. Management of a neonate with necrotizing enterocolitis and eight prolapsed stomas in a dehisced wound. *J Wound Ostomy Continence Nurs.* 1999;26:214; Garvin G. Caring for children with ostomies and wounds. In: Wise B, McKenna C, Garvin G, et al., eds. *Nursing Care of the General Pediatric Surgical Patient.* Gaithersburg, MD: Aspen; 2000:261; Metcalfe P, Schwarz R. Bladder exstrophy: neonatal care and surgical approaches. *Wound Ostomy Continence Nurs.* 2004;31:284; Wound Ostomy and Continence Nurses Society. *Pediatric Ostomy Care: Best Practice for Clinicians.* Mount Laurel, NJ: Wound Ostomy and Continence Nurses Society, 2011.

care of normal newborns (4). Occasionally, skin breakdown does occur; it can be treated with moisture barrier products and frequent diaper changes.

Gastrostomy Tubes

A. Indications

For indications and insertion technique, see Chapter 41.

B. Types of Tubes

See Table 42.4.

C. Gastrostomy Care

1. Assessment
   a. The health care provider must know if the patient has undergone a Nissen fundoplication or other antireflux procedure together with the gastrostomy.
   b. Tolerance to feedings
   c. Type and size of tube
   d. Insertion site
   e. Condition of the peristomal skin
2. Special considerations for patients with Nissen or other antireflux procedure
   a. Patient cannot vomit or burp.
   b. Vent tube after crying and at first sign of gagging, discomfort, or distress.
3. Gastrostomy tube site and routine skin care (6,10)
   a. Clean gastrostomy tube site two to three times per day in the postoperative period and once per day after the site has healed. Use normal saline and sterile cotton swabs in the early postoperative period. Use mild soap and water after the site has healed.

Diluted hydrogen peroxide (50% hydrogen peroxide and 50% water) is not recommended unless the site has dry, crusted blood (9).
   b. Ensure that the antimigration device is flush against skin and the gastrostomy tube has not migrated.
   c. Position tube at 90-degree angle.
   d. A bottle nipple placed over the tube with the flanges resting on the abdominal wall may also be used to keep the tube at a 90-degree angle; secure with tape (Fig. 41.5).
   e. Stabilize gastrostomy tube to prevent excess movement of tube, to decrease risk of stoma erosion, infection, bleeding, and development of granulation tissue.
   f. Use an anchoring device (e.g., Hollister Tube Drainage Attachment Device, Hollister Inc., Libertyville, Illinois) if the patient is allergic to tape or as a routine to secure the tube to skin.
   g. Rotate bolster, flange of nipple, or wings of button every 4 to 8 hours to prevent pressure necrosis of skin. Do not place gauze between skin and bolster. A tension tab can be created by placing tape on the tube and pinning it to the diaper. A one-piece shirt with snap enclosure or tubular elastic dressing can also be used to cover the tube.
   h. Assess site and peristomal skin for leaking, irritation, redness, rashes, or breakdown. Erythema and a minimal amount of clear drainage are to be expected in the first postoperative week.

D. Gastrostomy Tube Complications

Table 42.5 lists interventions for treating complications related to gastrostomy tubes.

TABLE 42.4 **Types of Gastrostomy Tubes**

Type	Description	Examples
Temporary/traditional	Most commonly used as initial tube following Stamm procedure; long, self-retaining catheters of latex or silicone rubber with self-retaining devices (i.e., balloon)	Malecot (Bard, Covington, Georgia) (collapsible wings), dePezzer (mushroom)
Gastrostomy feeding tubes	Silicone catheter with antimigration device and end cap	MIC (Kimberly-Clark/Ballard Medical, Draper, Utah), CORFLO (CORPAK MedSystems, Wheeling, Illinois)
Skin surface devices	Intended for use in established gastrostomy tract; have self-retaining devices, antimigration devices, and antireflux valves; two types, balloon and "Malecot type"	Bard Button (Bard, Covington, Georgia), MIC-KEY (Kimberly Clark/Ballard Medical, Draper, Utah)

Data from Borokowski S. Pediatric stomas, tubes, and appliances. *Pediatr Clin North Am.* 1998;45:1419.

TABLE 42.5 Interventions for Gastrostomy Tube Complications

Complication	Interventions
Leaking at insertion site	Ensure that tube is properly situated in stomach; pull back gently until resistance is met.
Stoma enlargement	Check water volume if balloon-type catheter. Confirm that it is water not Saline or Air Ensure that tube is firmly secured to prevent erosion of mucosal lining and skin. Use proper feeding attachment. Ensure that tube is properly flushed and cleaned. Protect skin with skin barrier (e.g., Stomahesive wafer or powder [ConvaTec, Skillman, New Jersey], Cavilon No Sting [3M, St. Paul, Minnesota]; or hydrocolloid dressing). Use foam dressing (e.g., Hydrasorb [ConvaTec, Skillman, New Jersey], Allevyn [Smith and Nephew, London, UK; Memphis, TN], Mepilex [Mölnlycke, Gothenburg, Sweden]) rather than gauze to "wick" moisture away from skin. If not contraindicated, consider H_2-blocker and prokinetic agent. Placing larger-size tube may temporarily control leakage but will not amend problem and is contraindicated. Place smaller tube and secure well to allow stoma to contract around the tube.
Dislodgement	Do not reinsert if <2 wks postop. Contact surgeon immediately. If >2 wks postop, replace as soon as possible (see Chapter 41).
Bilious residuals	Assess for migration of tube (particularly if Foley is being used).
Bilious vomiting Abdominal distention	Migration results from inadequate stabilization. Tube may migrate upward, causing vomiting and potential aspiration, or downward, causing gastric outlet obstruction. Migration into the small intestine can cause "dumping syndrome." When using a balloon catheter and migration is not recognized, inflation of the balloon can lead to esophageal, duodenal, or small bowel perforation.
Pain	Pull back, if migrated, and secure. Vent tube. Consult surgeon if problem does not resolve.
Granulation tissue	Normal finding; caused by proliferation of granulation epithelial tissue in response to inflammation and irritation by foreign body. Prevent by stabilizing the tube. Treat by cauterizing with silver nitrate. For large amount of granulation tissue, consider applying triamcinolone cream 0.5% 2–3 times daily until resolved.
Bleeding	Apply gentle pressure to site. Stabilize the tube. If granulation tissue is present, treat appropriately.
Irritant dermatitis	Protect skin with skin barrier (e.g., Stomahesive wafer, paste, or powder [ConvaTec, Skillman, New Jersey], Allevyn [Smith and Nephew, London, UK; Memphis, TN], iLEX paste [Medicon Biolab Technologies, Inc., Grafton, Massachusetts], or hydrocolloid dressing). Use foam dressing (e.g., Hydrasorb [ConvaTec, Skillman, New Jersey], Allevyn [Smith and Nephew, London, UK; Memphis, TN],) rather than gauze to "wick" moisture away from skin. Assess for sensitivity to products/latex.
Candida albicans	Apply topical antifungal to skin. Control leakage. Dry skin completely after cleaning. Patient should also be assessed for oral thrush.
Clogged tube	Flush well after medications with 5 mL lukewarm water. A small amount (3–5 mL) of carbonated soda or cranberry juice may also be poured into the tube. Allow to set for 10 min, then flush with water.
Infection	G-tube site infections are uncommon; cellulitis is treated with systemic antibiotics.

Data from Association of Women's Health, Obstetric and Neonatal Nurses, National Association of Neonatal Nurses. *Evidence-Based Clinical Practice Guideline: Neonatal Skin Care.* Washington, DC: AWHONN; 2001; Borkowski S. Gastrostomy surgery and tubes. *Sutureline.* 2000;8:1; Borkowski S. Gastrostomy tube stabilization and security. *Sutureline.* 2005;13:8; Borokowski S. Pediatric stomas, tubes, and appliances. *Pediatr Clin North Am.* 1998;45:1419; Colwell JC. A practical guide for the management of pediatric gastrostomy tubes based on 14 years of experience. *J Wound Ostomy Continence Nurs.* 2004;31:193; Craven DP, Fowler JS, Foster ME. Management of a neonate with necrotizing enterocolitis and eight prolapsed stomas in a dehisced wound. *J Wound Ostomy Continence Nurs.* 1999;26:214; Garvin G. Caring for children with ostomies and wounds. In: Wise B, McKenna C, Garvin G, et al., eds. *Nursing Care of the General Pediatric Surgical Patient.* Gaithersburg, MD: Aspen; 2000:261; Metcalfe P, Schwarz R. Bladder exstrophy: neonatal care and surgical approaches. *Wound Ostomy Continence Nurs.* 2004;31:284; Rogers VE. Managing preemie stomas: more than just the pouch. *J Wound Ostomy Continence Nurs.* 2003;30:100; Wound Ostomy and Continence Nurses Society. *Pediatric Ostomy Care: Best Practice for Clinicians.* Mount Laurel, NJ: Wound Ostomy and Continence Nurses Society, 2011.

References

1. Gauderer MWL. Stomas of the small and large intestine. In: O'Neil JA, Rowe MI, Grosfeld JL, et al., eds. *Pediatric Surgery.* 5th ed. St. Louis, MO: Mosby; 1998:1349.
2. Rogers VE. Managing preemie stomas: more than just the pouch. *J Wound Ostomy Continence Nurs.* 2003;30:100.
3. Metcalfe P, Schwarz R. Bladder exstrophy: neonatal care and surgical approaches. *Wound Ostomy Continence Nurs.* 2004;31: 284.
4. Wound Ostomy and Continence Nurses Society. *Pediatric Ostomy Care: Best Practice for Clinicians.* Mount Laurel, NJ: Wound Ostomy and Continence Nurses Society, 2011.
5. Craven DP, Fowler JS, Foster ME. Management of a neonate with necrotizing enterocolitis and eight prolapsed stomas in a dehisced wound. *J Wound Ostomy Continence Nurs.* 1999;26:214.
6. Borokowski S. Pediatric stomas, tubes, and appliances. *Pediatr Clin North Am.* 1998;45:1419.
7. Garvin G. Caring for children with ostomies and wounds. In: Wise B, McKenna C, Garvin G, et al., eds. *Nursing Care of the General Pediatric Surgical Patient.* Gaithersburg, MD: Aspen; 2000: 261.
8. Borkowski S. Gastrostomy tube stabilization and security. *Sutureline.* 2005;13:8.
9. Association of Women's Health, Obstetric and Neonatal Nurses, National Association of Neonatal Nurses. *Evidence-Based Clinical Practice Guideline: Neonatal Skin Care.* Washington, DC: AWHONN; 2001.
10. Borkowski S. Gastrostomy surgery and tubes. *Sutureline.* 2000;8:1.
11. Colwell JC. A practical guide for the management of pediatric gastrostomy tubes based on 14 years of experience. *J Wound Ostomy Continence Nurs.* 2004;31:193.

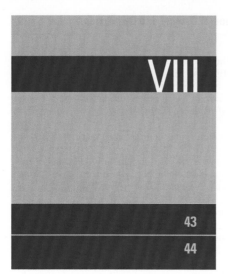

VIII Transfusions

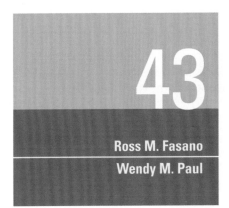

43

Transfusion of Blood and Blood Products

Ross M. Fasano

Wendy M. Paul

Overview

Blood Products Utilized in Neonates

A. Red blood cells (RBCs)
B. Whole or reconstituted whole blood
C. Platelet concentrates derived from whole blood or plateletpheresis
D. Fresh frozen plasma (FFP) or frozen thawed plasma
E. Cryoprecipitate
F. Granulocyte concentrates derived from granulocytapheresis

Sources of Blood Products

A. Banked donor blood
B. Directed donor transfusions
C. Autologous fetal blood transfusions

Indications, requirements, and transfusion techniques differ for each procedure and component. Simple transfusions are discussed in this chapter. Exchange transfusions are discussed in Chapter 44. Complications common to all blood products are listed later in this chapter.

A. Precautions (1)

1. Whenever possible, obtain informed consent prior to transfusions, delineating risks, benefits, and alternatives to transfusion.
2. Limit use of transfusions to justified indications.
3. Select blood product appropriate for infant's condition.
4. Confirm with proper identifiers at bedside that blood product is for correct patient. Maintain all records relevant to collection, preparation, transfusion, and clinical outcome.
5. Avoid excessive transfusion volume or rate unless acute blood loss or shock dictates faster transfusion.
6. Store blood and blood products appropriately. Freezing and lysis may occur if RBCs are stored in unmonitored refrigerators.
   a. Use blood bank refrigerator for storage of RBCs, whole blood, thawed FFP, and thawed cryoprecipitate.

b. Temperature should be controlled at 1°C to 6°C with constant temperature monitors and alarm systems.
   c. Refrigerator should be quality-controlled at least daily.
   d. Designated for blood products only
   e. Store platelets at 20°C to 24°C with continuous agitation.
7. RBCs and whole blood should be out of refrigeration for <4 hours to minimize risk of bacterial contamination and RBC hemolysis.
8. Use approved blood-warming devices for RBCs and whole blood. Syringes for aliquots must not be warmed in water baths because of the risk of contamination.
9. Stop transfusion or slow rate if baby manifests any adverse side effects.
   a. Tachycardia, bradycardia, or arrhythmia
   b. Tachypnea
   c. Systolic blood pressure increases of >15 mm Hg, unless this is the desired effect
   d. Temperature above 38°C and/or increase in temperature of ≥1°C
   e. Hyperglycemia or hypoglycemia
   f. Cyanosis
   g. Skin rash, hives, or flushing
   h. Hematuria/hemoglobinuria
   i. Hyperkalemia
10. Transfuse RBCs cautiously in infants with incipient or existing cardiac failure (2).
    a. Monitor heart rate, blood pressure, and peripheral perfusion.
    b. Consider partial exchange transfusion
       (1) With hemoglobin level <5 to 7 g/dL
       (2) With cord hemoglobin <10 g/dL
11. Prevent fluctuations in glucose during RBC transfusion
    a. In infants weighing <1,200 g or in other unstable infants, to prevent hypoglycemia
       (1) Do not discontinue parenteral glucose administration.
       (2) Establish separate IV line for blood administration.

b. When transfused blood has elevated glucose concentration, expect rebound hypoglycemia in infants with hyperinsulinism.

B. Pretransfusion Testing and Processing

1. Blood group and Rh type
   a. *Maternal ABO blood group and Rh type:* Screen maternal serum for atypical antibodies.
   b. *Baby's ABO blood group and Rh type:* Screen baby's serum for atypical antibodies if maternal blood is unavailable.
   c. Cord blood may be used for initial testing.
   d. Baby's blood group is determined from the red cells alone, because the corresponding anti-A and anti-B isoagglutinins are usually weak or absent in neonatal serum.
2. Cross-matching
   a. Compatible blood may be low-anti-A, anti-B titer group O Rh-negative blood or, blood of the infant's ABO group and Rh type (except in alloimmune hemolytic disease of the newborn).
   b. Conventional cross-match is not required if infant <4 months old and no atypical antibodies are detected.
   c. Compatibility testing for repeated small-volume transfusions is usually unnecessary because formation of alloantibodies is extremely rare in the first 4 months of life.
   d. If antibody screen is indirect antiglobulin test (IAT)-positive in mother or baby
      (1) Serologic investigation to identify antibody(ies) is necessary.
      (2) Full compatibility testing is required.
      (3) If anti-A or anti-B detected in infant, infant should receive RBCs lacking A or B antigen until antibody screen is negative.
   e. If infant has received large volumes of plasma or platelets, passive acquisition of antibodies may occur; cross-matching is recommended.
   f. If directed donor blood from a parent is used, cross-matching is required.
3. Specially processed products
   a. Transfusion-transmitted disease testing with all donor collections (see "Complications" section)
   b. Cytomegalovirus (CMV)-seronegative or third-generation leukodepleted (LD) blood is recommended for infants with birthweight ≤1,200 g born to seronegative mothers or those with unknown serostatus (3).
   c. Use of universal LD and/or CMV seronegative products is institution-specific (4).
4. Irradiation to prevent transfusion-associated graft-versus-host disease (TA-GVHD)
   a. Whole blood, PRBCs, previously frozen RBCs, granulocyte and platelet concentrates, and fresh

TABLE 43.1	**Clinical Indications for Irradiated Blood Components (2,56)**

1. Intrauterine transfusion (IUT) or postnatal transfusion in neonate who had received IUT
2. Premature infants, variably defined by weight and postgestational age
3. Congenital immunodeficiency suspected or confirmed
4. Undergoing exchange transfusion for erythroblastosis
5. Hematologic/solid organ malignancy
6. Recipient of familial blood donation
7. Recipient of HLA-matched or cross-match–compatible platelets or granulocytes

From Josephson CD. Neonatal and pediatric transfusion practice. In: Roback JD, eds. *Technical Manual of the American Association of Blood Banks.* 16th ed. Bethesda, MD: American Association of Blood Banks; 2008:639; Roseff SD, Luban NL, Manno CS. Guidelines for assessing appropriateness of pediatric transfusion. *Transfusion.* 2002;42:1398.

plasma have been implicated in TA-GVHD; LD products have also been implicated.
   b. Clinical indications for irradiated blood components are listed in Table 43.1.
   c. Some institutions provide irradiated blood products to all neonates to avoid TA-GVHD in patients with undiagnosed immunodeficiency.

C. Equipment

1. Blood product (see Appendix C)
2. Cardiorespiratory monitor
3. *Blood:* All blood and blood components must be filtered immediately prior to transfusion despite prestorage LD. Many transfusion services supply RBCs and occasionally platelets and cryoprecipitate, prefiltered to the neonatal intensive care unit (NICU).
   a. Administration set with inline filter of 120- to 170-μm pore size to be used for all products
   b. Microaggregate filter, 20- to 40- μm pore size
      (1) Must follow manufacturer's instructions
      (2) Some function only if product is dripped
      (3) Not advisable for syringe administration
      (4) Usefulness questionable and unnecessary if LD and/or additive RBCs used
   c. Prestorage LD (2,4,5)
      (1) Removes 99.9% of white blood cells (WBCs), or 3 log LD
      (2) Must follow manufacturer's instructions
      (3) Attenuation/abrogation of CMV and other viruses such as Epstein–Barr virus (EBV) and human T-lymphotropic virus (HTLV) I/II harbored in WBCs
      (4) Prestorage LD (performed by collecting facility) preferred to post-storage (bedside) LD
4. Sterile syringe
5. Blood administration set
   a. May be manufactured with integral 120- to 170-μm filter

b. May not be needed if prefiltered product is dispensed from transfusion service

c. Blood warmer not needed

6. Automated syringe pump with appropriate tubing and needle (6–9)

   a. Least hemolysis occurs with straight syringe pumps

   b. *Vascular access*: RBCs may be transfused through 24-, 25-, or 27-gauge needles and short catheters but not through 27- or 28-gauge central venous catheters.

   c. The amount of hemolysis that results from infusion of RBCs is directly proportionate to the age of the blood and the rate of transfusion and inversely proportional to needle size.

   d. Hyperkalemia, hemoglobinuria, and renal dysfunction may result if hemolyzed blood is transfused.

7. Normal saline flush (1 mL or more) to clear IV solution from line.

Red Blood Cell Transfusions

A. Indications

1. Guidelines and justifications for transfusions are controversial because there are few studies that address the appropriateness of various transfusion triggers in neonates. Therefore, indications for RBC transfusion vary among different institutions.

2. Current guidelines for neonatal RBC transfusion therapy are given in Table 43.2 (10,11). In general

   a. Infants with significant cardiopulmonary disease require more RBC transfusion support.

   b. Infants receiving minimal cardiopulmonary support, with acceptable weight gain, and with minimal episodes of apnea and bradycardia, require less RBC support.

TABLE 43.2	**Guidelines for Transfusion of RBCs in Patients <4 Months of Age**

Clinical Status	Target Hematocrit
For severe cardiopulmonary disease (requiring mechanical ventilation with FiO_2 >0.35)	>40%–45%
For moderate cardiopulmonary disease	>30%–35%
For major surgery	>30%–35%
For infants with stable anemia with unexplained apnea/bradycardia, tachycardia, or poor growth	>20%–25%

Modified from Fasano RM, Luban NL. Blood Component Therapy for the Neonate. In: Martin R, Fanaroff A, eds. *Fanaroff & Martin's Neonatal-Perinatal Medicine.* 9th ed. St. Louis: Elsevier; 2010:1360; Strauss RG. How I transfuse red blood cells and platelets to infants with the anemia and thrombocytopenia of prematurity. *Transfusion.* 2008;48:209.
Definitions for level of severity of cardiopulmonary disease may be defined individually by institution.

3. Liberal versus conservative RBC transfusion

   a. Studies on liberal versus conservative RBC transfusion practices have demonstrated mixed results in terms of clinical benefit of liberal transfusion practices toward preventing apneic episodes and immediate neurologic sequelae (12,13).

   b. Long-term neurodevelopmental benefit has not been ascertained for either transfusion practice (14).

   c. Several studies have documented a temporal relationship of RBC transfusions with the occurrence of necrotizing enterocolitis (NEC) in premature infants, which supports a more restrictive transfusion practice (15–19). Withholding feeds during transfusion may have a protective effect from NEC (16).

   d. The relationship between RBC transfusions and NEC requires further evaluation in premature infants.

B. Contraindications

1. None absolute

2. *Exert caution in patient with:*

   a. Volume overload

   b. Congestive heart failure

   c. T-activation

   d. Increased risk for NEC (especially extremely low-birthweight infants)

C. Technique

1. Determine total amount of blood needed.

   a. Calculate volume of blood for transfusion. Most infants are transfused 10 to 15 mL/kg of RBCs, which will increase the hemoglobin by 3 g/dL.

   b. *RBC volume required*: [EBV × (Hct desired − Hct observed)] Hct of RBC unit

      (1) Hct is hematocrit

      (2) EBV is the estimated patient's blood volume 80 to 85 mL/kg in full-term infants and approximately 100 to 120 mL/kg in preterm infants

      (3) RBC units collected in citrate-phosphate-dextrose-adenine (CPDA-1) have a Hct of approximately 70%, RBCs in extended-storage AP solutions (AS-1) have a Hct ≤60%

2. Include volume of blood needed for dead space of tubing, filter, pump mechanism (varies from system to system; may be as much as 30 mL).

3. Obtain blood product (see Appendix C).

   a. Several studies have documented the safety of using PRBCs stored in extended-storage anticoagulant preservative (AP) solutions to outdate (20–22).

   b. Avoid use of RBCs stored in extended-storage AP solutions for massive transfusions, unless the additive is removed by inverted storage or centrifugation; risks of hyperosmolality, hyperglycemia, hypernatremia, hyperkalemia, hyperphosphatemia are postulated (21,23,24).

c. Small volume transfusion of ≤15 mL/kg of RBCs stored to maximum outdate, delivers approximately 0.3 mEq/kg of K^+, and does not pose a significant risk to most neonates when transfused slowly over 2 to 4 hours (2,24).

d. Use of split RBC packs effectively limit donor exposures, and are safe for use in neonatal small volume transfusions up to the outdate of 35 or 42 days (2,25,26). This practice requires sterile connecting devices, and either transfer packs or syringe sets that permit multiple aliquots to be removed (Figs. 43.1 and 43.2).

4. Verify whether cross-matched product is necessary or un–cross-matched product is adequate.

5. Confirm that restrictions have been adhered to on blood product and transfusion tag.
   a. *CMV: Tested/untested*
   b. *Irradiated: Yes/no*
   c. *Directed (familial) donation: Yes/no*
   d. *RBC antigen-negative: Yes/no*
   e. *Sickle tested-negative: Yes/no*
   f. *Other restrictions specified: Yes/no*

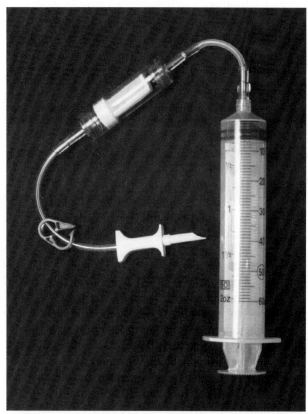

FIG. 43.1. Neonatal syringe set with filter. (Courtesy of Charter Medical Ltd., Winston-Salem, North Carolina). This system, when used with sterile connection technology, provides a closed delivery system that maintains primary unit outdate. Syringe blood aliquots (PRCBs, plasma) must be administered to the patient within 24 hours and syringe platelet aliquots within 4 hours.

6. Verify appropriateness of blood selected for patient by comparing blood product and unit tag (integral to blood unit) information and patient identification. Barcode reading devices are advisable.
   a. Blood unit tag and blood bag
   b. Patient hospital or medical record number
   c. Patient identification by armband or footband
   d. Blood group and type of both donor and recipient
   e. Expiration date and time and restrictions on unit and order
   f. Restrictions as ordered by physician or by institutional guidelines

7. Warming RBCs
   a. There is no need to warm small-volume PRBC aliquots, particularly if the transfusion is given over 2 to 3 hours.
   b. RBCs may be warmed by placing the syringe beside the infant in the warm-air incubator for 30 minutes prior to transfusion.
   c. Inappropriate warming by exposure of blood to heat lamps or phototherapy lights may produce hemolysis. Shielding the RBC component and tubing from UV light is recommended (27,28).

8. Adhere to sterile technique throughout procedure.

9. Some syringe sets have 150 micron inline filters attached such that they are filtered during the blood bank's aliquoting process (2). If prefiltered RBCs are provided by the blood bank in a syringe, attach tubing directly to syringe.

10. If RBCs are provided in a bag, use large-bore needle (18-gauge or larger) to withdraw volume into syringe. Filter should be placed between bag and syringe (Fig. 43.1).

11. Prime tubing with blood. Clear syringe and tubing of bubbles, and mount into infusion device.

12. Verify patency of vascular access.

13. Clear line into patient with normal saline.

14. Record and monitor vital signs.

15. Determine spot glucose test. Repeat hourly as needed.

16. *Begin transfusion at controlled rate*: 3 to 5 mL/kg/h.

17. Gently invert container of blood every 15 to 30 minutes to minimize sedimentation.

18. Stop transfusion if any adverse change in condition occurs.

19. At end of infusion, clear blood from line with saline.

20. Check recipient hemoglobin and hematocrit, if necessary, at least 2 hours after transfusion.

21. If posttransfusion hematocrit/hemoglobin is not up to expected level, consider
    a. Low hematocrit of RBC unit (extended-storage AP vs. CPDA-1 units)
    b. Inappropriate calculation of transfusion requirement
    c. Ongoing blood loss
    d. Transfusion reaction

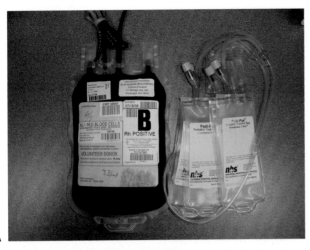

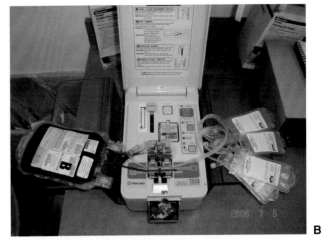

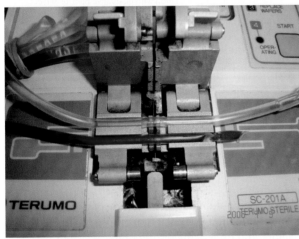

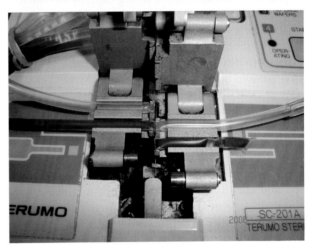

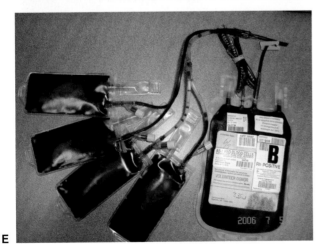

FIG. 43.2. Use of a sterile connecting device. **A:** An adult RBC unit is shown along with a set of pediatric transfer bags. The transfer bags can be attached by spiking the unit, causing it to expire in 24 hours; alternatively, the transfer bags can be connected using a sterile connection device. **B, C:** The separate tubings are loaded into the tubing holders of the device. The covers are closed. **D:** A welding wafer heated to about 500°F melts through the tubing. The tubing holders realign and the welding wafer retracts allowing the tubing ends to fuse together. **E:** The unit can now be aliquoted as needed. Because a functionally closed system has been maintained, the expiration date of the blood has not changed.

   e. Hemolysis due to ABO or other RBC incompatibility
     (1) Infant has circulating anti-A, anti-B, and anti-AB, which is bound to A or B antigens on transfused RBCs.
     (2) Direct antiglobulin test negative initially but now positive

     (3) Unexpected increase in bilirubin
     (4) Infant has RBC antibody other than ABO.
     (5) Hemolysis from extrinsic damage (mechanical) to RBCs or donor has hemolytic disorder.
     (6) Hemolysis from T-activation

Whole or Reconstituted Whole Blood Transfusions

A whole blood (WB) unit contains approximately 450 to 500 mL of blood and 70 mL of AP solution. WB stored longer than 48 hours has decreasing levels of coagulation factors V and VIII, does not contain functional platelets or granulocytes, and concentration of K^+ is high. Reconstituted WB is prepared by adding a unit of RBCs to a compatible unit of FFP and is preferable to the use of stored WB (29,30).

A. Indications

1. Massive transfusion as in acute blood loss, in excess of 25% of total blood volume (TBV) when restoration of blood volume and oxygen-carrying capacity are needed simultaneously.
2. Exchange transfusions
3. Cardiopulmonary bypass (CPB)
4. Extracorporeal membrane oxygenation
5. Continuous hemofiltration
6. There currently exists no consensus within the United States on the use of fresh WB, reconstituted WB, or reconstituted *fresh* WB (RFWB) for CPB pump priming or postoperative transfusion support in neonates with congenital heart disease.
   a. Recent studies have questioned the use of WB (31) and have suggested an advantage in clinical outcomes in infants with congenital heart disease receiving RFWB during CPB surgery (32).
   b. Additional prospective studies are warranted to determine optimal age of reconstituted WB units for neonates undergoing CPB surgery.
   c. Fresh WB (<48 hours old) is not universally available.

B. Precautions

1. Not suitable for simple transfusion for anemia
2. Not suitable for correction of coagulation factor deficiencies
3. Hyperkalemia may result from rapid transfusion of large volumes (24).
4. Anticoagulant (citrate) effects must be considered for large volume transfusion (21,24).

C. Equipment and Technique

1. Same as for RBCs
2. The rate of transfusion may be increased to 10 to 20 mL/kg/h to replace acute blood loss.
3. 120 to 150 micron inline filters often used for complex mechanical procedure.

Platelet Transfusions

A. Indications (Table 43.3)

The platelet count at which transfusion is recommended has to be individualized because hemostatic competence is

---

TABLE 43.3   **Guidelines for Platelet Transfusion in Neonates**

With Thrombocytopenia

1. Platelet count $<30 \times 10^9$/L in neonate with failure of platelet production
2. Platelet count $<50 \times 10^9$/L in stable premature infant:
   With active bleeding
   Invasive procedure with failure of platelet production
   Extremely low-birthweight (<1,000 g) infants within the first week of life
3. Platelet count $<50 \times 10^9$/L in neonates with (or presumed) NAIT*
4. Platelet count $<100 \times 10^9$/L in sick premature infant:
   With active bleeding
   Invasive procedure in patient with disseminated intravascular coagulation

Without Thrombocytopenia

1. Active bleeding in association with qualitative platelet defect
2. Unexplained, excessive bleeding in a patient undergoing cardiopulmonary bypass
3. Patient undergoing extracorporeal membrane oxygenation:
   With a platelet count of $<100 \times 10^9$/L
   With higher platelet counts and bleeding

Adapted from Josephson CD. Neonatal and pediatric transfusion practice. In: Roback JD, eds. *Technical Manual of the American Association of Blood Banks*. 16th ed. Bethesda, MD: American Association of Blood Banks; 2008:639; Wong EC, Paul WM. Intrauterine, neonatal, and pediatric transfusion therapy. In: Mintz PD, eds. *Transfusion Therapy: Clinical Principles and Practice*. Bethesda, MD: American Association of Blood Banks; 2011:209.
*NAIT, Neonatal Alloimmune Thrombocytopenia.

---

determined not only by the quantity of platelets but also by platelet function, vascular integrity, levels of coagulation factors, and underlying disorder/disease.

B. Contraindications (33)

1. Autoimmune thrombocytopenic purpura (neonatal ITP)
2. Heparin-induced thrombocytopenia (HIT)
3. Bleeding due to coagulopathy only (i.e., vitamin K deficiency)
4. Bleeding due to anatomic defect
5. Bleeding controllable with direct pressure/local measures (i.e., surgical bleeding)

C. Precautions

1. Use type-specific (Rh-negative) platelets when potential for sensitization is present (i.e., in Rh-negative female). Although platelets do not have Rh antigens, all products have some RBC contamination (less in platelet-pheresis), which may cause Rh sensitization (34).
2. Use platelets from donor with ABO-compatible plasma. Isohemagglutinins in ABO-incompatible plasma may result in hemolysis, a positive direct antiglobulin test, and poorer in vivo platelet survival than anticipated.
3. Transfuse platelets as soon after preparation as possible. Platelets should never be refrigerator-stored or warmed.
4. Platelets should not be infused through arterial lines.

D. Equipment and Technique

1. Platelets
   a. Random donor platelet concentrate (5.5×10^{10} platelets in 40 to 70 mL of plasma)
      (1) Separated from WB by centrifugation within 8 hours of blood draw and resuspended in plasma
      (2) Shelf life of 5 days
   b. Volume-reduced platelets
      (1) Standard platelet concentrate further concentrated to a volume of 15 to 20 mL by centrifugation
      (2) Associated with loss of platelets and possible decrease in platelet function
      (3) Shelf life reduced to 4 hours
      (4) Use only if infant has oliguria, severe volume load sensitivity
   c. Apheresis platelets (3×10^{11} platelets in volume of 250 mL plasma)
      (1) Removes only platelets, returns RBCs and plasma to donor
      (2) Usually LD before storage
      (3) Permits repeated donations from same donor every 48 hours under select circumstances
      (4) High yield of platelets
      (5) More expensive product
      (6) Useful when multiple platelet transfusions of a particular antigen specificity are required, as in neonatal alloimmune thrombocytopenia (NAIT) or for infants on extracorporeal membrane oxygenation needing multiple platelet transfusions.
      (7) May be HLA-typed or typed for HPA-1 or other specific platelet antigen in case of NAIT.
      (8) Maternal plateletpheresis product is preferred for NAIT. Use maternal antigen-negative platelets, washed, irradiated, and resuspended in ABO group-compatible plasma or saline.
2. Calculate volume of platelets to transfuse based on type of product.
   a. 10 to 15 mL/kg of random platelet provides 10×10^9 platelets/kg and should increase platelet count by approximately 50×10^9/L in the absence of ongoing consumption. Can use same calculations for apheresis platelets, but studies do not confirm posttransfusion increments.
   b. Advise use of equivalent unit (EU) calculations and not mL/kg for dosing apheresis platelets.
   c. 1 EU is the volume of a platelet aliquot that has a minimum platelet content of 5.5×10^{10} platelets (approximately 1 random donor platelet concentrate).
   d. The standard dose based on this method is 1 EU/5 to 10 kg, with a minimum dose of 1 EU. Volume reduction may be necessary for some extremely low-birthweight infants.
   e. Other products (HLA-matched, cross-matched platelets) used for platelet refractoriness; washed platelets if using HPA-matched maternal apheresis platelets.
3. Blood administration set with 120- to 170-μm inline filter, unless platelets have been prefiltered while drawing into a syringe. Specific sets designed for plasma/platelets have inline filters with reduced surface area to increase platelet transfusion efficacy.
4. Sterile syringe for automated pump infusion. Use of syringe technique will increase damage to platelets. Administer by drip if clinically feasible.
5. Automated syringe pump
6. Connecting IV tubing
7. IV access, preferably through 23-gauge or larger needle or through umbilical venous catheter
8. Normal saline flush solution

E. Technique for Platelet Administration by Automated Syringe

1. Estimate by weight the volume of platelets in a single bag to determine fluid load to infant.
2. Confirm correct platelet product.
   a. Infant and unit identification
   b. Infant and donor blood group, and Rh type
   c. *Check other restrictions*: CMV negative, irradiated, etc.
3. Attach, aseptically, in sequence
   a. Platelet concentrate or bag aliquot
   b. Platelet administration set, including filter
   c. Three-way stopcock
   d. Transfusion syringe
4. Draw volume of platelets for transfusion and tubing dead space into syringe. Clear air bubbles.
5. Remove syringe from three-way stopcock and attach to connecting tubing.
6. Establish IV access. If infant is at risk for hypoglycemia with interruption of continuous glucose source, start new IV or monitor closely throughout infusion.
7. Clear IV of glucose solution with 1 mL or more of normal saline.
8. Attach connecting tubing and syringe to IV line.
9. Monitor patient's vital signs.
10. Infuse platelets over 1- to 2-hour period, faster if tolerated by infant.
11. After infusion is complete, flush IV line with 1 mL of normal saline before restarting glucose solution.
12. Determine survival time of transfused platelets by obtaining platelet counts at 1 and/or 24 hours if concern for platelet refractoriness.

F. Complications

1. Accentuated hemolysis in sensitized but indirect antiglobulin test–negative ABO setup
2. Rh sensitization in Rh-negative recipient (34)
3. Volume overload
4. Allergic reactions, including hypotension

5. Transfusion-related lung injury (TRALI) (35)
6. Increased morbidity in NEC (36)

Complications discussed in more detail in "Complications of Blood Products" section.

Granulocyte Transfusions

A. Indications

1. Granulocyte transfusions are used infrequently because of improvements in antimicrobial medications, supportive care, and the occasional use of granulocyte- and granulocyte/macrophage-stimulating factors.
2. Granulocyte transfusion may be considered in the following conditions; however, reduction in morbidity or mortality have not been confirmed in randomized trials (37).
   a. Neonates <14 days old with bacterial sepsis and absolute neutrophil count (ANC) (+ band count) $<3 \times 10^9$/L, and older neonates with bacterial sepsis and ANC (+ band count) $<0.5 \times 10^9$/L
   b. Neutropenic neonates with fungal disease not responsive to standard antifungal therapy.

B. Equipment and Technique

1. Granulocyte concentrates for neonatal use are prepared by automated granulocytapheresis, and should contain 1 to 2×10^9 neutrophils/kg in a volume of 10- to 15-mL/kg. Steroid- and G-CSF-mobilized donor preferred.
2. Daily transfusions may be necessary until there is clinical improvement and evidence of recovery of neutrophil counts.
3. Component must be ABO- and Rh-compatible with recipient, and cross-match–compatible.
4. Product should be irradiated, CMV-negative, and infused as soon as possible after collection.
5. The product should not be refrigerated or warmed above room temperature.
6. Standard 120- to 170-μm filters should be used for infusion; microaggregate and LD filters must be avoided.

C. Precautions

1. Storage of product for >8 hours is associated with a rapid decrease in WBC function, making this a less than useful product.
2. Fever, alloimmunization, TRALI, and CMV infection have all been reported complications.

Fresh Frozen Plasma, Frozen Thawed Plasma, and Cryoprecipitate

A. Indications (2,38)

1. FFP, Frozen Thawed Plasma

   Clinically significant bleeding or for correction of hemostatic defects prior to invasive procedures in the presence of

   a. Complex factor deficiency unresponsive to vitamin K
   b. Isolated congenital factor deficiency for which virus-inactivated-plasma-derived or recombinant factor concentrates are unavailable
   c. Support during the management of disseminated intravascular coagulation
2. Cryoprecipitate
   a. Congenital or acquired dys- or hypofibrinogenemia*
   b. Congenital FXIII deficiency in the absence of FXIII concentrate*
   c. Bleeding associated with von Willebrand disease, hemophilia A when virally inactivated plasma-derived or recombinant factor products are unavailable.

B. Contraindications

1. None absolute
2. Exert caution when possibility of volume overload exists.
3. Use with caution in the setting of NEC and/or T-activation as it may aggravate hemolysis (39).
4. Not indicated for hypovolemic shock in the absence of bleeding, nutritional support, treatment of immunodeficiency, or prevention of intraventricular hemorrhage.

C. Equipment and Technique

See Platelet Transfusion.

1. Cross-matching is not required because type-specific or AB-negative product is usually issued.
2. Dose of FFP is 10 to 20 mL/kg; multiple transfusions may be required until the underlying condition resolves.
3. Once thawed, FFP should be transfused within 6 hours for labile factor replacement.
4. In cases for which repeated FFP transfusions are required, a thawed unit from a single donor may be divided into smaller aliquots and used within 24 hours if stored between 1°C and 6°C.
5. A dose of 1 U/5 kg of cryoprecipitate will increase the total fibrinogen by approximately 100 mg/dL in the absence of ongoing consumption.
6. 1 U of cryoprecipitate equals approximately 12 to 20 mL.

Directed Donor Transfusions

A. Potential Problems

Directed donations provide no known benefit in terms of increased safety and may pose unique immunologic and serologic risks to the neonate (30,40).

---

*In the presence of active bleeding or planned invasive procedures.

1. Possible increased risk of transmitting infectious disease because directed donors are often first-time or infrequent donors with no track record of safety, unlike established volunteer donors, whose screening tests are negative repeatedly.
2. Possibility of serologic incompatibility between the recipient baby and the family donors.
   a. Maternal plasma may contain alloantibodies directed against paternal RBC, leukocyte, platelet, and HLA antigens, which may result in significant hemolytic, thrombocytopenic, or pulmonary reactions (41).
   b. Paternal blood cells may express antigens to which the neonate may have been passively immunized by transplacental transfer of maternal antibodies.
   c. Routine pretransfusion testing may not detect these serologic incompatibilities.
3. Although biologic parents may be interested in donating for their infants, many are likely to be ineligible for medical or serologic reasons.

B. Precautions

1. Directed donations must be screened as stringently as volunteer donations.
2. If maternal RBCs or platelets are transfused, they should be given as washed cells or should be plasma reduced and irradiated.
3. Fathers and paternal blood relatives should preferably not serve as donors for blood components containing cellular elements (RBCs, platelets, or granulocytes); if their use is unavoidable, a full antiglobulin cross-match should be performed to detect incompatibilities.
4. All blood components obtained from first- or second-degree relatives should be irradiated prior to transfusion of the neonate to prevent TA-GVHD.

Autologous Fetal Blood Transfusions

The placenta contains 75 to 125 mL of blood at birth depending on the gestational age of the infant. Autologous transfusion in an infant can occur by collection, storage, and reinfusion of autologous cord blood, or by delaying cord clamping, a successful variation of autologous transfusion. Both maneuvers potentially provide a substantial volume of fetal blood for the neonate, eliminating the potential risks of transfusion transmitted diseases and TA-GVHD (42). Protocols for proper collection of autologous cord blood with appropriate anticoagulation, without bacterial contamination, are still being refined for these indications.

A. Indications

1. Autologous cord blood is a convenient source of autologous RBCs for elective transfusion to preterm infants.
2. Delivery room resuscitation of infants with shock and profound anemia, when O Rh-negative RBCs are not immediately available. Delaying cord clamping has

been shown to instantly increase RBC mass and circulating blood volume, while decreasing the immediate need of RBC transfusions and possibly the incidence of intraventricular hemorrhage in the preterm infant (43–45).
3. Source of cord blood for freezing for hematopoietic reconstitution.

B. Contraindications

1. Maternal infection
2. Chorioamnionitis
3. Sepsis
4. Hepatitis, HIV
5. Prolonged rupture of membranes >24 hours

C. Complications

1. Bacterial sepsis from contaminated collection (46).
2. Insufficient collection volumes from infants <1,000 g.
3. Over-/undercollection for volume of anticoagulant used
4. Volume overload to the neonate (delaying cord clamping)

Complications of Blood Transfusions

Transfusions are safer now than ever before, but they are not risk-free.

1. *Transmission of infectious diseases*: The potential risk of transfusion-transmitted infections in the United States has been dramatically reduced by extensive donor screening and laboratory testing. Current transfusion-transmitted disease testing for allogeneic blood donation include: Hepatitis B surface antigen (HBsAg) and core antibody (anti-HBc); anti–hepatitis C (anti-HCV), HIV-1/HIV-2 (anti-HIV-1/2), and HTLV-I/HTLV-II syphilis (FTA-Abs) and *Trypanosoma cruzi* antibodies; and nucleic acid testing (NAT) for HIV-1, HIV2, HCV, and West Nile virus (47).
   a. *Viruses*: Risk varies geographically (48–51)
      (1) *HIV*: Estimated potential risk in United States from a blood donor with negative serologic tests is 1 in 2.3 million (49).
      (2) *HTLV I and II*: Risk estimated at 1 in 2.9 million U transfused (51).
      (3) *Hepatitis B virus*: Risk 1 in 220,000 U transfused (50)
      (4) *Hepatitis C virus*: Risk 1 in 1.8 million (49)
      (5) *Hepatitis A virus*: Risk <1 in 1 million, asymptomatic in newborn, but may cause symptomatic infection in adults who are in contact with infected neonates.
      (6) *CMV*: Transmitted by cellular blood products, (not FFP or cryoprecipitate). Risk factors for neonatal transfusion-acquired CMV (TA-CMV) include birthweight <1,200 g, exposure to

≥50 mL of blood, and maternal CMV seronega-tivity. Risk of TA-CMV from CMV-seronegative or effectively leukoreduced components is <1% to 4% (47,52).

(7) Hepatitis G, parvovirus B-19, EBV

b. *Bacteria*

(1) Platelet concentrates and RBCs most often implicated

(2) *Frequency:*

Approximately 1 per 38,500 U transfused with low prevalence of septic reactions (1 in 250,000) for RBCs.

Approximately 1 per 5,000 U transfused with septic reactions in 1 in 116,000 for platelets, when pretransfusion bacterial screening (i.e., BacT/ALERT system) is employed. Lower bac-terial contamination rates and septic reactions exist for apheresis platelets compared to WB-derived platelets (53).

(3) *Organisms:*

Common RBC contaminants include *Yersinia enterocolitica, Serratia*

Spp., and *Pseudomonas* spp., *Enterobacter* spp., *Campylobacter* spp., and *Escherichia coli.* All have the potential to cause endotoxin-mediated shock in recipients.

Common platelet contaminants include *Staphylococcus aureus,*

Staphylococcus epidermidis, Bacillus spp. diphtheroid bacilli and Streptococci. Most fatal cases of bacterial contaminated platelets involve gram-negative organisms.

(4) *Treponema pallidum:* No new transfusion-transmitted cases reported in >30 years (48).

c. Protozoa

(1) *Malaria:* Rare in the United States but reported even in nonendemic areas (45)

(2) Babesiosis

(3) Chagas disease (*Trypanosoma cruzi*)

d. *Prions:* Creutzfeldt—Jakob

(1) Few proven cases of transfusion-transmitted new-variant Creutzfeldt–Jakob disease at pres-ent. Those described have been in the United Kingdom (54).

(2) Most blood collection centers attempt to mini-mize the risk by excluding donors considered to be at higher risk for possibly harboring the infec-tion, by family and travel history and specific medical history (47).

2. **Hemolytic reactions**

a. *Acute hemolytic immunologic reactions:* Rare, because of absence in infant of naturally occurring anti-A or anti-B antibodies, and infrequent posttrans-fusion red cell alloimmunization despite multiple transfusions.

b. *T-activation:* A form of immune-mediated hemolysis associated with the transfusion of adult blood con-taining naturally occurring anti-T antibodies, into neonates with exposure of a normally masked Thomsen–Friedenreich (T) cryptantigen on their RBC surface. T-activation can present with evidence of intravascular hemolysis following transfusion of blood products, or unexplained failure to achieve the expected posttransfusion hemoglobin increment (24,30).

(1) Commonly observed in premature infants with NEC and/or sepsis (39)

(2) Suspect T-activation in neonates at risk with intravascular hemolysis, hemoglobinuria, hemo-globinemia following transfusion of blood prod-ucts, or unexpected failure to achieve posttrans-fusion hemoglobin increment.

(3) Routine cross-matching techniques will not detect T-activation when monoclonal ABO anti-serum is used.

(4) *Diagnosis:* Minor cross-match of neonatal T-activated red cells with donor anti–T-containing serum, discrepancies in forward and reverse blood grouping, confirmed by specific agglutination tests using peanut lectins *Arachis hypogea* and *Glycine soja.*

(5) Use washed red cells, platelets, and low-titer anti-T plasma (if available) only when hemoly-sis is confirmed.

3. **Nonimmunologic causes of hemolysis**

a. Mechanical, through excessive infusion pressure through small needles or 20- to 40-μm filters

b. Accidental overheating or freezing of blood

c. Simultaneous administration of incompatible drugs and fluids

d. Transfusion of abnormal donor cells (glucose 6-phosphate dehydrogenase deficiency, hereditary spherocytosis)

4. **Other immunologic/nonimmunologic reactions**

a. TA-GVHD (See processing with irradiation for risk factors and prevention page 306)

(1) Seen 3 to 30 days following transfusion of a cel-lular component. Symptoms include fever; gen-eralized, erythematous rash with/without pro-gression to desquamation; diarrhea; hepatitis (mild to fulminant liver failure); respiratory dis-tress; and severe pancytopenia

(2) High mortality rate (80% to 100%)

b. *TRALI:*

(1) Secondary to transfusion of donor blood con-taining anti-HLA or neutrophil antibodies directed against recipient leukocytes, causing complement activation with microvascular lung injury and capillary leak.

(2) Presents within 4 hours of transfusion with respi-ratory distress due to noncardiogenic pulmonary

edema, hypotension, fever, and severe hypoxemia.

   (3) Reported only rarely in neonates due to the difficulty in distinguishing TRALI from other causes of respiratory deterioration in sick infants; however, it is documented in the setting of a designated blood transfusion between mother and infant (55).

  c. Transfusion-associated circulatory overload

   (1) Nonimmune alteration in pulmonary compliance and blood pressure due to volume overload

   (2) Presents with respiratory distress, cardiogenic pulmonary edema, and hypertension

5. Adverse metabolic effects

  a. Hyperkalemia

   (1) Blood that is irradiated and then refrigerator-stored may have K^+ levels of 30 to 50 mEq/L or higher in the supernatant plasma.

   (2) Small-volume transfusions of stored red cells do not cause clinically significant elevations in serum K^+ levels.

   (3) Life-threatening hyperkalemia has been described in sick infants and in those receiving rapid infusions of large volumes of stored red cells (24).

   (4) Washed or fresh (<14 days) red cells are recommended for infants with profound hyperkalemia, renal failure, or when large volumes are transfused rapidly.

  b. Hypoglycemia or hyperglycemia

  c. Hypocalcemia

  d. Alterations in acid–base balance with large transfusions

References

1. Carson TH, ed. *Standards for Blood Banks and Transfusion services.* 27th ed. Bethesda, MD: American Association of Blood Banks; 2011.
2. Josephson CD. Neonatal and pediatric transfusion practice. In: Roback JD, eds. *Technical Manual of the American Association of Blood Banks.* 16th ed. Bethesda, MD: American Association of Blood Banks; 2008:639.
3. Wong EC, Paul WM. Intrauterine, Neonatal, and Pediatric Transfusion Therapy. In: Mintz PD, eds. *Transfusion Therapy: Clinical Principles and Practice.* Bethesda, MD: American Association of Blood Banks; 2011:209.
4. Ferguson D, Hebert PC, Lee SK, et al. Clinical outcomes following institution of universal leukoreduction of blood transfusions of premature infants. *JAMA.* 2003;289:1950.
5. Strauss RG. Data-driven blood banking practices for neonatal RBC transfusions. *Transfusion.* 2000;40:1528.
6. Wong EC, Schreiber S, Criss VR, et al. Feasibility of red blood cell transfusion through small bore central venous catheters used in neonates. *Pediatr Crit Care Med.* 2004;5:69.
7. Nakamura KT, Sato Y, Erenberg A. Evaluation of a percutaneously placed 27-gauge central venous catheter in neonates weighing less than 1200 grams. *Jpen.* 1990;14:295.
8. Oloya RO, Feick HJ, Bozynski ME. Impact of venous catheters on packed red blood cells. *Am J Perinatol.* 1991;8:280.
9. Frey B, Eber S, Weiss M. Changes in red blood cell integrity related to infusion pumps: a comparison of three different pump mechanisms. *Pediatr Crit Care Med.* 2003;4:465.
10. Strauss RG. How I transfuse red blood cells and platelets to infants with the anemia and thrombocytopenia of prematurity. *Transfusion.* 2008;48:209.
11. Widness JA. Treatment and prevention of neonatal anemia. *NeoReveiws.* 2008;9:e526.
12. Kirpalani H, Whyte RK, Andersen C, et al. The Premature Infants in Need of Transfusion (PINT) study: a randomized, controlled trial of a restrictive (low) versus liberal (high) transfusion threshold for extremely low birth weight infants. *J Pediatr.* 2006;149:301.
13. Bell EF, Strauss RG, Widness JA, et al. Randomized trial of liberal versus restrictive guidelines for red blood cell transfusion in preterm infants. *Pediatrics.* 2005;115:1685.
14. Whyte RK, Kirpalani H, Asztalos EV, et al. Neurodevelopmental outcome of extremely low birth weight infants randomly assigned to restrictive or liberal hemoglobin thresholds for blood transfusion. *Pediatrics.* 2009;123:207.
15. Blau J, Calo JM, Dozor D, et al. Transfusion-related acute gut injury: necrotizing enterocolitis in very low birth weight neonates after packed red blood cell transfusion. *J Pediatr.* 2011;158:403.
16. El-Dib M, Narang S, Lee E, et al. Red blood cell transfusion, feeding and necrotizing enterocolitis in preterm infants. *J Perinatol.* 2011;31:183.
17. Paul DA, Mackley A, Novitsky A, et al. Increased odds of necrotizing enterocolitis after transfusion of red blood cells in premature infants. *Pediatrics.* 2011;127:635.
18. Singh R, Visintainer PF, Frantz ID 3rd, et al. Association of necrotizing enterocolitis with anemia and packed red blood cell transfusions in preterm infants. *J Perinatol.* 2011;31:176.
19. Josephson CD, Wesolowski A, Bao G, et al. Do red cell transfusions increase the risk of necrotizing enterocolitis in premature infants?. *J Pediatr.* 2010;157:972.
20. Jain R, Jarosz C. Safety and efficacy of AS-1 red blood cell use in neonates. *Transfus Apher Sci.* 2001;24:111.
21. Luban NL, Strauss RG, Hume HA. Commentary on the safety of red cells preserved in extended-storage media for neonatal transfusions. *Transfusion.* 1991;31:229.
22. Strauss RG, Burmeister LF, Johnson K, et al. Feasibility and safety of AS-3 red blood cells for neonatal transfusions. *J Pediatr.* 2000;136:215.
23. Luban NL. Massive transfusion in the neonate. *Transfus Med Rev.* 1995;9:200.
24. Pisciotto PT, Luban NLC. Complications of Neonatal Transfusion. In: Popovsky MA, eds. *Transfusion Reactions.* 3rd ed. Bethesda, MD: American Association of Blood Banks Press; 2007:459.
25. Luban NL. Neonatal red blood cell transfusions. *Vox Sang.* 2004;87:184.
26. Mangel J, Goldman M, Garcia C, et al. Reduction of donor exposures in premature infants by the use of designated adenine-saline preserved split red blood cell packs. *J Perinatol.* 2001;21:363.
27. Luban NL, Mikesell G, Sacher RA. Techniques for warming red blood cells packaged in different containers for neonatal use. *Clin Pediatr (Phila).* 1985;24:642.
28. Strauss RG, Bell EF, Snyder EL, et al. Effects of environmental warming on blood components dispensed in syringes for neonatal transfusions. *J Pediatr.* 1986;109:109.
29. Blood components. In: Gottschall J, eds. *Blood Transfusion Therapy: A Physician's Handbook.* 8th ed. Bethesda, MD: American Association of Blood Banks; 2005.
30. Fasano RM, Luban NL. Blood Component Therapy for the Neonate. In: Martin R, Fanaroff A, eds. *Fanaroff & Martin's Neonatal-Perinatal Medicine.* 9th ed. St. Louis: Elsevier; 2010:1360.

31. Mou SS, Giroir BP, Molitor-Kirsch EA, et al. Fresh whole blood versus reconstituted blood for pump priming in heart surgery in infants. *N Engl J Med.* 2004;351:1635.

32. Gruenwald CE, McCrindle BW, Crawford-Lean L, et al. Reconstituted fresh whole blood improves clinical outcomes compared with stored component blood therapy for neonates undergoing cardiopulmonary bypass for cardiac surgery: a randomized controlled trial. *J Thorac Cardiovasc Surg.* 2008;136:1442.

33. Blood components. In: Roseff SD, eds. *Pediatric Transfusion: A Physician's Handbook.* 3rd ed. Bethesda, MD: American Association of Blood Banks; 2009:1.

34. Cid J, Lozano M. Risk of Rh(D) alloimmunization after transfusion of platelets from D+ donors to D− recipients. *Transfusion.* 2005;3:453.

35. Sanchez R, Toy P. Transfusion related acute lung injury: a pediatric perspective. *Pediatr Blood Cancer.* 2005;45:248.

36. Kenton AB, Hegemier S, Smith EO, et al. Platelet transfusions in infants with necrotizing enterocolitis do not lower mortality but may increase morbidity. *J Perinatol.* 2005;25:173.

37. Mohan P, Brocklehurst P. Granulocyte transfusions for neonates with confirmed or suspected sepsis and neutropaenia. *Cochrane Database Syst Rev.* 2003;CD003956.

38. Poterjoy BS, Josephson CD. Platelets, frozen plasma, and cryoprecipitate: what is the clinical evidence for their use in the neonatal intensive care unit? *Semin Perinatol.* 2009;33:66.

39. Ramasethu J, Luban N. T activation. *Br J Haematol.* 2001;112:259.

40. Blood components. In: Roseff SD, eds. *Pediatric Transfusion: A Physician's Handbook.* 2nd ed. Bethesda, MD: American Association of Blood Banks; 2006:1.

41. Elbert C, Strauss RG, Barrett F, et al. Biological mothers may be dangerous blood donors for their neonates. *Acta Haematol.* 1991;85:189.

42. Luban NL. Management of anemia in the newborn. *Early Hum Dev.* 2008;84:493.

43. Aladangady N, McHugh S, Aitchison TC, et al. Infants' blood volume in a controlled trial of placental transfusion at preterm delivery. *Pediatrics.* 2006;117:93.

44. Rabe H, Reynolds G, Diaz-Rossello J. A systematic review and meta-analysis of a brief delay in clamping the umbilical cord of preterm infants. *Neonatology.* 2008;93:138.

45. Rabe H, Reynolds G, Diaz-Rossello J. Early versus delayed umbilical cord clamping in preterm infants. *Cochrane Database Syst Rev.* 2004;CD003248.

46. Eichler H, Schaible T, Richter E, et al. Cord blood as a source of autologous RBCs for transfusion to preterm infants. *Transfusion.* 2000;40:1111.

47. Nichols WG, Price TH, Gooley T, et al. Transfusion-transmitted cytomegalovirus infection after receipt of leukoreduced blood products. *Blood.* 2003;101:4195.

48. Fiebig EH, Busch MP. Infectious disease screening. In: Roback JD, eds. *Technical Manual of the American Association of Blood Banks.* 16th ed. Bethesda, MD: American Association of Blood Banks; 2008:241.

49. Busch MP, Glynn SA, Stramer SL, et al. A new strategy for estimating risks of transfusion-transmitted viral infections based on rates of detection of recently infected donors. *Transfusion.* 2005;45:254.

50. Busch MP, Kleinman SH, Nemo GJ. Current and emerging infectious risks of blood transfusions. *JAMA.* 2003;289:959.

51. Dodd RY. Current risk for transfusion transmitted infections. *Curr Opin Hematol.* 2007;14:671.

52. Bowden RA, Slichter SJ, Sayers M, et al. A comparison of filtered leukocyte-reduced and cytomegalovirus (CMV) seronegative blood products for the prevention of transfusion-associated CMV infection after marrow transplant. *Blood.* 1995;86:3598.

53. Fang CT, Chambers LA, Kennedy J, et al. Detection of bacterial contamination in apheresis platelet products: American Red Cross experience, 2004. *Transfusion.* 2005;45:1845.

54. Ludlam CA, Turner ML. Managing the risk of transmission of variant Creutzfeldt Jakob disease by blood products. *Br J Haematol.* 2006;132:13.

55. Yang X, Ahmed S, Chandrasekaran V. Transfusion-related acute lung injury resulting from designated blood transfusion between mother and child: a report of two cases. *Am J Clin Pathol.* 2004;121:590.

56. Roseff SD, Luban NL, Manno CS. Guidelines for assessing appropriateness of pediatric transfusion. *Transfusion.* 2002;42:1398.

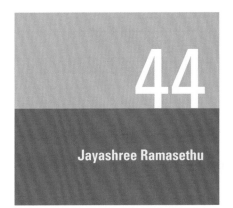

44

Exchange Transfusions

Jayashree Ramasethu

Advances in prenatal and postnatal care have led a marked decline in the frequency of exchange transfusions (ETs) in United States (1), resulting in significantly less experience in personnel performing the procedure (1). The reemergence of kernicterus as a public health problem underscores the importance of ET as a treatment modality that could potentially prevent devastating neurodevelopmental complications (2). In developing countries, ETs remain a vital therapeutic intervention (3,4).

A. Definitions

ET: Replacing the infant's blood with donor blood by repeatedly exchanging small aliquots of blood over a short time period.

B. Indications

1. Significant unconjugated hyperbilirubinemia in the newborn due to any cause, when intensive phototherapy fails or there is risk of acute bilirubin encephalopathy (5).
   a. Immediate ET may avert brain injury even when there are intermediate or advanced signs of acute bilirubin encephalopathy (6).
   b. Figure 44.1 indicates the total serum bilirubin levels at which ET is recommended for infants of 35 or more weeks' gestation.
   c. Indications for ET in more immature infants are variable and highly individualized, although some countries have attempted to establish uniform guidelines (7,8) (see Table 49.1).
2. Alloimmune hemolytic disease of the newborn (HDN) (9)
   a. For correction of severe anemia and hyperbilirubinemia
   b. In addition, in infants with alloimmune HDN, ET replaces antibody-coated neonatal red cells with antigen-negative red cells that should have normal in vivo survival and removes free maternal antibody in plasma

3. Severe anemia with congestive cardiac failure or hypervolemia (10)
4. Polycythemia
   Although partial exchange transfusion reduces the packed cell volume and hyperviscosity in neonates with polycythemia, there is no evidence of long-term benefit from the procedure (11).
5. Uncommon indications for which ET has been used
   a. Congenital leukemia (12)
   b. Extreme thrombocytosis (13)
   c. Neonatal hemochromatosis (14)
   d. Hyperammonemia (15)
   e. Organic acidemia (16)
   f. Lead poisoning (17)
   g. Renal failure (18)
   h. Drug overdose or toxicity (19)
   i. Removal of antibodies and abnormal proteins (20)
   j. Neonatal sepsis or malaria (21,22)

C. Contraindications

1. When alternatives such as simple transfusion or phototherapy would be just as effective with less risk
2. When patient is unstable and the risk of the procedure outweighs the possible benefit.
   Partial ET, particularly to correct severe anemia associated with cardiac failure or hypervolemia, can be used to stabilize the patient's condition before a complete or double volume ET is performed.
3. When a contraindication to placement of necessary lines outweighs indication for ET. Alternative access should be sought if ET is imperative.

D. Equipment

1. Infant care center (see Chapter 3)
   a. Automatic and manually controlled heat source
   b. Temperature monitor
   c. Cardiorespiratory monitor
   d. Pulse oximeter for oxygen saturation monitoring

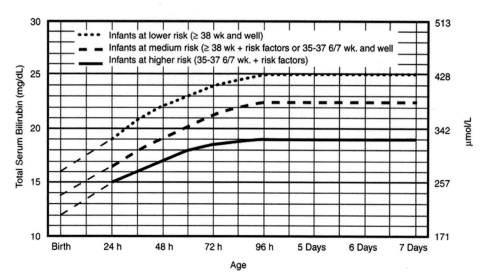

- The dashed lines for the first 24 hours indicate uncertainty due to a wide range of clinical circumstances and a range of responses to phototherapy.
- Immediate exchange transfusion is recommended if infant shows signs of acute bilirubin encephalopathy (hypertonia, arching, retrocollis, opisthotonos, fever, high pitched cry) or if TSB is ≥5 mg/dL (85 µmol/L) above these lines.
- Risk factors - isoimmune hemolytic disease, G6PD deficiency, asphyxia, significant lethargy, temperature instability, sepsis, acidosis.
- Measure serum albumin and calculate B/A ratio (See legend)
- Use total bilirubin. Do not subtract direct reacting or conjugated bilirubin
- If infant is well and 35-37 6/7 wk (median risk) can individualize TSB levels for exchange based on actual gestational age.

FIG. 44.1. Guidelines for exchange transfusion in infants 35 or more weeks gestation. (From American Academy of Pediatrics. Subcommittee on Hyperbiliru-binemia. Clinical Practice Guideline. Management of hyperbilirubinemia in the newborn infant 35 or more weeks gestation. *Pediatrics.* 2004;114:297.)

2. Resuscitation equipment and medication (immediately available)
3. Infant restraints
4. Orogastric tube
5. Suctioning equipment
6. Equipment for central and peripheral vascular access
7. Blood warmer and appropriate cartridge (see E7)
8. Sterile exchange transfusion equipment
   a. Preassembled disposable set with special four-way stopcock *or*
   b. Nonassembled
      (1) Two three-way stopcocks with locking connections
      (2) 5-, 10-, or 20-mL syringes
      (3) Waste receptacle (empty IV bottle or bag)
      (4) IV connecting tubing
9. Appropriate blood product
10. Syringes and tubes for pre- and postexchange blood tests

E. Precautions

1. Stabilize infant before initiating exchange procedure.
2. Do not start exchange procedure until personnel are available for monitoring and as backup for other emergencies.
3. Monitor infant closely during and after procedure.
4. Do not rush procedure.
   a. May necessitate repeat if efficacy is decreased by haste
   b. Stop or slow if patient becomes unstable.

5. Use blood product appropriate to clinical indication. Use freshest blood available, preferably <5 to 7 days.
6. Check potassium level of donor blood if patient has hyperkalemia or renal compromise.
7. Use only thermostatically controlled blood-warming device that has passed quality control for temperature and alarms. Be sure to review operating and safety procedures for specific blood warmer. Do not overheat blood (i.e., beyond 38°C).
8. Do not apply excessive suction if it becomes difficult to draw blood from line. Reposition line or replace syringes, stopcocks, and any adapters connected to line.
9. Leave anticoagulated, banked blood in line or clear line with heparinized saline if the procedure is interrupted.
10. Clear line with heparinized saline if administering calcium.

F. Preparation for Total or Partial Exchange Transfusion

1. Blood Product and Volume

Blood Product

   a. Communicate with blood bank or transfusion medicine specialist to determine most appropriate blood product for transfusion.
      (1) Plasma reduced whole blood or packed red cells reconstituted with plasma may be used (23).

(2) Blood may be anticoagulated with citrate phosphate dextrose (CPD or CPDA1) or heparin (heparinized blood is not licensed for use in the United States). Additive anticoagulant solutions are generally avoided; if there is no other option, packed red cells stored in additive solutions may be washed or hard packed prior to reconstitution for ET (24).

(3) Hematocrit (Hct) may be adjusted within the range of 45% to 60%, depending on desired end result.

(4) Blood should be as fresh as possible (<7 days)

(5) Irradiated blood is recommended for all ET to prevent graft-versus-host disease. There is a significant increase in potassium concentration in stored irradiated units, so irradiation should be performed as close to the transfusion as possible (<24 hours).

(6) Standard blood-bank screening is particularly important, including sickle cell preparation, HIV, hepatitis B, and CMV.

(7) Donor blood should be screened for G-6-PD deficiency and HbS in populations endemic for these conditions (25).

b. In presence of alloimmunization (e.g., Rh, ABO) special attention to compatibility testing is necessary (9)

(1) If delivery of an infant with severe HDN is anticipated, O Rh-negative blood cross-matched against the mother may be prepared before the baby is born.

(2) Donor blood prepared after the infant's birth should be negative for the antigen responsible for the hemolytic disease and should be cross-matched against the infant.

(3) In ABO HDN, the blood must be type O and either Rh-negative or Rh-compatible with the mother and the infant. The blood should be washed free of plasma or have a low titer of anti-A or anti-B antibodies. Type O cells may be used with AB plasma, but this results in two donor exposures per ET.

(4) In Rh HDN, the blood should be Rh-negative and may be O group or the same group as the infant.

c. In infants with polycythemia, the optimal dilutional fluid is isotonic saline rather than plasma or albumin (26).

Volume of Donor Blood Required

a. Whenever possible, use no more than the equivalent of one whole unit of blood for each procedure, to decrease donor exposure.

b. Quantity needed for total procedure = volume for the actual ET plus volume for tubing dead space and blood warmer (usually an additional 25 to 30 mL)

c. Double volume ET for removal of bilirubin, antibodies, etc.

$$2 \times \text{infant's blood volume} = 2 \times 80 - 120 \text{ mL/kg}$$

(Infant's blood volume in preterm infant $\cong$100 to 120 mL/kg, in term infant $\cong$80 to 85 mL/kg)

Exchanges approximately 85% of infant's blood volume (Fig. 44.2)

d. *Single-volume ET*: Exchanges approximately 60% of infant's blood volume (Fig. 44.2)

e. Partial ET for correction of severe anemia

$$\text{Volume (mL)} = \frac{\text{Infants blood volume} \times (\text{Hb desired} - \text{Hb initial})}{\text{Hb of PRBC} - \text{Hb initial}}$$

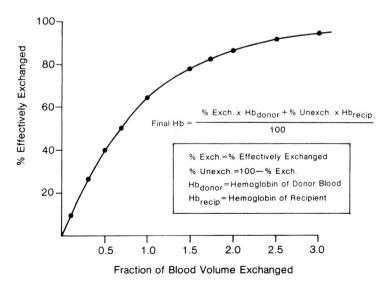

FIG. 44.2. Graph depicting the effectiveness of exchange transfusion against the fraction of blood volume exchanged. The formula permits the calculation of the final hemoglobin.

f. Single-volume or partial ET for correction of poly-cythemia

Volume (mL) =

$$\frac{\text{Infants blood volume} \times \text{desired HCT change}}{\text{Initial HCT}}$$

4. Preparation of Infant

a. Place infant on warmer with total accessibility and controlled environment. ET on small preterm infants may be performed in warm incubators, provided a sterile field can be maintained and lines are easily accessible.

b. Restrain infant suitably. Sedation and pain relief are not usually required. Conscious infants may suck on a pacifier during the procedure.

c. Connect physiologic monitors and establish baseline values (temperature, respiratory and heart rates, oxygen saturation by pulse oximetry).

d. Empty infant's stomach.
   (1) Do not feed for 4 hours prior to procedure, if possible.
   (2) Place orogastric tube, remove gastric contents, and leave on open drainage.

e. Start peripheral IV line for glucose and medication infusion.
   (1) If exchange procedure interrupts previous essential infusion rate
   (2) If prolonged lack of enteral feeds or parenteral glucose will lead to hypoglycemia
   (3) Extra IV line may be necessary for emergency medications.

f. Stabilize infant prior to starting exchange procedure (e.g., give packed-cell transfusion when severe hypovolemia and anemia are present); modify ventilator or ambient oxygen as required.

g. The use of albumin infusions prior to ET to improve bilirubin binding remains controversial (27).

3. Establish Access for ET

a. *Push–pull technique:* Central access—usually through umbilical venous catheter (UVC).

b. Isovolumetric exchange with simultaneous infusion of donor blood through venous line and removal of baby's blood through arterial line. This technique may be better tolerated in sick or unstable neonates because there is less fluctuation of blood pressure and cerebral hemodynamics (28). The technique is also favored when only peripheral vascular access is available or it is preferred for various reasons (29,30).
   (1) Infusion of donor blood may be through UVC or peripheral IV catheter.
   (2) Removal of baby's blood may be from umbilical arterial or venous catheter, or peripheral arterial catheter, usually a radial arterial line.

4. Laboratory Tests on Infants Blood Pre-exchange

Tests are based on clinical indications.

a. Pre-exchange diagnostic studies. Note that diagnostic serological tests on the infant, such as studies to evaluate unexplained hemolysis, antiviral antibody titers, neonatal metabolic screening, or genetic tests should be drawn prior to the ET.

b. Hemoglobin, hematocrit, platelets

c. Electrolytes, calcium, blood gas

d. Glucose

e. Bilirubin

f. Coagulation profile

5. Prepare Blood

a. Verify identification of blood product (see Chapter 43).
   (1) Type and cross-match data
   (2) Expiration date
   (3) Donor and recipient identities

b. Attach blood administration set to blood-warmer tubing and to blood bag.

c. Allow blood to run through blood warmer.

G. Technique (See also Website for Procedure Video)

Exchange Transfusion by Push–Pull Technique through Special Stopcock with Preassembled Tray

1. Read instructions provided by manufacturer carefully.

2. Wear head cover and mask. Scrub as for major procedure. Wear sterile gown and gloves.

3. Open preassembled equipment tray, using aseptic technique.

4. Identify positions on special stopcock in clockwise rotation (Figs. 44.3 and 44.4). The direction that the handle is pointing indicates the port that is open to syringe. The special stopcock allows clockwise rotation in the order used: (a) withdraw from patient, (b) clear to waste bag, (c) draw new blood, (d) inject into patient. Always rotate in clockwise direction to follow proper sequence, and keep connections tight.
   a. Male adapter to umbilical or peripheral line
   b. Female adapter to the extension tubing to which waste bag will be attached.
   c. Connection to tubing for attachment to blood-warmer coil
   d. Neutral "off" position in which additives may be administered through rubber stopper (180 degrees from waste-receptacle port)

5. Follow steps as illustrated by manufacturer to make all connections to blood and waste bags.

6. With stopcock open to blood source, clear all air into syringe. Turn in clockwise direction 270 degrees and evacuate into waste.

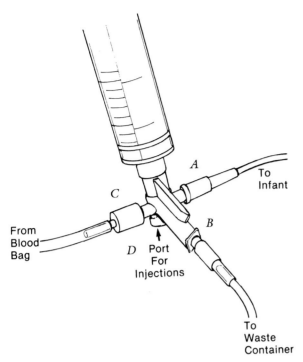

FIG. 44.3. Special four-way stopcock. **A:** Male adapter to infant line. **B:** Female adapter to waste container. **C:** Attachment to blood tubing. **D:** "Off" position (180 degrees from adapter to waste container), allowing injection through rubber-stoppered port "below" syringe. The stopcock is used in clockwise rotation when correctly assembled.

7. Turn stopcock to "off," and replace onto sterile field.
8. Use pre-existing umbilical venous line or insert UVC, as described in Chapter 30.
   a. Place a single-lumen UVC whenever possible. The internal lumen of a double-lumen UVC is smaller and makes it more difficult to perform the ET.
   b. Consider central venous pressure (CVP) measurement, using pressure transducer, in unstable baby.
   c. Place catheter in inferior vena cava (IVC) and verify position by radiograph.
   d. If catheter cannot be positioned in IVC, it may still be used cautiously in an emergency, when placed in the umbilical vein, if adequate blood return is obtained.
9. Have an assistant document all vital signs, in and out volumes, and other data, on the exchange record.
10. Check peripheral glucose levels every 30 to 60 minutes. Monitor cardiorespiratory status, continuous pulse oximetry. Determine blood gases as often as indicated by pre-existing clinical condition and stability.
11. Draw blood for diagnostic studies.
12. Usual rate of removal and replacement of blood during the ET is 5 mL/kg over a 2- to 4-minute cycle.
13. If infant is hypovolemic or has low CVP, start exchange with transfusion of aliquot into catheter. If infant is hypervolemic or has high CVP, start by withdrawing precalculated aliquot.
14. Remeasure CVP if indicated. Expect rise as plasma oncotic pressure increases, if CVP low at start.
15. Ensure that the stages of drawing and infusing blood from and into the infant are done slowly, taking at least a minute each to avoid fluctuations in blood pressure. Rapid fluctuations in arterial pressure in the push–pull technique may be accompanied by changes in intracranial pressure (28). Rapid withdrawal from the umbilical vein induces a negative pressure that may be transmitted to the mesenteric veins and contribute to the high incidence of ischemic bowel complications.
16. Gently agitate the blood bag every 10 to 15 minutes to prevent red cell sedimentation, which may lead to exchange with relatively anemic blood toward the end of the exchange.
17. Consider giving calcium supplement.
   a. When hypocalcemia is documented

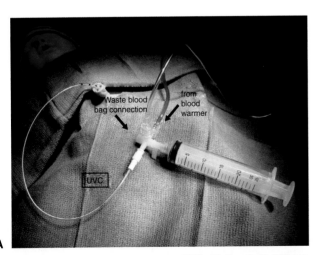

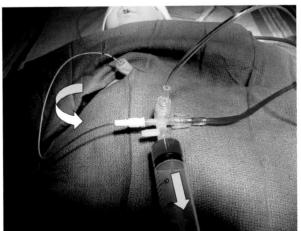

FIG. 44.4. **A, B:** ET using special four-way stopcock.

b. With symptoms or signs of hypocalcemia
   (1) Change in QTc interval
   (2) *Agitation and tachycardia:* These symptoms are not reliably correlated with ionized calcium levels.

   It is rarely necessary or advantageous to give calcium during an ET if the infant is normocalcemic. When administered, the effect may last only a few minutes. Calcium will reverse the effect of the anticoagulant in the donor blood and may cause clotting of the line, so administration through a peripheral IV line is preferred. If calcium is given through the UVC, prior to administration, clear the line of donor blood with 0.9% NaCl. Give 1 mL of 10% calcium gluconate per kilogram body weight. Administer slowly, with careful observation of heart rate and rhythm. Clear line again with 0.9% NaCl.

18. Perform calculated number of passes, until desired volume has been exchanged.
19. Be sure there is adequate volume of donor blood remaining to infuse after last withdrawal, if a positive intravascular balance is desired.
20. Clear umbilical line of banked blood and withdraw amount of infant's blood needed for laboratory testing, including re-cross-matching.
21. Infuse IV fluids with 0.5 to 1 U heparin/mL of fluid through UVC if further ETs are anticipated.

22. *Total duration for double volume ET:* 90 to 120 minutes.
23. Document procedure in patient's hospital record.

Exchange Transfusion Using a Single Umbilical Line and Two Three-Way Stopcocks in Tandem

The principles and techniques for using either the special stopcock or two three-way stopcocks in tandem are the same. It is important to ensure that all junctions are tight to produce a closed, sterile system. It is also essential to understand the working positions of the stopcocks before starting the exchange.

1. Scrub as for major procedure. Wear sterile gown and gloves.
2. Attach stopcock and tubing in sequence (Fig. 44.5).
   a. Proximal stopcock
      (1) Umbilical catheter
      (2) IV extension tubing to sterile waste container
   b. Distal stopcock
      (1) Tubing from blood-warming coil
      (2) 10- or 20-mL syringe
3. Clear lines of air bubbles.
4. Start exchange record.
5. Follow steps of push–pull technique until exchange is completed.

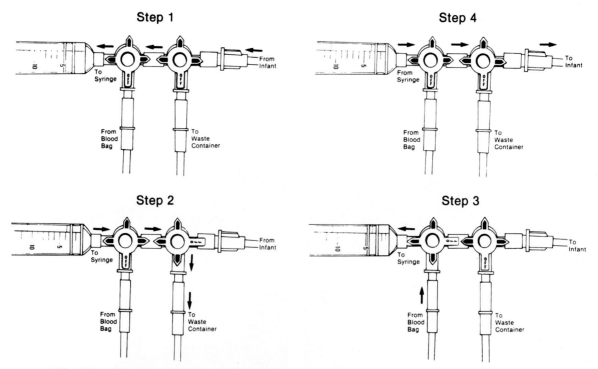

FIG. 44.5. Three-way stopcocks in tandem. *Step 1:* Stopcocks positioned for withdrawing blood from infant. *Step 2:* Stopcocks positioned for emptying withdrawn blood to waste container. *Step 3:* Stopcocks positioned for filling syringe from blood bag. *Step 4:* Stopcocks positioned for injecting blood into infant line.

Exchange Transfusion by Isovolumetric Technique (Central or Peripheral Lines)

1. Scrub as for major procedure.
2. Select two sites for line placement, and insert (See page 320).
   a. Venous for infusion
      (1) UVC or
      (2) Peripheral IV that is at least 23 gauge
   b. Arterial for removal
      (1) Umbilical artery catheter
      (2) Peripheral, usually radial if infant's size permits
3. Connect arterial line to three-way stopcock.
   a. Use short, connecting IV tubing to extend peripheral line.
   b. Attach additional connecting tubing to stopcock and place into sterile waste container.
   c. Attach empty 3- to 10-mL syringe to stopcock, for withdrawal of blood.

      An additional stopcock may also be placed on this port so that a syringe of heparinized saline (5 U/mL) may be attached for use as needed. Be cautious about total volume infused.
4. Connect venous line to single, three-way stopcock, which in turn connects to empty 5- to 10-mL syringe and to blood-warming coil.
5. Start exchange-transfusion record.
6. Withdraw and discard blood from arterial side at rate of 2 to 3 mL/kg/min, and infuse at same rate into venous side. Keep flow as steady as possible, and volumetrically equal for infusion and removal.
7. Intermittently, flush arterial line with heparinized saline to clear.

   The heparin solution remaining in tubing will be removed with next withdrawal, thus reducing significantly the total heparin dose actually received by the patient.
8. Follow steps as for push–pull technique until exchange is complete.
9. *Total duration for isovolumetric ET:* 45 to 60 minutes, may be longer in sick, unstable infant.

H. Postexchange for All Techniques

1. Continue to monitor vital signs closely for at least 4 to 6 hours.
2. *Rewrite orders:* Adjust any drug dosages as needed to compensate for removal by exchange.
3. Keep infant NPO for at least 4 hours. Restart feeds if clinically stable. Monitor abdominal girth and bowel sounds every 3 to 4 hours for next 24 hours if exchange has been performed using umbilical vascular lines. Observe for signs of feeding intolerance.
4. Monitor serum glucose levels every 2 to 4 hours for 24 hours.
5. Repeat blood gases as often as clinically indicated.
6. Measure serum ionized calcium levels and platelet counts in sick infants immediately after the ET and then as indicated.
7. Repeat hemoglobin, hematocrit, and bilirubin measurements approximately 4 hours after exchange, and further as clinically indicated. A double-volume ET replaces 85% of the infant's blood volume but eliminates only about 50% of the intravascular bilirubin. Equilibration of intra- and extravascular bilirubin and continued breakdown of sensitized and newly formed red cells by persisting maternal antibody results in a rebound of bilirubin levels following initial ET and may necessitate repeated ET in severe HDN.

I. Complications

1. Risk of death or permanent serious sequelae is estimated to be <1% in healthy infants, but as high as 12% in sick infants. There may be some uncertainty in ascribing adverse events to the ET in infants who are already critically ill (1,31)
2. Many of the adverse events are hematologic or biochemical laboratory abnormalities which may be asymptomatic. The most common adverse effects noted during or soon after the ET, usually in infants who are preterm and/or sick.
   a. Apnea and/or bradycardia
   b. Hypocalcemia
   c. Thrombocytopenia (<50,000 in 10% of healthy infants, up to 67% in infants <32 weeks' gestational age)
   d. Metabolic acidosis
   e. Vascular spasm
3. Complications reported from ET are related to the blood transfusion and to complications of vascular access (see Chapters 29, 30, and 43).
4. Potential complications include
   a. *Metabolic:* Hypocalcemia, hypo- or hyperglycemia, hyperkalemia
   b. *Cardiorespiratory:* Apnea, bradycardia, hypotension, hypertension
   c. *Hematologic:* Thrombocytopenia, dilutional coagulopathy, neutropenia, disseminated intravascular coagulation
   d. *Vascular catheter related:* Vasospasm, thrombosis, embolization
   e. *Gastrointestinal:* Feeding intolerance, ischemic injury, necrotizing enterocolitis
   f. *Infection:* Omphalitis, septicemia

References

1. Steiner LA, Bizzarro MJ, Ehrenkrantz RA, et al. A decline in the frequency of neonatal exchange transfusions and its effect on exchange transfusion related morbidity and mortality. *Pediatrics.* 2007;120:27.
2. Johnson L, Bhutani VK, Karp K, et al. Clinical report from the pilot USA Kernicterus Registry (1992 to 2004). *J Perinatol.* 2009; 29:S25.

3. Owa JA, Ogunlesi TA. Why are we still doing so many exchange blood transfusions for neonatal jaundice in Nigeria. *World J Pediatr.* 2009;5:51.

4. Gamaleldin R, Iskander I, Seoud I, et al. Risk factors for neurotoxicity in newborns with severe neonatal hyperbilirubinemia. *Pediatrics.* 2011;128:e925.

5. American Academy of Pediatrics. Subcommittee on Hyperbilirubinemia. Clinical Practice Guideline. Management of hyperbilirubinemia in the newborn infant 35 or more weeks gestation. *Pediatrics.* 2004;114:297.

6. Hansen TW, Nietsch L, Norman E, et al. Reversibility of acute intermediate phase bilirubin encephalopathy. *Acta Paediatr.* 2009;98:1689.

7. Watchko JF, Maisels J. Enduring controversies in the management of hyperbilirubinemia in preterm neonates. *Semin Fetal Neonatal Med.* 2010;15:136.

8. Van Imhoff DE, Dijk PH, Hulzebos CV, BARTrial study group, Netherlands Neonatal research Network. Uniform treatment thresholds for hyperbilirubinemia in preterm infants: background and synopsis of a national guideline. *Early Hum Dev.* 2011;87:521.

9. Ramasethu J, Luban NLC. Alloimmune hemolytic disease of the newborn. In: Kaushansky K, Lichtman MA, Beutler E, et al., eds. *Williams' Hematology.* 8th ed. New York: McGraw-Hill; 2010:799.

10. Naulaers G, Barten S, Vanhole C, et al. Management of severe neonatal anemia due to fetomaternal transfusion. *Am J Perinatol.* 1999;16:193.

11. Ozek E, Soll R, Schimmel MS. Partial exchange transfusion to prevent neurodevelopmental disability in infants with polycythemia. *Cochrane Database Syst Rev.* 2010;20:CD005089.

12. Sugiura T, Goto K, Nichonji T et al. Cytokine profiles before and after exchange transfusion in a neonate with transient myeloproliferative disorder and hepatic fibrosis. *J Pediatr Hematol Oncol.* 2010;32:e164.

13. Park ES, Kim SY, Yeom JS, et al. Extreme thrombocytosis associated with transient myeloproliferative disorder with Down syndrome with t(11;17)(q13;q21). *Pediatr Blood Cancer.* 2008;50:643.

14. Rand EB, Karpen SJ, Kelly S, et al. Treatment of neonatal hemochromatosis with exchange transfusion and intravenous immunoglobulin. *J Pediatr.* 2009;155:566.

15. Chen CY, Chen YC, Fang JT, et al. Continuous arteriovenous hemodiafiltration in the acute treatment of hyperammonemia due to ornithine transcarbamylase deficiency. *Ren Fail.* 2000;22:823.

16. Aikoh H, Sasaki M, Sugai K, et al. Effective immunoglobulin therapy for brief tonic seizures in methylmalonic acidemia. *Brain Dev.* 1997;19:502.

17. Chinnakaruppan NR, Marcus SM. Asymptomatic congenital lead poisoning- case report. *Clin Toxicol (Phila).* 2010;48:563.

18. Demirel G, Erdeve O, Utras N, et al. Exchange transfusion as rescue therapy in a severely premature child with acute renal failure. *Pediatr Nephrol.* 2011;26:821.

19. Sancak R, Kucukoduk S, Tasdemir HA, et al. Exchange transfusion treatment in a newborn with phenobarbital intoxication. *Pediatr Emerg Care.* 1999;15:268.

20. Dolfin T, Pomerance A, Korzets Z, et al. Acute renal failure in a neonate caused by the transplacental transfer of a nephrotoxic paraprotein: successful resolution by exchange transfusion. *Am J Kidney Dis.* 1999;34:1129.

21. Gunes T, Koklu E, Buyukkayhan D, et al. Exchange transfusion or intravenous immunoglobulin therapy as an adjunct to antibiotics for neonatal sepsis in developing countries: a pilot study. *Ann Trop Paediatr.* 2006;26:39.

22. Virdi VS, Goraya JS, Khadwal A, et al. Neonatal transfusion malaria requiring exchange transfusion. *Ann Trop Pediatr.* 2003;23:205.

23. Carson TH, ed. *Standards for Blood Banks and Transfusion services.* 27th ed. Bethesda, MD: American Association of Blood Banks; 2011.

24. Win N, Amess P, Needs M, et al. Use of red cells preserved in extended storage media for exchange transfusion in anti-k haemolytic disease of the newborn. *Transfus Med.* 2005;15:157.

25. Samanta S, Kumar P, Kishore SS, et al. Donor blood glucose 6-phosphate dehydrogenase deficiency reduces the efficacy of exchange transfusion in neonatal hyperbilirubinemia. *Pediatrics.* 2009;123:e96.

26. De Waal KA, Baerts W, Offringa M. Systematic review of the optimal fluid for dilutional exchange transfusion in neonatal polycythemia. *Arch Dis Child Fetal Neonatal Ed.* 2006;91:F7.

27. Mitra S, Samantha M, Sarkar M, et al. Pre- exchange 5% albumin infusion in low birth weight neonates with intensive phototherapy failure—a randomized controlled trial. *J Trop Pediatr.* 2011;57:217.

28. Murakami Y, Yamashita Y, Nishimi T, et al. Changes in cerebral hemodynamics and oxygenation in unstable septic newborns during exchange transfusion. *Kurume Med J.* 1998;45:321.

29. Weng YH, Chiu YW. Comparison of efficacy and safety of exchange transfusion through different catheterizations: femoral vein versus umbilical vein versus umbilical artery/vein. *Pediatr Crit Care Med.* 2011;12:61.

30. Chen HN, Lee ML, Tsao LY. Exchange transfusion using peripheral vessels is safe and effective in newborn infants. *Pediatrics.* 2008;122:e905.

31. Patra K, Storfer- Isser A, Siner B, et al. Adverse events associated with neonatal exchange transfusion in the 1990s. *J Pediatr.* 2004;144:626.

IX Miscellaneous Procedures

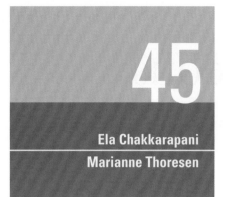

45

Brain and Whole Body Cooling

Ela Chakkarapani

Marianne Thoresen

Moderate therapeutic hypothermia (HT; rectal or esophageal temperature 33.5°C) initiated within 6 hours and continued for 72 hours reduces death or disability (NNT 6, 95% CI 5 to 9) and increases the number of survivors with normal neurology after perinatal asphyxia (NNT 8, 95% CI 5 to 17) (1–6). HT is delivered in newborn infants as whole body cooling (WBC) using different types of mattresses or wraps around the body, or as selective head cooling (SHC) using a "coolcap" around the head (1–3).

A. Indications

To decrease death or disability in the following group of infants (1–3)
  a. ≥36 weeks' gestation newborn infants <6 hours of age
  b. Evidence of asphyxia (at least one of the four criteria below must be met)
    (1) Apgar score at 10 minutes of age ≤5
    (2) Worst arterial or capillary or venous pH within 60 minutes of life <7
    (3) Arterial or capillary or venous base deficit within 60 minutes of life ≥12 or 16
    (4) Ventilated or resuscitated for at least the first 10 minutes after birth
and c **or** d
  c. Moderate or severe encephalopathy characterized by
    (1) Abnormal consciousness—lethargy or stupor or coma **and**
    (2) Hypotonia or abnormal reflexes (including oculomotor or pupillary abnormalities), or decreased/absent spontaneous activity, or abnormal (distal flexion/complete extension/decerebrate) posture, or absent/weak suck, or incomplete/absent moro **or**
  d. Clinical seizures
and
  e. 30 minutes abnormal background activity or seizures in amplitude-integrated electroencephalogram (aEEG) (Fig. 45.1)
    If aEEG is unavailable or not used as entry criteria (2), offer therapeutic HT to infants satisfying criteria a, b, and c or d.

B. Contraindications

1. Major congenital anomalies. However, local guidelines might differ. Some centers offer therapeutic HT to term infants with surgical, cardiac, chromosomal or sudden unexpected postnatal collapse, who have suffered significant perinatal asphyxial encephalopathy and whose intensive care will be continued (e.g., infant with surgical condition, ventilated asphyxiated infant with tracheoesophageal fistula requiring imminent surgery) (7), have a cardiac condition (e.g., infant with transposition of great arteries with tight atrial septum leading to hypoxic-ischemic encephalopathy), have a chromosomal condition (e.g., infant with trisomy 21 with perinatal asphyxia), and infants suffering postnatal collapse (e.g., sudden unexpected neonatal cardiorespiratory arrest leading to hypoxic-ischemic encephalopathy) unless HT might adversely influence the effect(s) of other required treatment (8).
2. Syndromes involving brain dysgenesis
3. Infants in moribund state.

C. Cooling at Birth

If the infant fulfills criteria (b) in Section A by 10 minutes of age, initiate passive HT.
  a. Switch off heater in the Resuscitaire/transport incubator.
  b. Do not wrap or cover the head with hat (9).
  c. Insert rectal or esophageal temperature probe as early as possible.

D. Cooling During Transport

1. Refer the infant to a center offering therapeutic HT as soon as possible.
2. Provide the required cardiorespiratory support, and use passive or other (see G–I) cooling method to achieve the target temperature early and maintain target temperature during transport (10).

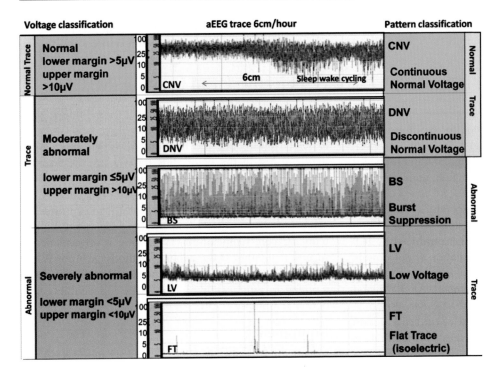

Voltage classification	aEEG trace 6cm/hour	Pattern classification	
Normal Trace — **Normal** lower margin >5μV upper margin >10μV	CNV ← 6cm → Sleep wake cycling	**CNV** **Continuous Normal Voltage**	**Normal Trace**
Trace — **Moderately abnormal**	DNV	**DNV** **Discontinuous Normal Voltage**	
lower margin ≤5μV upper margin >10μV	BS	**BS** **Burst Suppression**	**Abnormal Trace**
Abnormal — **Severely abnormal**	LV	**LV** **Low Voltage**	
lower margin <5μV upper margin <10μV	FT	**FT** **Flat Trace (isoelectric)**	

FIG. 45.1. Amplitude integrated electroencephalogram trace showing both voltage and pattern classification. Both infants with moderately and severely abnormal tracings will be eligible for cooling (from ref 13).

E. Securing Rectal Temperature Sensor

1. Measure and mark the rectal temperature sensor (tape bridge) (Fig. 45.2A).
2. Insert to 6 cm into the infant's rectum, after lubricating the tip of the sensor (Fig. 45.2B).

3. Secure the bridge to the infant's buttocks with tape (Fig. 45.2C).
4. Secure a DuoDERM/Tegaderm dressing (4 × 4 cm) on the infant's thigh and fix the sensor over the DuoDERM/Tegaderm with tape (Fig. 45.2E).
5. Insert a second rectal probe to 6 cm (Fig. 45.2 F), to be connected to the patient monitor to double check the

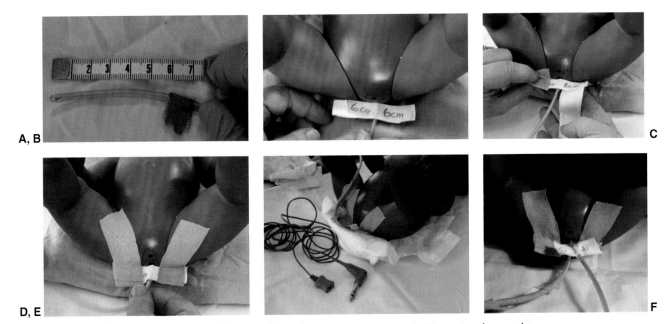

FIG. 45.2. Insertion and fixation of rectal temperature sensors. **A:** Measuring the rectal temperature sensor probe to 6 cm and marking with tape. **B:** The 6-cm mark on the rectal temperature sensor is identified by a bridge of tape. **C, D:** Securing the bridge on the rectal temperature sensor onto the buttock of the infant. **E:** Securing the rectal temperature sensor to the thigh. **F:** Insertion of the second rectal probe.

readings from the rectal probe connected to the cooling machine.

F. Supportive Intensive Care with HT

1. *Provide airway support and monitoring:* Appropriate respiratory support with ventilator or continuous positive airway pressure, and monitoring of transcutaneous oxygen saturation, pulmonary function, end-tidal CO_2, and arterial blood gases.
2. Maintain PCO_2 corrected for temperature >35 mm Hg (11) (PCO_2 at 33.5°C is approximately PCO_2 at 37°C × 0.83). The reduction in metabolism induced by HT can result in hypocapnia if ventilation is not closely monitored.
3. *Provide cardiac monitoring and support:* Arterial blood pressure, cardiac output, systemic vascular resistance monitoring, and adequate support of cardiac function and perfusion with inotropes, if necessary. Heart rate is reduced by approximately 10 beats/1°C during HT.

    Expected heart rate for cooled infants will be 80 to 100 beats per minute; however, inotropic support will increase the heart rate (12).
4. *Provide aEEG and EEG monitoring:* Use single- or two-channel aEEG recording to assess the background activity and monitor the time to normalization of background activity (13), identify seizures, and monitor the effect of anticonvulsants.
5. Actively monitor and treat clinical and electrical seizures, because seizures worsen neurodevelopmental outcome independent of the severity of hypoxic-ischemic brain injury (14). The serum drug levels of anticonvulsants should be monitored closely because HT reduces metabolism of drugs by the liver.
6. Monitor blood glucose and treat hypoglycemia. Hypoglycemia is common in severely asphyxiated infants, particularly within the first 24 hours (15).
7. Monitor serum electrolytes and maintain serum magnesium ≥1 mmol/L, as this may improve the neuroprotection (16).
8. Treat coagulopathy.
9. Sedate the cooled infants with appropriate sedatives to avoid cold stress.

    Experimental evidence shows that lack of sedation during HT may abolish the neuroprotective effect (17).
10. Monitor urine output. Catheterization may be necessary to maintain accurate fluid balance in sedated cooled infants.
11. Monitor core, surface, and scalp temperature (if on head cooling) every 15 minutes during induction and maintenance phases of HT, and during rewarming in manual modes. In servo modes, core, surface, and scalp temperatures can be monitored every 30 minutes during maintenance phase of HT.
12. Monitor skin for changes, and change the position of the infant every 8 hours to avoid pressure sores.

G. Selective Head Cooling (SHC)

SHC with mild systemic hypothermia (rectal temperature 34°C to 35°C) was the first method in clinical use and aims to selectively reduce the temperature of the brain more than the rest of the body, thus minimizing the systemic adverse effects of HT (18). It is currently not feasible to accurately measure temperature in different parts of the brain, and the large size of the infant's head can preclude achieving significant cooling in the deep brain without reducing core temperature (19). There is no evidence to suggest that either of the cooling methods (SHC or WBC) is superior to the other. SHC with mild HT has been reported to significantly reduce death and disability after perinatal asphyxia (1,20).

Equipment

1. Olympic Cool-Cap system (Figs. 45.3 and 45.4) (Natus Medical Incorporated, San Carlos, California)
    a. Olympic Cool-Cap system (control unit and cooling unit) (Fig. 45.3)
    b. Radiant warmer with skin/servo temperature sensor (Fig. 45.4)
    c. Bag of sterile water, 1 L (Fig. 45.3)
    d. *Cool-Cap:* Soft cap with water circulating channels (Fig. 45.5A, B)
    e. *Water cap retainer:* Ensures maximum surface area contact between the water cap and the infant's scalp (Fig. 45.5C)
    f. *Outer insulator cap:* Reflects external heat from the radiant warmer (Fig. 45.6A)
    g. *Heat shield:* Reflective shield to place over head and neck to block heat from the radiant warmer (Fig. 45.6B)
    h. *Connecting tubes:* Main hose pumps water in and out of the cooling unit (Fig. 45.3); cap connector tubes connect the cap to the main hose and feed water in and out of the water cap (Fig. 45.5A, B).
    i. Main hose support (Fig. 45.4)
    j. Spiked fill tube (Fig. 45.3)
    k. Cap tube support (optional) (Fig. 45.4)
    l. Disposable module clips
    m. Temperature sensor module (TSM) (Fig. 45.4)
    n. *Temperature probes:* To monitor rectal, scalp, and skin temperature, Tempheart shields (Fig. 45.4)
    o. DuoDERM/Tegaderm or comparable dressing
    p. Adhesive tape
    q. Rectal lubricant
    r. *Optional sensors:* Yellow Springs Instrument Co. (YSI)-compatible temperature sensors, esophageal, nasopharyngeal

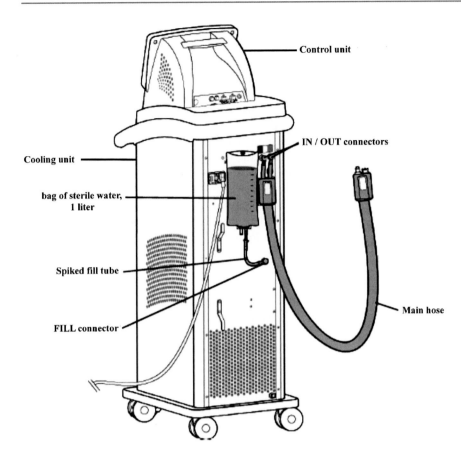

FIG. 45.3. CoolCap (Olympic) system—rear side showing control and cooling unit.

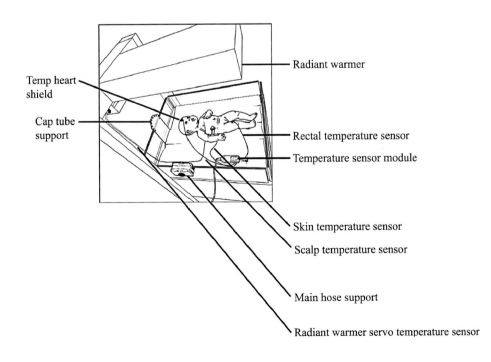

FIG. 45.4. Infant preparation for CoolCap. Infant placed in a radiant warmer bed with core, skin, radiant warmer, and scalp temperature sensor connected to the infant and the temperature sensor module.

Technique

1. Place infant in open crib with appropriate cardiorespiratory support and diaper removed (Fig. 45.4).
2. Place the radiant warmer bed in a flat horizontal position (Fig. 45.4), with the warmer turned off.
3. Lock the caster brakes on the cooling unit.
4. Plug in the power cord, and press the power switch to the *on* position.
5. Touch *set up* in the control unit (Fig. 45.3).
6. Enter *Patient information* for the setup wizard displays.
   a. *Required infant data:* Weight and *gestational* age.
   b. *Optional data (can be entered during treatment):* Patient name, ID, date and time of birth, clinical data and names of the optional sensors in use (see Equipment, above).
   c. Touch *Next.*
7. Connect *Temperature sensors,* for the setup wizard displays.
   a. Connect the TSM to the control unit aligning the red dots, then attach the TSM to the infant's bedding using the TSM clip (Figs. 45.3 and 45.4).
   b. Connect the *rectal temperature sensor* to the module.
   c. Secure rectal temperature sensor (see E).
   d. Connect the *scalp temperature sensor* to the TSM (Fig. 45.4).
   e. Position the tip of the sensor lateral to the anterior fontanel to allow cerebral ultrasound.
   f. Apply DuoDERM/Tegaderm over the sensor.
   g. Apply Tempheart shield (supplied with Cool-Cap equipment), with the tip pointing toward the back of infant's head. Any generic sensor shield can be used.
   h. Plug the *skin temperature* sensor into the TSM (Fig. 45.4).
   i. Position the tip of the skin sensor over the liver on the anterior abdominal wall.
   j. Plug the radiant warmer temperature servo probe into the radiant warmer.
   k. Place the tip of the radiant warmer servo probe by the side of the skin probe.
   l. Apply Tempheart shields over the skin and radiant warmer servo probes.
   m. Connect optional temperature sensors, such as esophageal, nasopharyngeal, or tympanic sensors, to the TSM.
   n. After confirming that each task is complete, touch *next.*
8. Enter *Cap temperature,* for the setup wizard displays (see Table 45.1).

   a. Cap temperature might have to be set higher, depending on infant's general condition (e.g., administration of drugs such as anticonvulsants, cardiac impairment requiring inotropes) to avoid overshooting of core temperature.
   b. Touch ▲ to increase or ▼ to decrease the water temperature. Each touch will increase or decrease the desired cap water temperature by 0.1°C.
   c. When the desired cap water temperature displays, touch *next.*
9. *Make the water connections,* for the setup wizard displays.
   a. *Installing main hose support (Figs. 45.3 and 45.4)*
      (1) Place the main hose support on the wall of the warmer bed, with the black inner foam contacting the wall.
      (2) Rotate the knob clockwise to tighten the support.
      (3) Position the main hose support so that there is an easy access to the back of the cooling unit.
   b. *Placing Cap tube support (Fig. 45.4):* Slide the cap tube support as far under the mattress as possible.
   c. *Filling the cooling unit with sterile water (Fig. 45.3)*
      (1) Spike a new 1-L sterile water bag with fill tube.
      (2) Hang the bag on the back of the cooling unit.
      (3) Connect the spiked fill tube to the FILL connector.
      (4) Clear any kinks in the tube.
   d. *Making main hose connections (Figs. 45.3 and 45.4)*
      (1) Slide the dovetail of the main hose into the dovetail slot on the back of the cooling unit.
      (2) Connect the main hose to the cooling unit—red to *In,* blue to *Out.*
      (3) Slide the dovetail of the distal end of the main hose into the dovetail slot of the main hose support.
   e. *Making Cap connections*
      (1) Select the appropriate cap size based on weight and head circumference (Table 45.2).
      (2) Slide the cap connector tubes fully onto the water cap flanges; red to red, blue to blue (Fig. 45.5A).
      (3) Connect the cap connector tubes to the main hose using the male/female connectors.
      (4) After all the tasks are complete, press *Next.*
   f. Setting up *fill cycle,* for the setup wizard displays
      (1) Check the hose and tube connections, then start filling the system.

TABLE 45.1	Recommended Initial Cap Water Temperatures	
Infant Size	**Infant Weight**	**Recommended Initial Cap Water Temperature**
Small	≥1.8–<2.5 kg	12–15°C
Medium	2.5–4 kg	10–12°C
Large	>4 kg	8–10°C

TABLE 45.2	Determination of Cap Size	
Cap Size	**Infant Weight**	**Head Circumference**
Small	≥1.8–<2.5 kg	<32 cm
Medium	2.5–4 kg	32–37 cm
Large	>4 kg	>37 cm

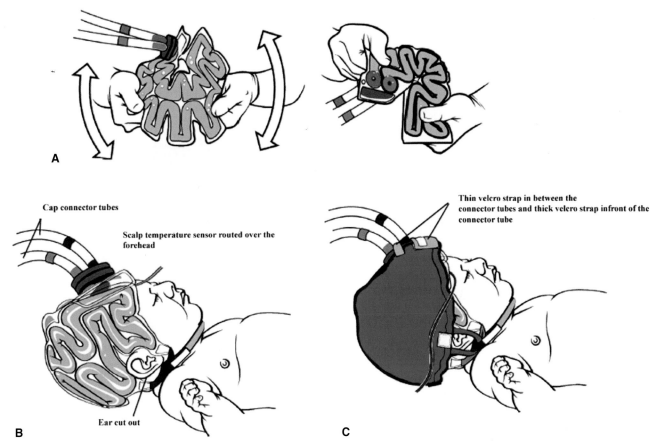

FIG. 45.5. Water cap (**A**), Water cap (**B**), and Water cap retainer (**C**) placement on the infant. **A:** Rocking, massaging, and inverting the water cap to remove any air bubbles from the crevices. **B:** Securing the water cap on the infant's head. **C:** Securing the water cap retainer over the water cap.

(2) After the system has filled, gently rock, massage, and invert the water cap to remove any air bubbles from the cap crevices (Fig. 45.5 A).

(3) After the tasks are complete, touch *Next*.

g. Placing *Caps and Shield*, for the setup wizard displays

(1) Position the *water cap* (Fig. 45.5B) on the infant's head, with the opening anterior, centered on the hairline and with the forehead exposed.

(2) Position the ear cutouts above the ears.

(3) Place the ear straps under the ears.

(4) Route the scalp temperature sensor wire out of the cap, over the infant's forehead.

(5) Place the cap connector tubes in the cap tube support.

(6) Place the *blue water cap retainer* (Fig. 45.5C) over the water cap.

(7) Slide the chin strap of the water cap through the ear straps of both water cap and the water cap retainer, and fasten the right and left Velcro fasteners.

(8) Place the large Velcro fastener on top of the infant's head, in front of the red cap tube, and the small Velcro fastener between the cap tubes.

(9) Place the *silver insulating cap* (Fig. 45.6A) over the water cap retainer.

(10) Secure the three Velcro fasteners on the inside of the water cap retainer to the patches on the inside of the insulating cap.

(11) Secure the Velcro fastener of the insulating cap in front of the cap connect tubes.

(12) Place the *heat shield* over the infant's head, aligning with the chin, and resting evenly and directly on the mattress (Fig. 45.6B).

(13) After each task is complete, touch *Cool* to start the system's cooling timer and main display screen.

h. Once the rectal temperature reaches 35.5°C, switch on the radiant warmer.

i. Set the servo control temperature on the radiant warmer to 37°C.

j. Adjust the water cap temperature to maintain the rectal temperature between 34°C and 35°C.

k. Continue cooling for 72 hours.

l. Commence rewarming after 72 hours and follow instructions on the screen for automated rewarming at 0.5°C/h. Switch off the cooling unit.

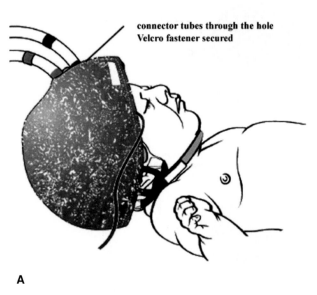

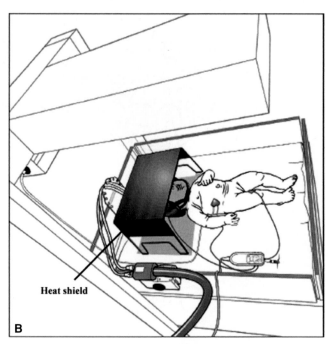

connector tubes through the hole
Velcro fastener secured

Heat shield

A

B

FIG. 45.6. **A:** Placement of insulating cap over the water cap retainer. The patches in the interior of the insulating cap attach to the Velcro fasteners on the exterior of the water cap retainer. **B:** Heat shield placed over the face and head of the infant.

Precautions

1. Use only sterile water.
2. Monitor for scalp changes every 12 hours.
3. SHC may not be appropriate for babies weighing <1.8 kg, due to reduced effectiveness of cooling in small for gestational age infants (21).
4. Avoid having the straps on the blue Lycra cap too tight to avoid swelling of the neck (Fig. 45.7).

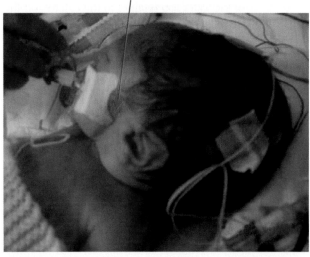

Neck swelling & impression caused by tight water cap retainer strap

FIG. 45.7. Neck swelling and impression caused by placing the strap of the water cap retainer too tightly.

Disadvantages

1. Involves repeated adjustments of the radiant warmer output and Cool-Cap water temperature.
2. It is not possible to store temperature data.
3. Rewarming rate cannot be individualized to infant.

H. Whole Body Cooling (WBC)

WBC can be achieved by

1. Passive cooling.
2. Cooling with simple adjuncts such as water bottles, gloves filled with water, gels, or fan.

   These methods are effective, but they are more difficult to use and are labor intensive. It is difficult to achieve stable temperature over a long period.
3. Manually controlled cooling machine and mattress
4. Servocontrolled cooling machines with body wrap or mattress.*

   Temperature, blood pressure, and heart rate variation during cooling with manual and servocontrolled WBC and manual SHC is shown in Figure 45.8.

Passive Cooling

After perinatal asphyxia, the metabolism of infants is naturally low, and the core temperature will fall unless active warming is commenced (22). When perinatal asphyxia is

---

*Each of these methods will be described with the corresponding figures.

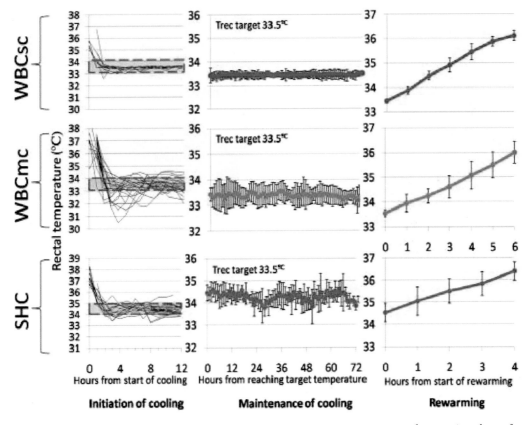

FIG. 45.8. Variability in the rectal temperature during initiation, maintenance, and rewarming phase of HT. SHC, selective head cooling manual (CoolCap n = 21); WBCmc, whole body cooling manual control (Tecotherm n = 25); WBCsc, whole body cooling servocontrolled (CritiCool n = 28).

likely in an infant at birth, passive cooling should be initiated as soon as ventilation is established (23). This method of cooling can be effective for days, depending on the environmental temperature, but it is usually used only until active cooling equipment is available (24).

Technique

1. No radiant warmer or other methods of warming should be initiated.
2. Keep the infant uncovered (small diaper may remain in place).
3. Monitor core temperature with rectal or esophageal probe. If overcooling occurs, infant can be rewarmed slowly with a heat source (e.g., warm water bottles, overhead heating [with heat shield to the head]) (Fig. 45.21).
4. Maintain ambient temperature below 26°C.
5. On completion of a 72-hour course of cooling, achieve rewarming at a rate of 0.5°C/h (i.e., from 33.5°C to 36.5°C in 6 hours).

Pitfalls

1. Core temperature monitoring is required to avoid excessive cooling (24,25).
2. Variability of core temperature during passive HT is high (23,24).

Cooling with Adjuncts

1. Gloves/Bottles Filled with Tap Water (Fig. 45.9)

Technique

a. Expose the infant fully and place in an open crib.
b. Remove all heat sources.
c. Maintain ambient temperature between 25°C and 26°C.
d. Use three rubber water bottles, filled with cold tap water, to form a mattress **and/or**
e. Place rubber gloves filled with water at approxima-tely 10°C next to the groins, axillae, and neck (26).
f. Monitor core temperature (rectal or esophageal) for 72 hours duration of HT.
g. Apply blankets and change gloves and/or water bottles as frequently as necessary to maintain core temperature at 33.5 ± 0.5°C.
h. Rewarming can be achieved passively by discontinuing active cooling and monitoring the rise in core temperature.
i. Gradual rewarming using external heat source, as for passive cooling, can be used with appropriate shield to protect the head (Figs. 45.6B, 45.21).

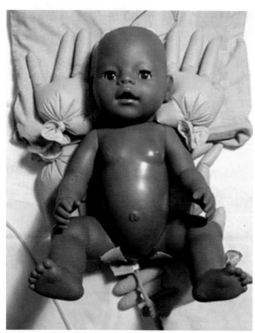

FIG. 45.9. Cooling with adjuncts. Gloves filled with cold water are placed around the head, trunk, and legs to cool the infant, along with rectal temperature monitoring.

Pitfalls

    a. There should be minimal variation in ambient temperature.

    b. Some, but relatively less, variability in core temperature compared with passive cooling.

    c. Frequent monitoring is required to determine when the gloves/water bottles need replacing.

2 Gels (5) (Fig. 45.10)

Technique

    a. Expose the infant to the ambient temperature in an open crib with an overhead warmer turned off.

    b. Apply two refrigerated gel packs (12 cm × 12 cm, at 7°C to 10°C) across the chest and/or under the head and shoulders.

    c. Remove one gel pack when the core temperature falls below 35°C.

    d. Remove the next gel pack when the core temperature falls below 34.5°C.

    e. Turn on the radiant warmer and manually adjust the heater output every 15 to 30 minutes if the core temperature falls below 33.5°C and use appropriate shield to protect the head (Fig. 45.21).

    f. Reapply gel packs if core temperature rises above 34°C.

    g. After 72 hours, increase the radiant warmer heater output to achieve rewarming by 0.5°C every 1 hour.

Pitfalls

  1. High variability of core temperature.

  2. Intensive monitoring and support required to maintain the desired core temperature.

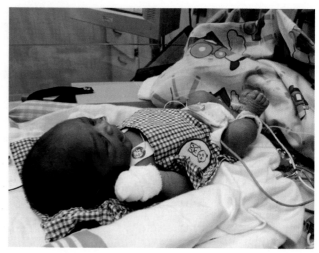

FIG. 45.10. Cooling with refrigerated gel packs placed under the head and across the chest and trunk.

3. Servocontrolled fan (27)

WBC is achieved using a custom-made, servocontrolled fan, which directs airflow cephalocaudally over the infant.

The fan unit consists of a Perspex box (30 × 15 × 10 cm) containing three fans. The fans are noiseless and are placed at the head of the infant. The unit produces an airflow of 105 ft/min at 100% power, and is powered on 12V direct current via a custom-made power supply. The fans are activated when the rectal temperature is at or above the preset activation temperature, and the power of the fans automatically increase or decrease with fluctuations in the rectal temperature.

Technique

    a. Place the infant in the supine position, with small diaper on, in an open crib with overhead radiant warmer turned off.

    b. Insert a rectal temperature probe to 6 cm, as described previously.

    c. Connect the rectal temperature probe to the radiant warmer temperature input.

       Serial output from the radiant warmer provides temperature data to the fan unit, via computer. The software (Labview for Windows, National Instruments Ltd, Austin, Texas) servo controls the power of the fans within the fan unit.

    d. Set the activation temperature of the fan manually, well below the target core temperature (33.5°C), and set the radiant warmer target temperature at 33.7°C. This allows the fan unit to consistently blow at low power, while the warmer provides heat as necessary to maintain the target rectal temperature.

    e. After completing 72 hours of HT, rewarm by turning off the fan and progressively increasing the target temperature on the radiant warmer to achieve rewarming at a rate ≤0.5°C/h. Shield the head from direct overhead heating (Fig. 45.21).

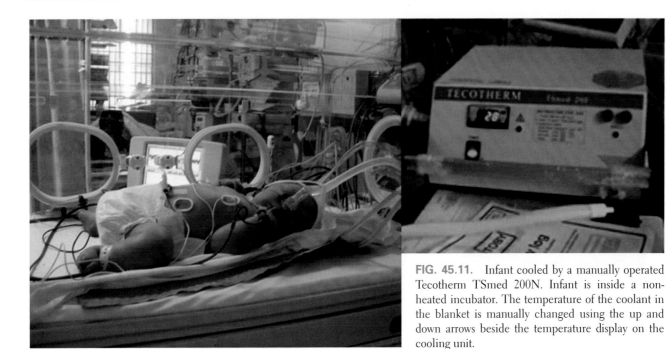

FIG. 45.11. Infant cooled by a manually operated Tecotherm TSmed 200N. Infant is inside a non-heated incubator. The temperature of the coolant in the blanket is manually changed using the up and down arrows beside the temperature display on the cooling unit.

Pitfalls

Shivering can occur with higher fan speeds.

Cooling Using a Manual Control Cooling Machine

Equipment

1. Tecotherm TSmed 200 N (TECCOM GmbH, Halle/Salle, Germany) (Fig. 45.11)
2. Power cable
3. Cooling unit
4. Dual lumen connecting hoses
5. Cooling mattress (AquaPad mattress)
6. Coolant (Thermal fluid TECOmed)
7. Fill-up set

Technique (3)

1. Switch on the cooling unit after plugging in the power cable.
2. Set the coolant temperature in the cooling unit to 20°C.
3. Place the mattress inside an incubator with power turned off.
4. Undress the infant down to small diaper to maximize skin contact with mattress for optimal heat exchange.
5. Secure a rectal temperature probe to 6 cm (see Fig. 45.2E).
6. Place the infant on the mattress inside the incubator.
7. When the rectal temperature reaches 35°C, increase the set temperature in the cooling machine to 25°C.
8. To maintain the rectal temperature between 33°C and 34°C, set temperature in the cooling machine to between 25°C and 30°C. This will vary with the body weight and heat production of the infant.
9. To rewarm the infant at 0.5°C/h, increase the set fluid temperature in the cooling machine by approximately 0.3°C/30 minutes. The core temperature will increase with increases in the mattress temperature. This is very difficult to get "right" and requires experience.
10. When core temperature of (36.5°C) has been reached, set the incubator temperature to maintain normothermia.
11. Remove the mattress.
12. Monitor rectal temperature for at least 24 hours after achieving normothermia (36.5°C) (28).

Pitfalls

1. Intermittent manual adjustment of coolant fluid temperature is required.
2. Overshoot of core temperature during induction of hypothermia.
3. Large swings in rectal temperature (29) (Fig. 45.11).

Cooling Using a Servocontrolled Cooling Machine

The servocontrolled cooling systems cool and maintain the core temperature by altering the temperature of the cooling fluid automatically, based on the core and surface temperature feedback to the system. The infant can be placed inside an incubator or preferably in an open bed.

1. *The CritiCool (Fig. 45.12) (MTRE Advanced Technologies Ltd, Yavne, Israel). Temperature Management Unit*

Other Equipment

  a. Power cable
  b. Connecting tubes
  c. Cure wrap (MTRE Advanced Technologies Ltd, Yavne, Israel)

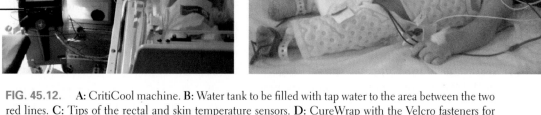

Green surface temperature sensor

Grey core (rectal) temperature sensor

Connecting tubes to temperature management unit

A

Water tank

B

Surface temperature sensor tip

Rectal temperature sensor tip

C

Curewrap

> 3.5kg

< 3.5kg

D

Female end of connecting tube to curewrap

E

Cooling during transport

F

FIG. 45.12.   A: CritiCool machine. **B:** Water tank to be filled with tap water to the area between the two red lines. **C:** Tips of the rectal and skin temperature sensors. **D:** CureWrap with the Velcro fasteners for infants 3.5 kg < and >3.5 kg. **E:** Connecting tube ends for insertion over the male connector of the CureWrap.

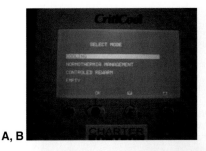
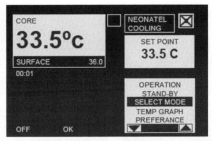
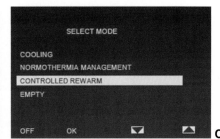

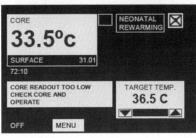
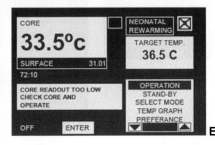

FIG. 45.13. Setting up CritiCool for neonatal cooling and automatic rewarming mode. **A–E** show the LCD display on the CritiCool.

d. Tap water

e. Rectal temperature probe ×2 (reusable) or adapter with single-use rectal probes

f. Skin temperature probe (reusable) or adapter with single-use probes

g. Layered bubble wrap pillow.

Technique

a. Position CritiCool unit and lock front wheels.

b. Fill tank of the temperature management unit with tap water to between the two red lines (Fig. 45.12A, B).

c. Select the size of the CureWrap ("cooling jacket") appropriate to the size of the infant (<3.5 kg and >3.5 kg) (Fig. 45.12D).

d. Connect the connecting tubes to the temperature management unit and the CureWrap (Fig. 45.12A).

e. Pull the collar off the female end of the connecting tube and insert over the male connector to the CureWrap.

f. Connect the connecting tubes to the metallic sockets in front of the temperature management unit.

g. Switch on the temperature management unit after connecting the power cable.

A prompt to confirm mode will appear with an audio alarm.

h. Cure wrap will fill with water; ensure the CureWrap is filled with water prior to wrapping and securing on infant.

i. Confirm neonatal cooling mode (Fig. 45.13A).

The default set core temperature in the management unit is 33.5°C. Water will not flow in the wrap without a valid core temperature reading.

j. Connect grey temperature sensor into Core socket and green temperature sensor into Surface socket. (Fig. 45.12A).

k. Circulation is confirmed when the "flow icon" (top right of display) is rotating (Fig. 45.13B).

l. Place the infant in the supine position on the CureWrap (which is shaped to fit the infant) in an open crib/bed.

m. Undress the infant down to a small diaper.

n. Insert the rectal temperature probe (grey sensor) supplied with the equipment 6 cm into the rectum (see E) (Fig. 45.2A).

o. Insert a second calibrated rectal probe to 6 cm, alongside the previous probe. The second probe is connected to a separate patient monitor to serve as a means to double check the rectal temperature.

p. Secure both the rectal temperature sensors (see E).

q. Cover the infant's legs and the trunk with the CureWrap, and secure with the Velcro straps (Fig. 45.14D).

r. Expose the umbilicus to allow insertion of umbilical lines and monitoring for bleeding (Fig. 45.14D).

s. Place six layers of bubble wrap between the head and the head portion of the wrap (Fig. 45.14B, C). This insulates the head from the cycling temperature in the CureWrap (30). Keeping the head exposed in an open bed maintains the superficial brain colder (29). The experimental evidence indicates that the fluctuation in the mattress temperature every 12 minutes induces similar fluctuations in the superficial brain temperature.

t. Secure the surface temperature probe to the forehead with tape (Fig. 45.14D).

u. Monitor core and surface temperature every 15 minutes during induction of HT and rewarming, and every 30 minutes during maintenance phase of HT.

v. After 72 hours of HT, rewarm using either the *manual* or *controlled* mode.

(1) During the *manual mode*, the user increases the set core temperature in the CritiCool by 0.2°C to 0.3°C per 30 minutes to increase the core temperature by 0.4°C to 0.5°C per hour. Rewarming

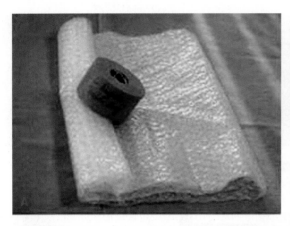

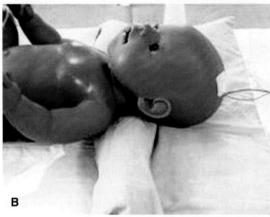

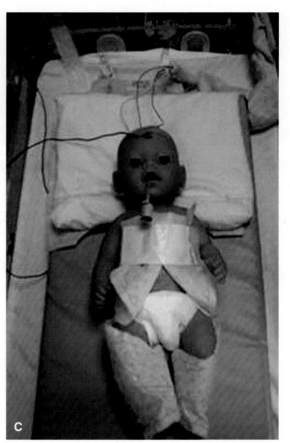

FIG. 45.14.   Insulating the head with bubble wrap. **A:** Pillow is prepared with six layers of bubble wrap. **B:** The layers of bubble wrap are rolled at one end to form a neck roll. **C:** CureWrap placed around the doll; bubble wrap pillow is covered with sheet; the neck rests on the neck roll; aEEG electrode is fixed in the parietal (P3) position.

degree and duration can be individualized to infant's clinical condition in this mode.

(2) To select *controlled rewarm mode*, press *menu*, select *mode*, press ▲ to move up or to move down, and highlight the controlled rewarm option. Press OK (Fig. 45.13C).

The message "CORE readout too low check core and operate" will appear (Fig. 45.13D).

Core, skin, and target temperatures are shown on the monitor of the temperature management unit (Fig. 45.13D). The water will no longer be circulating in the wrap. The default target temperature is 36.5°C; however, the set target temperature can be varied between 36°C and 38°C, using the ▲ or ▼ arrows below the target temperature read out (Fig. 45.13D).

(a) To start controlled rewarming, press *menu* and use the ▲ or ▼ arrows to select *Operation* (Fig. 45.13E).

(b) Once *Operation* is highlighted, press the *Enter* button to confirm (Fig. 45.13E).

(c) Once normothermia achieved, leave the infant on the wrap for 12 hours.

(d) If the infant is in a crib in which the temperature of the mattress can be increased, increase the temperature of the mattress to 1°C above the infant core temperature at the end of the 12-hour period and remove the wrap.

(e) Keep the infant's head uncovered and placed on the bubble wrap pillow to insulate the head from the heated mattress.

(f) Infant may be dressed in one layer of clothing.

(g) Monitor the rectal temperature for 24 hours after achieving normothermia (approximately 36.5°C rectal) to avoid hypo- or hyperthermia.

Precautions

a. The CureWrap must be applied loosely (allow a space of a finger width between the skin and the wrap) around the trunk to avoid impeding ventilation and pressure on the skin from the monitoring leads between the wrap and skin (Fig. 45.15).

b. Skin care must be performed a minimum of every 8 hours.

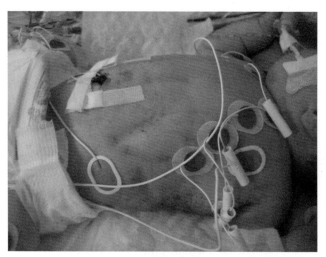

FIG. 45.15. Impressions on the skin produced by ECG leads under the wrap, which are the result of applying the CureWrap too tightly.

c. An alarm will alert the user if the rectal or surface probes become dislodged.
d. An alarm will sound if there is insufficient water in the temperature management unit.

Advantages (29)

a. Rapid initiation of HT
b. No overshoot of core temperature during induction
c. Variability of core temperature during maintenance and rewarming phase is minimal.
d. Better hemodynamic stability in terms of blood pressure and heart rate than manual cooling (Fig. 45.11, upper panel).

e. Equipment suitable to be secured in ambulance and used during transport.
f. Easy downloading of all temperature data.

2. Tecotherm Neo (Fig. 45.16) (TECCOM GmbH, Halle/Salle, Germany)

Equipment

a. Mains cable
b. Tecotherm Neo cooling unit
c. Cooling mattress
d. Mattress connecting hoses
e. Rectal temperature probe × 2
f. Lubricating jelly
g. Skin temperature probe × 1
h. Coolant fluid
i. Coolant fill-up set
j. Pillow of six-layered bubble wrap

Technique

a. Connect the mains cable to the power and switch on.
b. Connect the fill-up set to the cooling unit (Fig. 45.16B).
c. Keep the fill-up set above the cooling unit so that the coolant fills up the cooling unit.
d. Connect the mattress to the cooling unit with the connecting hose (Fig. 45.16A, C).
e. Connect the rectal temperature probe and the skin temperature probe to the cooling unit (Fig. 45.16C).
f. Set the Tecotherm Neo to programmable servocontrolled mode (this completes the induction and

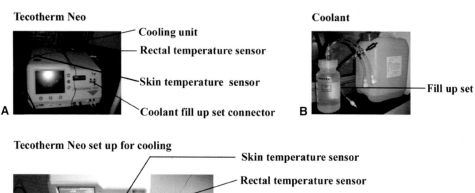

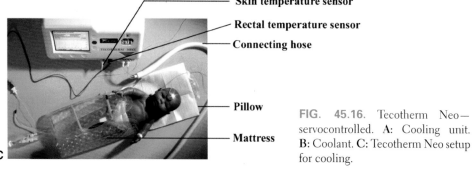

FIG. 45.16. Tecotherm Neo—servocontrolled. **A:** Cooling unit. **B:** Coolant. **C:** Tecotherm Neo setup for cooling.

maintains the temperature at the target of 33.5°C for 72 hours, followed by servocontrolled rewarming to 37°C over 7 hours).

g. Undress the infant down to small diaper.

h. Secure two rectal temperature probes to 6 cm (Fig. 45.2), and tape to the side of the thigh as previously described in E.

i. Secure the skin temperature probe on the forehead.

j. Place the infant supine on the mattress and encircle the baby with the mattress, in a closed unheated incubator or an open crib/bed (Figs. 45.16 and 45.17)

k. Secure the mattress at the front of the infant with the supplied ties (Figs. 45.16C and 45.17).

l. Place the pillow between the head and the mattress (30) (Fig. 45.17). Alarms are activated if there is no power, low fluid, no flow of fluid, rectal temperature is out of range by 0.5°C, and for system failure.

Precautions

Avoid tight wrapping of mattress. This can lead to excessive pressure on the skin. *(Fig. 45.17)*

Advantages (28)

a. Rapid initiation of HT

b. No overshoot of core temperature during induction

c. Variability of core temperature during maintenance and rewarming phase is minimal.

d. Easy downloading of all temperature data with memory stick.

3. *Blanketrol III* (Cincinnati Sub-Zero Products, Inc., Cincinnati, Ohio) (Fig. 45.18)

Equipment

a. BLANKETROL III unit

b. Hyper-hypothermia blanket

c. Dry sheet, bath blanket or DISPOSA-Cover

d. Connecting hose

e. 400 series probe

f. Lubricating jelly

g. Connector cable for the disposable probes

h. Distilled water
   Different modes of cooling are available.

a. *Manual mode (Fig. 45.19B):* Operation based on temperature of circulating water relative to the set blanket/water temperature.

b. *Auto Control (Fig. 45.19F):* Monitors patient temperature and delivers maximum heating or cooling therapy to bring patient's temperature to the set point.

c. *Gradient 10C (Fig. 45.19G):* Heats or cools the patient with water 10°C above or below the patient's temperature, until the patient reaches the desired set temperature.

d. *Gradient 10C Smart (Fig. 45.19G, I):* Heats or cools the patient with water 10°C above or below the patient's temperature and increases the gradient 5°C until set temperature is reached. When the patient's temperature deviates from set point after having reached the target temperature, the gradient returns to 10°C.

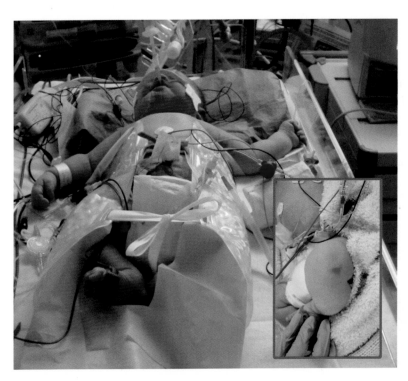

FIG. 45.17. Tecotherm Neo servocontrolled cooling. Reusable cooling mattress was wrapped around the lower body. Insert shows red pressure area on the knee, where the mattress was wrapped too tight.

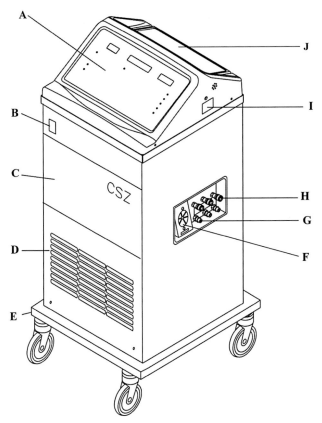

FIG. 45.18. Blanketrol III. A, control panel; B, power switch (I–on; O–off); C, storage drawer; D, grill; E, protective bumper; F, water flow indicator; G, male outlet coupling; H, female return coupling; I, patient probe jack; J, water fill tank.

e. *Gradient Variable (Fig. 45.19H):* Same as Gradient 10C mode, except that the gradient can be determined by user. Smart mode can be added to Gradient.

f. *Variable:* The gradient increases by 5°C beyond the specified gradient until the set temperature is reached. When the infant's temperature deviates from set point after having reached the target temperature, the gradient returns to the specified gradient.

g. *Monitor Only (Fig. 45.19J):* Displays the patient temperature without heating or cooling or circulating the water.

The cooling system is activated by pressing *Temp Set* and setting the target temperature, followed by pressing the mode selector. To change to *Monitor Only*, press the appropriately labeled button (Fig. 45.19J).

WBC with Gradient Variable Mode is Described Below

Technique

(1) Place the Blanketrol III unit in the patient area, accessible to the correct power source.

(2) Check the level of the distilled water in the reservoir. Lift the cover of the water fill opening and check that the water is visibly touching the strainer (Fig. 45.18J).

(3) Check that the power switch is in the *off* position (Fig. 45.18B).

(4) Insert the plug into a properly grounded receptacle.

(5) Lay the hyper-hypothermia blanket flat (Fig. 45.20) with the hose routed, without kinks, toward the unit.

(6) Cover the blanket with a dry sheet or disposable cover (Fig. 45.20), if single patient use blanket such as MAXI-THERM (Cincinnati Sub-Zero Products, Inc., Cincinnati, Ohio) is used.

(7) *Connect the blanket to the Blanketrol III unit:* Attach the quick-disconnect female coupling of the connecting hose to the male outlet coupling

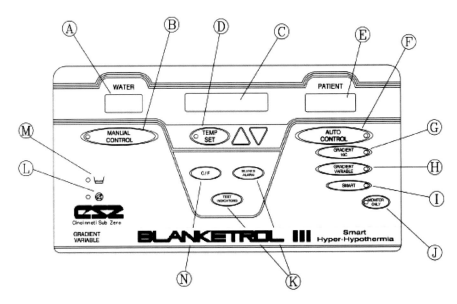

FIG. 45.19. Blanketrol III membrane control panel (115-volt unit). A, water temperature; B, manual control of circulating water temperature; C, LCD status display; D, temperature set button; E, patient temperature; F, auto control mode; G, gradient 10c mode; H, gradient variable mode; I, smart function; J, monitor patient temperature; K, test indicator (confirm all the indicators are working) and silence alarm; L, power failure (LED on the side flashes with audible alarm when power has been interrupted); M, low water symbol; N, Celsius or Fahrenheit.

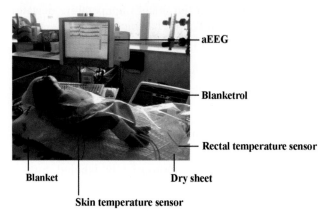

aEEG

Blanketrol

Rectal temperature sensor

Blanket

Dry sheet

Skin temperature sensor

FIG. 45.20.   Blanketrol III setup for cooling.

on the cooling unit (Fig. 45.18G) and the male coupling to the female return coupling (Fig. 45.18H) by pushing back the collar of the female coupling while connecting to the male coupling, followed by releasing the collar.

(8) Gently pull the connecting hose to ensure a positive connection, that there are no twists in the connecting hose, and that the blanket is flat.

(9) *Initiate precooling:* Precooling may not be necessary if the infant's temperature has already been lowered (e.g., by passive hypothermia during transport).

 (a) Switch on the cooling machine (Fig. 45.18B).

 (b) Press *Temp Set* (Fig. 45.19D).

 (c) Use the up (Δ) or down (∇) arrows by the side of *Set Temp* (Fig. 45.19) and set the temperature to 33.5°C.

 (d) Press *Manual Control* (Fig. 45.19B).

 (e) Listen for the compressor to activate.

 (f) Check the water flow indicator (Fig. 45.18, F) to confirm that water is circulating.

 (g) Place the infant on the blanket (Fig. 45.20).

 (h) Place patient temperature monitoring probes.

Rectal Temperature Sensor

(1) Mark a 400 series probe at 6 cm from the tip with tape/indelible pen (Fig. 45.2).

(2) Insert rectal probe 6 cm into the rectum, and secure to leg using DuoDERM/Tegaderm and tape, as described in E (Fig. 45.2).

Esophageal Temperature

(1) Measure a 400 series probe from nose/midline of the mouth to ear and then to an imaginary line between the nipples.

(2) Mark this position on the probe with tape/indelible pen.

(3) Insert the probe via mouth or nose up to the mark.

(4) Secure the probe to the upper lip.

 (a) Connect the rectal or esophageal probe to black cable jack.

 (b) Connect black cable to probe outlet in Blanketrol (Fig, 45.18I).

 (c) Initiate **induction** of HT (*Gradient Variable* mode)

(5) After 1 minute, press *Temp Set* (Fig. 45.18D).

(6) Press the Δ/∇ (Fig. 45.18) button to set the temperature to **33.5°C**.

 The status display (Fig. 45.19C) will read **33.5°C**.

(7) Press *Gradient Variable* (Fig. 45.19H).

(8) Press Δ/∇ (Fig. 45.16) to **20°C**.

(9) Press the *Gradient Variable* (Fig. 45.19H) again.

(10) Listen for the activation of the pump.

(11) Check that the water flow indicator (Fig. 45.18F) is rotating.

(12) Place the dry sheet or disposable cover over the infant, to decrease convection losses and fluctuations in water temperature in blanket (Fig. 45.20).

(13) Monitor temperature displays. The *Patient* display (Fig. 45.19E) will show the infant's actual temperature.

 The *Water* display (Fig. 45.19A) will show the actual temperature of the circulating water.

 The *Status* display (Fig. 45.19C) will show the mode of operation and set temperature.

 Monitor core temperature every 15 minutes to determine when the target temperature is reached.

Maintain HT (*Gradient Variable* Mode)

1. Press *Temp Set* (Fig. 45.19D).
2. Press the Δ/∇ (Fig. 45.19) button to maintain core temperature at **33.5°C**.
3. Press *Gradient Variable* (Fig. 45.19H).
4. Press the Δ/∇ (Fig. 45.19) button to **5°C** to minimize the temperature fluctuations between the patient and the water in the cooling blanket.
5. Press the *Gradient Variable* (Fig. 45.19H) again.
6. Listen for the activation of the pump.
7. Check that the water flow indicator (Fig. 45.18F) is rotating.

Initiate Manual Rewarming after 72 hours of HT

1. Press *Temp Set* (Fig. 45.19D).
2. Press Δ button to **0.5°C**.
3. Increase 0.5°C every hour until the core temperature is 36.5°C.
4. Press *Gradient Variable* (Fig. 45.19H).
5. Press Δ to 5°C to minimize the temperature fluctuations between the patient and the water in the cooling blanket.
6. Press *Gradient Variable* (Fig. 45.19H).

7. Listen for the activation of the pump.
8. Check that the water flow indicator (Fig. 45.18F) is rotating.

Initiate Post-Rewarming Care

When the rectal temperature has been 36.5°C for 60 minutes, the Blanketrol can be set to *Monitor Only* and the infant can be kept normothermic (36.5 ± 0.2 °C) with a servocontrolled overhead radiant warmer and overhead reflective shield (Fig. 45.21).

1. Press *Monitor Only* (Fig. 45.19J).
2. Keep core temperature probe in place for 24 hours after completion of cooling.
3. For radiant warmer, use servo control.
   Place the skin probe over the liver, right upper quadrant, below ribs.
   Set servo to achieve axillary temperature of 36.5 ± 0.2°C.
4. Cover the face and head with a reflective shield to prevent elevation of the superficial brain temperature (Fig. 45.21)
   Alternatively, the infant can be warmed in a Babytherm infant warmer (Dräger Medical Inc., Telford, Pennsylvania) or any "hot cot," which has the option of increasing the temperature of the mattress, by setting the temperature of the cot at the same temperature that the water in the Blanketrol was set at to maintain the infant normothermic.

a. Place a six-layered bubble wrap "pillow" between the infant's head and the hot cot, to prevent elevation of the superficial brain temperature (Fig. 45.14B, D).
b. Discontinue hourly core temperature monitoring after 24 hours, and resume routine 4 hourly temperature monitoring.

Precautions

1. Do not use deionized water. The majority of deionizers do not maintain a neutral pH of 7.
   This results in acidification of water, which can deteriorate the battery and the copper refrigeration line, ultimately leading to a leak in the refrigeration system.
2. Do not use alcohol, as it may cause blanket deterioration.
3. Do not overfill the reservoir in Blanketrol.
4. Check for leaks in the blanket and hose. Water leaks can be a risk for infection.
5. If the *Check Probe* alarm activates, confirm that the core temperature probe has not fallen out.
   If the core temperature probe is in place, consider changing the temperature cable rather than the temperature probe.
   a. Connect new temperature cable to Blanketrol (Fig. 45.18I) and to the temperature probe.
   b. Turn the machine off and back on.
   c. Press the *Temp Set* switch (Fig. 45.19D).
   d. Press **ΔV** until most recent set point is reached.
   e. Press *Auto Control* (Fig. 45.19F).

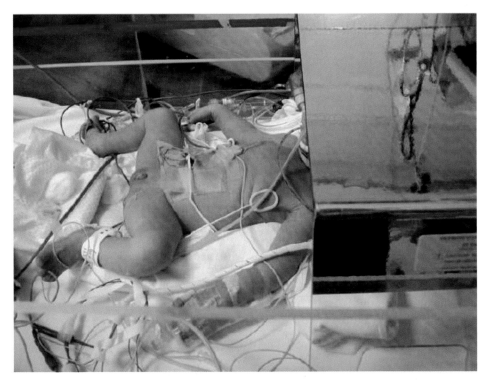

FIG. 45.21. Baby with head under heat shield to protect the head from direct overhead heating.

I. Rewarming

1. Rewarming is carried out after 72 hours of hypothermia.
2. Rewarming is generally achieved at a rate of 0.5°C/h, when it is carried out with a cooling unit.
3. Rewarming without cooling equipment (covering with blanket or warm gloves, etc.) should be undertaken with continuous monitoring of rectal temperature to ensure it does not occur faster than 0.5°C/h.
4. If seizures occur during rewarming (31), temporarily suspend rewarming until seizures cease with anticonvulsants; if the seizures are refractory to anticonvulsants, cooling again by 0.5 to 1°C may be necessary (this may decrease the mismatch between cerebral oxygen delivery and consumption [32] and prevent further seizures). The rewarming can be continued at a rate of 0.2°C/h after a seizure-free period (28).

J. Post-Rewarming Care

1. Monitor core temperature for 24 hours to avoid hyper- or hypothermia.
2. Protect the infant's head from heat source with a bubble-wrap pillow (in case of a heated crib or mattress) and a head shield (if a radiant warmer is used.)
3. Avoid placing the infant in an incubator, as this may cause an increase in superficial brain temperature.

K. Complications of Hypothermia

1. Increased levels of sedatives, anticonvulsants, and neuromuscular blocking agents due to individually decreased clearance of drugs metabolized in the liver (28,33)
2. Infants who are not well sedated will be uncomfortable due to the cold stress, and cooling may be painful. Therefore, cooled babies should be well sedated. Stress may reduce the effectiveness of cooling (17).
3. Thrombocytopenia (34)
4. Subcutaneous fat necrosis (35). This complication is rare and should be avoidable. This may be due to lack of adequate postural changes, keeping the skin cold, under pressure, and with poor perfusion.
5. Most predictors of outcome (except MRI) after perinatal asphyxia that are validated for normothermic infants are less predictive for cooled infants; hence, cutoff values and interpretations are different (13,36–39).

Acknowledgements

Dr. Sonia Bonifacio, University of California San Francisco, who kindly shared experience with Blanketrol cooling equipment and provided Figures 45.18, 45.19, and 45.20, and Dr. Terrie Inder, Washington University, St.Louis, MO, who provided Figure 45.10.

References

1. Gluckman PD, Wyatt JS, Azzopardi D, et al. Selective head cooling with mild systemic hypothermia after neonatal encephalopathy: Multicentre randomised trial. *Lancet*. 2005;365:663.
2. Shankaran S, Laptook AR, Ehrenkranz RA, et al. Whole-body hypothermia for neonates with hypoxic-ischemic encephalopathy. *N Engl J Med*. 2005;353:1574.
3. Azzopardi DV, Strohm B, Edwards AD, et al. Moderate hypothermia to treat perinatal asphyxial encephalopathy. *N Engl J Med*. 2009;361:1349.
4. Simbruner G, Mittal RA, Rohlmann F, et al. Systemic hypothermia after neonatal encephalopathy: Outcomes of neo.nEURO. network RCT. *Pediatrics*. 2010;126:e771.
5. Jacobs SE, Morley CJ, Inder TE, et al. Whole-body hypothermia for term and near-term newborns with hypoxic-ischemic encephalopathy: A randomized controlled trial. *Arch Pediatr Adolescent Med*. 2011;165:692.
6. Edwards AD, Brocklehurst P, Gunn AJ, et al. Neurological outcomes at 18 months of age after moderate hypothermia for perinatal hypoxic ischaemic encephalopathy: synthesis and meta-analysis of trial data. *BMJ*. 2010;340:c363.
7. Chakkarapani E, Harding D, Stoddart P, et al Therapeutic hypothermia: surgical infant with neonatal encephalopathy. *Acta Paediatr*. 2009;98:1844.
8. Thoresen M. Hypothermia after perinatal asphyxia: selection for treatment and cooling protocol. *J Pediatr*. 2011;158:e45.
9. Liu X, Chakkarapani E, Hoque N, et al. Environmental cooling of the newborn pig brain during whole-body cooling. *Acta Paediatr*. 2011;100:29.
10. O'Reilly KM, Tooley J, Winterbottom S. Therapeutic hypothermia during neonatal transport. *Acta Paediatr*. 2011;100:1084.
11. Pappas A, Shankaran S, Laptook AR, et al. Hypocarbia and adverse outcome in neonatal hypoxic-ischemic encephalopathy. *J Pediatr*. 2011;158:752.
12. Chakkarapani E, Thoresen M, Liu X, et al. Xenon offers stable haemodynamics independent of induced hypothermia after hypoxia-ischaemia in newborn pigs. *Intensive Care Med*. 2011; 38:316.
13. Thoresen M, Hellstrom-Westas L, Liu X, et al. Effect of hypothermia on amplitude-integrated electroencephalogram in infants with asphyxia. *Pediatrics*. 2010;126:e131.
14. Glass HC, Glidden D, Jeremy RJ, et al. Clinical neonatal seizures are independently associated with outcome in infants at risk for hypoxic-ischemic brain injury. *J Pediatr*. 2009;155:318.
15. Nadeem M, Murray DM, Boylan GB, et al. Early blood glucose profile and neurodevelopmental outcome at two years in neonatal hypoxic-ischaemic encephalopathy. *BMC Pediatr*. 2011; 11:10.
16. Bhat MA, Charoo BA, Bhat JI, et al. Magnesium sulfate in severe perinatal asphyxia: A randomized, placebo-controlled trial. *Pediatrics*. 2009;123:e764.
17. Thoresen M, Satas S, Loberg EM, et al. Twenty-four hours of mild hypothermia in unsedated newborn pigs starting after a severe global hypoxic-ischemic insult is not neuroprotective. *Pediatr Res*. 2001;50:405.
18. Thoresen M, Simmonds M, Satas S, et al. Effective selective head cooling during posthypoxic hypothermia in newborn piglets. *Pediatr Res*. 2001;49:594.
19. Van Leeuwen GM, Hand JW, Lagendijk JJ, et al. Numerical modeling of temperature distributions within the neonatal head. *Pediatr Res*. 2000;48:351.
20. Gunn AJ, Gluckman P, Wyatt JS, et al. Selective head cooling after neonatal encephalopathy - author's reply. *Lancet*. 2005;365:1619.
21. Wyatt JS, Gluckman PD, Liu PY, et al. Determinants of outcomes after head cooling for neonatal encephalopathy. *Pediatrics*. 2007; 119:912.
22. Burnard ED, Cross KW. Rectal temperature in the newborn after birth asphyxia. *BM J*. 1958;2:1197.

23. Chakkarapani E, Thoresen M. Use of hypothermia in the asphyxiated infant. *Perinatology.* 2010;1:20.
24. Hallberg B, Olson L, Bartocci M, et al. Passive induction of hypothermia during transport of asphyxiated infants: A risk of excessive cooling. *Acta Paediatr.* 2009;98:942.
25. Kendall GS, Kapetanakis A, Ratnavel N, et al. Passive cooling for initiation of therapeutic hypothermia in neonatal encephalopathy. *Arch Dis Child.* 2010;95:F408.
26. Thoresen M, Whitelaw A. Cardiovascular changes during mild therapeutic hypothermia and re-warming in infants with hypoxic-ischemic encephalopathy. *Pediatrics.* 2000;106:92.
27. Horn A, Thompson C, Woods D, et al. Induced hypothermia for infants with hypoxic- ischemic encephalopathy using a servo-controlled fan: An exploratory pilot study. *Pediatrics.* 2009; 123:e1090.
28. Thoresen M. Supportive care during neuroprotective hypothermia in the term newborn: Adverse effects and their prevention. *Clin Perinatol.* 2008;35:749.
29. Hoque N, Chakkarapani E, Liu X, et al. A comparison of cooling methods used in therapeutic hypothermia for perinatal asphyxia. *Pediatrics.* 2010;126:e124.
30. Liu X, Chakkarapani E, Hoque N, et al. Environmental cooling of the newborn pig brain during whole-body cooling. *Acta Paediatr.* 2010;100:29.
31. Battin M, Bennet L, Gunn AJ. Rebound seizures during rewarming. *Pediatrics.* 2004;114:1369.
32. Van der Linden J, Ekroth R, Lincoln C, et al. Is cerebral blood flow/metabolic mismatch during rewarming a risk factor after profound hypothermic procedures in small children? *Eur J Cardiothorac Surg.* 1989;3:209.
33. Roka A, Melinda KT, Vasarhelyi B, et al. Elevated morphine concentrations in neonates treated with morphine and prolonged hypothermia for hypoxic ischemic encephalopathy. *Pediatrics.* 2008;121:e844.
34. Jacobs S, Hunt R, Tarnow-Mordi W, et al. Cooling for newborns with hypoxic ischaemic encephalopathy. *Cochrane Database Syst Rev.* 2007:CD003311.
35. Strohm B, Hobson A, Brocklehurst P, et al. Subcutaneous fat necrosis after moderate therapeutic hypothermia in neonates. *Pediatrics.* 2011;128:e450.
36. Gunn AJ, Wyatt JS, Whitelaw A, et al. Therapeutic hypothermia changes the prognostic value of clinical evaluation of neonatal encephalopathy. *J Pediatr.* 2008;152:55.
37. Rutherford M, Ramenghi LA, Edwards AD, et al. Assessment of brain tissue injury after moderate hypothermia in neonates with hypoxic-ischemic encephalopathy: a nested substudy of a randomised controlled trial. *Lancet Neurol.* 2010;9:39.
38. Thoresen M. Patient selection and prognostication with hypothermia treatment. *Semin Fetal Neonatal Med.* 2010;15:247.
39. Elstad M, Whitelaw A, Thoresen M. Cerebral Resistance Index is less predictive in hypothermia encephalopathic newborns. *Acta Paediatr.* 2011;100:1344.

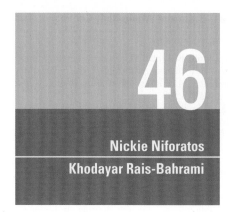

46

Nickie Niforatos
Khodayar Rais-Bahrami

Removal of Extra Digits and Skin Tags

A. Indications

Removal of Nonfunctional Extra Digit

1. Prevention of accidental avulsion or torsion around narrow base
2. Cosmetic correction at parental request
3. Consider surgical excision as an alternative to prevent the development of amputation neuromas (1,2)

B. Contraindications

1. Concomitant illness in infant
   This is an elective procedure that is painful when the clamp is applied. To prevent accidental avulsion of appendage if extra digit on a narrow base were to become entangled, apply a soft dressing or adhesive bandage until infant is stable enough for removal.
2. Bleeding diathesis
3. Additional anomalies where further surgical correction may be necessary (3)
4. Base of extra digit >2 mm wide
5. Bone crossing the isthmus between extra digit and hand

C. Equipment

All Sterile

1. Antiseptic solution and swabs appropriate for major procedure
2. Straight mosquito hemostat
3. Surgical silk suture, 3-0 or 4-0
4. Fine or delicate scissors
5. Adhesive bandage
6. Local anesthetic cream

D. Precautions

1. Perform procedure only on stable, healthy infant
2. Consider surgical evaluation for any questionable digit.
   a. When base is >2 mm wide
   b. When extra digit is on radial side of hand or is a duplicated thumb

   c. When clamping will not crush base to a thin, translucent, layer indicative of hemostasis after excision
   d. When there appears to be a joint at the base
   e. When bony structures are present in the digit as confirmed by radiography (4)
3. Consider surgical evaluation for any questionable skin tag.
   a. When tag may be used for ear or nasal deformity reconstruction (5)
   b. When tag is large or in critical areas
4. Apply hemostat to base of extra digit prior to placing ligature.
   a. Allows closer amputation without residual bump
   b. Allows faster autoamputation or removal of most of digit within a few hours

E. Technique

Removal of Nonfunctional Digit (Fig. 46.1)

1. Apply local anesthetic cream to appendage and base.
2. Cleanse digit and the surrounding skin with antiseptic. Allow to dry.
3. Clamp hemostat as close to the base of extra digit as possible but without drawing up extra skin (Fig. 46.2A).
4. Tightly tie suture around digit between hemostat and hand.
5. Keep clamp in place until digit has turned white (at least 5 minutes).
6. Using as a cutting guide the edge of the hemostat farther from the hand, excise the digit (Fig. 46.2B).
7. Remove hemostat and observe for hemostasis, leaving ligature in place. If there is any bleeding, reapply hemostat and ligature.
8. Cover with an adhesive bandage until residual stump autoamputates.

Removal of Skin Tags (Fig. 46.3)

The removal of small skin tags follows essentially the same technique as for extra digits: Clamp close to base of lesion to achieve hemostasis, and apply ligature between hemostat and normal area. If the lesions are large or in critical areas, removal is best delayed beyond the neonatal period. Consider other diagnoses associated with skin tags (6).

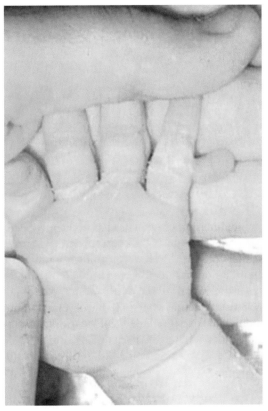

FIG. 46.1. Nonfunctional extra digit on ulnar side of left hand (note wide base; surgical excision is preferred).

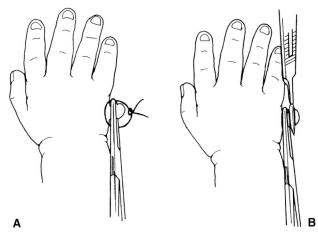

A **B**

FIG. 46.2. **A:** Place fine hemostat as close to base of extra digit as possible, and firmly secure ligature between clamp and hand. **B:** After finger turns white, excise digit tag outside hemostat, leaving ligature in place for autoamputation of residual stump.

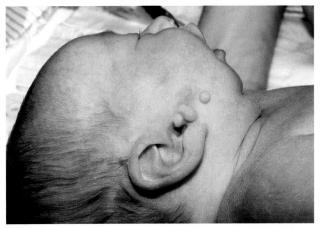

FIG. 46.3. Skin tags of right ear and cheek. Removal of tags this large requires surgical excision rather than ligation for best result and may be associated with other malformations.

F. Complications

1. Hemorrhage
   a. Failure to achieve complete hemostasis prior to excision
   b. Loosening of ligature before blood supply is retracted
2. Infection
3. Inappropriate removal of digit or tag in presence of related anomalies
4. Incomplete ligation leading to traumatic neuroma (1,2)

References

1. Leber GE. Surgical excision of pedunculated supernumerary digits prevents traumatic amputation neuromas. *Pediatr Dermatol.* 2003;20:108.
2. Mullick S, Borschel GH. A selective approach to treatment of ulnar polydactyly: preventing painful neuroma and incomplete excision. *Pediatr Dermatol.* 2010;27(1):39.
3. Horii E, Hattori T, Koh S et al. Reconstruction for Wassel type III radial polydactyly with two digits equal in size. *J Hand Surg Am.* 2009;34(10):1802.
4. Gomella TL, Cunningham MD, Eyal FG, et al. Newborn physical exam. In: Gomella TL, ed. *Neonatology: Management, Procedures, On-Call Problems, Diseases, and Drugs.* 4th ed. Stanford, CT: Appleton & Lange; 2004:35.
5. Jones KL. Preauricular tags or pits: frequent in. In: Jones KL, eds. *Smith's Recognizable Patterns of Human Malformations.* 6th ed. Philadelphia: Elsevier Saunders; 2006;899.
6. Eley KA, Pleat JM, Wall SA. Reconstruction of a congenital nasal deformity using skin tags as a chondrocutaneous composite graft. *J Craniofac Surg.* 2009;20(2):573.

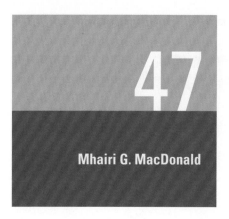

47

Circumcision

Mhairi G. MacDonald

A. Indications

Newborn male circumcision, one of the oldest formally recorded surgical procedures, remains controversial (1–3). Many physicians and lay people consider circumcision routine, but complications, although relatively rare, can be severe. Therefore, despite the perceived simplicity of the procedure, meticulous attention to anatomic landmarks, wound care, and follow-up is necessary.

B. Contraindications

1. Age <1 day (i.e., before complete physical adaptation to extrauterine life has occurred)
2. Any current illness
3. Prematurity (<37 weeks' gestation)
4. Bleeding diathesis or family history of bleeding disorder
5. Abnormality of urethra or penile shaft (foreskin may be essential for later reconstruction [e.g., hypospadias, chordee, very small penis])
6. Local infection
7. Lack of truly "informed" parental consent (see Chapter 2)

C. Equipment (4–7)

1. Necessary for all Methods

Sterile

a. Gown and gloves
b. Cup with antiseptic
c. 4- × 4-inch gauze pads
d. Small, flexible, blunt probe
e. Two straight mosquito hemostats
f. Large, straight hemostat
g. Tissue scissors

Nonsterile

Materials for restraint

2. Equipment for Analgesia

a. *Local anesthetic:* 1% lidocaine hydrochloride without epinephrine in a tuberculin syringe with a 1.2-cm × 27-gauge needle

Circumcision of neonates has frequently been used as a model to study the response of the newborn to pain (see Chapter 6) (8) However, until recently, neonatal circumcision has been performed without anesthesia. Since the initial report by Kirya and Werthmann in 1978 (9), there have been reports of several controlled studies that have concluded that the use of dorsal penile nerve block is both effective and safe

The effectiveness of EMLA (eutectic mixture of local anesthetics; lidocaine and prilocaine) 5% cream has also been studied. Conclusions from meta-analysis of data from several sources has led to the conclusion that EMLA cannot be recommended over other analgesic techniques with proven efficacy, such as regional nerve block with lidocaine.

3. Optional Equipment

a. Sterile fine-tipped marking pen
b. Sterile gauze impregnated with petroleum jelly (e.g., Vaseline)

4. Additional equipment for Use with Gomco Clamp

All equipment is sterile.

a. Gomco circumcision clamp (Gomco Surgical Manufacturing Corp., Buffalo, New York) (4), size 1 to 2 cm for average newborn glans (size range 1 to 3.5 cm)

   Be sure to use a size that is large enough to protect the glans (10).
b. No. 11 scalpel blade and holder
c. A small safety pin

5. Additional Equipment for Use with Plastibell

All equipment is sterile.

a. Plastibell plastic cone (Hollister, Libertyville, Illinois); available in presterilized packs; size range based on size of glans penis: 1.1, 1.3, and 1.5 cm. A linen suture is included in the pack (Fig. 47.1). When selecting size, make sure that it is not so large that it allows proximal migration of the bell and excessive loss of penile skin, nor so small that it could impair penile circulation.
b. Scissors capable of cutting through plastic

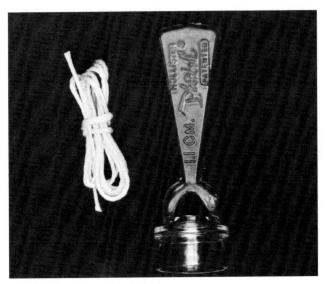

FIG. 47.1. Plastibell with linen suture.

D. Precautions

1. Obtain fully informed consent (see Chapter 2).
   a. Explain expected course of circumcision to parents. When Plastibell is used, parents should be told to call their physician if ring has not fallen off within 10 days.
   b. Be aware of laws pertaining to ritual circumcision (e.g., Jewish *brit milah*) and the complications of the practice of orally suctioning the blood after cutting the foreskin (oral *metzitzah*) (11).
2. Never circumcise at time of delivery. Circumcise long enough before discharge to allow adequate wound observation.
3. Do not use local anesthetic containing epinephrine.
4. Specifically locate coronal sulcus and urethral meatus.
5. Make sure that inner epithelium is completely separated from glans penis and that prepuce can be retracted to visualize entire circumference of coronal sulcus.
6. Never use electrocautery.
7. Do not use circumferential dressing.
8. Recheck wound prior to discharging patient and 1 to 2 weeks after circumcision. Residual skin should retract completely, and the entire coronal sulcus must be visible to avoid postcircumcision adhesions, the most common complication.

E. Technique

A complete description of formal surgical excision has been excluded from this edition because of the requirement to use sutures and the associated increased risk of bleeding compared with methods that involve crushing of tissue.

Ritual circumcisions are most commonly performed using a Mogen clamp. The method involves no dorsal incision or sutures (5); however, because the glans is not visible

at the time of excision of the prepuce, there is potential for damage to the glans and urethra.

1. Immobilize infant in supine position.
2. Put on cap and mask.
3. Scrub as for major procedure.
4. Put on gown and gloves.
5. Prepare skin with antiseptic, and drape.
6. Perform penile dorsal nerve block if desired.
   a. Be familiar with anatomy of dorsal nerves of penis (Fig. 47.2) (9). Although only the two dorsal penile nerves are targeted by the injection of lidocaine, the ventral penile nerve is also blocked by infiltration through the subcutaneous tissue. Some have advocated additional anesthesia ventrally, blocking the perineal nerves (a branch of the pudendal nerve)
   b. Identify dorsal nerve roots at 10- and 2-o'clock positions.
   c. Identify by palpation the symphysis pubis and corpora cavernosa at the penile base.
   d. Estimate depth of pubic bone from penile base to indicate necessary depth of injection (should not exceed 0.5 cm).
      Although the ideal area for infiltration corresponds to the 2- and 10-o'clock positions, 1 cm distal to the penile base, if the base is buried in pubic fat, the injection must be done at the junction of pubic and pelvic skin.
   e. Stabilize organ, with gentle traction, at angle of 20 to 25 degrees from midline.
   f. Pierce skin over one of dorsal nerves at penile root, and advance carefully posteromedially (0.25 to 0.5 cm) (Fig. 47.2) into subcutaneous tissue to avoid lodging in the erectile tissue. After entering skin, needle should not meet resistance and tip should

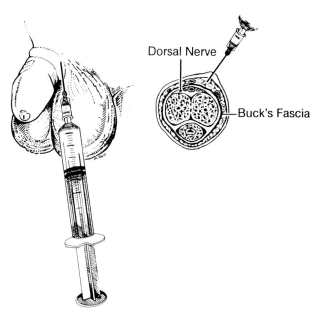

FIG. 47.2. Penis is stabilized at angle of 20 to 25 degrees from midline. The formation of a lidocaine ring is shown (see text).

remain freely movable. If the tip of the needle is not freely mobile, it is probably embedded in the corpora cavernosum beneath the dorsal nerve and should be withdrawn slightly.

g. Aspirate to rule out intravascular position.

h. Slowly infiltrate area with 0.2 to 0.4 mL of lidocaine (never infiltrate as needle is advanced or withdrawn).

i. Repeat procedure at other dorsolateral position.

After infiltration, a small lidocaine ring forms (Fig. 47.2). The swelling is minimal and does not interfere with the circumcision procedure.

j. Wait 3 to 5 minutes for analgesia.

Analgesia is usually obtained after 3 minutes and typically disappears within 20 to 30 minutes. However, there is individual variation, and testing of the prepuce with a hemostat is suggested prior to dissection.

7. Locate coronal sulcus (Fig. 47.3A). Marking the position of the sulcus with ink on the skin of the penile shaft, prior to the procedure, is helpful in demarcating this vital landmark.

8. Use mosquito hemostat to dilate preputial ring (Fig. 47.3B).

9. Use blunt probe to separate inner epithelium of prepuce from glans penis (Fig. 47.3C).

Failure to do this completely may result in a concealed penis (see G3c and G14).

10. Perform dorsal slit if desired.

This step is not mandatory as long as there is adequate separation of the glans from the prepuce.

a. Grasp rim of prepuce on dorsal aspect with mosquito hemostats, approximately 2 to 4 mm apart (Fig. 47.3D).

b. Visualize urethra.

c. Place lower blade of large, straight hemostat between prepuce and glans to within 3 to 4 mm of corona, making sure to avoid urethra.

d. Close hemostat for 5 to 10 seconds to crush foreskin in dorsal midline.

e. Use tissue scissors to cut prepuce along crush line (Fig. 47.3E).

f. Check that prepuce is freed from entire surface of glans. Complete separation if necessary.

11. Complete circumcision using method of choice.

a. Use of circumcision clamp

(1) Check clamp to ensure that all parts are present, fit well, and are in good working order.

(2) Assemble clamp, ensuring that yolk (arm) articulates correctly with baseplate.

(3) Draw prepuce backward gently to expose entire glans penis.

(4) Break down all residual adhesions, and observe position of meatus. If meatus is abnormal, cease at this point.

(5) Sponge glans dry with gauze swabs.

(6) Select stud (bell) of adequate size (see C), and place over glans (Fig. 47.4A).

(7) Pull prepuce over stud.

(a) Approximate edge of dorsal slit. (A sterile safety pin may be used.)

(b) Observe amount of skin remaining under baseplate for accuracy.

Proper placement of prepuce over stud is essential. Pulling too taut may lead to removal of excessive penile skin. Insufficient tension may lead to incomplete circumcision.

(8) Place baseplate of clamp over stud (with pin perpendicular to shaft of penis) so that prepuce is sandwiched between them (Fig. 47.4B).

(9) Continue to pull upward on stud until entire prepuce is drawn through baseplate and stud engages with baseplate.

(10) Hook yoke (arm) of clamp under side arms on shaft of stud and bolt firmly to baseplate, after checking position of prepuce between stud and baseplate (Fig. 47.4C).

(11) Remove safety pin.

(12) Wait 10 minutes.

Hemostasis is produced by pressure between baseplate and rim of stud. If the clamp is removed before 10 minutes has elapsed, wound edge hemostasis may be inadequate. If significant bleeding occurs during the procedure, remove the device and search for bleeding vessel—avoid blindly placing sutures.

(13) Remove prepuce with scalpel held parallel to and flush with upper surface of baseplate. Never use electrocautery; however, use of an ultrasound dissection scalpel has been described as a safe alternative to electrocautery (6).

(14) Loosen bolt on clamp and remove.

(15) *Optional:* Dress with loose, noncircumferential sterile gauze impregnated with Vaseline.

Gough and Lawton (7) have shown that the addition of tincture of benzoin to the dressing adversely affected wound healing and the addition of topical antibiotic did not produce better results than those achieved with ordinary paraffin gauze.

(16) Apply tight diaper for 1 hour.

(17) For 24 hours after circumcision, check (or instruct parents to check) for bleeding, excessive swelling, and difficulty voiding.

(18) Until circumcised area is completely healed, do not immerse in water; give sponge bath.

b. Use of Plastibell

(1) Follow steps 3 to 5 of E11a.

(2) Select bell of correct size (see C).

(3) Cone should fit snugly without pressure on glans.

(4) Grooved rim of bell should be just distal to apex of dorsal slit.

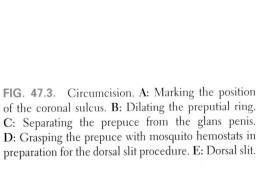

A

B

C

D

E

FIG. 47.3. Circumcision. **A:** Marking the position of the coronal sulcus. **B:** Dilating the preputial ring. **C:** Separating the prepuce from the glans penis. **D:** Grasping the prepuce with mosquito hemostats in preparation for the dorsal slit procedure. **E:** Dorsal slit.

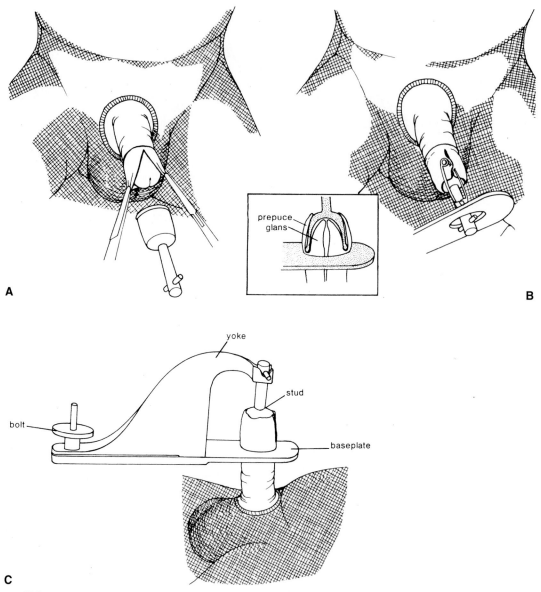

FIG. 47.4. Circumcision with a Gomco clamp. **A:** Placing the stud over the glans. **B:** Placing the baseplate of the clamp over the stud until the stud engages with the baseplate (*inset*). **C:** Gomco clamp in position for circumcision.

(5) If necessary, cut small segment out of cone so that it clears frenulum.

(6) Hold prepuce firmly in place over cone (Fig. 47.5A).

(7) Tie suture tightly around rim of bell so that prepuce is firmly compressed into groove.

(8) Trim prepuce distal to ligature with tissue scissors. Use outer rim of cone as guide.

(9) Break off cone handle. Tissue beneath ligature will atrophy and separate from bell in 5 to 8 days (maximum 10 to 12 days) (Fig. 47.5B).

c. Observe and care for circumcision as in steps 17 and 18 of Gomco clamp (E11a).

F. Management of Postoperative Bleeding

Postoperative bleeding usually stems from inadequate hemostasis (e.g., unrecognized neonatal hepatitis (14) or hereditary clotting disorders). Rarely, anomalous vessels are responsible.

Continuous Ooze

1. Apply manual pressure for 5 to 10 minutes.
   Check that the string on the Plastibell is in place and is sufficiently tight.

2. Assess bleeding site. If continued oozing

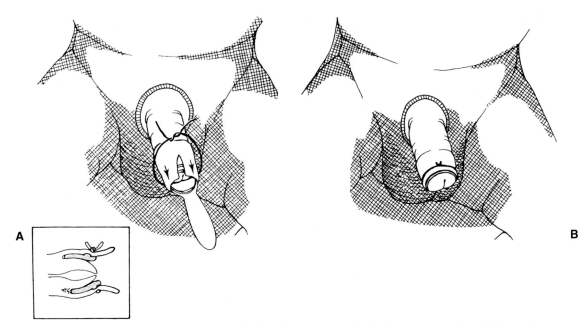

FIG. 47.5. Circumcision with a Plastibell. **A:** The prepuce is pulled forward onto the bell. **Inset:** The prepuce is compressed into the groove by the circumferential suture. **B:** Appearance of the completed circumcision.

a. Apply topical thrombin (Thrombostat) on absorbable gelatin sponge (Gelfoam) or oxidized cellulose (Oxycel, Surgicel); do not use circumferential dressing.

b. Silver nitrate and epinephrine have also been used topically to control bleeding. To avoid local ischemia or systemic effects, do not exceed a 1:100,000 concentration of epinephrine.

Active Hemorrhage or Uncontrolled Ooze

1. Surgical assessment—ligation of bleeding vessel
2. Consider underlying coagulopathy.

G. Complications (Fig. 47.6)

The overall incidence of complications associated with circumcision ranges from approximately 0.2% to 7% (10–30)

1. Hemorrhage (14)
2. Infection (11,16,17)
   More common with the Plastibell. Most are mild and respond to wet to dry dressings and Sitz baths, but fatalities have been reported
   a. Local
   b. Systemic (16)
   c. Necrotizing fasciitis (17)
3. Incomplete circumcision (most common complication)
   a. Phimosis
   b. Skin bridge between penile shaft and glans (commonly due to inadequate skin removal and failure to visualize the corona on follow-up examination)
   c. Concealed penis (see also G14) (18)

4. Trauma
   a. Urethral laceration during dorsal slit procedure (avoided by keeping urethra in view at all times during the procedure)
   b. Loss of penis (most commonly due to injuries related to cautery) (20) /amputation of glans (10,12)
   c. Hypospadias/epispadias
   d. Cyanosis/necrosis of glans penis caused by overly tight Plastibell, misplaced sutures, or overtight circumferential bandage (7,13)
   e. Urethrocutaneous fistula associated with use of Gomco clamp or Plastibell (most commonly caused by using a Plastibell or clamp of incorrect size or failure to recognize congenital megaloureter) (19)
5. Urinary retention (22)
   a. Tight (or occlusive) dressing or glanular prolapse through ring of Plastibell (21)
   b. Meatal stenosis resulting from urethral meatitis (23)
6. Inflammation/ulceration of meatus (9,23)
7. Circumcision of hypospadias
8. Chordee most commonly is the result of dense ventral scarring from inflammation; may be due to removal of excess skin from shaft or secondary to a skin bridge
9. Inclusion cyst of prepuce
10. Lymphedema (24)
11. Venous stasis (25)
12. Displacement with lodging of Plastibell around penile shaft or glans penis (9)
13. Death
    a. Anesthetic (1)

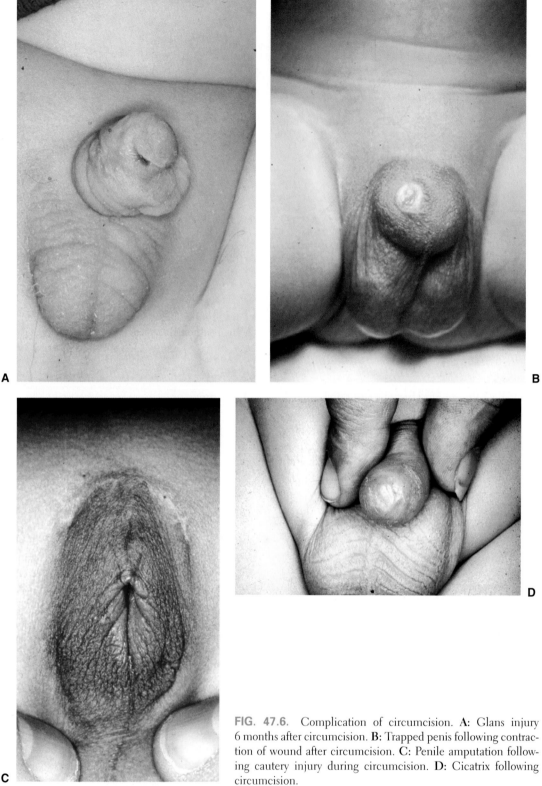

FIG. 47.6. Complication of circumcision. **A:** Glans injury 6 months after circumcision. **B:** Trapped penis following contraction of wound after circumcision. **C:** Penile amputation following cautery injury during circumcision. **D:** Cicatrix following circumcision.

b. Infection

c. Hemorrhage (14)

14. Wound separation/removal of excess skin (Fig. 47.6) (26)
    Buried penis is usually the result of inappropriate circumcision in a chubby baby with a small or concealed penis. Excessive removal of skin should be treated with application of antiseptic (iodophor) daily and not with grafting or burying the penis in scrotum. The skin will grow back.

15. Recurrence of pneumothorax (27)

16. Reaction to epinephrine used to control bleeding
    a. Tachycardia
    b. Local vasospasm (may lead to necrosis of the glans)

17. Complications due to local anesthetic
    a. Methemoglobinemia has been reported following exposure to prilocaine, procaine, benzocaine, and lidocaine (28).
    b. Hematoma; those reported in neonates have resolved spontaneously.
    c. Seizures (29)

18. Mechanical problems with Gomco clamp (30)
    a. Loss of a part
    b. Warping of the plate after multiple use
    c. Breakage of arm during tightening
    d. Grooves and nicks in bell at junction of bell and plate

References

1. Gairdner D. The fate of the foreskin—a study of circumcision. *Br Med J.* 1949;2:1433.
2. History of circumcision: a religious obligation or a medical necessity. *J Nephrol.* 2011;Suppl 17:S100.
3. Farley SJ. Neonatal circumcision: the controversy rages on. *Nat Clin Pract Urol.* 2009;6(2):59
4. Yellen HS. Bloodless circumcision of the newborn. *Am J Obstet Gynecol.* 1935;30:146.
5. Dubrisin R, Zaprudsky P. Circumcising neonates with the Mogen clamp. *Contemp OB/Gyn.* 1991;36:79.
6. Fette A, Schleef J, Haberlik A, et al. Circumcision in pediatric surgery using an ultrasound dissection scalpel. *Technol Health Care.* 2000;8:75.
7. Gough DCS, Lawton N. Circumcision—which dressing?. *Br J Urol.* 1990;65:418.
8. Garry DJ, Swoboda E, Elimian A, et al. A video study of pain relief during newborn male circumcision. *J Perinatol.* 2006;26:106.
9. Kirya C, Werthmann MW Jr. Neonatal circumcision and penile dorsal nerve block—a painless procedure. *J Pediatr.* 1978;92:998.
10. Essid A, Hamazaoui M, Sahli S, et al. Glans reimplantation after circumcision accident. *Prog Urol.* 2005;15:745.
11. Gesundheit B, Grisaru-Soen G, Greenberg D, et al. Neonatal genital herpes simplex type 1 infection after Jewish ritual circumcision: modern medicine and religious tradition. *Pediatrics.* 2004;114:e259.
12. Barnes S, Ben Chaim J, Kessler A. Postcircumcision necrosis of the glans penis: gray scale and color Doppler sonographic findings. *J Clin Ultrasound.* 2007;35(2):105.
13. Bode CO, Ikhisemojie S, Ademuyiwa AO. Penile Injuries from proximal migration of the Plastibell circumcision ring. *J Pediatr Urol.* 2010;6(1):23.
14. Hiss J, Horowitz A, Kahana T. Fatal haemorrhage following male ritual circumcision. *J Clin Forensic Med.* 2000;7:32.
15. Pieretti RV, Goldstein AM, Pieretti-Varmacke R. Late complications of newborn circumcision: a common and avoidable problem. *Pediatr Surg Int.* 2010;26(5):515.
16. Kirkpatrick BV, Eitzman DV. Neonatal septicemia after circumcision. *Clin Pediatr.* 1974;13:767.
17. Woodside JR. Necrotizing fasciitis after neonatal circumcision. *Am J Dis Child.* 1980;134:301.
18. Trier WC, Drach GW. Concealed penis—another complication of circumcision. *Am J Dis Child.* 1973;125:6.
19. Limaye RD, Hancock RA. Penile urethral fistula as a complication of circumcision. *J Pediatr.* 1968;72:105.
20. Cook A, Koury AE, Bagli DJ, et al. Use of buccal mucosa to simulate the coronal sulcus after traumatic penile amputation. *Urol.* 2005;66:1109.
21. Horowitz J, Sussheim A, Scalettar HE. Abdominal distention following ritual circumcision. *Pediatrics.* 1976;57:579.
22. Pearce I. Retention of urine: an unusual complication of the Plastibell device. *Br J Urol Int.* 2000;85:560.
23. Mackenzie AR. Meatal ulceration following neonatal circumcision. *Obstet Gynecol.* 1966;28:221.
24. Yildirim S, Taylan G, Akoz T. Circumcision as an unusual cause of penile lymphedema. *Ann Plast Surg.* 2003;50:665.
25. Ly L, Sankaran K. Acute venous stasis and swelling of the lower abdomen and extremities in an infant after circumcision. *Can Med Assoc J.* 2003;169:216.
26. Van Duyn J, Warr WS. Excessive penile skin loss from circumcision. *J Med Assoc Ga.* 1962;51:394.
27. Auerbach MR, Scanlon JW. Recurrence of pneumothorax as a possible complication of elective circumcision. *Am J Obstet Gynecol.* 1978;132:583.
28. Peker E, Cagan E, Dogan M. et al. Methemoglobinemia due to local anesthesia with prilocaine for circumcision. *J Pediatr Child Health.* 2010;46(6):362.
29. Moran LR, Hossain T, Insoft RM. Neonatal seizures following lidocaine administration for elective circumcision. *J Perinatol.* 2004;24:395.
30. Feinberg AN, Blazek MA. Mechanical complications of circumcision with a Gomco clamp. *Am J Dis Child.* 1988;142:813.

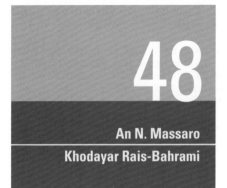

48 Drainage of Superficial Abscesses

An N. Massaro

Khodayar Rais-Bahrami

A. Definitions

A Superficial abscess is

1. A localized collection of pus resulting from bacterial organisms that cause necrosis, liquefaction, accumulation of leukocytes and debris, which presents as a fluctuant soft tissue swelling that may have associated erythema and induration (Fig. 48.1) (1–5)
2. In newborns, usually caused by invasion of local bacterial flora (2), direct inoculation, (e.g., animal bites) (6) or skin piercing (7)

B. Indications

1. To establish free drainage of contents from a superficial abscess

   Surgical incision and drainage is the definitive treatment for soft tissue abscesses. Antibiotic therapy alone is ineffective in the setting of localized abscess (1,2,8–11)
2. To identify pathogens and direct antimicrobial therapy if needed (2,12–16)
3. To differentiate infectious from noninfectious lesions (15,17,18)

C. Contraindications

1. Carefully identify and avoid
   a. Cephalohematoma
   b. Hemangioma
   c. Cystic hygroma
   d. Encephalocele
2. Avoid premature incision and drainage of abscesses that have not yet fully matured (i.e., in the initial stages of induration and inflammation prior to formation of pus) (4). This may lead to
   a. A noncurative intervention
   b. Possible extension of infectious process
   c. Bacteremia
      Premature incision may be avoided by the use of ultrasound with or without diagnostic needle aspiration (19,20).

D. Equipment

Sterile

1. Gloves and gown
2. Antiseptic swabs or cup containing antiseptic solution
3. 1-mL syringe
4. Nonbacteriostatic, isotonic saline without preservative
5. 23-gauge needle
6. 2- × 2-inch gauze squares
7. Scalpel with no. 11 blade
8. Cotton-tipped culture swab
9. Mosquito hemostat
10. 0.5-inch, fine-mesh, plain gauze

Nonsterile

1. Ethyl chloride spray as topical anesthetic. (For larger lesions, local anesthesia with lidocaine may be used.)
2. Mask and cap
3. Adhesive tape

E. Precautions

1. Use appropriate isolation techniques to safeguard other infants.
2. Obtain blood cultures after drainage.
3. Do not suture abscess cavity following incision and drainage.
4. Débride all tissue undergoing putrefaction and digestion thoroughly (3).
5. Make skin incisions:
   a. Conform with skin creases/natural folds to minimize scar formation
   b. Large enough to allow for proper débridement and drainage
   c. Simple linear–cruciate or elliptical skin incisions may result in more unsightly scar formation (4).
6. For abscesses in cosmetic areas, areas under significant skin tension (i.e., extensor surfaces), or areas with extensive scar tissue (i.e., sites of prior drainage procedures), a stab incision or needle aspiration alone may be preferable. (This may require multiple decompressions and/or

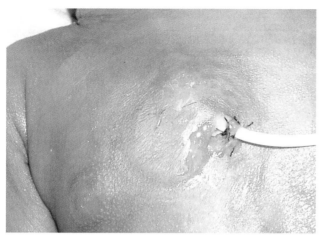

FIG. 48.1. Superficial abscess in the site of a Broviac central venous line insertion in the left anterior chest wall.

delayed complete incision and drainage if reaccumulation occurs.)

7. Care should be taken in areas with abundant vascular and neural structures, such as the groin, posterior knee, antecubital fossa, and neck (5).

8. If foreign body is suspected, a radiograph should be obtained (4).

F. Technique (2–5)

1. Spray roof of abscess with ethyl chloride until skin becomes white. (If local anesthesia is required, lidocaine can be injected subcutaneously with a 25-gauge needle into the dome of the abscess.)

2. Prepare as for major procedure if abscess is to be drained, or for minor procedure if needle aspiration alone is to be performed (see Chapter 5).

3. Prepare local area with antiseptic (e.g., iodophor).

4. Aspiration (may be performed in combination with incision and drainage for confirmation of presence of pus and collection of material for culture, or alone if abscess is in area where incision is not preferable [see E6]).

   a. Attach sterile needle to syringe.

   b. Insert needle into pustule, abscess cavity, or advancing border of cellulitis.

   c. Aspirate the material deep within the lesion.

   d. If no material is aspirated, inject 0.1 to 0.2 mL of nonbacteriostatic saline and withdraw immediately.

   e. *Process aspirated material immediately:* Gram stain and culture for anaerobic and aerobic organisms; Giemsa stain for suspected herpes. Perform other special stains as warranted.

5. Incision and drainage

   a. Insert scalpel blade and incise at point of maximum fluctuance. The size of the incision should be as small as possible yet allow for continued adequate drainage (i.e., length of the abscess cavity).

   b. Obtain specimen for culture with cotton-tipped applicator, if not obtained by prior aspiration with syringe and needle.

   c. Evacuate exudate from abscess with gentle pressure from finger or hemostat wrapped in gauze. Use caution when probing abscess with finger in cases of suspected retained foreign bodies or fragments—for this reason, hemostat wrapped in gauze is the preferred method (4).

   d. If necessary, insert mosquito hemostat into abscess cavity and spread blades to break septa and to release remaining collections of pus (Fig. 48.2A). Recognize that this may cause discomfort and should be done rapidly.

6. Lavage area with sterile saline to remove residual pus (optional).

7. If indicated, insert plain, 0.5-inch gauze into abscess cavity to stop bleeding and/or to serve as a wick to promote drainage (Fig. 48.2B).

8. Apply dry, sterile dressing.

9. Remove half of gauze packing in 24 hours and remainder within 48 hours. (Some larger wounds may require multiple packing changes.)

10. Check abscess wound, and apply sterile warm soaks for 20 to 30 minutes, three times a day, until healing has commenced, as indicated by

    a. Cessation of drainage

    b. Formation of granulation tissue

    c. Resolution of local tissue inflammation

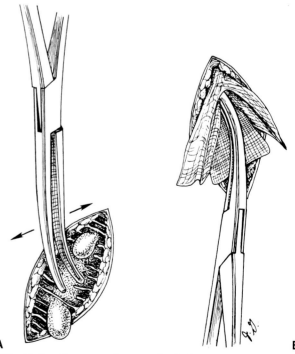

FIG. 48.2. Drainage of a superficial abscess. **A:** Breaking the septa with a clamp. **B:** Packing the wound.

G. Complications

1. Introduction of infection into sterile abscess or hematoma
2. Local bleeding
3. Injury to blood vessels, nerves, or tendons (deep to abscess cavity) (5)
4. Incomplete drainage with recurrent abscess formation (1,3)
5. Systemic infection (21,22)
6. Scar formation at drainage site, requiring skin graft (23)
7. Reduction of breast size following incomplete drainage of breast abscess (24)

References

1. Meislin HW, Lerner SA, Graves MH, et al. Cutaneous abscesses. Anaerobic and aerobic bacteriology and outpatient management. *Ann Intern Med.* 1977;87:145.
2. Meislin HW, McGehee MD, Rosen P. Management and microbiology of cutaneous abscesses. *JACEP.* 1978;7:186.
3. Macfie J, Harvey J. The treatment of acute superficial abscesses: a prospective clinical trial. *Br J Surg.*1977;64:264.
4. Butler KH. Incision and drainage. In: Roberts JR, Hedges JR, eds. *Clinical Procedures in Emergency Medicine.* 4th ed. Philadelphia: WB Saunders; 2004:717.
5. Albom MJ. Surgical gems. Surgical management of a superficial cutaneous abscess. *J Dermatol Surg.* 1976;2:120.
6. Brook I. Microbiology and management of human and animal bite wound infections. *Prim Care.*2003;30:25.
7. Folz BJ, Lippert BM, Kuelkens C, et al. Hazards of piercing and facial body art: a report of three patients and literature review. *Ann Plast Surg.* 2000;45:374.
8. Duong M, Markwell S, Peter J, et al. Randomized, controlled trial of antibiotics in the management of community-acquired skin abscesses in the pediatric patient. *Ann Emerg Med.* 2010;55:401.
9. Lee MC, Rios AM, Aten MF, et al. Management and outcome of children with skin and soft tissue abscesses caused by community-acquired methicillin-resistant Staphylococcus aureus. *Pediatr Infect Dis J.* 2004;23:123.
10. Llera JL, Levy RC. Treatment of cutaneous abscess: a double-blind clinical study. *Ann Emerg Med.* 1985;14:15.
11. Rajendran PM, Young D, Maurer T, et al. Randomized, double-blind, placebo-controlled trial of cephalexin for treatment of uncomplicated skin abscesses in a population at risk for community-acquired methicillin-resistant Staphylococcus aureus infection. *Antimicrob Agents Chemother.* 2007;51:4044.
12. Zetola N, Francis JS, Nuermberger EL, et al. Community-acquired methicillin-resistant Staphylococcus aureus: an emerging threat. *Lancet Infect Dis.* 2005;5:275.
13. Halvorson GD, Halvorson JE, Iserson KV. Abscess incision and drainage in the emergency department–Part I. *J Emerg Med.* 1985;3:227.
14. Fridkin SK, Hageman JC, Morrison M, et al. Methicillin-resistant Staphylococcus aureus disease in three communities. *N Engl J Med.* 2005;352:1436.
15. Rudoy RC, Nakashima G. Diagnostic value of needle aspiration in Haemophilus influenzae type b cellulitis. *J Pediatr.*1979;94:924.
16. Garcea G, Lloyd T, Jacobs M, et al. Role of microbiological investigations in the management of non-perineal cutaneous abscesses. *Postgrad Med J.* 2003;79:519.
17. Jarratt M, Ramsdell W. Infantile acropustulosis. *Arch Dermatol.* 1979;115:834.
18. Kahn G, Rywlin AM. Acropustulosis of infancy. *Arch Dermatol.* 1979;115:831.
19. Loyer EM, DuBrow RA, David CL, et al. Imaging of superficial soft-tissue infections: sonographic findings in cases of cellulitis and abscess. *Am J Roentgenol.* 1996;166:149.
20. Cardinal E, Bureau NJ, Aubin B, et al. Role of ultrasound in musculoskeletal infections. *Radiol Clin North Am.* 2001; 39:191.
21. Blick PW, Flowers MW, Marsden AK, et al. Antibiotics in surgical treatment of acute abscesses. *Br Med J.* 1980;281:111.
22. Fine BC, Sheckman PR, Bartlett JC. Incision and drainage of soft-tissue abscesses and bacteremia. *Ann Intern Med.* 1985; 103:645.
23. Feder HM Jr, MacLean WC, Moxon R. Scalp abscess secondary to fetal scalp electrode. *J Pediatr.* 1976;89:808.
24. Rudoy RC, Nelson JD. Breast abscess during the neonatal period. A review. *Am J Dis Child.* 1975;129:1031.

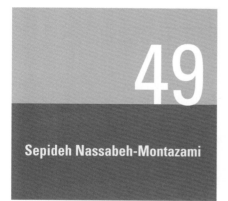

49

Phototherapy

Sepideh Nassabeh-Montazami

Phototherapy is the most common therapeutic intervention used for the treatment of hyperbilirubinemia (1). Phototherapy causes three reactions: configurational and structural isomerization of the bilirubin molecule and photo-oxidation, leading to polar, water-soluble photoproducts that can be excreted in bile and urine without the need for conjugation or further metabolism (2).

The aim of phototherapy is to reduce serum bilirubin levels to decrease the risk of acute bilirubin encephalopathy and the more chronic sequel of bilirubin toxicity, kernicterus (1). High-intensity phototherapy significantly reduces the *total serum bilirubin* (TSB) and decreases the need for exchange transfusion (3).

A. Indications

1. Clinically significant indirect hyperbilirubinemia. Indications to start phototherapy in babies with hyperbilirubinemia vary depending on gestational age, birthweight, hours of life, presence of hemolysis, and other risk factors such as acidosis and sepsis (1,4).
2. The TSB level must be considered when making the decision to commence treatment, as there is significant variability in laboratory measurement of direct bilirubin levels (5).
3. The American Academy of Pediatrics has published clinical practice guidelines for phototherapy in newborn infants at 35 weeks' or more gestation (1) (Fig. 49.1).
4. These guidelines do not apply to preterm infants <35 weeks' gestation. Preterm infants are at higher risk of developing hyperbilirubinemia compared to term infants. Although guidelines have been proposed, the decision to initiate phototherapy in this group of infants remains variable and highly individualized (4,6) (Table 49.1).

B. Contraindications

1. Congenital porphyria or a family history of porphyria is an absolute contraindication to the use of phototherapy. Severe purpuric bullous eruptions have been described in neonates with congenital erythropoietic porphyria treated with phototherapy (7).
2. Concomitant use of drugs or agents that are photosensitizers is also an absolute contraindication (8).
3. Concurrent therapy with metalloporphyrin heme oxygenase inhibitors has been reported to result in mild transient erythema (9).
4. Although infants with cholestatic jaundice may develop the "bronze baby syndrome" when exposed to phototherapy (see H), the presence of direct hyperbilirubinemia is not considered to be a contraindication (1). However, because the products of phototherapy are excreted in the bile, the presence of cholestasis may decrease the effectiveness of phototherapy.

C. Equipment

In order to have an understanding of the equipment available for phototherapy, it is necessary to be familiar with the terminology involved (10).

1. *Spectral qualities* of the delivered light (wavelength range and peak). Bilirubin absorbs visible light within the wavelength range of 400 to 500 nm, with peak absorption at 460 ± 10 nm considered to be the most effective (2).
2. *Irradiance* (intensity of light), expressed as watts per square centimeter (W/cm^2), refers to the number of photons received per square centimeter of exposed body surface area.
3. *Spectral irradiance* is irradiance that is quantitated within the effective wavelength range for efficacy and is expressed as $\mu W/cm^2/nm$. This is measured by various commercially available radiometers. Specific radiometers are generally recommended for each phototherapy system, because measurements of irradiance may vary depending on the radiometer and the light source (1,10).

A variety of phototherapy equipment devices exist and may be free-standing, attached to a radiant warmer, wall-mounted, suspended from the ceiling, or fiberoptic systems. These in turn may contain various light sources

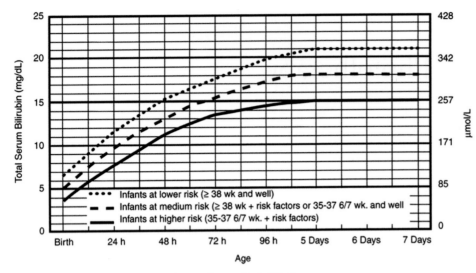

• Use total bilirubin. Do not subtract direct reacting or conjugated bilirubin.
• Risk factors = isoimmune hemolytic disease, G6PD deficiency, asphyxia, significant lethargy, temperature instability, sepsis, acidosis, or albumin < 3.0g/dL (if measured)
• For well infants 35-37 6/7 wk can adjust TSB levels for intervention around the medium risk line. It is an option to intervene at lower TSB levels for infants closer to 35 wks and at higher TSB levels for those closer to 37 6/7 wk.
• It is an option to provide conventional phototherapy in hospital or at home at TSB levels 2-3 mg/dL (35-50mmol/L) below those shown but home phototherapy should not be used in any infant with risk factors.

FIG. 49.1. Guidelines for phototherapy in hospitalized infants of 35 or more weeks' gestation. (From American Academy of Pediatrics Subcommittee on Hyperbilirubinemia. Management of hyperbilirubinemia in the newborn infant 35 or more weeks of gestation. *Pediatrics.* 2004;114: 297.)

to deliver the phototherapy. The clinician is, therefore, faced with a vast array of equipment to choose from and must be aware of advantages and disadvantages of each type. Table 49.2 describes some of the phototherapy devices commonly used in the United States.

4. Fluorescent tubes
   a. "Special blue" tubes, such as F20 T12/BB, provide more irradiance in the blue spectrum than other tubes and are the most effective fluorescent light source. (2). The "special blue F20 T12/BB" tubes provide much greater irradiance than regular blue tubes, labeled F20T12/B. The flickering glare of the blue light has been reported to cause giddiness, nausea, and temporary blurring of vision in nursing personnel (11). One way to overcome this has been to use cool white light in conjunction with the special blue, but this combination can decrease efficacy by as much as 50%, depending on the proportion of cool white light used (12).
   b. Green/turquoise lamps penetrate the skin to a greater depth, but the advantage over blue light is unclear (13–15).
   c. Cool white lamps may be inadequate in sufficiently decreasing total bilirubin levels unless the lights are positioned in close proximity to the infant (13). As mentioned previously, this type of light has also been used together with special blue tubes.
   d. Daylight lamps, like cool white lamps, have a wider wavelength spectrum and are less effective than blue light (12).

5. Halogen lamps
   a. Halogen spotlight systems utilize single or multiple metal halide lamps as the light source and can provide high irradiance over a small surface area (>20 μW/cm^2/nm).
   b. These units can generate considerable heat, with the potential of causing thermal skin injury; therefore, they must not be in close proximity to the patient.
   c. The variable positioning with respect to the distance from the infant as well as heterogeneity of the irradiance can lead to unreliable dosing and unpredictable clinical responses. In addition, they are more expensive than fluorescent bulbs (2).

6. Fiberoptic systems
   a. UV-filtered light from a tungsten–halogen bulb enters a fiberoptic cable and is emitted from the sides and end of fiberoptic fibers inside a plastic pad.

TABLE 49.1	Guidelines for the Use of Phototherapy and Exchange Transfusion in Preterm Infants Based on Gestational Age		
	Total Bilirubin Level (mg/dL/μmol/L)		
		Exchange Transfusion	
Gestational Age (wk)	**Phototherapy**	**Sick**[a]	**Well**
36	14.6 (250)	17.5 (300)	20.5 (350)
32	8.8 (150)	14.6 (250)	17.5 (300)
28	5.8 (100)	11.7 (200)	14.6 (250)
24	4.7 (80)	8.8 (150)	11.7 (200)

[a]Rhesus disease, perinatal asphyxia, hypoxia, acidosis, hypercapnia.
From Maisels MJ, Watchko JF. Treatment of jaundice in low birthweight infants. *Arch Dis Child Fetal Neonatal Ed.* 2003;88:F459.

TABLE 49.2	Phototherapy Devices Commonly Used in the United States, and Their Performance Characteristics

Device	Manufacturer	Distance to Patient (cm)	Treatable Body Surface Area (%)	Spectrum, Total (nm)	Bandwidth[a] (nm)	Peak (nm)	Footprint Irradiance (μW/cm^2/nm) Mean ± SD
Light Emitting Diodes NeoBLUE	Natus Medical, San Carlos, CA	30	100	420–450	20	462	30 ± 7
Fluorescent BiliLite CW/BB	Olympic Medical, San Carlos, CA	45	100	380–720	69	578	8 ± 1
BiliLite BB	Olympic Medical, San Carlos, CA	45	100	400–550	35	445	17 ± 2
BiliLite TL52	Olympic Medical, San Carlos, CA	45	100	400–626	69	437	19 ± 3
BiliBed	Medela, McHenry, IL	0	71	400–560	80	450	36 ± 2
Halogen MiniBiliLite	Olympic Medical, San Carlos, CA	45	54	350–800	190	580	7 ± 5
Phototherapy Lite	Philips Inc, Andover, MA	45	54	370–850	200	590	5 ± 5
Halogen fiberoptic Biliblanket	Ohmeda, Fairfield, CT	0	24	390–600	70	533	20 ± 6
Wallaby II Preterm	Philips, Inc, Andover, MA	0	19	400–560	45	513	16 ± 6
WallabyII Term	Philips, Inc, Andover, MA	0	53	400–560	45	513	8 ± 1
SpotLight 1000	Philips, Inc, Andover, MA	45	54	400–560	45	513	6 ± 3
PEP Model 2000	PEP Fryeburg, ME	23	100	400–717	63	445	28 ± 11
BiliSoft	GE Healthcare, Laurel, MD	0	71	400–670	40	453	25 ± 16

[a]Spectral bandwidth defined as the width of the emission spectrum in nm at 50% of peak light intensity.
From Bhutani VK, the Committee on Fetus and Newborn. Phototherapy to prevent severe neonatal hyperbilirubinemia in the newborn infant 35 or more weeks of gestation. *Pediatrics.* 2011;128:e1046.

b. The pad emits insignificant levels of heat, so it can be placed in direct contact with the infant to deliver up to 35 μW/cm^2/nm of spectral irradiance, mainly in the blue–green range (16).

c. The orientation of the fiberoptic fibers determines the uniformity of emission and is unique to each of the commercially available devices.

d. The main advantages of these systems are that, while receiving phototherapy, the infant can be held and/or nursed, thereby minimizing infant–parent separation. In addition, covering the infant's eyes is not necessary, preventing further parental anxiety.

e. The main disadvantage of the fiberoptic pads is that they cover a relatively small surface area and, therefore, have less efficacy compared to overhead sources. They should not be used as the sole means of providing phototherapy in an infant with significant hyperbilirubinemia (1,2,11).

f. These devices are often used as an adjunct to conventional overhead application of phototherapy to provide "double" phototherapy (circumferential phototherapy), which has greater efficacy because greater body surface area is exposed to the light (10,16).

7. Gallium nitride light-emitting diodes (LEDs)

a. These systems are semiconductor phototherapy devices capable of delivering high spectral irradi-ance levels of >200 μW/cm^2/nm with very little generation of heat within a very narrow emission spectrum in the blue range (460 to 485 nm), with low infrared emission and no ultraviolet emission (10,17,18).

b. LEDs have a longer lifetime (>20,000 hours) and have become cost-effective for use in phototherapy devices. LEDs and compact fluorescent tubes are equally efficacious in the management of hyperbilirubinemia (19).

D. Technique (Conventional Phototherapy)

Intensive phototherapy is defined as the use of light in the 430- to 490-nm band delivered at 30 μW/cm^2/nm or higher to the greatest body surface area possible (1,10).

1. Position the phototherapy unit over the infant to obtain desired irradiance (10 to 40 μW/cm^2/nm). The maximal amount of irradiance achieved by the standard technique is generally 30 to 50 μW/cm^2/nm. The distance of the light from the infant has a significant effect on the intensity of phototherapy, and to achieve maximal intensity, the lights should be positioned as close as possible to the infant. Fluorescent tubes may be brought within approximately 10 cm of term infants

without causing overheating, but halogen spot phototherapy lamps should not be positioned closer to the infant than recommended by the manufacturer, because of the risk of burns (10).

2. If increased irradiance is required, add additional units or place a fiberoptic phototherapy pad under the infant (10,16). Additional surface area may be exposed to phototherapy by lining the sides of the bassinet with aluminum foil or a white cloth (20).

3. Keep the photoradiometer calibrated and perform periodic checks of phototherapy units to make sure that adequate irradiance is being delivered (10).

4. Maintain an intact acrylic/safety glass shield over phototherapy light bulbs to block ultraviolet radiation and to protect the infant from accidental bulb breakage.

5. Provide ventilation to the phototherapy unit to prevent overheating light bulbs.

6. Maintain cleanliness and electrical safety.

E. Technique (Fiberoptic Phototherapy)

Fiberoptic phototherapy can be used as the sole source of phototherapy or as an adjunct to conventional treatment.

1. Insert the panel into disposable cover so that it is flat and directed toward the infant.

2. Place the covered panel around the infant's back or chest and secure in position. The phototherapy blanket/pad must be positioned directly next to the infant's skin to be effective. Avoid constriction and skin irritation under the infant's arms if the panel is wrapped around the infant.

3. Discard disposable covers after each treatment and when soiled.

4. Use eye patches if there is any direct exposure to lights in panel or if used with conventional phototherapy for double-sided effect.

5. Ensure stability and adequate ventilation of the illuminator unit by placing it on a secure surface.

6. Connect the fiberoptic panel to illuminator.

7. Keep the fiberoptic panel and illuminator clean and dry.

8. Allow the lamp to cool for 10 to 20 minutes before moving the illuminator. Do not place sharp or heavy objects on the panel or cable.

Care of the Infant Receiving Phototherapy

1. Monitor temperature, particularly of infants in an incubator, who may develop hyperthermia.

2. Monitor intake, output, and weight. Fluid supplementation may be necessary secondary to increased insensible losses and frequent stooling. Encourage breastfeeding. Healthy term breast-fed infants may be supplemented with milk-based formula if maternal milk supply is inadequate. IV fluids are rarely required.

Milk feeding inhibits the enterohepatic circulation of bilirubin (1).

3. The use of eye protection in the form of eye patches is necessary for infants receiving overhead phototherapy. Masks adhering directly to Velcro tabs on the temples are preferable to circumferential headbands.

4. Maximize skin exposure to phototherapy source by using the smallest possible diapers as well as keeping blanket rolls from blocking light.

5. Avoid fully occlusive dressings, bandages, topical skin ointments, and plastic in direct contact with the infant's skin, to prevent burns.

6. Remove plastic heat shields and plastic wrap that decrease irradiance delivered to the skin (21).

7. If in use, shield the oxygen saturation monitor probe from the phototherapy light.

8. Encourage parents to continue feeding, caring for, and visiting their infant.

F. Home Phototherapy

Home phototherapy decreases costs of hospitalization and eliminates separation of mother and infant. It is safe and effective for selected infants. Home phototherapy should be used only in infants whose bilirubin levels are in the "optional phototherapy" range (Fig. 49.1).

1. Make arrangements to measure the infant's serum bilirubin every 12 to 24 hours, depending on the previous concentration and rate of rise. The infant should be examined daily by a visiting nurse or at an office.

2. The supervising physician should be in contact with the family daily during the period of treatment.

3. The infant should be rehospitalized if he or she shows signs of illness or if the serum bilirubin concentration exceeds 18 mg/dL.

G. Efficacy of Phototherapy

The clinical impact of effective phototherapy should be evident within 4 to 6 hours of initiation, with a decrease of more than 2 mg/dL (34 μmol/L) in serum bilirubin concentration. The clinical response depends on the rates of bilirubin production, tissue deposition and elimination, and photochemical reactions of bilirubin. The therapeutic efficacy of phototherapy depends on several factors.

1. *Exposed body surface area:* The greater the area exposed, the greater the rate of bilirubin decline.

2. Distance of the infant from the light source

3. Skin thickness and pigmentation

4. Total bilirubin at clinical presentation

5. Duration of exposure to phototherapy

H. Discontinuation of Phototherapy and Follow-Up

1. There is no single standard for discontinuing phototherapy. The total serum bilirubin (TSB) level that determines the discontinuation of phototherapy depends on the age of the infant, the age and bilirubin level at which treatment was initiated, and the etiology of the hyperbilirubinemia (1,22).
2. For infants who are readmitted to the hospital (usually for TSB levels of 18 mg/dL or higher), phototherapy may be discontinued when the serum bilirubin level falls below 13 to 14 mg/dL.
3. For infants who are readmitted with hyperbilirubinemia and then discharged, significant rebound is uncommon, but may still occur. In cases of prematurity, positive direct antiglobulin (Coombs) test, and for babies treated <72 hours, the likelihood of rebound is much higher, and these risk factors should be taken into account when planning postphototherapy follow-up (23). Generally, a follow-up bilirubin measurement within 24 hours after discharge is recommended (1).

I. Complications of Phototherapy

"Phototherapy has been used in millions of infants for more than 30 years, and reports of significant toxicity are exceptionally rare" (1).

Complications include the following.

1. "Bronze baby syndrome" occurs in some infants with cholestatic jaundice who are exposed to phototherapy, as a result of accumulation in the skin and serum of porphyrins. The bronzing disappears in most infants within 2 months (24). Rare complications of purpuric eruptions due to transient porphyrinemia have been described in infants with severe cholestasis who receive phototherapy (25).
2. Diarrhea or loose stools (26)
3. Dehydration secondary to insensible water loss
4. Skin changes ranging from minor erythema, increased pigmentation, and skin burns, to rare and more severe blistering and photosensitivity in infants with porphyria and hemolytic disease. Concerns about an increase in the number of melanocytic nevi have not been substantiated (27).
5. Although there is a risk of potential retinal damage from light exposure, adverse effects have not been reported in neonates because eye patches are used routinely (28).
6. Separation of mother and infant and interference with bonding.

References

1. American Academy of Pediatrics Subcommittee on Hyperbilirubinemia. Management of hyperbilirubinemia in the newborn infant 35 or more weeks of gestation. *Pediatrics*. 2004; 114:297.
2. McDonagh AF, Lighter DA. Phototherapy and the photobiology of bilirubin. *Semin Liver Dis*. 1988;8:272.
3. De Carvalho M, Mochdece C, Moreira ME. High intensity phototherapy for the treatment of severe nonhemolytic neonatal hyperbilirubinemia. *Acta Pediatrica*. 2011;100:620.
4. Watchko J, Maisels MJ. Enduring controversies in the management of hyperbilirubinemia in preterm neonates. *Semin Fetal Neonatal Med*. 2010;15:136.
5. Davis A, Rosenthal P, Newman T. Interpreting conjugated bilirubin levels in newborns. *J Pediatr*. 2011;35:134.
6. van Imhoff DE, Dijk PH, Hulzebos CV, et al. Uniform treatment thresholds for hyperbilirubinemia in preterm infants: background and synopsis of a national guideline. *Early Hum Dev*. 2011;87: 521.
7. Soylu A, Kavukcu S, Turkmen M. Phototherapy sequela in a child with congenital erythropoietic porphyria. *Eur J Pediatr*. 1999;158:526.
8. Kearns GL, Williams BJ, Timmons OD. Fluorescein phototoxicity in a premature infant. *J Pediatr*. 1985;107:796.
9. Valaez T, Petmezaki S, Henschke C, et al. Control of jaundice in preterm newborns by an inhibitor of bilirubin production: studies with tin-mesoporphyrin. *Pediatrics*. 1994;93:1.
10. Bhutani VK, the Committee on Fetus and Newborn. Phototherapy to prevent severe neonatal hyperbilirubinemia in the newborn infant 35 or more weeks of gestation. *Pediatrics*. 2011;128: e1046.
11. Sarici SU, Alpay F, Unay B, et al. Comparison of the efficacy of conventional special blue light phototherapy and fiberoptic phototherapy in the management of neonatal hyperbilirubinemia. *Acta Paediatr*. 1999;88:1249.
12. De Carvalho M, De Carvalho D, Trzmielina S, et al. Intensified phototherapy using daylight fluorescent lamps. *Acta Pediatr*. 1999;88:768.
13. Ebbesen F, Agati G, Pratesi R. Phototherapy with turquoise versus blue light. *Arch Dis Child Fetal Neonatal Ed*. 2003;88:F430.
14. Seidman DS, Moise J, Ergaz Z. A prospective randomised controlled study of phototherapy using blue and blue-green light emitting devices and conventional halogen quartz phototherapy. *J Perinatol*. 2003;23:123.
15. Roll EB, Christensen T. Formation of photoproducts and cytotoxicity of bilirubin irradiated with turquoise and blue phototherapy light. *Acta Pediatr*. 2005;94:1448.
16. Tan KL. Comparison of the efficacy of fiberoptic and conventional phototherapy for neonatal hyperbilirubinemia. *J Pediatr*. 1994;125:607.
17. Vreman HJ, Wong RJ, Stevenson DK, et al. Light emitting diodes: a novel light source for phototherapy. *Pediatr Res*. 1998;44:804.
18. Seidman DS, Moise J, Ergaz Z, et al. A new blue light emitting phototherapy device: a prospective randomized controlled study. *J Pediatr*. 2000;136:771.
19. Kumar p, Murki S, Chawla D, et al. Light emitting diodes vs compact fluorescent tubes for phototherapy in neonatal jaundice: a multicenter randomized controlled trial. *Indian Pediatr*. 2010;47:131.
20. Eggert P, Stick C, Schroder H. On the distribution of irradiation intensity in phototherapy. Measurements of effective irradiance in an incubator. *Eur J Pediatr*. 1984;142:58.
21. Kardson J, Schothorst A, Ruys JH, et al. Plastic blankets and heat shields decrease transmission of phototherapy light. *Acta Paediatr Scand*. 1986;75:555.
22. Maisels MJ, Kring E. Bilirubin rebound following intensive phototherapy. *Arch Pediatr Adolesc Med*. 2002;156:669.

23. Kaplan M, Kaplan E, Hammerman C, et al. Post phototherapy neonatal rebound: a potential cause of significant hyperbilirubinemia. *Arch Dis Child.* 2006;91:31.

24. Rubaltelli F, Da Riol R, D'Amore ES, et al. The bronze baby syndrome: evidence of increased tissue concentration of copper porphyrins. *Acta Pediatr.* 1996;85:381.

25. Paller AS, Eramo LR, Farrell EE, et al. Purpuric phototherapy induced eruption in transfused neonates: relation to transient porphyrinemia. *Pediatrics.* 1997;100:360.

26. DeCurtis M, Guandalini S, Fasano A, et al. Diarrhea in jaundiced neonates treated with phototherapy: role of intestinal secretion. *Arch Dis Child.* 1989:64:1161.

27. Mahe E, Beauchet A, Aegerter P, et al. Neonatal blue light phototherapy does not increase nevus count in 9 year old children. *Pediatrics.* 2009;123:e896.

28. Hunter JJ, Morgan JL, Merigan WH, et al. The susceptibility of the retina to photochemical damage from visible light. *Prog Retin Eye Res.* 2012;31:28.

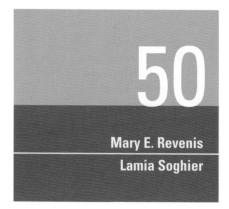

50

Mary E. Revenis

Lamia Soghier

Intraosseous Infusions

A. Indications

1. Emergency IV access when other venous access is not readily available; to restore intravascular volume so that peripheral venous access becomes possible. See Table 50.1 for categories of fluid and medications that have been infused (1–6).

B. Contraindications (3,5,6)

1. Bone without cortical integrity (fracture, previous penetration): Extravasation of infusate
2. *Sternal site*: Potential damage to heart and lungs (7)
3. Overlying soft tissue infection
4. Osteogenesis imperfecta
5. Obliterative diseases of marrow such as osteopetrosis

C. Equipment (Fig. 50.1)

Sterile

1. Surgical gloves
2. Antiseptic swabs
3. Gauze squares
4. Aperture drape
5. 1% lidocaine in 1-mL syringe with a 25-gauge needle
6. Needle, in order of preference (1–3,10)
   a. Bone marrow or intraosseous needle (18-gauge) (stylet and adjustable depth indicator preferred)
   b. Short spinal needle with stylet (18- or 20-gauge)
   c. Short hypodermic needle (18- or 20-gauge)
   d. Butterfly needle (16- to 19-gauge) (8)
7. 5-mL syringe on a three-way stopcock and IV extension set with clamp
8. IV-infusion set and IV fluid
9. 5-mL syringes with saline flush solution

Optional

Intraosseous needle placement device (intended for use at the proximal tibial location). Devices approved for newborns are the battery operated driver EZ-IO PD (Pediatric) (Vidacare, San Antonio, Texas) (approved for 3 kg or larger), and the spring-activated B.I.G. Bone Injection Gun (WaisMed,

Houston, Texas). There are company-provided reports of use in delivery rooms and intensive care nurseries. Published information on use of these devices in small premature infants is scarce. There is limited information on the incidence of success or complications when using these devices, as compared with manual insertion of the intraosseous needle (9).

Nonsterile

1. Small sand bag or rolled towel to aid in stabilizing limb
2. Tape
3. Armboard
4. Disposable plastic cup

D. Precautions

1. Limit use to emergency vascular access, when peripheral or central venous access is not feasible (11).
2. Avoid inserting needle through infected skin or subcutaneous tissue.
3. Stabilize limb with counterpressure, with sand bag or towel roll directly opposite proposed site of penetration, to avoid bone fracture.
4. If hand is also used to stabilize limb, do not position hand directly opposite puncture site, to avoid inadvertent puncture of hand by the intraosseous needle if it goes through the limb. This is true regardless of whether a sand bag or towel is used. Limit needle size to decrease risk of bone fracture.
5. Administer drugs in the usual doses for IV administration; however, when possible, to reduce the risk of bone marrow damage, dilute hypertonic or strongly alkaline solutions prior to infusion (2).
6. Discontinue intraosseous infusion as soon as alternative venous access is established, to reduce risk of osteomyelitis.

E. Technique

Proximal Tibia (1–3,12) (Fig. 50.2)

1. Position patient supine.
2. Place sand bag or towel roll behind knee to provide countersupport behind puncture site.

TABLE 50.1	Types of Intraosseous Infusates Reported in the Literature (4,5,17,19,23)

1. Fluids
    a. Normal saline
    b. Crystalloids
    c. Glucose (dilute if possible when using D50) (17,24)
    d. Ringer's lactate (19)
2. Blood and blood products
3. Medications
    a. Anesthetic agents
    b. Antibiotics
    c. Atropine (19)
    d. Calcium gluconate
    e. Dexamethasone (19)
    f. Diazepam(19)
    g. Diazoxide (19); phenytoin (25)
    h. Dobutamine (23)
    i. Dopamine (23,24,26)
    j. Ephedrine (27)
    k. Epinephrine (27)
    l. Heparin (19)
    m. Insulin
    n. Isoproterenol (26)
    o. Lidocaine
    p. Morphine
    q. Sodium bicarbonate (dilute if possible) (17,28)
4. Contrast material (29)

3. Clean proximal tibia with antiseptic solution.
4. Put on sterile gloves.
5. Apply aperture drape.
6. If appropriate, inject lidocaine into skin, soft tissue, and periosteum (13).

7. *Determine penetration depth on needle:* Rarely more than 1 cm in infants or 0.5 cm in small premature infants.
    a. For needle or bone needle injection device with adjustable depth indicator, adjust sheath to allow desired penetration.
    b. For needle without an adjustable depth indicator, hold the needle in the dominant hand with blunt end supported by the palm and the index finger approximately 1 cm from the bevel of the needle to avoid pushing it past this mark.
8. Palpate tibial tuberosity with index finger (Fig. 50.3).
9. Hold the thigh and knee above and lateral to the insertion site with the palm of the nondominant hand. Wrap fingers and thumb around, but not behind, the knee to stabilize the proximal tibia.
10. Insert needle on the flat, anteromedial surface of the tibia, 1 to 2 cm below and 1 cm medial to the tibial tuberosity. If the tibial tuberosity is not palpable, estimate penetration site 15 to 20 mm distal to the patella and medial along the flat aspect of the tibia.
11. Direct needle at a 90-degree angle (11).
12. Advance needle.
    a. For manual insertion, advance needle using firm pressure with a twisting motion until there is a sudden, slight decrease in resistance, indicating puncture of the cortex.
    b. If an automatic spring-activated intraosseous needle injection device is used, turn the device to the "0" line to insert 0.5 cm. Hold the cylinder against the puncture site at a 90-degree angle with one hand. Release the safety latch on the cylinder with the

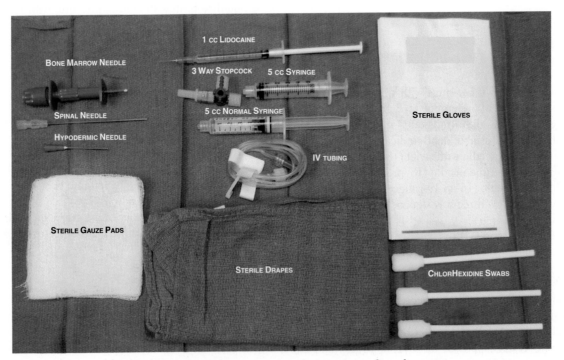

FIG. 50.1. Sterile equipment necessary for intraosseous line placement.

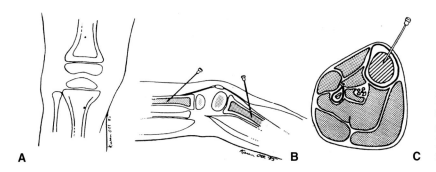

FIG. 50.2. A: Anterior view. **B:** Sagittal section. **C:** Cross section through tibia. (Reproduced with permission from Hodge D. Intraosseous infusions: a review. *Pediatr Emerg Care.* 1985;1:215.)

other hand. Depress the cylinder, as with a syringe, without the use of force.

c. If a battery-operated driver with attached needle is utilized, hold the driver in the dominant hand. Position the needle against the puncture site at a 90-degree angle. Depress the trigger to activate the driver. Do not force the driver, but apply firm, steady pressure, allowing the driver to insert the needle. Stop when there is a sudden decrease in resistance.

13. Do not advance the needle beyond cortical puncture.
14. Remove the stylet.
15. Confirm the position of the needle in the marrow cavity.
    a. Needle should stand without support in larger patients, but should never be left unsupported. (Fig. 50.4)
    b. Securely attach a 5-mL syringe and attempt to aspirate blood or marrow. Aspiration is not always successful when using an 18- or 20-gauge needle.
       If bone marrow is aspirated, it can be analyzed for blood chemistry values, partial pressure of arterial carbon dioxide, pH, hemoglobin level (14,15), type and cross-match, or cultured (15).
    c. Attach syringe of saline flush solution and infuse 2 to 3 mL slowly, while palpating the tissue adjacent

to the insertion site and beneath the extremity to detect extravasation. There should be only mild resistance to fluid infusion.

16. If marrow cannot be aspirated and significant resistance to fluid infusion is met
    a. The hollow bore needle may be obstructed by small bone plugs.
       (1) Reintroduce the stylet, or
       (2) Introduce a smaller-gauge needle through the original needle.
       (3) Attach syringe of saline flush and flush 2 to 3 mL of fluid.
    b. The bevel of the needle may not have penetrated the cortex.
       (1) Redetermine estimated depth needed.
       (2) Advance.
       (3) Flush with saline.
    c. The bevel of the needle may be lodged against the opposite cortex.
       (1) Withdraw needle slightly.
       (2) Flush with saline.
17. Observe the site for extravasation of fluid, indicating that
    a. The placement is too superficial, or
    b. The bone has been penetrated completely.

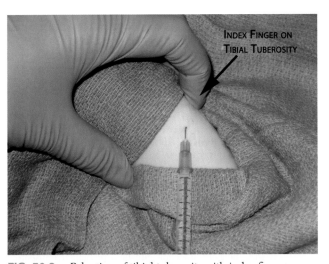

FIG. 50.3. Palpation of tibial tuberosity with index finger.

INDEX FINGER ON TIBIAL TUBEROSITY

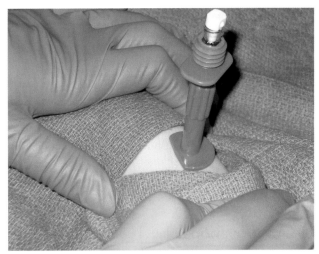

FIG. 50.4. Intraosseous needle in place should stand without support.

c. If extravasation occurs, withdraw needle and select a different bone.

18. When needle position is confirmed
    a. Attach syringe and infuse medications or fluid directly into the needle or via an IV extension set with clamp. Clear medications with saline flush.
    b. For continuous infusion, attach a standard IV infusion set with an infusion pump to the intraosseous needle and administer at the same rate as for IV infusion (2).

19. Secure intraosseous needle and maintain a clean infusion site while the needle is in place.
    a. Tape the flanges of the needle to the skin to prevent dislodgement. If a needle safety latch is provided, attach the latch and then apply tape.
    b. If desired, cover the exposed end of the needle with a disposable cup, taping the cover down. Cutting off the bottom of the cup will aid in visualization of the site for monitoring.

20. Secure IV tubing with tape to the leg.
21. Secure the leg to the armboard.
22. Obtain radiograph to confirm position of needle and to rule out fracture.
23. Monitor frequently for fluid extravasation.
24. Discontinue intraosseous infusion as soon as alternative IV access is achieved.

    In an infant with hypotension/hypovolemia, infusion via the interosseous route can restore peripheral perfusion to a point at which venous access is possible in well under 30 minutes.
    a. Remove needle gently, with slight rotation motion if needed.
    b. Apply a sterile dressing over the puncture site.
    c. Apply pressure to the dressing for 5 minutes.

Distal Tibia (2,10,11) (Fig. 50.5)

1. Position patient supine.
2. Prepare site and needle as for proximal tibia.
3. Insert needle in the medial surface of the distal tibia just proximal to the medial malleolus.
4. Direct needle cephalad away from the joint space.
5. Proceed as for proximal tibia.

Distal Femur (1) (Fig. 50.2)

1. Position patient supine.
2. Place sand bag or towel roll behind knee.
3. Prepare site and needle as for proximal tibia.
4. Insert needle 1 to 3 cm above the external condyles in the anterior midline.
5. Direct needle cephalad at an angle of 10 to 15 degrees.
6. Proceed as for proximal tibia.

F. Complications (1,4,16,17)

1. Fracture of bone (18)
2. Complete penetration of bone (19)

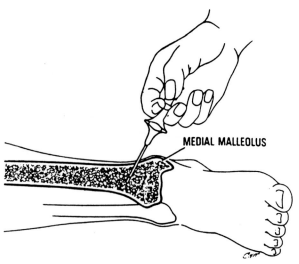

FIG. 50.5. Intraosseous infusion into the distal tibia. (Reproduced with permission from Spivey WH. Intraosseous infusions. *J Pediatr.* 1987;111:639.)

3. Osteomyelitis (16,17)
4. Periostitis (17)
5. Subcutaneous abscess
6. Cellulitis
7. Sepsis
8. Extravasation of fluid from the puncture site
9. Subperiosteal or subcutaneous infiltration or hematoma
10. Compartment syndrome (20)
11. Subcutaneous sloughing
12. Death (reported only with sternal bone site) (7)
13. Theoretical (as yet unreported) (21,22)
    a. Embolization of bone fragments or fat
    b. Damage to bone marrow
    c. Damage to growth plate

References

1. Fiser D. Intraosseous infusion. *N Engl J Med.* 1990;322:1579.
2. Spivey W. Intraosseous infusions. *J Pediatr.* 1987;111:639.
3. De Boers S, Russell T, Seaver M, et al. Infant intraosseous infusion. *Neonatal Netw.* 2008;27:25.
4. Ellemunter H, Simma B, Trawoger R, et al. Intraosseous lines in preterm and full term neonates. *Arch Dis Child Fetal Neonatal Ed.* 1999;80:F74.
5. Engle WA. Intraosseous access for administration of medications in neonates. *Clin Perinatol.* 2006;33:161ix.
6. deCaen A. Venous access in the critically ill child; when the peripheral intravenous fails! *Pediatr Emerg Care.* 2007;23:422.
7. Turkel H. Deaths following sternal puncture. *JAMA.* 1954;156:992.
8. Lake W, Emmerson AJ. Use of a butterfly as an intraosseous needle in an oedematous preterm infant. *Arch Dis Child Fetal Neonatal Ed.* 2003;88:F409.
9. Geritse BM, Scheffer GJ, Draaisma JM. Prehospital intraosseous access with the bone injection gun by a helicopter transported emergency medical team. *J Trauma.* 2009;66:1730.

10. Iserson K, Criss E. Intraosseous infusions: a usable technique. *Am J Emerg Med.* 1986;4:540.

11. Sommer A, Weis M, Deanovic D, et al. Intraosseous infusion in the pediatric emergency medical service. Analysis of emergency medical missions 1990–2009. *Anaesthesist.* 2011;60:125.

12. Boon J, Gorry D, Meiring J. Finding an ideal site for intraosseous infusion of the tibia; An anatomical study. *Clin Anat.* 2003; 16:15.

13. Mofenson HC, Tascone A, Caraccio TR. Guidelines for intraosseous infusions. *J Emerg Med.* 1988;6:143.

14. Johnson L, Kissoon N, Fiallos M, et al. Use of intraosseous blood to assess blood chemistries and hemoglobin during cardiopulmonary resuscitation with drug infusions. *Crit Care Med.* 1999;27: 1147.

15. Orlowski JP, Porembka DT, Gallagher JM, et al. The bone marrow as a source of laboratory studies. *Ann Emerg Med.* 1989; 18:1348.

16. Rosetti V, Thompson B, Miller J, et al. Intraosseous infusion: an alternative route of pediatric intravascular access. *Ann Emerg Med.* 1985;14:885.

17. Heinild S, Sondergaard J, Tudvad F. Bone marrow infusions in childhood: experiences from a thousand infusions. *J Pediatr.* 1947;30:400.

18. La Fleche F, Slepin M, Vargas J, et al. Iatrogenic bilateral tibial fractures after intraosseous infusion attempts in a 3-month-old infant. *Ann Emerg Med.* 1989;18:1099.

19. Valdes MM. Intraosseous administration in emergencies. *Lancet.* 1977;1:1235.

20. Vidal R, Kissoon N, Gayle M. Compartment syndrome following intraosseous infusion. *Pediatrics.* 1993;91:1201.

21. Pediatric Forum. Emergency bone marrow infusions. *Am J Dis Child.* 1985;139:438.

22. Fiser RT, Walker WM, Seibert JJ, et al. Tibial length following intraosseous infusion: a prospective, radiographic analysis. *Pediatr Emerg Care.* 1997;13:186.

23. Berg RA. Emergency infusion of catecholamines into bone marrow. *Am J Dis Child.* 1984;138:810.

24. Neish SR, Macon MG, Moore JW, et al. Intraosseous infusion of hypertonic glucose and dopamine. *Am J Dis Child.* 1988;142:878.

25. Walsh-Kelly C, Berens R, Glaeser P, et al. Intraosseous infusion of phenytoin. *Am J Emerg Med.* 1986;4:523.

26. Bilello JF, O'Hair KC, Kirby WC, et al. Intraosseous infusion of dobutamine and isoproterenol. *Am J Dis Child.* 1991;145:165.

27. Shoor PM, Berrynill RE, Benumof JL. Intraosseous infusion: pressure-flow relationship and pharmacokinetics. *J Trauma.* 1979; 19:772.

28. Spivey WH. Comparison of intraosseous, central and peripheral routes of sodium bicarbonate administration during CPR in pigs. *Ann Emerg Med.* 1985;14:1135.

29. Cambray EJ, Donaldson JS, Shore RM. Intraosseous contrast infusion: efficacy and associated findings. *Pediatr Radiol.* 1997;27:892.

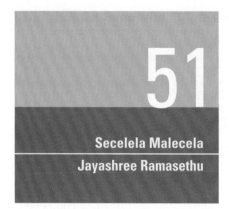

51

Tapping a Ventricular Reservoir

Secelela Malecela

Jayashree Ramasethu

The subcutaneous ventricular access device or ventricular reservoir (Fig. 51.1) is used to drain cerebrospinal fluid (CSF) in preterm infants with posthemorrhagic hydrocephalus and occasionally in term infants with obstructive hydrocephalus following intracranial hemorrhage (1–5). The ventricular reservoir is inserted in preterm infants who are too small or too unstable to have a ventriculoperitoneal (VP) shunt and may abrogate the need for a VP shunt in some infants. It also allows drainage and clearing of CSF which may be bloody and have a high protein content, thus decreasing the risk of blockage when a VP shunt is inserted (2,3,6).

The reservoir is usually tapped immediately following insertion, by the neurosurgeon, to ensure proper placement and to drain excess CSF. Subsequent taps are performed in the neonatal intensive care unit (NICU), aiming to remove enough CSF to prevent further ventriculomegaly and maintain normal head growth (2,7).

A. Indications

1. Rapidly increasing head circumference, more than 2 mm/day (7)
2. Clinical signs of raised intracranial pressure, such as a full or tense anterior fontanelle, separation of the sutures, apnea and bradycardia, poor feeding or vomiting
3. Ultrasound or radiologic evidence of progressive ventriculomegaly

B. Contraindications

1. Low circulating blood volume
2. Cellulitis or abrasion over the reservoir site
3. Sunken fontanelle or overlapping sutures
4. Severe coagulopathy

C. Equipment (other than the cap and mask, all equipment is sterile)

1. Mask, cap, gloves
2. Standard infant lumbar puncture set
3. Povidine–iodine surgical scrub and prep solution
4. An aperture drape

5. Scalp-vein needle (25- or 27-gauge)
6. 20-mL syringe

D. Precautions

1. Use strict aseptic technique.
2. Maintain continuous cardiorespiratory monitoring during the procedure.
3. Do not use local anesthetic.
4. Do not place IV lines on the same side of the scalp.
5. Do not shave the operative area.
6. Always use a fresh site for insertion of the needle with every tap.
7. Insert needle just far enough into the reservoir to obtain CSF; inserting the needle too deep may damage the reservoir base.

E. Technique

1. Infant should be restrained and comfortable, with the head in neutral position.
2. Clip any long hair, but do not shave the operative area.
3. Clean skin over the reservoir and a radius of at least 5 cm of the surrounding skin using surgical scrub for 2 to 5 minutes. Use light but firm contact.
4. Dry with blotting pads.
5. Don mask and cap.
6. Scrub hands and put on sterile gloves.
7. Paint area with povidone–iodine solution and allow area to dry.
8. Drape area while maintaining patient visibility.
9. Insert scalp-vein needle at an angle of 30 to 45 degrees through the skin into the reservoir bladder.
10. Aspirate fluid at a rate of 1 to 2 mL/min (Fig. 51.2). Remove no more than 10 to 15 mL/kg. Some authors advocate letting the CSF drain spontaneously, rather than aspirating, in order to reduce fresh bleeding into the ventricles (8).
11. Remove needle and hold firm pressure for 2 minutes, until CSF leakage stops.
12. Clean area with sterile saline to remove the povidone–iodine.
13. Remove the restraints.

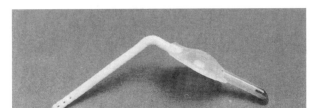
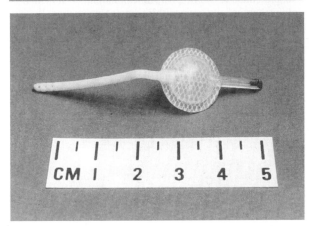

FIG. 51.1. McComb reservoir. Ventricular access device: lateral (*top*) and superior (*bottom*) views.

14. Send CSF sample for culture, cell count, glucose, and protein (the frequency of testing CSF varies among institutions from daily to weekly). If fluid is dark and bloody, it is reasonable to send only a culture sample.

F. A Successful Tap

1. At the end of the procedure, the anterior fontanelle should be soft and flat (not sunken), and the cranial bones should be approximated well at the sutures.
2. If sufficient volume is removed, the fontanelle may be full 24 hours later, but the sutures should not be separated.
3. If the fontanelle remains flat, the interval for tapping may be lengthened to every other day and/or the amount of CSF removed at each tap reduced.

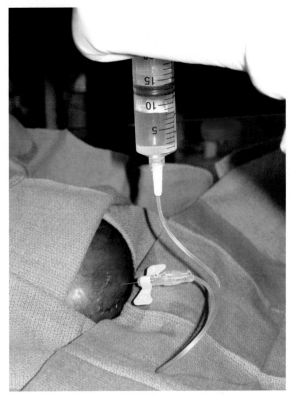

FIG. 51.2. Tapping a ventricular reservoir.

G. Follow-Up

1. Assess clinical response to taps, daily head circumference, and weekly cranial ultrasonography.
2. Interval between taps may range from twice a day to once every 2 to 3 days.
3. Taps should be continued until the infant weighs 2 kg and is a suitable candidate for shunt placement or until the hydrocephalus resolves.

H. Complications

See Table 51.1 (4,7–9)

TABLE 51.1 Complications of Ventricular Reservoir Drainage

Problem (Incidence)	What To Do
Hyponatremia (20%–60%)	Monitor serum electrolytes every other day and supplement sodium intake.
Hypoproteinemia (15%)	Ensure adequate protein intake. Monitor serum albumin weekly.
Infection (0%–8%)	A combination of intravenous and intrareservoir antibiotics may rarely be successful. Removal of the reservoir is usually necessary.
Subgaleal CSF collection (0%–9%)	Percutaneous aspiration of fluid using a different needle at the same time as the reservoir is tapped. Tap larger volume of CSF from the reservoir or increase frequency of taps to reduce pressure.
CSF leaks through incision (0%–3%)	Increase frequency of reservoir taps.
Ventricular access device occlusion (0%–10%)	Replace reservoir.
Trapped contralateral ventricle (6%)	Place second reservoir.
Fresh bleeding into the ventricle (0%–40%)	Prevent by using 25- or 27-gauge needle, aspirate slowly or let CSF drain spontaneously rather than aspirating.
Bradycardia, pallor, hypotension (rare)	Stop aspiration. Infuse 10–15 mL/kg of normal saline IV rapidly. Remove a smaller volume at a slower rate at next tap.
Skin breakdown over reservoir (rare)	Avoid abraded skin when tapping the reservoir. Avoid excoriating skin while prepping site.

References

1. McComb JG, Ramos AD, Platzker AC, et al. Management of hydrocephalus secondary to intraventricular hemorrhage in the preterm infant with a subcutaneous ventricular catheter reservoir. *Neurosurgery.* 1983;13:295.

2. Limbrick DD Jr, Mathur A, Johnston JM. Neurosurgical treatment of progressive posthemorrhagic ventricular dilation in preterm infants: a 10 year single institution study. *J Neurosurg Pediatr.* 2010;6:224.

3. Willis B, Javalkar V, Vannemreddy P, et al. Ventricular reservoir and ventriculoperitoneal shunts for premature infants with posthemorrhagic hydrocephalus: an institutional experience. *J Neurosurg Pediatr.* 2009;3:94.

4. Peretta P, Ragazzi P, Carlino CF, et al. The role of the Ommaya reservoir and endoscopic third ventriculostomy in the management of post-hemorrhagic hydrocephalus of prematurity. *Childs Nerv Syst.* 2007;23:765.

5. Brouwer AJ, Groenendaal F, Koopman C, et al. Intracranial hemorrhage in full term newborns: a hospital based cohort study. *Neuroradiology.* 2010;52:567.

6. Wellons JC III, Shannon CN, Kulkarni AV, et al. A multicenter retrospective comparison of conversion from temporary to permanent cerebrospinal fluid diversion in very low birth weight infants with posthemorrhagic hydrocephalus. *J Neurosurg Pediat.r* 2009;4:50.

7. Whitelaw A, Evans D, Carter M, et al. Randomized clinical trial of prevention of hydrocephalus after intraventricular hemorrhage in preterm infants: brain-washing versus tapping fluid. *Pediatrics.* 2007;119:e1071.

8. Moghal NE, Quinn MW, Levene MI, et al. Intraventricular hemorrhage after aspiration of ventricular reservoirs. *Arch Dis Child.* 1992;67:448.

9. Kormanik K, Praca J, Gorton HJL, et al. Repeated tapping of ventricular reservoir in preterm infants with post-hemorrhagic ventricular dilatation does not increase the risk of reservoir infection. *J Perinatol.* 2010;30:218.

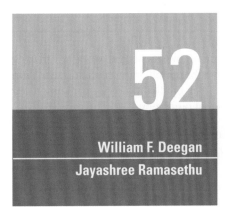

52 Treatment of Retinopathy of Prematurity

William F. Deegan

Jayashree Ramasethu

Retinopathy of prematurity (ROP), a disorder of developing retinal blood vessels in the preterm infant, may lead to poor visual acuity or blindness. Screening and timely treatment improves visual outcomes.

A. Screening for ROP (1–3)

Guidelines for screening preterm infants for ROP are published and updated regularly (1–3). Recommendations for screening in the United States are (1)

1. Infants with a birth weight of <1,500 g or a gestational age of 30 weeks or less (as defined by the attending neonatologist).
2. Selected infants with a birth weight between 1,500 and 2,000 g or gestational age of more than 30 weeks with an unstable clinical course, including those requiring cardiopulmonary support and who are believed by their attending pediatrician or neonatologist to be a high risk.
3. The timing of the first exam varies with gestational age. The initial examination for infants born between 22 and 27 weeks' gestational age is at 31 weeks' postconceptional age (gestational age at birth plus chronological age). Infants born later than 27 weeks' should be screened initially 4 weeks after birth.
4. Follow-up exams depend on the retinal findings as classified by the International Classification of ROP (4). Table 52.1 has been adapted from the joint policy statement of the American Academies of Pediatrics and Ophthalmology, and the American Association for Pediatric Ophthalmology and Strabismus (1).
5. Babies whose clinical condition deteriorates should be followed closely (i.e., weekly), as late reactivation and worsening are possible.
6. Binocular indirect ophthalmoscopy with scleral depression after pupillary dilation remains the gold standard to accurately screen and monitor babies with ROP. The exams are done at the bedside with the assistance of the baby's nurse.
7. Telemedicine screening with wide-field imaging has been shown to have excellent sensitivity and specificity in some centers (5).

B. Classification of ROP (4)

1. *Location:* Three zones based on concentric circles, centered on the optic disc (Fig. 52.1)
   a. *Zone I:* Circle whose center is the optic disc and whose radius is twice the distance from the optic disc to the center of the macula
   b. *Zone II:* Circle whose radius extends from the optic disc to the nasal ora serrata and is peripheral to Zone I
   c. *Zone III:* Temporal crescent of retina anterior to Zone II
2. Extent of disease
   The retina is divided into 12 equal segments, or clock hours. The extent of retinopathy specifies the number of clock hours involved.
3. Staging the disease (1,4) (Figs. 52.2 and 52.3)
   a. *Stage 1—Demarcation line:* A flat white line in the plane of the retina, separating avascular retina anteriorly from vascularized retina posteriorly
   b. *Stage 2—Ridge:* Elevated fibrovascular tissue extending out of the plane of the retina and separating the vascularized and avascular retina.
   c. *Stage 3—Extraretinal fibrovascular proliferation:* Neovascularization extending from the ridge into the vitreous. This tissue may cause the ridge to appear ragged or "fuzzy" (Fig. 52.2).
   d. *Stage 4—Partial retinal detachment:* A separation of the retina from the underlying choroid. Traction by the vitreous, through the presence of neovascular tissue, pulls the retina away from its underlying attachments. The intervening (subretinal) space fills with a proteinaceous fluid.
      (1) *Stage 4A:* Detachment spares the macula.
      (2) *Stage 4B:* Involves the macula
   e. *Stage 5—Total retinal detachment:* Retinal tissue becomes inextricably bound to reactive vitreous and is pulled by the vitreous into the retrolental space (hence the older term, retrolental fibroplasia).
4. Additional signs indicating severity of active ROP
   a. *"Plus" disease:* Dilation and tortuosity of retinal vessels in at least two quadrants of the eye. This is seen

TABLE 52.1	Follow-up Examination Schedule

Findings	Follow-up
Stage 1–2 in Zone 1 Stage 3 in Zone II	1 wk or less
Immature retina (no ROP) in Zone I Stage 2 in Zone II Regressing ROP in Zone I	1–2 wk
Stage 1 in Zone II Regressing ROP in Zone I	2 wk
Immature retina (no ROP) in Zone II Regressing or Stage 1–2 in Zone III	2–3 wk

From Section on Ophthalmology, American Academy of Pediatrics, American Academy of Ophthalmology, American Association for Pediatric Ophthalmology and Strabismus. Screening examinations of premature infants for retinopathy of prematurity. *Pediatrics.* 2006;117:572. Erratum Pediatrics 2006;118:1324.

best in the posterior pole. A + symbol is added to the ROP stage number to designate the presence.

b. *"Preplus" disease:* More arterial tortuosity and more venous dilation than normal, but insufficient for diagnosis of "plus"disease; may progress to frank "plus"disease.

c. *Aggressive posterior ROP:* Also called type "II ROP" or "rush disease."This is an uncommon, severe form of ROP, characterized by its posterior location, prominent plus disease in all four quadrants, out of proportion to the peripheral retinopathy, and rapid progression.

5. Additional features
   a. Iris vascular engorgement (Fig. 52.3) and pupillary rigidity (manifested by poor dilation after mydriatic instillation) are harbingers of active, advanced ROP(6).
   b. Corneal and lenticular opacity may be present in the eyes of any premature infant regardless of the presence of ROP (7).

C. Laser Treatment of ROP (8,9)

Ablation of the avascular portion of the retina decreases the production of angiogenic growth factors and reduces the risk of retinal detachment. In patients with ROP, cryotherapy has been replaced with transpupillary laser photocoagulation delivered via an indirect ophthalmoscope, with improved structural and functional outcomes.

1. Indications for Laser Treatment

Early Treatment for Retinopathy of Prematurity Study guidelines (10,11):
   a. Peripheral retinal ablation should be considered for any eye with type I ROP:
      (1) *Zone I:* Any stage of ROP with plus disease
      (2) *Zone I:* Stage 3 ROP with or without plus disease
      (3) *Zone II:* Stage 2 or 3 ROP with plus disease
   b. Consider close monitoring (serial examinations) as opposed to retinal ablation for any eye with type 2 ROP, as defined below. Regression of ROP can occur in about 50% of these patients without treatment (10); treatment should be considered if progression to type 1 status occurs.
      (4) *Zone 1:* Stage 1 or 2 ROP without plus disease
      (5) *Zone 2:* Stage 3 ROP without plus disease
   c. Treatment is recommended within 72 hours of detection of a stage of ROP requiring ablative therapy, when possible, in order to minimize the risk of retinal detachment.

2. Contraindications

   a. Stage 4 to 5 ROP, in which case laser may be done (intraoperatively) in conjunction with incisional surgery (scleral buckle, vitrectomy, or both) (12)
   b. Vitreous hemorrhage sufficient to obscure a view of the retina
   c. Instability of medical condition sufficient to make the stress of sedation and laser inadvisable
   d. Lethal medical illness

3. Personnel

   a. Ophthalmologist
      (1) Determines the need for treatment

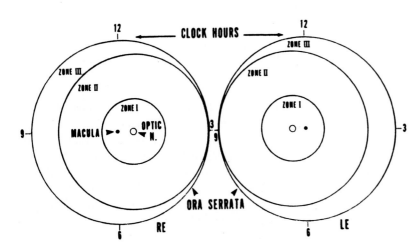

FIG. 52.1. Scheme of retina of right eye (RE) and left eye (LE), showing zone borders and clock hours employed to describe location and extent of retinopathy of prematurity. (From Committee for Classification of Retinopathy of Prematurity. An international classification of retinopathy of prematurity. *Arch Ophthalmol.* 1984;102:1130, with permission.)

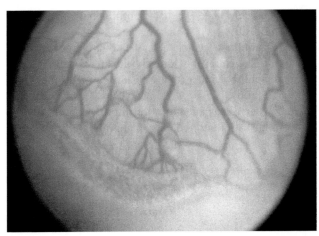

FIG. 52.2. Dilated, tortuous vessels end in vascular shunts at a thickened ridge of fibrovascular tissue. Avascular retina lies anterior to the ridge.

(2) Administers topical anesthetic
(3) Ensures that all personnel present at the treatment are wearing laser safety goggles
(4) Performs the laser
(5) Watches for and treats ocular complications that may arise during and after the procedure
(6) Follows the baby postoperatively until ROP is resolved
  b. Neonatology fellow, attending neonatologist, or pediatric anesthesiologist
    (1) Administers systemic sedative agents (midazolam, fentanyl, ketamine, or a combination)

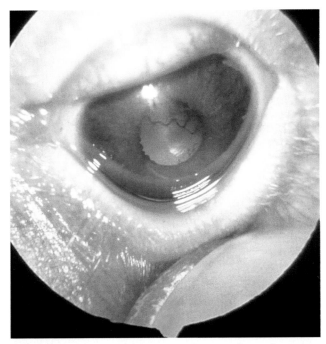

FIG. 52.3. Dilation and tortuosity of iris vessels may be seen in severe threshold retinopathy of prematurity.

(2) Monitors patient for and treats any systemic complications that develop during or after treatment
(3) Provides information to the ophthalmologist regarding the patient's overall condition throughout the procedure
  c. Assistant to the ophthalmologist
    (1) Helps with laser and instruments
    (2) Records the treatment parameters used during treatment
  d. Neonatal nurse
    (1) Instills dilating drops several times in the hour preceding treatment
    (2) Immobilizes the patient during treatment

4. Equipment

  a. Cardiorespiratory, blood pressure, and pulse oximeter
  b. Appropriate respiratory support (ventilator, laryngoscope and endotracheal tubes, face mask, self-inflating resuscitation bag, suction, and oxygen source)
  c. Emergency medications (atropine, epinephrine, bicarbonate, calcium, phenobarbital)
    Note: Precalculation of weight-appropriate doses is helpful.
  d. Topical ocular anesthetic (e.g., tetracaine, proparacaine)
  e. *Cycloplegic/mydriatic eye drops:* Cyclomydril (Alcon Laboratories, Fort Worth, Texas) (cyclopentolate hydrochloride 0.2% and phenylephrine hydrochloride 1%) or 0.5% cyclopentolate and 1% or 2.5% phenylephrine
  f. Calcium alginate-tipped nasopharyngeal applicators or Flynn depressor (Fig. 52.4), for scleral depression
  g. Balanced salt solution for rewetting cornea during procedure
  h. Neonatal eyelid speculum (Fig. 52.4)
  i. 28- and 20-diopter lenses

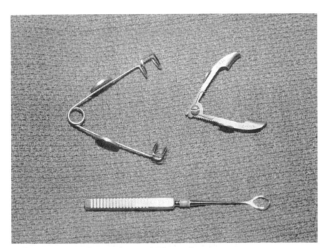

FIG. 52.4. Lid speculae and Flynn depressor.

j. Portable argon or diode laser (9) with indirect (head-lamp) delivery system

k. Appropriate laser safety goggles

5. Precautions and Complications (Table 52.2)

a. Ensure that laser is fully functional.

b. If the infant is at high risk for an adverse event that would terminate treatment prematurely, treat the more advanced eye first (assuming both have threshold ROP).

c. Discontinue feedings at least 4 hours before the procedure, or empty the stomach with an orogastric tube.

d. Establish IV access for infusions of medications and IV fluids.

e. Observe oxygen saturation monitor carefully, and adjust administered oxygen appropriately.

TABLE 52.2	**Complications of Laser for Retinopathy**
Complication	**Treatment/Action**
Systemic: Intra- and immediately postop	
Bradycardia	Interrupt treatment. Assess airway, oxygen delivery. Atropine 0.1 mg IV
Hypoxia/cyanosis	Evaluate airway. Administer supplemental oxygen.
Apnea	Evaluate airway. Gentle stimulation. Administer supplemental oxygen. Hand-ventilate (self-inflating resuscitation bag, face mask).
Tachycardia	Assess pain control. Administer additional analgesic. Monitor blood pressure and perfusion.
Hypertension	Assess pain control. Administer additional analgesic. If moderate, observe. If severe, consider hydralazine 0.1 mg/kg IV
Arrhythmia	Manage as appropriate for arrhythmia.
Seizure (mechanism uncertain: ? anticholinergic effect)	Supportive care. Phenobarbital.
Ocular: Intraop	
Closure of central artery	Relieve pressure on globe (stop scleral depression).
Corneal clouding/abrasion	Rinse with balanced salt solution/saline. Interrupt treatment.
Retinal/vitreous/choroidal hemorrhage	Gentle pressure on globe (until arterial pulsations visible). Avoid lasering blood. May have to terminate treatment if extensive.
Ocular: Postop	
Conjunctival hemorrhage	Observation.
Conjunctival laceration	Antibiotic ointment t.i.d. for 3–4 d.
Corneal abrasion	Antibiotic ointment t.i.d. for 3–4 d. Follow with slit lamp exam with fluorescein.
Hyphema	Topical cycloplegic and steroids. Follow intraocular pressure closely. Consider washout if high pressure, no resolution in 7–10 d.
Retinal/vitreous/choroidal hemorrhage	Close follow-up.
Ocular: Late	
Amblyopia, strabismus, myopia	Pediatric ophthalmology assessment 3–4 mo after treatment(s). Educate parents prior to discharge regarding need for regular ophthalmology follow-up.

t.i.d., three times per day.

f. *Stabilize the infant:* Correct electrolyte imbalances, platelet deficiency, etc.

g. Use only 1% phenylephrine if there is a history of hypertension.

h. Wipe off any excess drops spilling onto the skin to avoid transcutaneous absorption (skin vessel blanching occurs with phenylephrine).

6. Technique

a. General preparation

   (1) Instill eyedrops (per orders from ophthalmologist) into both eyes in the hour prior to procedure. Maximal dilation is critical for optimum laser; therefore, several (three or four) instillations of drops may be required, especially in eyes with neovascularization/vascular engorgement of the iris.

   (2) Transport the patient to surgical suite or designated procedure room in the nursery.

   (3) Ensure monitors are attached and functioning.

b. *Immobilize infant:* Swaddle in a clean towel or blanket to immobilize arms and legs.

c. Ensure that the IV tubing is accessible.

d. Administer IV sedation.

   If local anesthesia is to be used, a combination of topical (e.g., tetracaine, proparacaine) and systemic analgesic/sedative (e.g., IV morphine) medications are administered prior to injection.

e. Distribute laser safety goggles and dim overhead lights.

f. Retract lids.

g. *Perform laser:* Cover the avascular retina with confluent gray–white burns (Fig. 52.5).

h. Have an assistant count and record the number of spots and the duration and power of each spot.

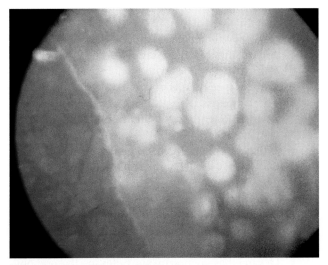

FIG. 52.5.   Freshly lasered avascular retina.

7. Postoperative Care

a. Instill 0.25% scopolamine hydrobromide in treated eye(s) daily for 3 to 5 days.

b. Apply antibiotic–steroid preparation (e.g., tobramycin–dexamethasone) to treated eye(s) three to four times daily for 5 to 7 days.

c. Monitor the patient with a cardiorespiratory monitor for 24 to 72 hours.

d. Perform a dilated retinal exam 1 to 2 weeks after treatment.

e. If opaque media are present at the time of laser, or if the pupil does not dilate adequately, complete treatment of the avascular retina may be impossible, and "skip areas" may be visible in the weeks after treatment. Treatment of these areas should be considered if there is not marked resolution of the adjacent plus disease and/or neovascularization.

f. Follow the infant every 1 to 2 weeks until the ROP resolves completely. If at the time of discharge ROP is still present, ensure that the parents and the physicians responsible for the care of the infant after discharge are aware of the extreme importance of maintaining a regular schedule of outpatient examinations. Once the ROP has resolved completely, the baby should be seen by a pediatric ophthalmologist within 1 to 2 months to assess vision, ocular alignment and motility, refractive status, etc.

g. Long-term follow-up over several years is necessary. See outcomes and postdischarge follow-up below.

D. Intravitreal Injection for ROP

1. Background

Recently, the efficacy of anti-VEGF drug bevacizumab for use in ROP has been reported (13). The drug halts the development of new vessels and halts disease progression. Intravitreal injections of anti-VEGF agents have been used to treat wet (neovascular) age-related macular degeneration (AMD), proliferative diabetic retinopathy, neovascular glaucoma, etc. Although there is considerable debate and no consensus on its use in ROP, this section is being included in the Atlas for completeness, and to provide additional treatment options if laser therapy is not possible (14–16).

2. Precautions

a. The major concern with bevacizumab in premature infants with ROP is systemic absorption and its effect on the developing infant. Bevacizumab is absorbed systemically after intravitreal injection. The risks of systemic effects on developing neonates have not been established.

b. The optimal and safe dose of bevacizumab in ROP has not been determined; the current dose (0.625 mg) is extrapolated from that used in adults with ocular neovascular disease (1.25 mg), and may represent a several-fold increase in drug delivered/body weight over adults (17).

c. No protocol for near- and long-term monitoring of bevacizumab in neonates has been developed.

d. The informed consent process for the use of intravitreal bevacizumab for ROP must reflect the uncertain status of the treatment, the off-label use of the drug, and the lack of long-term results, including the possibility of unknown systemic side effects.

3. Indications

a. Threshold ROP in posterior Zone 1 disease. An early report showed benefit over laser in posterior (Zone 1) disease (13).

b. In unstable infants in whom laser may be contraindicated
   (1) Intravitreal injection does not require systemic sedation/anesthesia; in this regard, the procedure may be preferable to laser in unstable infants.

c. As salvage therapy if laser treatment has not been effective (16).

4. Contraindications

a. Infection in or around the eyes

b. Lethal medical illness

c. Failure of consensus between parent(s), treating physicians, and hospital personnel about the uncertain nature of intravitreal bevacizumab in ROP and the risks of intravitreal injection (informed consent)

5. Personnel

a. Ophthalmologist
   (1) Determines the need for treatment
   (2) Participates in informed consent process
   (3) Administers topical anesthetic
   (4) Performs the injection
   (5) Performs indirect ophthalmoscopy after the injection(s)

(6) Follows the baby for ocular complications and resolution of ROP

b. Neonatologist
   (1) Provides information about the status of the infants to the treating ophthalmologist
   (2) Participates in the informed consent process
   (3) Monitors infant for systemic complications during and after treatment

c. Nurse/assistant at bedside
   (1) Helps prepare the baby for injection (i.e., swaddles the baby)
   (2) Helps prepare the instruments at the bedside

6. Equipment

a. Topical anesthetic

b. Sterile lid speculum (one per eye)

c. Caliper (one per eye)

d. Sterile cotton-tipped applicators (CTA)

e. Sterile gloves

f. Topical Betadine

g. Topical antibiotic drops (ciprofloxacin 0.3%) and ointment

h. Sterile syringe of bevacizumab (0.625 mg in 0.025 mL) with 30-gauge needle (one per eye)

7. Complications (Table 52.3)

a. The most worrisome risk is postinjection infection (endophthalmitis). Babies with active or recent ocular surface or lid infections (e.g., conjunctivitis) should not have intravitreal injection

b. The risk of adverse systemic side effects (bradycardia, oxygen desaturation) is mitigated by the absence of systemic sedation/anesthesia, and the rapid nature of the procedure. However, it is reasonable to follow those precautions listed for laser treatment in Section F4.

8. Technique

a. The baby's eyes are dilated according to the standard dilation protocol.

b. Sterile towels are placed around the baby's head.

c. Topical anesthetics are instilled.

d. The lids are prepped with Betadine.

e. Wire lid speculum is placed.

f. The caliper is used to mark a spot on the sclera 1.7 mm posterior to the limbus in the inferotemporal quadrant.

g. A Betadine-soaked CTA is gently pressed over the mark and excess Betadine is allowed to collect in the inferior fornix.

h. The injection is given.

i. A topical antibiotic drop is given.

j. The ophthalmologist performs binocular indirect ophthalmoscopy.

k. Dexamethasone/polymyxin B/dexamethasone ointment may be instilled.

TABLE 52.3	Ocular Complications of Intravitreal Injection
Complication	**Treatment**
Immediate	
Closure of central retinal artery	Paracentesis (withdrawal of fluid from anterior chamber with needle)
Conjunctival hemorrhage	Observation
Vitreous hemorrhage	Observation and re-evaluation (with ultrasonography if hemorrhage obscures view of retina) in 3–5 d
Within days/weeks	
Infection/endophthalmitis	Prompt treatment with intravitreal antibiotics (vancomycin and ceftazidime)
Vitreous hemorrhage	As above
Retinal detachment	Incisional surgery (vitrectomy)

9. Postinjection Care/Concerns

a. Topical antibiotic drops should be instilled 3 to 4 times a day for 3 days.

b. Portable slit-lamp examination should be performed 48 to 72 hours postinjection

c. Any signs of infection (lid edema and erythema, conjunctival injection, clouding of the cornea) should be reported *immediately* to the treating ophthalmologist.

d. Examination by treating ophthalmologist in 1 week.

E. Postdischarge Care

A critical component of treatment of ROP is postdischarge care.

1. No baby with any ROP, or who has regressed ROP after treatment, should leave the neonatal intensive care unit (NICU) without a scheduled follow-up examination (1,18).

2. It is imperative that infants who develop any stage of ROP, especially those with prethreshold stage 3 or those that have received treatment, are seen within 1 to 2 weeks of discharge, or as directed by the ophthalmologist involved in the baby's care.

3. A careful, reproducible tracking system for arranging follow-up should be established by every NICU. A member of the staff of each NICU should be responsible for maintaining and periodically auditing this system.

4. Verbal and written instructions for follow-up should be given to the parents. Parents should be given a discharge form indicating their baby's *scheduled* follow-up among their discharge instructions. The importance of scheduled follow-up should be prominently stated on the form.

F. Outcome

1. Early treatment for type I high-risk prethreshold ROP has been shown to improve retinal structural outcome and visual acuity outcomes at 6 years of age (11).

2. Favorable outcome with vision of 20/40 or better was noted in 35% of treated eyes.

3. However, 65% of eyes receiving early treatment develop visual acuity worse than 20/40.

4. *Unfavorable outcome despite treatment:* Visual acuity 20/200 in 15%; blindness or low vision in 9%.

5. The outcome for eyes with Zone I disease, although poor, has improved with laser and incisional surgery (vitrectomy). Specifically, laser treatment of the posterior avascular retina can be accomplished easily and without necessitating conjunctival incisions, as in cryotherapy.

6. Treated eyes carry a risk of retinal dystopia, myopia, and subsequent strabismus and amblyopia (11,19). To minimize the effect of refractive errors and strabismus, careful follow-up by a pediatric ophthalmologist is mandatory.

7. Premature infants are at risk for intracranial pathologies that may limit visual function. Pediatric ophthalmologists, neurologists, and others involved in the care of former preemies should be in frequent contact in order to address the often complex and changing visual deficits present in these children.

References

1. Section on Ophthalmology, American Academy of Pediatrics, American Academy of Ophthalmology, American Association for Pediatric Ophthalmology and Strabismus. Screening examinations of premature infants for retinopathy of prematurity. *Pediatrics.* 2006;117:572. Erratum Pediatrics 2006;118:1324.

2. Wilkinson AR, Haines L, Head K, et al. UK retinopathy of prematurity guidelines. *Early Hum Dev.* 2008;84:71.

3. Jefferies AL, Canadian Pediatric Society; Fetus and Newborn Committee. Retinopathy of prematurity: recommendations for screening. *Paediatr Child Health.* 2010;15:667.

4. An International Committee for the Classification of Retinopathy of Prematurity. The international classification of retinopathy of prematurity revisited. *Arch Ophthalmol.* 2005;123:991.

5. Silva RA, Murakami Y, Lad EM, et al. Stanford University network for diagnosis of retinopathy of prematurity (SUNDROP): 36 month experience with telemedicine screening. *Ophthalmic Surg Lasers Imaging.* 2011;42:12.

6. Kivlin JD, Biglan AW, Gordon RA, et al. For Cryotherapy for Retinopathy of Prematurity Group. Early retinal vessel development and iris vessel dilatation as factors in retinopathy of prematurity. *Arch Ophthalmol.* 1996;114:150.

7. Marcus I, Salchow DJ, Stoessel KM, et al. An ROP screening dilemma: hereditary cataracts developing in a premature infant after birth. *J Pediatr Ophthalmol Strabismus.* 2012;14:49;e1.

8. Simpson JL, Melia M, Yang MB. A report by the American Academy of Ophthalmology. Current role of cryotherapy in retinopathy of prematurity. *Ophthalmology.* 2012;119:873.

9. Houston SK, Wykoff CC, Berrocal AM, et al. Laser treatment for retinopathy of prematurity. *Lasers Med Sci.* 2011 Dec 2. [Epub ahead of print].

10. Early Treatment for Retinopathy of Prematurity Cooperative Group. Revised indications for the treatment of retinopathy of prematurity: results of the Early Treatment for retinopathy of Prematurity randomized trial. *Arch Ophthalmol.* 2003;121:1684.

11. Early Treatment for Retinopathy of Prematurity Cooperative Group. Final visual acuity results in the Early Treatment for Retinopathy of Prematurity Study. *Arch Ophthalmol.* 2010;128: 663.

12. Hubbard GB. Surgical management of retinopathy of prematurity. *Curr Opin Ophthalmol.* 2008;19:384.

13. Mintz-Hittner HA, Kennedy KA, Chuang AZ, et al. Efficacy of intravitreal bevacizumab for stage 3+ retinopathy of prematurity. *N Engl J Med.* 2011;364:603.

14. Darlow BA, Ellis AL, Gilbert CE, et al. Are we there yet? Bevacizumab therapy for retinopathy of prematurity. *Arch Dis Child Fetal Neonatal Ed.* 2011 Dec 30. [Epub ahead of print].

15. Tolentino M. Systemic and ocular safety of intravitreal anti-VEGF therapies for ocular neovascular disease. *Surv Ophthalmol.* 2011;56:95.

16. Spandau U, Tomic Z, Ewald U, et al. Time to consider a new treatment protocol for aggressive posterior retinopathy of prematurity? *Acta Ophthalmol.* 2012 Jan 23. [Epub ahead of print].

17. Lim LS, Mitchell P, Wong TY. Bevacizumab for retinopathy of prematurity: letter. *N Engl J Med.* 2011;364:2359.

18. Day S, Menke AM, Abbott RL. Retinopathy of prematurity malpractice claims: the Ophthalmic Mutual Insurance Company experience. *Arch Ophthalmol.* 2009;127:794.

19. Davitt BV, Quinn GE, Wallace DK, et al. Early Treatment for Retinopathy of Prematurity Cooperative Group. Astigmatism progression in the early treatment for retinopathy study to 6 years of age. *Ophthalmology.* 2011;118:2326.

53

Peritoneal Dialysis

Kathleen A. Marinelli
Majid Rasoulpour

Acute Peritoneal Dialysis (1–5)

In neonates, acute peritoneal dialysis (PD) is frequently preferred over hemodialysis (HD), continuous arteriovenous hemofiltration with or without dialysis (CAVH/D), and continuous venovenous hemofiltration with or without dialysis (CVVH/D), because it is technically easier to perform. Peritoneal surface area per kilogram of body weight is relatively larger in newborns and children than in adults. Therefore, PD usually allows adequate clearance and removal of excess fluid (6). In addition, PD avoids the need for anticoagulation and maintenance of adequate vascular access, which are required for the other methods (7).

A. Indications

1. Renal failure, when conservative management has failed to adequately control any of the following conditions (8,9).
   a. Hypervolemia
   b. Hyperkalemia
   c. Hyponatremia
   d. Refractory metabolic acidosis
   e. Hyperphosphatemia
   f. Azotemia
   g. Additional fluid space needed for delivering drugs and/or nutrition
2. Inherited disorders of organic and amino acid metabolism when HD or CVVH/D is unavailable (10,11)
   a. In hyperammonemic metabolic crisis, however, evidence suggests that ammonia is more efficiently removed by extracorporeal techniques than by PD (12,13).
   b. In babies with imminent or current intracranial hemorrhage, PD is considered the therapeutic option of choice, especially in nonhyperammonemic disorders (12).

B. Relative Contraindications

1. Acute abdomen
2. Abdominal adhesions

3. Immediately after abdominal surgery (14)
4. Diaphragmatic or abdominal wall disruptions

C. Equipment (Figs. 53.1 through 53.3)

Sterile

1. Masks, drapes, gowns, and gloves
2. Povidone–iodine
3. 1% lidocaine without epinephrine
4. 3-mL syringe with 25-gauge needle
5. IV cutdown tray with no. 11 surgical blade
6. 3-0 Prolene sutures (either as part of cutdown tray or separately)
7. 22-gauge angiocatheter or a femoral catheter with guidewire
8. A temporary catheter such as a 14-gauge angiocatheter or one of the commercially available temporary dialysis catheters, (e.g., a Trocath [Trocath Peritoneal Dialysis Center, Kendall McGaw Laboratories, Sabana Grande, Puerto Rico])
9. Dialysis solution (1.5%, 2.5%, or 4.25%)
   a. Other concentrations can be made by manual mixing of standard solutions
10. Heparin
11. Inline burette set
12. Ultra Set CAPD Disposable Disconnect Y-Set
13. MiniCap Extended Life PD Transfer Set with Twist Cap
14. Medicap with povidone–iodine solution
15. FlexiCap Disconnect Cap with povidone–iodine solution

Nonsterile

1. Waterproof tape
2. Baby weigh scale with low resolution (e.g., Medela, which has a resolution of 2 g from 0 to 6,000 g) (Fig. 53.2)

   An alternative approach is to utilize a pediatric cycler set. Experience in using this equipment is necessary. We recommend a commercially available cycler that provides a minimum fill volume of 50 mL with 10-mL increments.

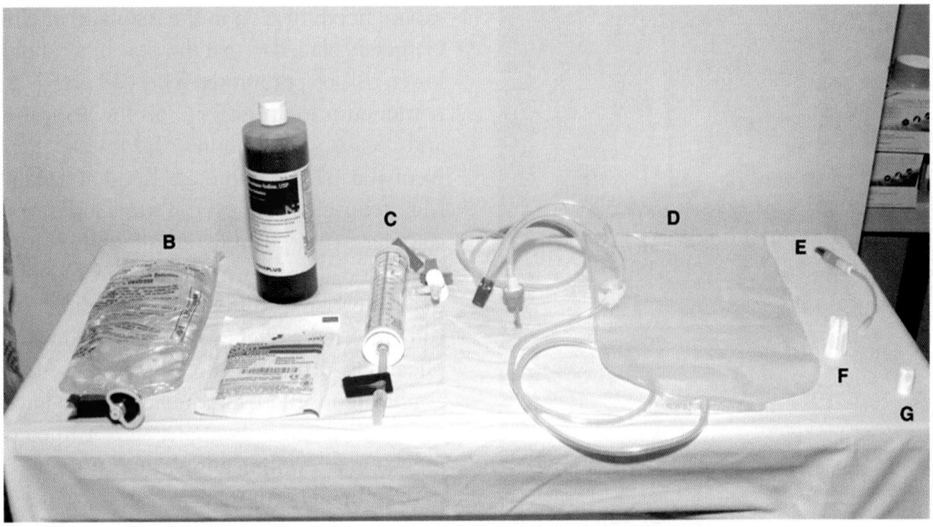

FIG. 53.1. *A*, IV pole (Fig. 53.3); *B*, Dianeal PD-2 Peritoneal Dialysis Solution (Baxter, Deerfield, Illinois); *C*, Inline Burette Set 150 mL (Abbott Laboratories, North Chicago, Illinois); *D*, Ultra Set CAPD Disposable Disconnect Y-Set (Baxter, Deerfield, Illinois); *E*, MiniCap Extended Life PD Transfer Set With Twist Clamp (Baxter, Deerfield, Illinois); *F*, Flexicap Disconnect Cap with povidone–iodine solution (Baxter, Deerfield, Illinois); *G*, Minicap with Povidone–Iodine Solution (Baxter, Deerfield, Illinois).

3. HomeChoice Automated PD System (Fig. 53.2) or any other reliable fluid warmer
4. IV pole

D. Preprocedure Care

1. Obtain informed consent.
2. Check body weight and abdominal girth.
3. Check for infection at the insertion site.
4. Decompress the stomach.
5. Catheterize the bladder.
6. Place preweighed diaper under the patient.
   Before assembly of system, wash hands and put on a mask. All connections should be made using sterile technique. Universal precautions should be observed

(Chapter 5). Keep all tubing clamped. See Fig. 53.3 for connections.

7. Add 500 U of heparin to each 1 L of the dialysis solution. Start with 1.5% dialysate.
8. Warm a liter bag of dialysate (Dianeal or other), or a larger bag if 1 L dialysate is not available, by resting it on the heating surface of the HomeChoice Automated PD System, or a reliable fluid warmer. The temperature can be set between 35°C and 37°C. For a newborn, keep the temperature at 37°C (in older pediatric patients, the temperature is usually set to 36°C, and occasionally to 35°C if the environmental temperature is high).
9. Spike the inline burette set (Abbott Laboratories, North Chicago, Illinois) into the dialysate (Dianeal or other) when the ideal temperature has been achieved.

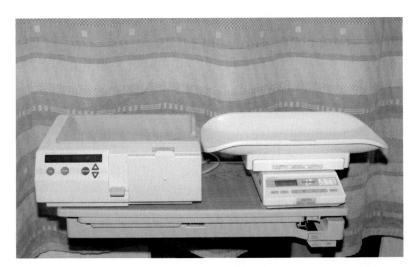

FIG. 53.2. **Right:** HomeChoice Automated PD System (Baxter, Deerfield, Illinois). **Left:** Medela BabyWeigh Scale (Medela, McHenry, Illinois).

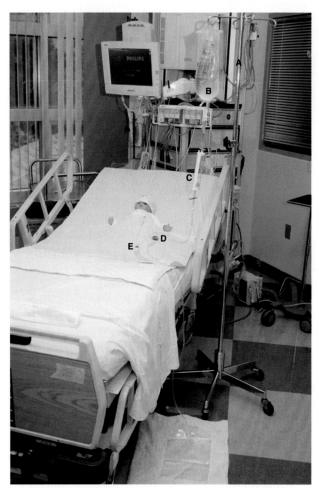

FIG. 53.3. An assembled peritoneal dialysis circuit illustrates an IV pole *(A)* and an inline burette *(C)* that is connected to an Ultra Set CAPD Y-Set *(D)*. The short limb of this Y-Set is connected to the transfer set *(E)*, which is connected to a Tenckhoff catheter exiting from the abdominal cavity of a doll, and the long limb has a bag at the end (located on the floor).

10. Connect the outlet of the burette set to the inflow line of the Ultra Set CAPD Disposable Disconnect Y-Set.
11. Connect the short arm end of the Y-Set to the twist clamp end of a MiniCap Extended Life PD Transfer Set with Twist Clamp (Baxter, Deerfield, Illinois). If the catheter is placed surgically, this transfer set is routinely connected by most surgeons to the Tenckhoff catheter, before assessment of patency, and you will be able to skip this step.
12. Prime the circuit in a sterile fashion, clamp, and cap the end of the transfer set, or the short limb of the Y-Set.

E. Procedure (Also Refer to Chapter 26 and Abdominal Paracentesis Video on the Procedures Website)

The ideal technique is surgical insertion of a permanent peritoneal dialysis catheter, which can be placed by an experienced surgeon in the neonatal intensive care unit (15). Catheters placed to exit the skin in a caudal direction. carry a lower risk of peritonitis. The catheter is tunneled from the peritoneum to an exit site on the skin; it usually works well and leaks infrequently (Quinton Pediatric Tenckhoff Neonatal 31-cm catheter, Kendall Healthcare, Mansfield, Massachusetts) However, if surgical insertion of a permanent catheter is not possible, an alternative approach is to utilize an angiocatheter or a temporary PD catheter for no longer than a few days to minimize infection risk. Note that surgically inserted catheters are associated with fewer acute complications (16). With catheters inserted at the bedside, guidewire-inserted femoral catheters have shown the least mechanical complications; IV catheters produce more mechanical complications than femoral catheters, but less than catheters with stylets (17,18).

1. Monitor vital signs.
2. Restrain infant in supine position.
3. Scrub.
4. Prepare the skin of the abdomen (Chapter 5).
5. Drape to expose the insertion site.
    The choice of insertion site is influenced by the preference of the physician and/or the presence of postoperative wounds, abdominal wall infection, or organomegaly. A location one-third the distance from the umbilicus to the symphysis pubis in the midline or a site lateral to the rectus sheath in either of the lower quadrants is preferred.
6. Infuse approximately 0.5 mL of lidocaine around the insertion point.
7. Select either a 14-gauge angiocatheter or a temporary dialysis catheter.
8. If you elect to use a 14-gauge angiocatheter
    a. Insert the angiocatheter at the insertion site.
    b. Remove the stylet.
    c. Infuse approximately 20 mL of normal saline to confirm a free flow. Clamp.
    d. Proceed to step 10.
9. If using a soft and flexible temporary catheter, such as a Cook catheter (Cook Critical Care, Bloomington, Indiana), follow the manufacturer's instructions. Then proceed to step 10.
10. Test patency.
    a. Temporary catheter
        (1) Unclamp. May observe flow of a few drops of saline. Connect the free end of the transfer set to the catheter.
        (2) Allow approximately 30 mL of dialysis solution to enter peritoneal cavity by gravity.
        (3) Clamp the short arm of the Y-Set (inflow).
        (4) Unclamp the long arm of the Y-Set (outflow).
        (5) Repeat steps a(2) through a(4) several times.
        (6) Secure the temporary catheter with a purse-string suture and tape if inflow and outflow occur readily.

TABLE 53.1	Complications of Peritoneal Dialysis
Problem (Risk)	**What to Do**
Perforation of bladder, bowel, or major vessels (3%–7%)	Surgical consultation
Puncture-site bleeding (3%–15%)	Apply pressure gently. Purse-string suture.
Blood-stained dialysis maintained after several cycles	Check hematocrit frequently. Continue heparin. Rule out major-vessel bleeding.
Leakage from exit site (2%–20%)	Reduce dwell volume until leakage stops.
Extravasation of dialysate into the anterior abdominal wall	Replace with new catheter.
More than 10% of solution retained in each of several consecutive cycles Reposition infant gently. (outflow obstruction) (15%–30%)	Reposition catheter by rotation and slight retraction. *Do not advance.* Remove if unchanged. Replace with new catheter.
Two-way obstruction (3%–20%)	Irrigate catheter with small amount of dialysate or saline aseptically. Reposition. Remove if unchanged.
Dislodgment of catheter (3%)	Replace with new catheter.
Hydrothorax (0%–10%)	Reposition infant, head and chest above level of abdomen. Decrease dwell volume.
Hyperglycemia (10%–60%)	Avoid high concentrations of dialysate unless outflow is inadequate. Low dose of insulin if needed.
Lactic acidosis	Use bicarbonate dialysate.[a]
Hyponatremia	Reduce fluid intake. Aim to increase outflow if secondary to fluid overload.
Hypernatremia	Increase fluid intake if secondary to excessive ultrafiltrate.
Exit site infection (4%–30%)	Systemic antibiotics.
Peritonitis (0.5%–30%)	Several rapid flushing exchanges. Blood culture. Systemic vancomycin plus ceftazidime or an aminoglycoside. For fungal peritonitis, systemic therapy is needed and catheter should be removed.
Hernia (inguinal or umbilical) (2%–13%)	Possible need for future repair.
Small bowel herniation and gangrene at catheter exit site (one case report)	Surgical consultation
Removal of therapeutic drugs	See Appendix E.

[a]1.5% bicarbonate dialysis solution: 140 mEq/L Na, 110 mEq/L Cl, 30 mEq/L HCO₃, 15 g of glucose; add sterile water to 1,000 mL.
Data from Kohli HS, Barkataky A, Kumar RSV, et al. Peritoneal dialysis for acute renal failure in infants: a comparison of three types of peritoneal access. *Ren Fail.* 1997;19:165; Kohli HS, Bhalla D, Sud K, et al. Acute peritoneal dialysis in neonates: comparison of two types of peritoneal access. *Pediatr Nephrol.* 1999;13:241; Matthews DE, West KW, Rescorla FJ, et al. Peritoneal dialysis in the first 60 days of life. *J Pediatr Surg.* 1990;25:110; Wong KKY, Lan LCL, Lin SCL, et al. Small bowel herniation and gangrene from peritoneal dialysis catheter exit site. *Pediatr Nephrol.* 2003;18:301.

b. Tenckhoff catheter
  (1) Unclamp the transfer set. Observe either saline or dialysis fluid, which was instilled at surgery, draining. Allow to drain to completion. Connect the short arm of the Y-Set to the transfer set.
  (2) Follow steps a(2) through a(5) of step 10 above.
      This procedure (step 10) usually results in a positive fluid balance (the volume drained is less than the volume infused). This retention is acceptable.

F. Management

1. Establish a cycle time. This is usually about 60 minutes and consists of a fill by gravity, dwell time of 45 minutes, and drain by gravity.
2. Establish a dialysis volume per pass. Starting volume is usually 20 to 30 mL/kg.
3. Clamp the long arm of the Y-Set (outflow line).
4. Unclamp the inflow line.
5. Allow the dialysate to flow in as quickly as possible, while carefully observing vital signs.
6. Clamp the inflow line.
7. Allow the fluid to dwell.
8. Unclamp the outflow when dwell time is completed.
9. Allow 5 to 10 minutes for draining.
10. Clamp the outflow line.
11. Repeat the cycle.
12. Increase the volume by 5 mL/kg/cycle slowly. Maximum volume is 40 mL/kg if tolerated, attained over 12 to 24 hours.
13. Continue to add 500 U of heparin/L of dialysate, until dialysate effluent return is clear, with no evidence of cloudiness.
14. Add 3 mEq/L of K if serum K level is ≤4 mEq/L.

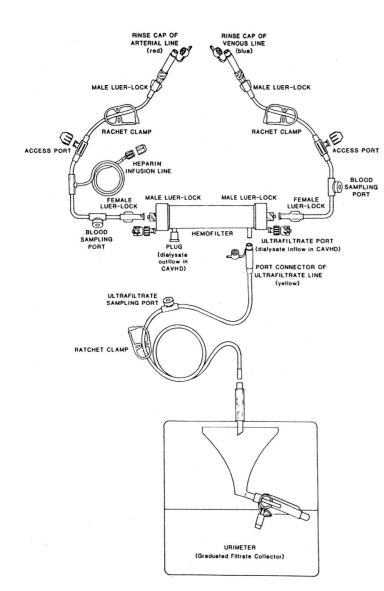

FIG. 53.4. A continuous arteriovenous hemofiltration circuit.

G. Monitoring

1. Maintain hourly PD flow sheet.
   a. Volume in
   b. Volume out
   c. Net/hr (+/–)
   d. Net over the course of dialysis (+/–)
   e. Intakes (enteral, parenteral)
   f. Outputs (urine, gastric, insensible water loss, etc.)
2. Establish a desired fluid balance. Increase volume slowly if negative balance is required. Reassess the state of hydration frequently.
3. Measure serum glucose and potassium every 4 hours for the first 24 hours or until stable, then twice a day. Obtain other serum electrolyte levels twice daily. Check blood urea nitrogen, serum creatinine, serum calcium, serum phosphorus, and serum magnesium once a day.
4. Obtain cell count, Gram stain, and culture of peritoneal effluent every 12 hours.
5. Recognize that some drug dosages may need adjustments (19–21) (see Appendix E).

H. Complications

See Table 53.1.

Continuous Arteriovenous Hemofiltration in Newborns
A short discussion of CAVH and CVVH is included for completeness. However, use of these modalities should be limited to regional centers and performed by those with the required expertise.

CAVH is an extracorporeal technique for removing plasma water and dissolved solutes of <50,000 Da over an extended period of time. With use of an arterial access line of the largest possible diameter and a venous access line, blood enters the extracorporeal circuit (arterial tubing, hemofilter, and venous tubing) by way of the arterial line and returns to the patient by way of the venous line (Fig. 53.4). The arteriovenous pressure gradient frequently produces adequate blood flow through the circuit; however, the addition of a blood pump may be necessary. As blood flows through the extracorporeal device, plasma water and dissolved solutes are filtered out (ultrafiltered) through the pores of a hemofilter. A hemofilter is composed of many fine capillaries of highly water-permeable membranes, located within a cylindric case. The filtered-off fluid (ultrafiltrate) is drained out by way of an exit incorporated on the surface of the hemofilter. The fluid removed has all the characteristics of an ultrafiltrate of plasma water.

Except when it is incorporated in an extracorporeal membrane oxygenation circuit for ultrafiltration, CAVH has been widely replaced by CVVH/D. It is used effectively in neonates with inborn errors of metabolism (33). Two single-lumen catheters (or one double-lumen venous catheter) are used for vascular access in CVVH/D. Blood flow is maintained by a pump and is, therefore, independent of the

patient's systemic blood pressure. Several brands of CVVH machines are currently available for CVVH/D (34).

References

1. Blatz S, Paes B, Steele B. Peritoneal dialysis in the neonate. *Neonatal Netw.* 1990;8:41.
2. Stapleton FB, Jones DP, Green RS. Acute renal failure in neonates: incidence, etiology and outcome. *Pediatr Nephrol.* 1987; 1:1314.
3. Meeks ACG, Sims DG. Treatment of renal failure in neonates. *Arch Dis Child.* 1988;63:1372.
4. Matthews DE, West KW, Rescorla FJ, et al. Peritoneal dialysis in the first 60 days of life. *J Pediatr Surg.* 1990;25:110.
5. Fischbach M. Peritoneal dialysis prescription for neonates. *Peritoneal Dial Int.* 1996;16:S512.
6. Esperanca MJ, Collins DL. Peritoneal dialysis efficiency relation to body weight. *J Pediatr Surg.* 1966;1:162.
7. Chan KL, Ip P, Chiu CSW, et al. Peritoneal dialysis after surgery for congenital heart disease in infants and young children. *Ann Thorac Surg.* 2003;76:1443.
8. Anand SK. Acute renal failure in the neonate. *Pediatr Clin North Am.* 1982;29:791.
9. Moghal NE, Embleton ND. Management of acute renal failure in the newborn. *Semin Fetal Neonatal Med.* 2006;11:207.
10. Batshaw ML, Brusilow SW. Treatment of hyperammonemic coma caused by inborn errors of urea synthesis. *J Pediatr.* 1980;97:893.
11. Gartner L, Leupold D, Pohlandt F, et al. Peritoneal dialysis in the treatment of metabolic crises caused by inherited disorders of organic and amino acid metabolism. *Acta Paediatr Scand.* 1989; 78:706.
12. Daschner M, Schaefer F. Emergency dialysis in neonatal metabolic crises. *Adv Ren Replace Ther.* 2002;9:63.
13. Arbeiter AK, Kranz B, Wingen AM, et al. Continuous venovenous haemodialysis (CVVHD) and continuous peritoneal dialysis (CPD) in the acute management of 21 children with inborn error of metabolism. *Nephrol Dial Transplant.* 2010;25:1237.
14. Mattoo TK, Ahmad GS. Peritoneal dialysis in neonates after major abdominal surgery. *Am J Nephrol.* 1994;14:6.
15. Chadha V, Warady BA, Blowey DL, et al. Tenckhoff catheters prove superior to Cook catheters in pediatric acute peritoneal dialysis. *Am J Kidney Dis.* 2000;35:1111.
16. Kohli HS, Barkataky A, Kumar RSV, et al. Peritoneal dialysis for acute renal failure in infants: a comparison of three types of peritoneal access. *Ren Fail.* 1997;19:165.
17. Kohli HS, Bhalla D, Sud K, et al. Acute peritoneal dialysis in neonates: comparison of two types of peritoneal access. *Pediatr Nephrol.* 1999;13:241.
18. Ronnholm KAR, Holmberg C. Peritoneal dialysis in infants. *Pediatr Nephrol.* 2006;21:751.
19. Trompeter RS. A review of drug prescribing in children with end-stage renal failure. *Pediatr Nephrol.* 1987;1:183.
20. Aandgil A, Srivastava RN. Drug prescribing in children with renal failure. *Indian Pediatr.* 1989;26:693.
21. Bennett WM, Blyth WB. Use of drugs in patients with renal failure. In: Schrier RW, Gottschalk CW, eds. *Disease of the Kidney.* 4th ed. Boston: Little, Brown; 1988:3437.
22. Kohli HS, Arora P, Kher V, et al. Daily peritoneal dialysis using a surgically placed Tenckhoff catheter for acute renal failure in children. *Ren Fail.* 1995;17:51.
23. Bunchman T. Acute peritoneal dialysis access in infant renal failure. *Perit Dial Int.* 1996;16:S509.
24. Walle JV, Raes A, Castillo D, et al. New perspectives for PD in acute renal failure related to new catheter techniques and introduction of APD. *Adv Perit Dial.* 1997;13:190.
25. Blowey DL, McFarland K, Alon U, et al. Peritoneal dialysis in the neonatal period: outcome data. *J Perinatol.* 1993;13:59.

26. Sizun J, Giroux JD, Rubio S, et al. Peritoneal dialysis in the very-low-birth-weight neonate (less than 1000g). *Acta Paediatr.* 1993; 82:488.

27. Werner HA, Wensley DF, Lirenman DS, et al. Peritoneal dialysis in children after cardiopulmonary bypass. *J Thorac Cardiovasc Surg.* 1997;113:64.

28. Dittrich S, Dahnert I, Vogel M, et al. Peritoneal dialysis after infant open heart surgery: observations in 27 patients. *Ann Thorac Surg.* 1999;68:160.

29. Sorof JM, Stromberg D, Brewer ED, et al. Early initiation of peritoneal dialysis after surgical repair of congenital heart disease. *Pediatr Nephrol.* 1999;13:641.

30. Reznik VM, Griswold WR, Peterson BM, et al. Peritoneal dialysis for acute renal failure in children. *Pediatr Nephrol.* 1991;5:715.

31. Huber R, Fuchshuber A, Huber P. Acute peritoneal dialysis in preterm newborns and small infants: surgical management. *J Pediatr Surg.* 1994;29:400.

32. Wong KKY, Lan LCL, Lin SCL, et al. Small bowel herniation and gangrene from peritoneal dialysis catheter exit site. *Pediatr Nephrol.* 2003;18:301.

33. Westrope C, Morris K, Burford D, et al. Continuous hemofiltration in the control of neonatal hyperammonemia: a 10 year experience. *Pediatr Nephrol.* 2010;25:1725.

34. Menster M, Bunchman TE. Nephrology in pediatric intensive care unit. *Semin Nephrol.* 1998;18:330.

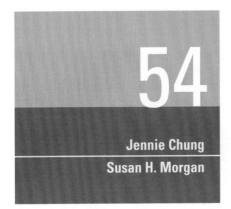

54 Neonatal Hearing Screening

Jennie Chung
Susan H. Morgan

A. Purpose

1. To identify hearing loss in the neonatal period in order to provide early intervention so that delay in speech and language development may be minimized.
2. To support accurate reporting by state of incidence of congenital hearing loss.

B. Background

1. The prevalence of congenital hearing loss in newborns is 1.4 (range 0 to 4.6) per 1,000 infants screened with 97% of newborns screened in the United States (1).
2. The risk of hearing loss can increase substantially when infants are exposed to certain perinatal risk factors (e.g., cytomegalovirus) or have medical conditions requiring certain interventions (e.g., extracorporeal membrane oxygenation) in intensive care nurseries (Table 54.1).
3. Early intervention for hearing loss can help maximize the child's potential (2). Delaying diagnosis of hearing loss can lead to significant problems in language and speech acquisition (3).

C. Indications

1. *Every newborn* should receive a hearing screen before discharge from the hospital (4,5).
   a. Currently, 47 states and the District of Columbia have passed legislation mandating universal newborn hearing screening for every infant regardless of background and risk factors (6).
   b. Every US state and territory has established an Early Hearing Detection and Intervention (EHDI) program to help insure infants receive hearing screening and intervention services (7).
   c. The Centers for Disease Control and Prevention's Early Hearing Detection and Intervention Program recommends that infants identified by a failed hearing screen be referred for a comprehensive audiology evaluation *as soon as possible and always before 3 months of age* (8).

2. Infants who meet **high-risk criteria** for acquiring hearing loss warrant immediate hearing screening, followed by ongoing monitoring. Table 54.1 lists factors known to be associated with permanent congenital, late-onset, or progressive hearing loss in childhood. *Even if they have passed their initial hearing screen,* it is critical that infants with any of these risk factors be referred to audiology after discharge so that they may continue to be monitored during the early years of language acquisition and development (5).

D. Types of Hearing Loss

1. *Conductive:* Resulting from impaired sound transmission through ear canal, tympanic membrane, and middle ear
2. *Sensorineural:* Due to cochlear or retrocochlear disorder
3. *Mixed:* Has a both conductive and sensorineural component
4. *Auditory neuropathy spectrum disorder:* A relatively new term used to describe auditory characteristics of patients who exhibit normal cochlear outer hair cell function but disordered or dyssynchronous neural conduction in other sites deep to the cochlea along the auditory pathway (9).

E. Types of Hearing Screen

1. *Otoacoustic emissions (OAE):* A noninvasive screening tool that measures sounds generated by a functioning cochlea. A probe containing a miniature microphone delivers a sound stimulus, either click or tone, into the ear canal and records the cochlear response that travels from the cochlea back into the ear canal. This assembly is coupled to a computer for analysis of the sound in the ear canal and for processing of the otoacoustic emission. Results may be automatically analyzed and interpreted as either "pass" or "refer" for each ear. Figure 54.1 shows an infant undergoing OAE screening. This screening tool evaluates the peripheral auditory system extending to cochlear function.

TABLE 54.1	High-Risk Registry Associated with Hearing Loss in Childhood

- Illness or condition that requires admission of 5 days or longer to NICU
- Exposure to any of the following treatment regardless of NICU duration of stay
  - Extracorporeal membrane oxygenation
  - Ventilator
  - Ototoxic medication
  - Loop diuretics
  - Hyperbilirubinemia requiring exchange transfusion
- Stigmata or other findings associated with a syndrome known to include sensorineural or permanent conductive hearing loss
- Family history of permanent childhood sensorineural hearing loss
- Craniofacial anomalies, including those with morphologic abnormalities of the pinna and ear canal and temporal bone anomalies
- In utero infection, such as cytomegalovirus, herpes, toxoplasmosis, or rubella
- Parental or caregiver concern regarding hearing, speech, language, and developmental delay
- Postnatal infections associated with sensorineural hearing loss, including bacterial meningitis
- Syndromes associated with progressive hearing loss, such as neurofibromatosis, osteopetrosis, and Usher syndrome
- Neurodegenerative disorders, such as Hunter syndrome, or sensory motor neuropathies, such as Friedreich ataxia and Charcot-Marie-Tooth syndrome
- Head trauma
- Chemotherapy

From American Academy of Pediatrics, Joint Committee on Infant Hearing. Year 2007 position statement: principles and guidelines for early hearing detection and intervention programs. *Pediatrics.* 2007;120:898.

2. *Automated auditory brainstem response (AABR):* Also a noninvasive screening tool that records auditory brainstem responses and compares them to a template representing typical results in neonates. Occlusive earphones cover the ears and emit sound stimuli into the ear canal. Electrodes are placed on the head and nape of neck to detect electrical activity from the auditory nerve and brainstem in response to the sound stimuli. A computer registers samples of the electrical activity over a fixed

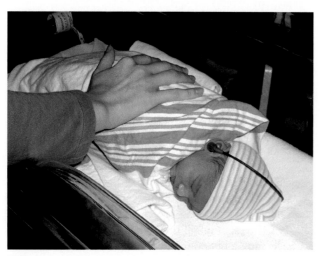

FIG. 54.1. An infant undergoing OAE screening.

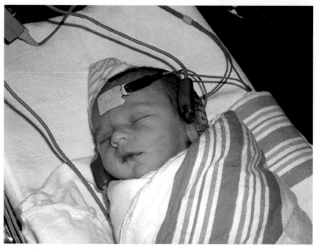

FIG. 54.2. An infant undergoing AABR screening.

period of time. The averaged responses are then compared to a normal newborn template to determine if the result is a "pass" or a "refer" for each ear. Figure 54.2 shows an infant undergoing AABR screening. In addition to assessing middle ear and cochlear activity, this test evaluates the function of the auditory nerve and auditory brainstem.

3. *Auditory brainstem response (ABR) also referred to as brainstem auditory evoked response (BAER):* Not typically used as the initial hearing screen tool, BAER is a diagnostic test used to predict type and severity of hearing loss. BAER testing is conducted after a failed screening measurement. Auditory brainstem responses are determined in each ear for both click and tone stimuli. These sounds are presented by air (earphone) as well as bone conduction. Severity of hearing loss is expressed in decibels and described as conductive, sensorineural, or mixed.

F. Techniques

1. *Both OAE and AABR screening systems can be automated:* An individual only needs to be appropriately trained to set up and apply the equipment. A computer processes the incoming information and gives a readout of the result, usually as "pass" or "refer."
2. Care should be taken to attempt screening in a relatively quiet environment, as well as ensuring that the infant is resting comfortably and the ear canals are free from obvious debris, to avoid false "refer" result.

G. Specific Protocols

1. *For infants admitted to neonatal intensive care unit (NICU) for more than 5 days:* the Joint Committee on Infant Hearing recommends ABR technology as the only appropriate screening technique for use in the

NICU (5). This specific population is at high risk for having auditory neuropathy, which is detected by AABR but not by OAE (9,10). Immediate and direct referral should be made to an audiologist if an infant does not pass AABR in the NICU.

2. *For well-nursery infants:* Although OAE is more often used than AABR, both methods are widely used in many hospitals, as there is no standardization of newborn hearing screening protocols for well infants. Some hospital programs screen neonatal hearing with OAE first. If infant does not pass OAE, AABR will be used to rescreen. There are advantages and disadvantages to using OAE as the first newborn hearing screen. Please refer to H for an explanation. For infants who do not pass AABR as the first screening test, a direct referral to an audiologist should be made as the infant might have a neuro auditory disorder, and OAE should not be used to rescreen (5).

3. *For infants **readmitted** to hospitals:* A repeat hearing screen is recommended for infants <1 month old, who were readmitted to hospital, if the medical condition is associated with increased risk of hearing loss (e.g., meningitis or hyperbilirubinemia requiring exchange transfusion) (5).

4. The following timeline is a goal objective in Healthy People 2020 (5,9,11)
   a. *By 1 month old:* All newborns to have hearing screened
   b. *By 3 months old:* Those that do not pass initial screening need to have a comprehensive evaluation by an audiologist.
   c. *By 6 months old:* Infants with confirmed hearing loss should receive appropriate interventions.

H. Limitations

1. Infant hearing screening can be compromised by environmental noise (such as a busy intensive care unit) or infant movement. OAE screening, more so than AABR, is particularly affected by vernix occluding the ear canal, or middle ear pathology such as effusion (12).

2. OAE screening, although less time-consuming to set up and conduct, has a higher "refer" (fail) rate than AABR. The refer rates for OAE screening alone have been cited in the literature as being between 5.8% and 6.5%, with refer rates using AABR screening around 3.2% (13,14). In particular, infants who are <48 hours old are more likely to have a "refer" result if screened with OAE, as the presence of vernix and debris in the ear canal can be a significant factor (15).

3. Some infants who pass newborn screening will later demonstrate permanent hearing loss. Although this loss may reflect delayed hearing loss, both ABR and OAE screening technology will miss some hearing loss (mild or isolated frequency losses) (5).

I. Contraindications

1. *Patient has significantly atretic or total lack of external ear canal:* Refer directly to pediatric audiologist.
2. Although it is certainly fair to rescreen an infant who has potentially failed screening because of excessive background noise, vernix in ear canal, etc., multiple rescreening attempts in hopes of eventually obtaining a "pass" are not recommended and can contribute to delayed identification of congenital hearing loss.

J. Special Circumstances

1. *Hearing parents whose infant does not pass a hearing screening:* Parents are often quite concerned to learn their infant has not passed a hearing screening. The result can be especially stress provoking for parents whose infant may have spent a good deal of time in a NICU and may be facing additional medical concerns upon discharge. It is extremely important to remember that *a failed hearing screening is not a definitive diagnosis of hearing loss.* It is an important indicator that the infant needs immediate referral to an audiologist for further detailed evaluation, which may or may not result in a formal diagnosis of hearing loss.

2. *Deaf parents whose infant does not pass a hearing screen:* Deaf parents, especially culturally deaf individuals who use American Sign Language and identify strongly with being members of the deaf community, are often thrilled to find out that their infant may have hearing loss. This is a cultural identification: These parents are rejoicing in the fact that their infant is like them and will have a cultural place of significance in their social world. This is often in direct opposition to the traditional medical perspective on hearing loss. The parental reaction can be frankly surprising for involved health care professionals. It is very important to realize that *these infants of culturally deaf parents are not facing the immediate crisis* of delayed language development referred to earlier. American Sign Language is a well-researched, intact language (16,17) that is immediately accessible to an infant of deaf parents. Although it is still extremely important to establish audiologic follow-up for these infants of deaf parents who fail a hearing screen, it is also critical to respect the potential cultural implication for such families. These parents may be celebrating in a manner very similar to hearing parents who are happy that their infant has passed the hearing screening.

K. Complications

OAE and AABR are considered to be noninvasive and safe procedures. Like any procedure that involves the application of electrode pads, mild superficial skin abrasions could possibly occur with the removal of the electrode pads after AABR testing.

References

1. Hearing Screen and Follow-up Survey, 2009. Centers for Disease Control and Prevention. Available at: http://www.cdc.gov/ncbddd/hearingloss/2009-Data/2009_EHDI_HSFS_Summary-508-OK.pdf Accessed August 27, 2011.

2. Holden-Pitt L, Diaz J. Thirty years of the annual survey of deaf and hard of hearing children and youth: a glance over the decades. *Am Ann Deaf*. 1998;143:72.

3. Yoshinaga-Itano C. From screening to early identification and intervention: discovering predictors to successful outcomes for children with significant hearing loss. *J Deaf Stud Deaf Educ*. 2003;8:11.

4. Early Identification of Hearing Impairment in Infants and Young Children. NIH Consensus Statement Online 1993. Available at: http://consensus.nih.gov/1993/1993HearingInfantsChildren092html.htm. Accessed August 24, 2011.

5. American Academy of Pediatrics, Joint Committee on Infant Hearing. Year 2007 position statement: principles and guidelines for early hearing detection and intervention programs. *Pediatrics*. 2007;120:898.

6. American Speech-Language-Hearing Association.. Status of State Early Hearing Detection and Intervention (EHDI) Laws. Available at: http://www.asha.org/Advocacy/state/bill_status/. Accessed August 24, 2011.

7. National Center for Hearing Assessment and Management Utah State University. State EHDI information. Available at: http://www.infanthearing.org/states_home/. Accessed August 24, 2011.

8. Centers for Disease Control and Prevention. Hearing Loss in Children: Recommendations and Guidelines. Available at: http://www.cdc.gov/ncbddd/hearingloss/recommendations.html. Accessed August 25, 2011.

9. Xoinis K, Weirather Y, Mavoori H, et al. Extremely low birth weight infants are at high risk for auditory neuropathy. *J Perinatol*. 2007;27:718.

10. D'Agostino J, Austin L. Auditory neuropathy: a potentially under-recognized neonatal intensive care unit sequel. *Adv Neonatal Care*. 2004;4:344.

11. US Department of Health and Human Services, Office of Disease Prevention and Health Promotion. Healthy People 2020 Topics and Objectives: Hearing and Other Sensory or Communication Disorders. July 18, 2011. Available at: http://healthypeople.gov/2020/topicsobjectives2020/objectiveslist.aspx?topicId=20. Accessed August 30, 2011.

12. De Michele A. Newborn hearing screening. *eMedicine*. 2005. Available at: www.emedicine.com/ent/topic576.htm. Accessed August 27, 2011.

13. Vohr B, Oh W, Stewart E, et al. Comparison of costs and referral rates of 3 universal newborn hearing screening protocols. *J Pediatr*. 2001;139:238.

14. Clarke P, Iqbal M, Mitchell S. A comparison of transient-evoked otoacoustic emissions and automated auditory brainstem responses for pre-discharge neonatal hearing screening. *Int J Audiol*. 2003;42:443.

15. Lin H, Shu M, Lee K, et al. Comparison of hearing screening programs between one step with transient evoked otoacoustic emissions (TEOAE) and two steps with TEOAE and automated auditory brainstem response (AABR). *Laryngoscope*. 2005;115:1957.

16. Stokoe W. *A Dictionary of American Sign Language on Linguistic Principles*. Washington, DC: Gallaudet Press; 1965, rev. ed. 1976.

17. Stokoe W. Sign language structure. *Ann Rev Anthropol*. 1980;9:365.

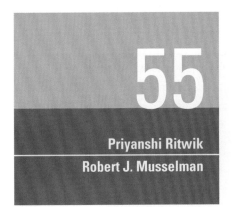

55

Management of Natal and Neonatal Teeth

Priyanshi Ritwik

Robert J. Musselman

The occurrence of teeth in the oral cavity at birth or within the first 30 days of life is uncommon. Such teeth have been called natal and neonatal teeth, respectively. This distinction, however, is temporal and artificial. Relevant clinical inferences can be made by further describing these teeth as mature or immature based on the quality of dental tissue and degree of dental development (1). Hebling et al. (2) classified natal teeth into four clinical categories (Table 55.1).

The reported incidence of natal and neonatal teeth varies; a range of 1 in 2,000 to 3,500 is widely accepted (3). Overall, natal teeth occur more frequently than neonatal teeth (3:1) (4). However, in a study of 18,155 infants, the reported incidence of natal and neonatal teeth was 1:716 (5). Most (85%) of natal and neonatal teeth are mandibular incisors (6,7). There are also case reports of natal teeth in the posterior regions of the alveolar process (3,8–10), thereby necessitating an examination of the posterior region of the alveolar processes at birth for the presence of teeth. Approximately, 95% of natal and neonatal teeth are a member of the normal complement of the deciduous dentition (11); this indicates that supernumerary natal and neonatal teeth are rare. Hence, natal and neonatal teeth should usually be retained.

A. Etiology

1. Superficial positioning of the primary tooth germ (12)
2. Infection and malnutrition (12)
3. Febrile illness (12)
4. Maternal exposure to toxins (polychlorinated bisphenol, polychlorinated dibenzofuran, polychlorinated dibenzo-p-dioxin) (13)
5. Syndrome/medical condition (Table 55.2) (12)

TABLE 55.1	Hebling Classification of Natal Teeth

1. Shell-shaped crown poorly fixed to the alveolus by gingival tissue with absence of a root
2. Solid crown poorly fixed to the alveolus by gingival tissue with little or no root
3. Eruption of the incisal margin of the crown through the gingival tissue
4. Edema of gingival tissue with an unerupted but palpable tooth

B. Clinical Presentation (Figs. 55.1 through 55.6)

There is variability in the presentation of natal and neonatal teeth. Although some have normal crown shape and color and are held firmly in the alveolar process, others present as discolored microdonts with hypermobility. The latter are the immature type of teeth. The management of the patient depends on the clinical presentation.

C. Clinical Assessment

Clinical assessment should include an assessment of the tooth, oral soft tissues, and the systemic disposition of the patient.

1. Dental assessment
   a. *Mobility:* Tooth mobility >1 mm is usually an indication for the extraction of the natal/neonatal tooth.
   b. *Color and shape of tooth:* Discoloration and abnormal morphology indicate an immature natal/neonatal tooth, which usually will require removal.
   c. *Root formation:* This can be assessed with a dental radiograph. However, a loose tooth is likely to be lacking in root structure and is likely to exfoliate spontaneously and early, with the risk of aspiration.
2. Soft tissue assessment
   a. *Ventral surface of the tongue:* Riga-Fede disease is the term given to an ulcerative granuloma formed

TABLE 55.2	Conditions Associated with Higher Incidence of Natal/Neonatal Teeth

Ellis-Van Creveld syndrome
Hallermann-Streiff syndrome
Craniofacial synostosis
Multiple steatocystoma
Congenital pachyonychia
Sotos syndrome
Cleft palate
Pierre Robin anomalad

on the ventral surface of the tongue. It results from irritation of the tongue by the sharp margins of the mandibular incisor.

b. *Gingival tissue:* Gingival tissue adjacent to the natal/neonatal tooth should be examined for presence of inflammation or granulomatous lesion, caused by irritation by the sharp cervical margins of an immature tooth.

3. General assessment

Table 55.2 lists the systemic conditions associated with higher incidence of natal/neonatal teeth. They should each be ruled out to ensure that a pre-existing medical condition is not overlooked.

D. Precautions

1. Keep in mind that the initial question in management of natal teeth is whether extraction is indicated. Indiscriminate extraction of natal/neonatal teeth is discouraged (14).
2. Natal and neonatal teeth should be differentiated from cystic lesions such as Bohn nodules and Epstein pearls, by palpation and location in the infant's mouth. Bohn nodules and Epstein pearls are firm and have a smooth, rounded surface. There will usually be several nodules/pearls, and they may be located on the posterior palate or mandibular ridge.
3. Prior to extraction, it must be confirmed that the patient has received the appropriate dose of vitamin K at birth (12). There has been one report of difficulty in achieving hemostasis by local pressure after the extraction of natal tooth. This patient received microfibrillar collagen hemostat over the extraction site (3). Current literature supports the extraction of the natal tooth at 10 days or later after birth, unless there is significant risk of aspiration (11).
4. A detailed family history should be obtained, to rule out inherited coagulopathy.
5. Following the extraction, the socket should be curetted to remove odontogenic tissue (see F).
6. *Long-term care:* Whether the patient receives conservative restorative treatment or extraction, the parents should be encouraged to maintain regular dental appointments with a pediatric dentist. This enables monitoring of the extraction site and parental guidance in oral hygiene practices for their infant.

E. Technique

Nonextraction Case

If the tooth is firm and appears of normal color and shape, extraction is not indicated.

1. Should the mother complain of discomfort while breast-feeding, the use of a breast pump and bottling of milk should be encouraged.

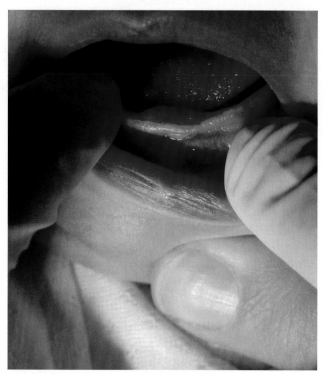

FIG. 55.1. Patient 1: Normal (edentulous) alveolar ridge in neonate.

2. If the patient presents with Riga-Fede disease, a pediatric dentist should be consulted. The sharp margins of the tooth can be smoothed using photopolymerized dental composite restorative resin. This results in spontaneous resolution of the tongue lesion (15).
3. Pain relief and faster healing may be accomplished by carefully applying Kenalog in Orabase (16).
4. If it is decided to not extract the teeth, the parents must receive guidance on infant oral health. The tooth/teeth should be brushed with a soft bristled toothbrush and a smear of fluoridated toothpaste in the morning and at

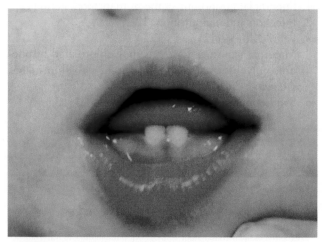

FIG. 55.2. Patient 2: Hebling classification #3 neonatal tooth; not indicated for extraction.

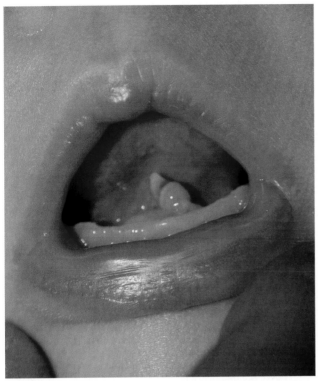

FIG. 55.3. Patient 3: Hebling classification #2 natal tooth; this tooth was extracted.

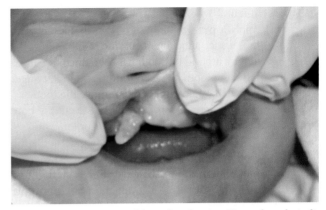

FIG. 55.5. Patient 4: Hebling classification #2 natal tooth; indicated for extraction. The natal tooth was present at the site of alveolar cleft in this 3-day-old Hispanic girl. This tooth was extracted with topical anesthetic.

night after the last feeding. The infant should not be put to sleep in a crib with a feeding bottle containing formula, milk, or juice.

Extraction Case

Extraction is indicated if there is hypermobility of the tooth or if the tooth is of the immature type (malformed, discolored, lacking root development). These would be classified as class 1 or 2 by Hebling et al. (2).

    a. Equipment
        (1) 2- × 2-inch gauze piece
        (2) Topical anesthetic
            Lidocaine 2% gel is the local anesthetic of choice. Topical oral anesthetic agents containing benzocaine should be avoided due to the risk of methemoglobinemia in children under 2 years of age (17).
        (3) Blunt-nosed sterile surgical scissors

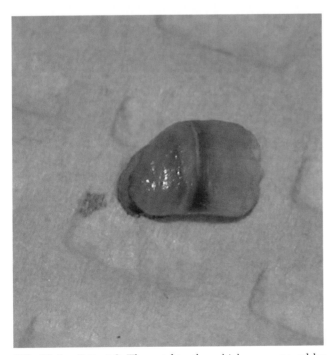

FIG. 55.4. Patient 3: The natal tooth—which was removed by grasping the tooth with gloved fingers—holding the tooth with a 2- × 2-inch gauze square.

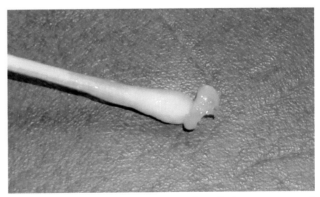

FIG. 55.6. Patient 4: Extracted natal tooth that was removed with 2- × 2-inch gauze after topical anesthetic application.

b. Technique
(1) Apply a pea-size amount of topical anesthesia to the tissue attachment of the tooth, after the gingiva around the tooth has been dried by gauze.
(2) Hold the tooth between thumb and index finger in gauze square and gently remove the tooth.
(3) Blunt-nosed scissors can be used to cut the connecting tissue if it is very fibrous or tenacious.

If in the physician's clinical judgment, the tooth cannot be removed by the above technique, then the infant needs to be referred to a pediatric dentist for evaluation and possible extraction.

F. Complications of Extraction

1. Tissue tags comprising dental papilla and/or Hertwig's epithelial root sheath remain in the extraction socket (18). These tissues may continue to form dental hard tissues, that is, dentin and root structure (18). These aberrant dental hard tissues may interfere with the normal eruption of adjacent primary teeth (18).
2. The development of postextraction pyogenic granuloma (19) and hamartoma (20) have been reported.
3. In 9% of patients with natal/neonatal teeth associated with alveolar cleft, a second toothlike structure may develop later. This emphasizes the necessity to maintain regular dental appointments for these patients.

References

1. Spouge JD, Feasby WH. Erupted teeth in the newborn. *Oral Surg Oral Med Oral Pathol.* 1966;22:198.
2. Hebling J, Zuanon ACC, Vianna DR. Dente natal—a case of natal teeth. *Odontol Clin.* 1997;7:37.
3. Brandt SK, Shapiro SD, Kittle PE. Immature primary molars in the newborn. *Pediatr Dent.* 1983;5:210.
4. Haberland C, Persing J. Neonatal teeth in a 6-week-old baby with bilateral cleft lip and palate: Case report and review of the literature. *Oral Surg Oral Med Oral Pathol Oral Radiol Endod.* 2010;110:e20.
5. Kates GA, Needleman HL, Holmes LB. Natal and neonatal teeth: a clinical study. *J Am Dent Assoc.* 1984;109:441.
6. Zhu J, King D. Natal and neonatal teeth: a review of 24 cases reported in literature. *J Pediatr.* 1950;36:349.
7. Badenhoff J, Gorlin RJ. Natal and neonatal teeth. *Pediatrics.* 1963;32:1087.
8. Friend GW, Mincer HH, Carruth KR, et al. Natal primary molar: case report. *Pediatr Dent.* 1991;13:173.
9. Masatomi Y, Abe K, Ooshima T. Unusual multiple natal teeth: case report. *Pediatr Dent.* 1991;13:170.
10. Kumar A, Grewal H, Verma M. Posterior natal teeth. *J Indian Soc Pedod Prev Dent.* 2011;29:68.
11. Howkins C. Congenital teeth. *Br Dent Assoc.* 1932;53:402.
12. Cunha RF, Boer FA, Torriani DD, Frossard WT. Natal and neonatal teeth: review of the literature. *Pediatr Dent.* 2001;23:158.
13. Alaluusua S, Kiviranta H, Leppaniemi A, et al. Natal and neonatal teeth in relation to environmental toxicants. *Pediatr Res.* 2002;52:652.
14. Watt J. Needless extractions. *Br Dent J.* 2004;197:170.
15. Slayton R. Treatment alternatives for sublingual traumatic ulceration (Riga-Fede disease). *Pediatr Dent.* 2000;22:413.
16. Seminario AL, Ivancakova R. Natal and neonatal teeth. *Acta Med (Hradec Kralove).* 2004;47:229.
17. U.S Food and Drug Administration. FDA Drug Safety Communication: Reports of a rate, but serious and potentially fatal adverse effect with the use of over-the-counter (OTC) benzocaine gels and liquids applied to the gums or mouth. Available at: http://www.fda.gov/Drugs/DrugSafety/ucm250024.htm. Accessed July 1, 2011.
18. Nedley MP, Stanley RT, Cohen DM. Extraction of natal teeth can leave odontogenic remnants. *Pediatr Dent.* 1995;17:457.
19. Muench MG, Layton S, Wright JM. Pyogenic granuloma associated with a natal tooth: case report. *Pediatr Dent.* 1992;14:265.
20. Oliveira LB, Tamay TK, Wanderley MT, et al. Gingival fibrous hamartoma associated with natal teeth. *J Clin Pediatr Dent.* 2005;29:249.

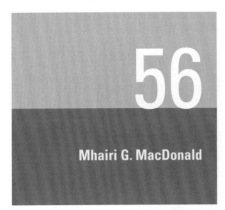

56 Relocation of a Dislocated Nasal Septum

Mhairi G. MacDonald

A. Indications

To avoid future surgery, breathing and feeding problems, epistaxis, malocclusion, and sinusitis.

Fetal compression sufficient to cause some degree of nasal deformation is a frequent physical finding on early newborn examination and normally resolves within 48 hours of birth (Fig. 56.1). In some instances, intrauterine forces or pressure applied during delivery cause a true septal dislocation (Fig. 56.2). The incidence of true septal dislocation ranges from 1% to 4% of births (1–8). The otolaryngology literature indicates that septal dislocation should be relocated within a few days of birth for the best outcome (2,4,9,10). To differentiate compression deformity from true septal dislocation, apply gentle pressure to the tip of the nose; a dislocated septum will move farther from the midline at the base, a compressed septum will not move from the midline at the base. A compressed nose can be restored to normal anatomy with gentle pressure; a nose with septal dislocation cannot.

B. Contraindications

1. Presence of other nasal or midline congenital anomalies requiring more extensive treatment
2. Posterior septal dislocation
3. Nasal orifice too small to easily admit smallest septal forceps

C. Equipment

1. Septal forceps—modified Walsham or other appropriately sized septal forceps (Fig. 56.3).

D. Precautions

1. Reduction should be performed within the first 3 to 4 days after birth.

2. Otolaryngology evaluation for refractory dislocations or associated facial abnormalities
3. Adequate restraint of infant, especially the head
4. Remember that many newborns are obligate nasal breathers; insertion of a large-bore nasogastric tube into the stomach or an oral airway, prior to the procedure, will serve to separate the tongue from the palate and to promote oral respiration.

E. Technique

1. Place septal forceps into the nares on the anterior aspect of the cartilaginous septum, posterior to columella. Advance blades gently, approximately 0.5 to 1 cm. Do not advance past the inferior aspect of the middle turbinate; *do not force* (Fig. 56.4A).
2. Gently close the forceps onto the septum.
3. Direct the pressure of the lower edges of the forceps blades toward the midline, to move the septum into alignment with the nasal groove on the vomer (spine)—a slight upward motion may be required to lift the inferior border of the septum over the side of the vomer into the spinal groove (can be compared to replacing a sliding door into the slider) (Fig. 56.4B,C).
4. Re-examine to ensure adequate reduction.

F. Complications

1. Hemorrhage
2. Damage to nasal structures (e.g., the turbinates, septum)
3. Damage to skull base—resulting in cerebrospinal fluid leak (if speculum inserted too far)
4. Persistent dislocation

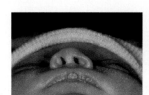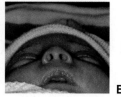

FIG. 56.1. Nasal compression without septal deviation. **A:** Shortly after birth, the nose is asymmetrical from simple compression with an angled septum at rest. **B:** The septum assumes its normal angle. (From Fletcher MA. *Physical Diagnosis in Neonatology.* Philadelphia: Lippincott-Raven; 1998:211.)

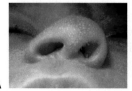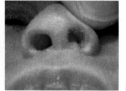

FIG. 56.2. **A:** At rest, it is difficult to distinguish a true deviation. **B:** Attempts to restore normal anatomy are unsuccessful as the septum remains deviated at the base. (From Fletcher MA. *Physical Diagnosis in Neonatology.* Philadelphia: Lippincott-Raven; 1998:211.)

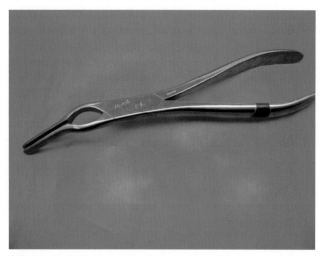

FIG. 56.3. Walsham septal forceps.

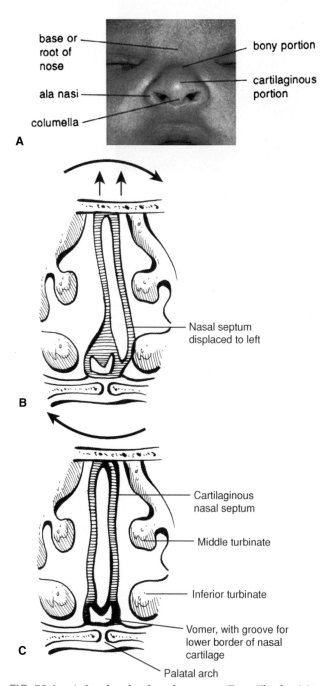

FIG. 56.4. **A:** Landmarks of nasal anatomy. (From Fletcher MA. *Physical Diagnosis in Neonatology.* Philadelphia: Lippincott-Raven; 1998:210.) **B:** The cartilaginous nasal septum displaced to the left from the ridge on the vomer. *Large arrows* indicate the direction of turn of the forceps blades needed to replace the septum into the groove; *small arrows* indicate the concurrent upward pull. **C:** The septum postreplacement.

References

1. Kawalski H, Spiewak P. How septum deformities in newborn occur. *Int J Pediatr Otorhinolaryngol.* 1998;44:23.
2. Tasca I, Compradretti GC. Immediate correction of nasal septum dislocation in newborns. *Am J Rhinol.* 2004;18:47.
3. Podoshin L, Gertner R, Fradis M, et al. Incidence and treatment of deviation of the nasal septum in newborns. *Ear Nose Throat J.* 1991;70:485.
4. Silverman SH, Leibow SG. Dislocation of the triangular cartilage of the nasal septum. *J Pediatr.* 1975;87:456.
5. Jeppesen F, Windfield J. Dislocation of nasal septal cartilage in the newborn. *Acta Obstet Gynecol Scand.* 1972;51:5.
6. Bhattacharjee A, Uddin S, Purkaystha P. Deviated nasal septum in the newborn—a 1 year study. *Indian J Otolaryngol Head Neck Surg.* 2005;57:304.
7. Kent SE, Rock WP, Nahl SS, et al. The relationship of nasal septal deformity and palatal asymmetry in neonates. *J Laryngol Oto.* 1991;105:424.
8. Kent SE, Reid AP, Brain DJ, et al. Neonatal septal deviations. *J R Soc Med.* 1988;81:132.
9. Pentz S, Pirsig W, Linders H. Long-term results of neonates with nasal deviation: a prospective study over 12 years. *Int J Pediatr Otorhinolaryngol.* 1994;28:183.
10. Gola R, Cheynet F, Guyot L, et al. Nasal injuries during labor and in early childhood. Etiopathogenesis, consequences, and therapeutic options. *Rev Stomatol Chir Maxillofac.* 2002;103:41.

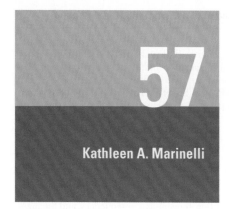

57 Lingual Frenotomy

Kathleen A. Marinelli

A. Definitions

1. Lingual frenulum—a fold of mucosa connecting the midline of the inferior surface of the tongue to the floor of the mouth (1)

   Generally thin, membranous, and avascular in the newborn (Fig. 57.1)
2. Ankyloglossia (tongue tie)—a congenital oral abnormality, characterized by an abnormally short, thick, and/or tight lingual frenulum (1–3)
   a. "Ankyloglossia" derives from the Greek *agkylos*—crooked, and *glossa*—tongue.
   b. Many different variations of tongue tie
   c. Differing degrees of severity
   d. May restrict mobility of the tongue tip
3. Anterior tongue tie—anterior position of the lingual frenulum, usually very thin and membranous, with resultant restricted tongue tip movement

   By far the most common (one study reports 94% of tongue ties) (4).
4. Posterior tongue tie—more subtle, and thus more difficult to diagnose, as anterior tongue tip usually has free movement (4,5) (Fig. 57.2).

   Thick fibrous band, which, if not visible, can be palpated with gloved finger as "bump" or thick band at the back of the tongue.

   Increasingly associated with breast-feeding difficulties. Reported incidence of posterior tongue tie in one series 6% of all tongue ties (4).
5. Lingual frenotomy (tongue clipping)—a minor surgical procedure, appropriate for treatment of significant ankyloglossia in infants
   a. "Frenotomy" means to cut—no tissue is removed
   b. Can be accomplished at the bedside in the neonatal intensive care unit or postpartum unit, or in an outpatient clinic setting by a trained physician or dentist (6–8)
6. Frenuloplasty or frenectomy—more complicated surgical procedures employing Z-plasty technique or with removal of tissue
   a. Reserved for older children, adults, or infants with a complicated lingual frenulum, such as a thickened frenulum containing genioglossus muscle or a "complete" ankyloglossia in which tongue is fused to the floor of the mouth
   b. Performed in the operating room, by an otolaryngologist or oral surgeon, under conscious sedation or general anesthesia

B. Purpose

1. Lingual frenotomy—performed when the presence of ankyloglossia restricts or impedes an infant's ability to suckle successfully
   a. Most common in breast-feeding infants
   b. Occasionally seen in infants using an artificial teat
2. Other problems related to ankyloglossia that may manifest in older children and adults, for which prophylactic frenotomy in infancy (when procedure is relatively simple and safe) should be considered (2,3,9–13).
   a. Mechanical problems

      Gingival recession, mandibular diastema, malocclusion, prognathism, difficulty with intraoral toilet (licking the lips, sweeping food debris off teeth)
   b. Articulation errors in speech
   c. Social effects
      (1) Difficulty playing a wind instrument, licking an ice cream cone or lollipop, social interactions (kissing, etc.)
      (2) Can lead to social embarrassment and the need for the more complicated frenuloplasty procedure outside the neonatal period

C. Background

1. There is much controversy surrounding ankyloglossia regarding.
   a. Definitions
      (1) Range from vague descriptions of a tongue that functions with a less than normal range of activity to specific description of a frenulum that is short, thick, muscular, or fibrotic (3) (Figs. 57.1 and 57.2)

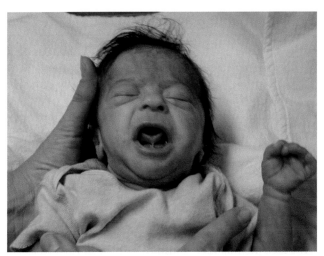

FIG. 57.1. Newborn with significant ankyloglossia. Note heart-shaped tongue, inability to raise tongue tip toward roof of mouth.

   (2) A range of methods to describe and quantify tongue tie have been proposed, including methods of measuring the anatomic differences and quantifying observations (2,14–17).

  b. Clinical significance (1,2,8,18,19)

   (1) Prior to the introduction and widespread use of breast milk substitutes in the early 20th century, breast-feeding was necessary for survival.

    (a) Release of tongue tie was commonly performed by the midwife at delivery (18,20).

    (b) Tongue tie does not generally pose a problem for the more passive process of bottle feeding.

    (c) With a decrease in breast-feeding rates, frenotomy became unnecessary for infant feeding.

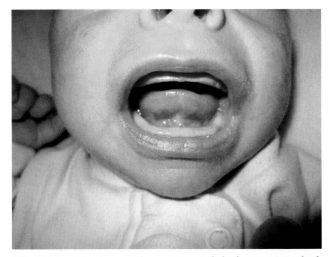

FIG. 57.2. Newborn with posterior Ankyloglossia. Note thick posterior fibrous band. (Photograph courtesy of Evelyn Jain, BA, BSc, MD, FCFP.)

   (2) With the current resurgence in breast-feeding and increasing knowledge of the risks of breast milk substitutes, tongue tie is again emerging as an entity that interferes with successful breast-feeding.

   (3) A recent article surveying >1,500 pediatricians, otolaryngologists, lactation consultants, and speech pathologists concluded that there is little consensus among and within these groups regarding the significance or management of ankyloglossia (21).

  c. Need for surgical intervention (2)

   (1) Some babies with tongue tie can breast-feed successfully with no surgical intervention (1,22).

   (2) Each breast-feeding dyad is a unique combination of many factors, including the infant's intraoral structures, adequacy of suckling, and the size, shape, and elasticity of maternal nipples.

   (3) An emerging body of literature suggests that, for those mother–baby dyads who are experiencing difficulty breast-feeding associated with the presence of tongue tie, frenotomy is a safe, effective, and immediate means of providing relief of symptoms and supporting breast-feeding (4,5, 18,19,22–28).

  d. *Timing of surgical intervention:* To facilitate breast-feeding, it can be performed in the first days of life, or anytime thereafter if problems emerge.

2. Incidence of tongue tie ranges from 0.02% to 4.8% in various studies (1,2,13,19,23,26,29).

  a. There appears to be a genetic predisposition in some families.

   (1) Frequently, when an infant presents for possible frenotomy, someone in the immediate family has a tongue tie.

  b. Most studies report an approximately 2:1 male predominance.

3. In a recent study, 22% of 425 North American pediatricians surveyed indicated they had performed frenotomies; however, only 10% reported being taught the technique during residency (21).

D. Indications

1. In the neonate, presence of ankyloglossia, usually in a breast-feeding infant, causing one or more of the following (4,5,13,22,23,27–30).

  a. Maternal nipple trauma, pain, nipple/breast infection

  b. Poor latch

  c. Ineffective suckling; continuous suckling

  d. Weight loss, poor infant weight gain, failure to thrive

  e. Early weaning

E. Contraindications

1. Presence of genioglossus muscle or vascular tissue in the frenulum, with no thin membranous tissue for incision

Refer to appropriate surgeon for consideration for frenuloplasty.

2. Known bleeding disorder (e.g., hemophilia)

Refer to otolaryngologist for repair in the operating room.

F. Limitations

1. If the difficulty with breast-feeding was not caused by the tongue tie, release of the tongue tie will not result in improvement.
2. Even when tongue tie is the cause, to ensure the best outcome attention must be paid to latch and suckling after release.

Postfrenotomy, it is not unusual for a period of suck training, by an appropriately trained lactation specialist, to be required to correct abnormal tongue movements. Follow-up with a trained lactation specialist is extremely important for breast-feeding success.

G. Equipment

Sterile

1. Iris scissors
2. Grooved retractor (optional—see below) (Fig. 57.3)
3. Gloves
4. Gauze pads
5. Topical anesthetic gel for oral use (optional—see below)
6. Cotton swab
7. Topical Neo-Synephrine, Gelfoam, or silver nitrate sticks (optional—see H, below)

Nonsterile

1. Blanket or towel for swaddling

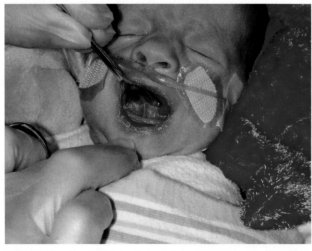

FIG. 57.3. Grooved retractor used to raise tongue and visualize the frenulum. Notice how thin and membranous the anterior edge is.

H. Precautions (Fig. 57.3)

1. Ensure, by careful examination of the frenulum, that there is no vascular or muscular tissue in the field of incision. Transillumination may be used to enhance visualization.
2. Avoid submandibular duct orifices lateral to the frenulum.
3. Avoid the thicker, most posterior, part of the frenulum, which carries the blood supply.

I. Technique (2,3,9,18,21,26,27) (Figs. 57.2 and 57.3)

1. Place the infant on a firm surface, or in caregiver's lap with head against caregiver's lower abdomen.
2. Firmly swaddle the infant in a blanket or towel (see Chapter 4).
3. Have an assistant standing at the head of the infant to stabilize the shoulders with their fingers while steadying the head with their palms, or have a caregiver do the same with the infant in their lap.
4. Stand on right side of infant if right-handed.
5. Visualize the frenulum by positioning light source to the left of the infant, allowing essentially transillumination of the frenulum.
6. Place two gloved fingers of the left hand below the tongue, on either side of the midline, or one gloved finger below the tongue to one side of midline, or position a grooved retractor (whichever you find most comfortable), to push the tongue up toward the roof of the mouth, exposing the frenulum (Fig. 57.3.). Inspect the frenulum for any vascular or muscular structures.
7. Frenotomy should be performed only if the frenulum is thin, transparent, and free of other structures.
8. Utilization of local anesthesia (optional)
   a. With no anesthesia, there is minimal, brief discomfort (8,13,18,21,26,30) because the frenulum is poorly innervated.

   Infants frequently squirm with positioning, but usually do not cry during procedure.
   b. Topical anesthetic gel can be applied to the frenulum with a cotton swab.
9. Divide the membranous frenulum with iris scissors (Fig. 57.4).

For Anterior Tongue Tie

a. Begin at the free border and proceed posteriorly, closer to the tongue than to the floor of the mouth.
b. In most cases, a single cut will free the tongue sufficiently.
c. Occasionally, 2 to 3 small, sequential cuts (1 to 3 mm) are required.
d. Each subsequent cut allows improved retraction and visualization for the next cut.

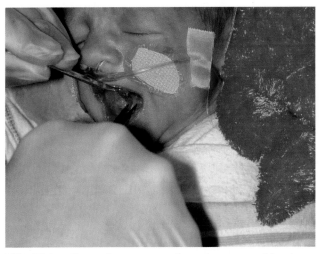

FIG. 57.4. Grooved retractor used to raise tongue. Iris scissors make incision.

e. Divide frenulum anterior to the vascular bundle, until the tongue is freed and can extend past lower alveolar ridge and lips and elevate to the roof of the mouth (equally important for breast-feeding) (Fig. 57.5).
f. Observe for posterior tongue tie, which may have been obscured by anterior tongue tie (Fig. 57.2). If present, the next step may be required.

For Posterior Tongue Tie (should be performed only by practitioners with experience in treating posterior tongue tie)

a. Visualize the sublingual area. A membranous small band may or may not be visible. (Fig. 57.2)
b. Diagnosis is made by palpation. With the index finger nail down push the midline posteriorly. A posterior tongue tie will feel like a vertical tight band under the mucous membrane.

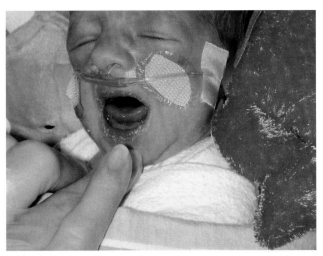

FIG. 57.5. After incision, minimal blood noted. Tongue now extends past lower alveolar ridge.

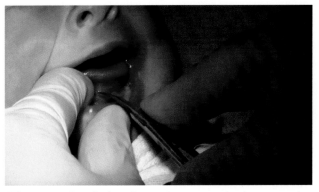

FIG. 57.6. Initial clip of posterior tongue tie, in very center. Note use of finger as an alternative to grooved retractor used in Figure 57.5. (Photograph courtesy of Evelyn Jain BA, BSc, MD, FCFP.)

c. Clip in center of band with iris scissors as narrowly as possible (Fig. 57.6), until diamond shape opens (Fig. 57.7).
d. Palpate edges of the "diamond." There can be taut edges laterally, which may need a clip of another millimeter until no longer taught and "diamond" is wide open (Fig. 57.8).
10. Control any bleeding (usually minimal) with direct pressure applied with a sterile gauze pad. There is generally more bleeding with posterior frenulum clipping. If excessive bleeding (more than 3 to 5 cc)
    a. Continue to apply pressure. Steps b, c, and d (below) are rarely required.
    b. Apply topical Neo-Synephrine (Afrin) as vasoconstrictor on cotton swab, *or*
    c. Apply small piece of Gelfoam *or*
    d. Dab with silver nitrate stick
11. Inform mother that breast-feeding may resume immediately.

Mothers frequently note an immediate and dramatic improvement in breast-feeding, with reduced

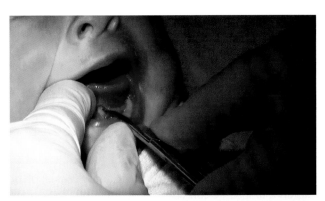

FIG. 57.7. A second, smaller, clip of posterior tongue tie to open the "diamond" and remove tautness laterally. (Photograph courtesy of Evelyn Jain BA, BSc, MD, FCFP.)

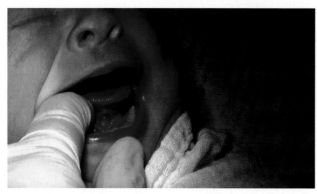

FIG. 57.8. Completed frenotomy of posterior tongue tie with open diamond evident. (Photograph courtesy of Evelyn Jain BA, BSc, MD, FCFP.)

discomfort, improved latch, stronger suckling, and absence of the clicking sounds frequently produced by the tongue-tied infant while breast-feeding (6,7,18,19,21–28).

If no improvement is noted, it is important to work with mother and baby in suck training and continue frequent re-evaluation.
12. Antibiotic therapy is not required.
13. Postoperatively, a white fibrin clot may form.

Reassure parents that this is not a sign of infection.
14. Arrange follow-up in 1 to 2 weeks to check healing of the incision.

J. Complications (2,6,13,18,19,24,26)

1. Extremely rare when performed by a practitioner familiar and comfortable with the procedure
   a. Excessive bleeding virtually never occurs unless deep lingual arteries and/or veins are severed.
   b. *Infection:* Extremely rare
   c. *Damage to tongue:* Extremely rare
   d. *Damage to submandibular ducts:* Extremely rare
   e. Recurrent ankyloglossia due to excessive scarring
      (1) Generally less severe than original presentation
      (2) Often amenable to revision surgery
   f. Glossoptosis (tongue swallowing) due to excessive tongue mobility
      Theoretical concern—has never been reported in modern literature.

Acknowledgement

Photographs and assistance with procedural information on posterior tongue tie courtesy of Evelyn Jain, BA, BSc, MD, FCFP, Clinical Assistant Professor, Department of Family Medicine, University of Calgary, Calgary, Alberta, Canada.

References

1. Hall DMB, Renfrew MJ. Tongue tie. *Arch Dis Child.* 2005; 90:1211.
2. Lalakea ML, Messner AH. Ankyloglossia: does it matter?. *Pediatr Clin North Am.* 2003;50:381.
3. Kupietzky A, Botzer E. Ankyloglossia in the infant and young child: clinical suggestions for diagnosis and management. *Pediatr Dent.* 2005;27:40.
4. Hong P, Lago D, Seargeant J, et al. Defining ankyloglossia: A case series of anterior and posterior tongue ties. *Int J Pediatr Otorhinolaryngol.* 2010;74:1003.
5. Chu MW, Bloom DC. Posterior Ankyloglossia: a case report. *Int J Pediatr Otorhinolaryngol.* 2009;73:881.
6. Hansen R, MacKinlay GA, Mansen WG. Ankyloglossia intervention in outpatients is safe: our experience [letter]. *Arch Dis Child.* 2006;91:541.
7. Naimer SA, Biton A, Vardy D, et al. Office treatment of congenital ankyloglossia. *Med Sci Monit.* 2003;9:CR432.
8. Wallace H, Clarke S. Tongue tie division in infants with breast-feeding difficulties. *Int J Pediatr Otorhinolaryngol.* 2006;70:1257.
9. Kummer AW. Ankyloglossia: to clip or not to clip? That's the question. *ASHA Leader.* 2005;10:30.
10. Lalakea ML, Messner AH. Ankyloglossia: the adolescent and adult perspective. *Otolaryngol Head Neck Surg.* 2003;128:746.
11. Lalakea ML, Messner AH. The effect of ankyloglossia on speech in children. *Otolaryngol Head Neck Surg.* 2002;127:539.
12. Marchesan IQ. Lingual frenulum: classification and speech interference. *Int J Orofacial Myol.* 2004;30:31.
13. Messner AH, Lalakea ML. Ankyloglossia: incidence and associated feeding difficulties. *Arch Otolaryngol Head Neck Surg.* 2000;126:36.
14. Hazelbaker AK. The assessment tool for lingual frenulum function. Master's thesis. Pasadena, CA: Pacific Oaks College; 1993.
15. Kotlow AL. Ankyloglossia (tongue-tie): a diagnostic and treatment quandary. *Quintessence Int.* 1999;30:259.
16. Williams WN, Waldron CM. Assessment of lingual function when ankyloglossia (tongue tie) is suspected. *J Am Dent Assoc.* 1985;110:353.
17. Ruffoli R, Giambelluca MA, Scavuzzo MC, et al. Ankyloglossia: a morphological investigation in children. *Oral Dis.* 2005;11:170.
18. Griffiths DM. Do tongue ties affect breastfeeding? *J Hum Lact.* 2004;20:409.
19. Wright JE. Tongue-tie. *J Paediatr Child Health.* 1995;31:276.
20. Horton CE, Crawford HH, Adamson JE, et al. Tongue-tie. *Cleft Palate J.* 1969;6:8.
21. Messner AH, Lalakea ML. Ankyloglossia: controversies in management. *Int J Pediatr Otorhinolaryngol.* 2000;54:123.
22. Hogan M, Westcott C, Griffiths M. Randomized, controlled trial of division of tongue tie in infants with feeding problems. *J Pediatr Child Health.* 2005;41:246.
23. Ricke LA, Baker NJ, Madlon-Kay DJ, et al. Newborn tongue tie: prevalence and effect on breast-feeding. *J Am Board Fam Pract.* 2005;18:1.
24. Marmet C, Shell E, Marmet R. Neonatal frenotomy may be necessary to correct breastfeeding problems. *J Hum Lact.* 1990;6:117.
25. Notestine G. The importance of the identification of ankyloglossia (short lingual frenulum) as a cause of breastfeeding problems. *J Hum Lact.* 1990;6:113.
26. Masaitis NS, Kaempf JW. Developing a frenotomy policy at one medical center: a case study approach. *J Hum Lact.* 1996;12:229.
27. Berry J, Griffiths M, Westcott C. A double-blind, randomized, controlled trial of tongue-tie division and its immediate effect on breastfeeding. *Breastfeed Med.* 2011 Oct 14. [Epub ahead of print],
28. Buryk M, Bloom D, Shope T. Efficacy of neonatal release of ankyloglossia: a randomized trial. *Pediatrics.* 2011;128:280.
29. Ballard JL, Auer CE, Khoury JC. Ankyloglossia: assessment, incidence, and effect of frenuloplasty on the breast-feeding dyad. *Pediatrics.* 2002;110:e63.
30. Amir LH, James PJ, Beatty J. Review of tongue-tie release at a tertiary maternity hospital. *J Pediatr Child Health.* 2005;41:243.

TABLE A.1	Neonatal Pain Scales

Scale	Assessment Parameters	Age Level (GA)	Pain Stimulus	Reliability Data	Scoring	Clinical Utility
Neonatal Infant Pain Scale (NIPS)	Behavioral	28–38 weeks	Procedural	Interrater reliability >0.92	0–7 with intervention suggested for pain scores ≥4	• Easy and fast to use
Neonatal Infant Pain, Agitation and Sedation Scale (NPASS)	Physiologic, Behavioral, Contextual	23–40 weeks	Acute, sedation, postoperative, ventilated	Interrater reliability >0.85	0–10 pain 0–10 sedation Intervention suggested for pain scores >3	• Combined pain and sedation scale • First neonatal combined pain and sedation scale; includes a premature pain assessment that adds to score based on GA
CRIES	Behavioral, Physiologic	32–60 weeks	Postoperative	Interrater reliability >0.72	0–10 with intervention suggested for pain score >4	• Easy to use
Premature Infant Pain Profile (PIPP)	Physiologic, Behavioral, Contextual	Term and pre-term neonates	Postoperative, Procedural	Inter- and intrarater reliability >0.93	Score ≥12 indicated moderate to severe pain	• Not fast to use • Scoring of infant occurs 15 seconds immediately before event and 30 seconds immediately after event • Modified PIPP scale has been developed for easier use. • Limited use in the intubated, paralyzed, and extremely premature neonate.
Scale for Use in the Newborn (SUN)	Behavioral, Physiologic	Term and pre-term neonates			0–28 Average baseline scores 10–14.	• Not an easy scale compared to NIPS
Neonatal Facial Coding System (NFCS)	Behavioral	25 weeks to term neonates	Procedural	Inter- and intrarater reliability >0.85		• Established as a scale to assess pain in newborns and infants
COVERS Neonatal Pain Scale	Physiologic, Behavioral	27–40 weeks	Designed to assess the needs of all infants in the NICU	Interrater reliability of >0.84 in preterm neonates and >0.95 in term neonates	0–18	• Cannot be used in paralyzed neonates. • Criteria used for scoring is applicable to a wider range of infants (e.g., visible crying in the intubated neonate as a behavioral response, looks at a change in need of oxygen).

| **TABLE A.2** | Sedative and Analgesic Agents Commonly Used in Pediatrics | | | | | |

Therapeutic Class	Medication	Mechanism of Action	Metabolism	Route of Administration (neonates)	Dose and Frequency	Reversal Agent	Comments
Nonopioid analgesic	Acetaminophen (paracetamol)	Inhibits peripheral pain impulse generation via serotonergic pathways.[a]	**Hepatic:** Cytochrome P450 (CYP) enzymes; sulfate and glucuronide metabolites CYP2E1, 1A2, 3A4 metabolize small amount to hepatotoxic NAPQI "detoxified" by glutathione conjugation.[b]	Oral, rectal, IV infusion 10-mg/mL. IV dose FDA labeled for >2 yr of age: 15 mg/kg q6h or 12.5 mg q4h *Limit: 75 mg/kg/d Infuse dose over 15 min.*	**GA 28–32 wk:** Oral: 10–12 mg/kg/dose q6–8h[c] **Rectal:** 20 mg/kg/dose q12h *Limit: 40 mg/kg/d* **GA 32–36 wk and term** ≤10 d: Oral: 10–15 mg/ kg/dose q6h. **Rectal:** 30 mg/kg then 15 mg/kg/ dose q8h *Limit: 60 mg/kg/d* **Term ≥10 d:** Oral: 10–15 mg/kg/dose q6h. **Rectal:** 30 mg/kg then 20 mg/kg/ dose q6–8h *Limit: 75 mg/kg/d*	None: GI decontamination/ acetylcysteine for toxicity	Inducers of CYP2E, 1A2, 3A4: (phenobarbital, phenytoin, rifampin) alter metabolism; ↑ hepatotoxicity Neonates: ↓ CYP activity; ↓ toxicity with ↑ serum concentrations. Additive analgesic effect with opioid. *Ineffective for acute procedural pain.* Rectal absorption slow and unreliable New IV form: OFIRMEV[d] 1,000 mg/100 mL AWP (USD) $12.90/vial[e] *Single-use vial Expiration 6 h*
Nonsteroidal antiinflammatory drugs (NSAIDs) Arylpropionic	Ibuprofen	Inhibition of cyclooxygenase enzyme and isoforms decreasing prostaglandin biosynthesis (PGI2) resulting in analgesia	**Hepatic:** Phase I and II enzyme biotransformation with urinary and biliary excretion. Metabolism primarily by CYP2C9 and CYP2C8. ↓ CYP2C9 activity in newborn, increasing over first year of life. Polymorphisms CYP2C9 may cause ADRs. Clearance ↑ after birth also affected by weight, age. $t_{1/2}$: 20–24 h (newborn) vs. 2 h (adults)	IV, Oral tablets, solutions	Oral: 4–10 mg q6–8h as needed *Limit: 40 mg/kg/d* IV: Ibuprofen lysine: 10 mg/kg then two doses: 5 mg/kg at 24 h and at 48 h "off label" for analgesia. *No data regarding use >3 d.*	None: Maintain hydration, avoid use of nephrotoxins. Discontinue anticoagulants, replace blood loss if needed, correct low platelets.	Oral solutions may contain benzoate— "*gasping syndrome*" in newborn. IV: No data for analgesic dosing for newborns IV ibuprofen lysine is labeled for PDA closure. *Limited data on use of ibuprofen analgesia for infants <3 mo of age; monitor urine output, renal function.* Calderol 400 mg/4 mL AWP (USD) $8.82/vial. *Not labeled for <17 yr of age.* IV ibuprofen.[f,g] **NSAID precautions:** Use lowest effective dose for shortest duration possible May displace bilirubin. Caution in asthma, renal or hepatic insufficiency, bleeding disorders, GI disease (bleeding or ulcers), and those patients receiving anticoagulants. Use of ≥1 NSAID not recommended. All NSAIDs have potential adverse cardiovascular effects. *High incidence of renal and GI side effects reported with use of ibuprofen to treat patent ductus arteriosus (PDA): NSAIDS not recommended for routine analgesic use in neonate.*

		Mechanism	Metabolism	Routes	Dosing	Antidote	Comments
Heteroaryl acetic acid NSAIDs:	Ketorolac	Inhibition of cyclooxygenase enzyme and isoforms decreasing prostaglandin biosynthesis (PGI2) resulting in analgesia	**Hepatic:** Phase I and II enzyme biotransformation with urinary and biliary excretion. Metabolism primarily by CYP2C9 and CYP2C8. ↓ CYP2C9 activity in newborn, increasing over first year of life.	IV, IM, Oral tablets,	**IV:** 0.5 mg/kg/dose q6-8h Infants >1 mo and children <2 y of age IM: Avoid — painful, erratic absorption	**None:** Maintain hydration, avoid use of nephrotoxins. Discontinue anticoagulants, replace blood loss if needed, correct low platelets.	No data for newborn on dosing for oral tablets or nasal spray. Not to exceed 48-72 h treatment Labeling for >2 y: Limit therapy to ≤5 d; ↑ adverse effects and no data.[h] Monitor: hematologic parameters (platelets, Hct, Hgb), clinical signs of bleeding, fluid status, BUN/Scr, urine output during therapy. **NSAID precautions as for ibuprofen.** *Not recommended for routine analgesic use in newborn.* Ophthalmic solution (Acular LS): ≥3 y of age for postop pain/inflammation nasal spray (Sprix)
Opioid Agonists (μμ) receptor	Morphine	Binds to Mu opiate receptors in CNS inhibiting ascending pain pathways; altering the perception of and response to pain; generalized CNS depression	**Hepatic:** Glucuronide conjugation to morphine-6-glucuronide (active) and morphine-3-glucuronide (inactive) Onset of action: 5 min (lower lipid solubility) Peak effect: 15 min Neonates: delayed maturation of CYP enzyme/conjugation resulting in a longer half-life, slower clearance, and longer elimination. Half-life: Preterm neonates: 10-20 h Neonates: 4.5-13.3 h	Oral, rectal, IM, intranasal, IV, SC, epidural	**IV:** 0.05-0.1 mg/kg/dose q1-4h **Continuous infusion:** 0.01-0.03 mg/kg/h **Intranasal:** 0.2 mg/kg/dose **Oral:** 0.3 mg/kg/dose q1-4h	**Naloxone:** Neonatal depression: 0.1 mg/kg/dose IV/IM/SC. May repeat q2-3 min minutes as needed Neonatal opiate intoxication: 0.1 mg/kg/dose IV	Use preservative free formulations (**PF**). *Neonates are more susceptible to respiratory depression (morphine-3-glucuronide—predominant metabolite in neonates).* Adult clearance values by 6 mo of age. Slower rates of dependence and withdrawal vs. fentanyl. May delay attainment of full enteral feeding in the preterm neonate. Long-term AE on neurologic system in preterm infants remains unclear. *Analgesic effect on acute pain in preterm neonates remains controversial.* Morphine considered safer than midazolam for neonates requiring sedation. *May require exceeding maximum dose in opioid tolerance with close monitoring.*
Semisynthetic opioid Mu opioid receptor agonists	Codeine	Binds to Mu opiate receptors in CNS inhibiting ascending pain pathways; altering the perception of and response to pain; generalized CNS depression; antitussive *Codeine has 1/10 of receptor affinity of morphine-"prodrug."*	**Hepatic:** Activation via CYP2D6 to morphine to morphine. Glucuronide conjugation to morphine-6-glucuronide (active) and morphine-3-glucuronide (inactive). *Ultra rapid metabolizers:* (≥2 copies CY2D6 alleles) risk opioid toxicity due to extensive conversion of codeine to morphine. 10% of dose eliminated in urine as parent drug Half-life: Neonates: 4.5 h Infants: 2.6 h	Oral, tablets, liquid, IM, SC injection Available with acetaminophen in elixir: 24 mg acetaminophen and 2.4 mg codeine per mL (refer to acetaminophen dosing for max limit for age)	0.5-1 mg/kg/dose q4-6h **IM:** Avoid — painful, erratic absorption. ***Do not administer IV; causes severe hypotension.***	**Naloxone:** Neonatal depression: 0.1 mg/kg/dose IV/IM/SC. May repeat q2-3 min as needed Neonatal opiate intoxication: 0.1 mg/kg/dose IV	**Analgesic effect dependent on conversion to morphine.** Codeine injection (not available in U.S., available in Canada): Codeine phosphate 15 mg; 30 mg/mL (may be given orally). *Contains sodium metabisulfite preservative* Highly constipating vs. morphine Consider possible impact of CYP2D6 polymorphisms.

(continued)

TABLE A.2 Sedative and Analgesic Agents Commonly Used in Pediatrics (*Continued*)

Therapeutic Class	Medication	Mechanism of Action	Metabolism	Route of Administration (neonates)	Dose and Frequency	Reversal Agent	Comments
Synthetic opioid agonists	Alfentanil	Binds with stereo-specific receptors at many sites within CNS, ↑s pain threshold, alters pain perception, inhibits ascending pain pathways	**Hepatic** Onset of action: <5 min Duration: <15–20 min	IV **IV Injection:** 500 mcg/mL preservative free (2 mg/5 mL vial)	10–20 mcg/kg for procedural analgesia	**Naloxone:** Neonatal depression: 0.1 mg/kg/dose. May repeat q2–3 min as needed Neonatal opiate intoxication: 0.1 mg/kg/dose IV	Chemical derivative of fentanyl—1/4 as potent as fentanyl Chest wall rigidity common in doses ≥20 mcg/kg. Administer slowly over 3–5 min. May produce more hypotension than fentanyl CYP3A4 polymorphisms may affect response to fentanyl, alfentanil, and sufentanil. Monitor for CYP3A4 drug interactions: e.g., inhibitors fluconazole, macrolide antibiotics. Consult reference/clinical pharmacist for updated information.
	Fentanyl	Binds with stereo-specific receptors at many sites within CNS, ↑s pain threshold, alters pain perception, inhibits ascending pain pathways	**Hepatic:** CYP3A4 oxidative N dealkylation to norfentanyl (>90%) and inactive metabolites. ↑ lipid solubility. Onset of action: 3 min Duration: 30 min Clearance 70% of adult values in term neonates, ↑s rapidly at birth.	Intranasal, IV	**IV:** Pain/sedation: 0.5–4 mcg/kg/dose slow IV q2–4h **Intranasal:** 1.5–2 mcg/kg/dose **Continuous IV:** 0.5–2 mcg/kg/h and titrate	**Naloxone:** Neuromuscular blocking agent (prevents chest wall rigidity)[i]	Rapid infusion of IV fentanyl can lead to chest wall rigidity.[i] Infuse slowly over 3–5 min. Less histamine release than morphine; more suitable for neonates with chronic lung disease (CLD) ↓s pulmonary vascular resistance—may be useful in persistent pulmonary hypertension (PPHN). Shows more rapid tolerance and withdrawal versus morphine (3–5 d fentanyl vs. 2 wk morphine).[i] Monitor for CYP3A4 drug interactions: e.g., inhibitors fluconazole, macrolide antibiotics. Consult reference/clinical pharmacist for updated information.
	Methadone	Binds to opiate receptors in CNS. These mu-receptors inhibit ascending pain pathways, which alter pain perception and response to pain. Causes generalized CNS depression. Desensitizes δ-opioid receptors, antagonizes NMDA receptors involved in pain sensitization.[k]	**Hepatic:** CYP3A4/CYP2D6 N-demethylated to an active metabolites Onset of action: 20 min IV, 30–60 min Oral (slow) Prolonged elimination halfLife (15–55 h) Half-life: ↑ variability when used for analgesia in neonates: (3.8–62 h)[k]	Oral (liquid, tablets), IV, IM, SC	Neonatal abstinence syndrome: 0.05–0.2 mg/kg/dose q12–24h	**Naloxone** Neonatal depression: 0.1 mg/kg/dose IV/IM/SC May repeat q2–3 min as needed Neonatal opiate intoxication: 0.1 mg/kg/dose IV	Difficult to titrate doses due to prolonged halfLife. *Oral solutions may contain propylene glycol or benzyl alcohol "gasping syndrome" in neonates.* Some references consider equipotent with morphine. Varies with age, disease state, and previous opioid exposure. Use caution as incomplete cross-tolerance has occurred with methadone and other opioids. Long-term effects of NMDA-receptor antagonism in the neonate is unknown. High oral bioavailability, low cost, minimal SE once optimal dose is achieved. Many drug interactions with CYP3A4, CYP2D6 substrates in the NICU (fluconazole, zidovudine, macrolides, phenobarbital, etc). Consult updated drug interaction databases.

Class	Drug	Action	Metabolism	Route	Dose	Antidote	Comments
α-adrenergic agonist analgesics	Clonidine	Stimulates alpha-2-adrenoreceptors in locus ceruleus, ↓s presynaptic calcium, inhibits NE release from sympathetic nerve endings reducing sympathetic outflow. (Useful in managing opioid withdrawal—activates K⁺ channel via G inhibitory protein as opioids.)	**Hepatic:** Primarily hydroxylation, via CYP2D6. **Onset of action:** Oral: 30–60 min IV	Oral, IV	**Oral:** 1 mcg/kg/dose q4–6h Maximum: 6 mcg/kg/dose **IV infusion:** 0.5 mcg/kg/h increasing to maximum: 3 mcg/kg/h	**None:** Discontinue Infusion/dose, Support respiration, cardiac function, Correct BP	Attenuates adrenergic hyperactivity; somatic and autonomic signs of withdrawal. Consider as adjunct for infants with persistent and severe signs of withdrawal (i.e., long-term continuous opioid/benzodiazepine IV infusions). *Hold doses for SBP <50 mm Hg or HR <100 bpm.* *Do not confuse with clonazepam (Klonopin).* Has been used for treating opioid induced myoclonus in neonates.
	Dexmedetomidine	Hypnotic, analgesic, sympatholytic. ↓ sympathetic response to pain; Selectively stimulates dorsal horn of spinal cord α_2-adrenergic receptors; produces sedation via α_1-effects in locus ceruleus, preserving spontaneous ventilation. ↑ intraoperative hemodynamic stability.	**Hepatic:** Primarily by CYP2A6 then N-glucuronidation and N-methylation. Clearance in newborn ≈30% of adult, ↑ to adults rates by 12 months of age.[l]	IV, IM (preservative-free solution) 100 mcg/mL (2 mL)	**IV:** 1 mcg/kg initial then 0.5 mcg/kg[l]	Most adverse effects respond to: DC infusion or ↓ rate. Treat bradycardia: atropine; hypotension; ↑ IVF or start vasopressor. Hypertension during load dose: ↓ rate.	Additive analgesic effect with ketamine, fentanyl. Sevoflurane for surgical procedures. Control of withdrawal with prolonged opioid use. Sedation during mechanical ventilation. Monitor pain scores; may cause significant ↓ body temperature[l] Avoid abrupt discontinuation—rapid awakening, anxiety, "fighting" ventilator, and withdrawal. ↓ dose in hepatic insufficiency Not labeled for use for <18 y
General anesthetics	Ketamine	Direct action on cortex and limbic system to produce dissociative anaesthesia. Blocks D-2 dopamine receptor. Noncompetitive agonist of NMDA. No effect on pharyngeal or laryngeal reflexes.[m]	**Hepatic:** N-dealkylation hydroxylation, glucuronide conjugation, dehydration of hydroxylated metabolites	IV	**IV:** 0.5–2 mg/kg Induction dose: 1–2 mg/kg **Continuous IV infusion** (sedation): 5–20 mcg/kg/min Titrate to desired level.[m]	**None** Discontinue infusion, Support respiration, cardiac function, Emergence reactions (pediatrics < adults)[m]	Provides sedation, analgesia, amnesia. Caution in GERD: ↑ vomiting, will ↑ICP, not adequate as sole anesthetic for surgical procedures of pharynx, larynx, bronchial tree or visceral pain pathways. Premedicate with IV atropine dose secondary to increased production of upper respiratory and salivary secretions. **Limited neonatal use due to potential ↑ ICP and neurotoxicity.**[m] Long-term effects are unknown Potential neuroprotective effects in animal models. Sedation in mechanically ventilated neonates, especially during suctioning,

(continued)

TABLE A.2 Sedative and Analgesic Agents Commonly Used in Pediatrics (*Continued*)

Therapeutic Class	Medication	Mechanism of Action	Metabolism	Route of Administration (neonates)	Dose and Frequency	Reversal Agent	Comments
	Propofol	Alkylphenol sedative–hypnotic. Increases responsiveness of GABA receptor to GABA, potentiating glycine activity (mediates response to noxious stimuli).	**Hepatic:** Extensive metabolism via CYP, with glucuronide and sulfate conjugation.	IV	IV: 200–300 mcg/kg/min initial dose.[n] Usual dose range[n]: 125–150 mcg/kg/min **Effective, safe dose range for neonates needs further study.**	None Discontinue infusion, Support respiration, cardiac function, correct acid-base status.	Advantages: Rapid onset, short $t_{1/2}$. SE: Pain at injection site, hypotension, apnea. Generics: Contain benzyl alcohol, sodium benzoate. **No analgesic properties/ assess sedative effect.** ↓ doses required when used with opioids.[n] Monitor lipids, metabolic status during infusion.
Benzodiazepines	Diazepam	Binds to GABA receptors in CNS decreasing excitability of neuronal cells	**Hepatic:** CYP P450 oxidation and demethylation to active metabolites (oxazepam). **Half-life:** Diazepam Infants (40–50 h) Neonates (50–100 h)	IV, Oral	IV: 0.1–0.3 mg/kg dose over 3–5 min, maximum total dose of 2 mg. Oral: 0.2–1 mg/kg q6–8h for NAS	Flumazenil 0.01 mg/kg IV (total dose 0.05 mg/kg)	Not first-line IV due to: benzoic acid, benzyl alcohol, sodium benzoate. Extravasation may cause necrosis. **Complications of: all benzodiazepines: myoclonic jerking, excessive sedation, respiratory depression.**
	Lorazepam	Binds to GABA receptors in CNS decreasing excitability of neuronal cells	**Hepatic:** Glucuronide conjugation to inactive metabolite: *lorazepam glucuronide*	IV, Oral	IV/Oral: 0.05–0.1 mg/kg q4–8h as needed. **IV continuous infusion:** 0.05–0.1 mg/kg/h Dilute with sterile water 1:1 prior to infusion	Flumazenil 0.01 mg/kg IV (total dose 0.05 mg/kg)	Risk of withdrawal (irritability, agitation, tremors, sleep problems) after long-term sedation with IV benzodiazepines. Slower BBB penetration vs. diazepam. Caution: Monitor for propylene glycol toxicity with continuous infusion. Oral solutions contain propylene glycol +/– benzyl alcohol ("gasping syndrome") ↓ dose for hepatic dysfunction. Incompatible with TPN
	Midazolam	Binds to GABA receptors in CNS decreasing excitability of neuronal cells	**Hepatic:** CYP-P450 hydroxylation followed by glucuronide conjugation, highly protein bound **Rapid onset:** 1–5 min IV <5 min intranasal **Peak sedative action:** <20 min	IV, Oral, intranasal	**IV (slow):** 0.05–0.15 mg/kg/dose **Intranasal:** 0.1–0.3 mg/kg/dose **Oral:** 0.15–0.45 mg/kg/dose **Continuous infusion:** 0.03–0.06 mg/kg/h = 0.5–1 mcg/kg/min	Flumazenil 0.01 mg/kg IV (total dose 0.05 mg/kg)	**No analgesic effect.** Anxiolytic, sedative, muscle relaxant, anticonvulsant **Not recommended for continuous intravenous infusion in neonates.** Caution in hepatic impairment. Monitor for hypotension, respiratory depression, and seizure-like activity. Decreases cerebral blood flow velocities Decrease dose in neonates with decreased cardiac output.

Agent	Mechanism	Metabolism	Route/Dose	Adverse effects	Comments
					More data needed to address safety and efficacy of midazolam in neonates. **Insufficient evidence to promote routine use of midazolam as sedative for neonates.[o]** Reports of serious neurologic and hemodynamic effects. Reports on effects of negative cerebral artery blood flow. Midazolam induces apoptosis and is concentration dependent via activation of mitochondrial pathway in neonatal animal models.
Sucrose analgesia — Oral sucrose solution	Activation of endogenous opioid system through taste[o]	**Carbohydrate Metabolism:** Undergoes gastric hydrolysis, utilized as a carbohydrate (3.94 kcal/g)	Oral	**None** Adverse effects ≤1.5%: Choking, spitting-up, vomiting after dose	Use 12%–24% sucrose or glucose 20%–30%. Administer 1–2 min prior to procedure. Concentrated preparations are hyperosmolar (up to 1000 mOsm/L). *Use with caution especially in preterm neonates.* Long-term safety and neurodevelopmental outcomes of repeated oral sucrose administration is not known. Coadministration of sucrose with non-nutritive sucking may be additive/synergistic. Place on tip of tongue (location of opioid receptors). Reduces pain during venipunctures/heelsticks Consider limiting total daily doses to <10 in term infants, safe number of doses unknown, especially in preterms. Tolerance may develop with repeated doses. Use in neonates of opioid-dependent mothers is controversial.
Topical anesthetics — Lidocaine 1 mg with epinephrine	Blocks initiation and conduction of nerve impulses via ↓ sodium permeability	**Hepatic/dermal:** CYP-450 and small amount of dermal metabolism to Monoethylglycinexylidide	**Subcutaneous (SC)** SC 2–5 mg/kg SC	**None** Mild swelling, bruising, and bleeding at site of injection. Systemic toxicity in neonate after inadvertent lidocaine intravascular injection during Dorsal Penile NerveBlock.[q]	Available with epinephrine (vasoconstrictor) for select procedures (e.g., suture).[p] *Examine labels closely—avoid error.* Consider adding sodium bicarbonate to buffer to ↓ pain or warming vial prior to injection to body temperature. Use SC (without EPI) for ring or nerve blocks.

(continued)

TABLE A.2	Sedative and Analgesic Agents Commonly Used in Pediatrics (Continued)

Therapeutic Class	Medication	Mechanism of Action	Metabolism	Route of Administration (neonates)	Dose and Frequency	Reversal Agent	Comments
	Lidocaine 4% liposomal cream	Blocks initiation and conduction of nerve impulses via ↓ sodium permeability	Hepatic/dermal: CYP-450 and small amount of dermal metabolism to Monoethyl-glycinexylidide	Topical	Topical:	Local skin reactions	Use in term infants for short term procedures. *Avoid use in premature infants: contains benzyl alcohol.* Avoid prolonged contact.[p]
	Lidocaine 2.5%/prilocaine 2.5% eutectic mixture cream	Blocks initiation and conduction of nerve impulses via ↓ sodium permeability	Hepatic/dermal: CYP-450 and small amount of dermal metabolism to Monoethyl-glycinexylidide	Topical	Topical 0.5–2 g under occlusive dressing 1 hr prior to procedure 2 g = Term infants 0.5 g = Preterm *Avoid applying over larger areas and for >2 h duration*	Local skin reactions Methemoglobinemia	Methemoglobinemia prolonged contact/large amounts in young infants/children.[q] Drugs predisposing to methemoglobinemia include: Sulfas, acetaminophen, benzocaine, nitrofurantoin, nitroglycerin, phenobarbital, phenytoin Has been used safely in preterms in small amounts once daily. Do not apply near or in open wounds. Do use in severe hepatic disease. Use with caution in infants receiving class I antiarrhythmics.

[a]Anderson BJ. Paracetamol (acetaminophen): mechanisms of action. *Paediatr Anaesth.* 2008;18(10):915.

[b]Section on Clinical Pharmacology and Therapeutics; Committee on Drugs, Sullivan JE, Farrar HC. Fever and antipyretic use in children. *Pediatrics.* 2011;127(3):580.

[c]van Lingen RA, Deinum JT, Quak JM, et al. Pharmacokinetics and metabolism of rectally administered paracetamol in preterm neonates. *Arch Dis Child Fetal Neonatal Ed.* 1991;80(1)F59.

[d]Ofirmev (acetaminophen). Injection package labeling. San Diego, CA: Cadence Pharmaceuticals, Inc.; 2010.

[e]Reuters T. *Red Book: Pharmacy's Fundamental Reference.* Los Angeles, CA: PDR Network; 2011.

[f]Taketomo CK, Hodding JH, Kraus DM. Pediatric Dosage Handbook. 18th ed. Hudson, OH: Lexi-Comp; 2011.

[g]Caldolor (ibuprofen). Injection package labeling. Nashville, TN: Cumberland Pharmaceuticals Inc.: 2009.

[h]Lei-Lai M, Kauffman R, Uy H, et al. A randomized comparison of ketorolac tromethamine to morphine for postoperative analgesia in critically ill children. *Crit Care Med.* 1999;27:2786.

[i]Fahnenstich H, Steffan J, Kau N, et al. Fentanyl-induced chest wall rigidity and laryngospasm in preterm and term infants. *Crit Care Med.* 2000;28:836.

[j]Arnold JH, Truog RD, Orav EJ, et al. Tolerance and dependence in neonates sedated with fentanyl during extracorporeal membrane oxygenation. *Anesthesiology.* 1990;73:1136.

[k]Chana SK, Anand KJS. Can we use methadone for analgesia in preterm infants? *Arch Dis Child Fetal Neonatal Ed.* 2001;85:F79.

[l]Ozcengiz D, Gunes Y, Atci M. Preliminary experience with dexmedetomidine in neonatal anesthesia. *J Anesthesa Clin Pharmacol.* 2011;27(1):17.

[m]Bhutta AT. Ketamine: a controversial drug for neonates. *Semin Perinatol.* 2007;31:303.

[n]Shah PS, Shah VS. Propofol for procedural sedation/anaesthesia in neonates. *Cochrane Database Syst Rev.* 2011;(3):CD007248.

[o]Anand KJ, Barton BA, McIntosh N, et al Analgesia and sedation in preterm infants who require ventilator support: results from the NOPAIN trial. *Arch Pediatr Adolesc Med.* 1999;153:331.

[p]Tutag Lehr V, Taddio A. Practical approach to topical anesthetics in the neonate. *Semin Perinatol.* 2007;(5):323.

[q]Guay J. Methemoglobinemia related to local anesthetics; a summary of 242 episodes. *Anesth Analg.* 2009;108:837.

TABLE B.1	Neonatal Surgical Tray

Quantity	Manufacturer	Catalog	Instrument Name
			Forceps
2	Aesculap	OC020R	Iris Forceps Straight 4″
2	Aesculap	OC022R	Iris Forceps Curved Serrated 4″
2	Aesculap	BD511R	Adson Forceps with teeth 4¾″
2	Aesculap	FB400R	DeBakey Forceps 2 mm × 6″
			Clamps
2	Aesculap	BH104R	Hartmann Mosquito Clamp Straight 4″
2	Aesculap	BH105R	Mosquito Clamp Curved 4″
2	Aesculap	BH110R	Halstead Mosquito Clamp Straight 5″
2	Aesculap	BH111R	Halstead Mosquito Clamp Curved 5″
			Needle Holders
1	Aesculap	BM204R	Derf Needle Holder
1	Aesculap	BM218R	Crile Wood Needle Holder 6″
			Scissors
1	Aesculap	BC210R	Iris Scissors Straight 4³/₈″
1	Aesculap	BC252R	Mayo Scissors Straight 6¾″
1	PW	35-2109	DeMartel Vascular Scissors 7¾″
			Retractors
1	Aesculap	BV010R	Alm Retractor 2¾″
1	Aesculap	BV011R	Alm Retractor 4″
2	Aesculap	OA338R	Blair Retractor Sharp 4-prongs × 5¾″
			Miscellaneous
4	Aesculap	BF431R	Towel Clip Small
1	Aesculap	MB603R	Eye Probe 5″
1	Aesculap	US063	Metal Iodine Cup 6 oz.
12	Kendall	9132	Sponge Gauze 2″ × 2″
12	Kendall	9024	Sponge Gauze 4″ × 4″
6	MediAction	706-B	OR Blue Towel
			Add to Tray after Sterilization
1	BD Eclipse	305780	BD Eclipse Needle 1 mL 25-gauge × 5/8″
2	BD Eclipse	305062	Syringe Luer-Lok 5 mL BD Needle 18-gauage × 1.5″
1	BD Eclipse	371615	Disposable Scalpel Blade #15
1	BD Eclipse	371611	Disposable Scalpel Blade #11
1	Misc	0607	Connector Tubing Plastic 5 in 1
3	Misc	0610	Rubber Band # 16
1	Cardinal	U11 T	Umbilical Tape
1	Cardinal	683G	Black Silk Suture 4-0
1	Cardinal	682	Black Silk Suture 5-0

NB. These are the contents of the Neonatal Surgical Tray used at Georgetown University Hospital, Washington, DC. Descriptors are given for ordering but are subject to individual preference. Disposable, single-use, or plastic instruments from commercially prepared trays are suitable for many procedures.

TABLE B.2	Selected Sutures Appropriate for Common Neonatal Procedures			
Type	**Raw Material**	**Tissue Use**	**Advantages**	**Disadvantages**
Vicryl or Dexon	Synthetic copolymers	Subcutaneous Fascia	Mild tissue reaction (2+) Low infectivity rate For absorbable suture or ligature Maintain knots	Cannot be used for approximation under stress 60% strength at 2 wk Safety in cardiovascular tissue not established Requires flat and square ties with extra throws
Silk	Braided protein filament from silk worm	Skin Fascia	Best knot holding Easiest to use Strong for size	High infectivity rate High tissue reaction
Nylon	Polyamide polymer Mono- or braided filament	Monofilament: skin closure and plastic surgery Braided: any tissue	Inert Least tissue reaction Lowest infectivity	Poor knot holding, requires at least six ties Not as easy to handle
Prolene	Polymer of propylene Monofilament	Skin Pull-out subcuticular	Inert Low tissue reaction (0–1+) Low infectivity Very strong for size Holds knot better than nylon	Remains encapsulated
Skin closure tape	Reinforced nylon filaments to back or porous paper tape	Skin superficial laceration or when subcuticular suture also used	Easy to place and remove Quick to apply No skin reactivity Least scarring No anesthetic required	Will not stick to wet or oily skin (wipe skin with alcohol first) Will not hold if wound is widely separated or under tension Cannot evert wound edges

TABLE C.1 Blood Products

Whole Blood Products

Product	Shelf Life	Advantages	Disadvantages	Comments
A. Whole blood Hct ~40%	CPD = 21 d Heparin = 24 – 48 h CPDA-1 = 35 d Additive solution (AS) = 42 d	1. Provides volume 2. Provides RBCs 3. Provides some coagulation factors	1. WBC, and platelets relatively nonfunctional unless fresh and unrefrigerated 2. Storage lesion defects (K^+) in plasma fraction	1. Used for exchange transfusion 2. PRBCs and FFP preferable for correction of massive blood loss 3. Heparinized blood not licensed for use in USA, but used in other countries
B. Reconstituted whole blood Hct variable	24 h	1. Allows preparation of whole blood from stored RBCs (packed or frozen) and FFP 2. Allows preparation of Group O cells with low-titer A and B antibody plasma	1. Time for preparation	1. Use for exchange transfusion 2. Hematocrit may be adjusted by formula 3. Provides replacement equivalent of fresh whole blood Formula for reconstitution: volume of plasma to add = volume PRBCs × (Hct PRBCs/Hct desired – 1).
D. Autologous fetal blood	1. Fresh heparinized <4 h 2. CPD = 21 d 3. CPDA = 35 d 4. AS = 42 d	1. Potential immediate availability in delivery room or from blood bank	1. Risk of bacterial contamination 2. Difficult to obtain correct anticoagulant blood ratio 3. Requires anticipatory preparation for best procedural control 4. Complicated procedure to perform in DR and maintain sterility	1. Information on advantages of autologous blood is limited 2. Properly prepared and tested banked blood a better choice if time permits 3. Developing countries exploring use 4. Competition for umbilical cord banking 5. Consider delaying cord clamping as alternative

Red Cell Products

Products	Volume (mL)	Shelf Life	Advantages	Disadvantages	Comments
A. PRBCs Hct 70%–75% in CPDA-1 Hct 55%–60% in additive solutions (AS)	1. CPDA-1 = 250 2. AS = 350	1. CPDA-1 = 35 d 2. AS = 42 d	1. Readily available 2. Easy to prepare	1. Accentuated storage lesion defects if unit is at end of shelf life 2. Less RBC mass/mL of transfused product, if PRBCs in additive solutions are used	1. Principal use for correction of anemia 2. With sterile connecting device, can remove aliquots for transfusion 3. If only AS products available, hard pack for massive transfusion or for exchange transfusion

(continued)

TABLE C.1 Blood Products (*Continued*)

Red Cell Products

Products	Volume (mL)	Shelf Life	Advantages	Disadvantages	Comments
B. Sedimented RBCs Hct 65%–80% (variable)	variable	As above	1. Does not require centrifugation 2. Contains less plasma than standard RBC units	1. Hct may not be as high as desired	An alternative to hard-packing without centrifugation
C. Quad pack collection Hct 55%–75%	Mother unit = 250–350 Each satellite unit ≤150	1. CPD = 21 d 2. CPDA-1 = 35 d 3. AS = 42 d	1. Allows multiple transfusions to one infant 2. Volume of each quad adjustable	1. Outdate rates high unless NICU has number of infants 2. Some wastage expected	Many neonatal units find this collection system valuable if they do not have sterile connecting equipment available.
D. Leukodepleted RBCs	1. CPDA-1 = 250 2. AS = 350	Depends on anticoagulant-Preservative solution as above	1. WBC count <1–5 × 10^6/product 2. Reduces risk of transmission of CMV	1. Prestorage LD preferred over bedside filters 2. Cannot LD a unit from sickle-trait donor 3. Leukodepletion failures occur	1. Indicated for prevention of febrile transfusion reactions and for leukocyte alloimmunization in older children, but these phenomena are rare in neonates 2. Does not prevent TA-GVHD
E. Washed RBCs	200	24 h	1. Removes 80% WBCs 2. Removes platelets, K, anticoagulant 3. Hct adjustable—less viscosity	1. Time required for preparation 2. Equipment not always available 3. Expires 24 h after washing as "open" system	1. Can wash portions of quad pack 2. May be combined with FFP for exchange transfusions. 3. Major indications include patients with hyperkalemia and T activation
E. Irradiated PRBCs	1. CPDA-1 = 250 2. AS = 350	Depends on anticoagulant preservative solution	1. Abrogates GVHD in susceptible infants	1. Storage limited to 28 d postirradiation or by original expiration date due to K^+ leak 2. Equipment not always available	1. Irradiation before issue preferable to long-term refrigerator storage postirradiation
F. Frozen deglycerolized RBCs	200	Frozen up to 10 yr After thawing/deglycerolizing 24 h	1. Maintenance of 2, 3-DPG and ATP 2. Removes >80% WBCs	1. Higher cost than other preparations 2. Equipment not always available 3. Expires 24 h after washing	1. RBCs frozen with glycerol, thawed, and deglycerolized by washing prior to transfusion, resuspended in 0.9% NaCl 2. Allows storage of rare types of blood

TABLE C.1 Blood Products (*Continued*)

Platelet Products

Products	Volume (mL)	Shelf Life	Advantages	Disadvantages	Comments
A. Platelet concentrate (random donor platelets)	45–60	5 d	Approximately 5.5×10^{10} platelets in 45–60 mL plasma	1. Contains some WBCs, few RBCs, and plasma 2. Rh D immunization possible	1. Use immediately on receipt from blood bank and never refrigerate 2. May be leukocyte-reduced but need 2–3 U. pool for efficient LD 3. Volume may be reduced by centrifugation for use when out of group or extreme volume restriction is necessary; changes expiration to 4 h
B. Single-donor apheresis platelets	250–300	5 d	1. $>3 \times 10^{11}$ platelets in 250–300 mL of plasma 2. Always LD with current collection equipment 3. If used over 5 d, can reduce donor exposures. 4. Repeated pheresis from some donor possible	1. Large volume; needs to be split or aliquoted into EUs.	1. Allows selection of HLA- and HPA-compatible donors 2. 1 EU = 5.5×10^{10} platelets 3. Std dose = 1 EU/5–10 kg with minimum dose of one EU (volume reduction may be necessary for ELBW infants)

Plasma Products

Products	Volume (mL)	Shelf Life	Advantages	Disadvantages	Comments
A. FFP	180–300	Frozen (–18 °C) = 1 yr Thawed = 24 h	1. Contains plasma proteins, coagulation factors, anticoagulant proteins, complement, and albumin	1. 20–45 min thawing time 2. Not for volume expansion or fibrinogen replacement	1. Separated from WB within 6–8 h collection 2. Must be ABO-compatible 3. Use blood filter 4. Confused with F24, now more commonly available
B. Cryoprecipitate	10–25	Frozen (–18 °C) = 1 yr Thawed = 4 h	1. Better source of fibrinogen and VWF than plasma products	1. Limited indications include F XIII and congenital/acquired fibrinogen deficiency	1. Must be ABO-compatible 2. Use blood filter 3. Transfuse immediately after thaw 4. Dose = 1 U/5–10 kg but small volume confusing
C. Albumin	5%	3 yr at room temperature	1. Heat-treated to reduce risk of infectious diseases 2. Requires no cross-match 3. Increases plasma oncotic pressure	1. Expense 2. Does not provide coagulation factors	1. Five micron filter required 2. Na 145 mEq/L 3. Osmolarity 300 MOs m/L
D. Albumin	25%	3 yr at room temperature	1. Requires no cross-match 2. Increases plasma oncotic pressure with low volume	1. Expense 2. Does not provide coagulation factors 3. Can produce pulmonary edema, and cardiac failure	1. Five micron filter required 2. Na 130–160 3. Osmolarity 1,500 MOs m/L

(continued)

TABLE C.1   Blood Products (*Continued*)

Plasma Products

Products	Volume (mL)	Shelf Life	Advantages	Disadvantages	Comments
E. Plasma frozen within 24 h (F24)	180–300	1 yr if frozen; 1–5 d postthawing	1. Contains plasma proteins, coagulation factors, anticoagulant proteins, complement, and albumin	1. May be less effective for FV, FVIII, and VWF replacement 2. Not indicated for volume expansion/fibrinogen replacement	1. Separated from WB and frozen with 24 h 2. Most commonly available from blood suppliers
F. Single source plasma	180–300		1. Contains plasma proteins, coagulation factors, anticoagulant proteins, complement, and albumin		1. From single-donor plasmapheresis 2. Can be aliquoted into small volumes and frozen for neonatal use
G. Recovered plasma	180–300		1. Contains plasma proteins, coagulation factors, anticoagulant proteins, complement, and albumin	1. May be less effective for FV, FVIII, and VWF replacement 2. Not indicated for volume expansion/fibrinogen replacement	1. Plasma recovered from WB without specialized time limit. 2. Quality of factors/anticoagulant proteins not well studied

Elective Change of Orotracheal Tube in Intubated Patient

This procedure allows continued ventilation through a pre-established airway whenever it is necessary to change an endotracheal (ET) tube or to place a nasotracheal tube. By maintaining the original airway as long as possible during the change, there is less need for haste and less stress to the patient. An obvious prerequisite is that the original ET tube be patent and correctly positioned in the trachea.

Rapid Replacement Method

1. Prepare equipment and patient as for initial orotracheal intubation.
2. Release tube fixation device without displacing tube.
3. Have assistant hold first ET tube in place at far left of the infant's mouth while continuing to ventilate infant.
4. Visualize glottis with laryngoscope.
5. Pass second orotracheal tube down far right of the mouth until it aligns with glottic opening.
6. When new tube is positioned for direct insertion, have assistant withdraw first tube carefully.
7. Advance new tube into position.
8. Verify position and secure tube as previously described.

Alternative Method: Insertion Over a Feeding Tube

Because of the narrow diameter of ET tubes in small infants, feeding tubes narrow enough to fit inside the ET lumen are often too flexible to stay within the trachea as the tubes are being changed. Be prepared to intubate directly should the feeding tube dislodge.

1. Prepare equipment and patient as for initial orotracheal intubation.
2. Release tube fixation device without displacing tube.
3. Select the largest feeding tube that will easily go through the current and new endotracheal tubes. Remove the flared end of feeding tube and the adaptor on the new tube.
4. Remove adaptor of currently in-place ET tube.
5. Quickly insert the feeding tube through the lumen to a depth not greater than the ET tube.

6. While holding feeding tube in place, pull ET tube out of trachea and off feeding tube.
7. Slide new ET tube over feeding tube into trachea.
8. Replace tube adaptor.
9. Verify position and secure tube as previously described.

Selective Left Endobronchial Intubation

The angles of the bronchi are such that more often than not a tube will seek the right mainstem bronchus. The exceptions will be conditions that push the left side down (left upper-lobe emphysema) or that pull the right side up (marked upper-lobe atelectasis or hypoplasia). Normally, successful right mainstem intubation simply requires a longer tube. Selective intubation of the left bronchus is a more difficult and dangerous procedure; therefore, following all precautions is especially important.

Place the ET tube under guidance by direct bronchoscopy or under fluoroscopy when these procedures are available without compromise to infants (1,2).

The following procedure is a simple, indirect method based on a modification that tends to make the ET tube bend toward the left when it meets resistance at the carina (3).

1. Cut an elliptical hole through half the diameter of ET tube 1 cm in length and 0.5 cm above the tip of the oblique distal end.
2. Perform an orotracheal intubation as above, keeping the cut hole directed toward the left lung.
3. Turn infant's head toward the right (4).
4. While auscultating the lung fields, advance the tube to 0.5 to 1 cm below the calculated depth of the carina or until differential breath sounds are heard.
5. If breath sounds diminish on the left, withdraw the ET tube until they return.
6. Take a chest radiograph to confirm left bronchial position.
7. Fix tube securely.
8. Reassess position frequently, as tube may dislodge from one mainstem into the other.
9. Follow patient closely for particular complications of
   a. Air leak of ventilated area
   b. Stasis pneumonia of nonventilated area

c. Dislodgement from left mainstem bronchus
d. Ventilatory insufficiency due to significant disease in the only lung being ventilated

Nonvisualized Oral Intubation

This technique has a higher risk of complications and is less often successful than when direct visualization is used. Reserve the blind oral intubation for true emergencies in small infants when there is equipment failure (e.g., laryngoscope light) and when ventilation by mask is contraindicated (e.g., thick meconium).

1. Stand at infant's feet.
2. Carefully slide first two fingers of gloved, left hand into back of oropharynx at the base of tongue, until reaching vallecula and epiglottis. Keep fingers in the center of the tongue.
3. Using index finger, pull epiglottis forward.
4. Keep infant's head in midline.
5. With right hand, guide ET tube, without stylet, along left middle finger, which is held just above index finger.
6. Advance tube carefully just beyond fingertips.
7. Avoid pushing against any obstruction.
8. If available, have assistant press gently on trachea in suprasternal notch and report when tube passes under finger.
9. Verify position, and fix tube as previously described.

Blind Nasotracheal Intubation (5)

Blind nasotracheal intubation is often used in adults. Because a stiff tube is needed, the chance of perforation in infants is greater if a stylet is used. Although an intubation under direct visualization is preferred, the presence of severe micrognathia or oral masses makes this approach valuable. It is critical not to push against any resistance.

1. Keep infant supine with neck flexed and shoulders supported by a small roll.
2. Shape a stylet so the tip of the endotracheal tube will curve anteriorly at 90 degrees. Be certain the tip of the stylet stays above the end of the ET tube. Alternately, freeze an ET tube in this configuration and remove stylet just prior to insertion.
3. Maintaining the curve in the tube anterior, insert the tube carefully through the nostril until its tip is in the oropharynx.
4. Pull the jaw forward into a sniff position with the head midline and put slight external pressure over the cricoid cartilage.
5. Advance the tube to a suitable depth unless there is any resistance.

6. Remove stylet and verify presence of exhaled humidity and equal breath sounds.

Intubation in Severe Cleft Defects

There are several possible modifications for ET tubes that are useful for fixation or elective intubation when there is a large cleft palate. For emergency intubations, the following modification using a standard tongue blade is usually immediately available (6). For techniques or difficult intubation alternatives, see above (7).

1. Open infant's mouth and lay sterile tongue blade flat across maxilla, with ends extending from corners mouth. Have assistant hold in place.
2. Follow steps for routine intubation, using tongue blade for support of laryngoscope as necessary.
3. After intubation, fix tube to padded tongue blade.
4. Recognize that tongue thrust on tube in absence of a normal palate may lead to extubation even without visible external lengthening of tube.

Emergency Retrograde Intubation (8)

When facial anomalies preclude other routes, retrograde intubation using a modified Seldinger technique is possible. Because the cartilaginous support of the trachea is so poor, needle puncture is far more difficult in neonates.

Equipment

1. Venous cannula with stylet, 14 or 16 gauge
2. Feeding catheter. Verify that the catheter will pass through the lumen of the angiocath.
   a. A 14-gauge cannula will admit a 5-French (Fr) feeding tube.
   b. A 16-gauge cannula will admit a 3.5-Fr feeding tube.
3. Hemostat
4. Endotracheal tube

Technique

1. Sedate infant if possible.
2. Clean skin over cricothyroid area.
3. At the level of the cricothyroid, puncture skin with cannula and stylet. Angle cannula at 45 degrees from the skin and directed toward the head.
4. Insert into lumen or trachea only until there is a give in resistance or air returns.
5. Remove the stylet.
6. Thread feeding tube through the lumen of the cannula until it can be retrieved from the nose or oropharynx.

7. Bring cephalic end of feeding tube out of the nose or mouth, leaving other end well outside skin insertion.
8. While feeding tube is in place, remove the cannula from the tracheal insertion site.
9. Clamp the feeding tube at its tracheal insertion so it will not be pulled into the trachea farther than desired.
10. At the upper end, slip the ET tube over the feeding tube and along its course until it has passed the proper distance into the trachea. Stabilize the ET tube.
11. Cut the feeding tube at its tracheal insertion.
12. While keeping the ET tube in place, pull the feeding tube through the ET tube.
13. Secure ET tube after verifying correct intratracheal position.

References

1. Georgeson K, Vain N. Intubation of the left main bronchus in the newborn infant: a new technique. *J Pediatr.* 1980;96:920.
2. Mathew O, Thach B. Selective bronchial obstruction for treatment of bullous interstitial emphysema. *J Pediatr.* 1980;96:475.
3. Weintraub Z, Oliven A, Weissman D, et al. A new method for selective left main bronchus intubation in premature infants. *J Pediatr Surg.* 1990;25:604.
4. Sivasubramanian K. Technique of selective intubation of the left bronchus in newborn infants. *J Pediatr.* 1979;94:479.
5. Williamson R. Blind nasal intubation of an apneic neonate. *Anesthesiology.* 1988;69(4):633.
6. Zawistowska J, Menzel M, Wytyczak M. Difficulties and modifications of intubation technique in infants with labial, alveolar and palatal clefts. *Anaesth Resusc Intens Ther.* 1973;1:211.
7. Stool SE. Intubation techniques of the difficult airway. *Pediatr Infect Dis J.* 1988;7:154.
8. Cooper CM, Murray-Wilson A. Retrograde intubation. Management of a 4.8 kg, 5 month infant. *Anaesthesia.* 1987;42:1197.

Appendix E

Chapter 53

TABLE E.1	Drugs Requiring Adjustment in Severe Renal Failure

Drug	Method	Adjustment	Elimination by PD
Acetaminophen	i	q8 h	No
Acyclovir	i	q48 h	No
Allopurinol	i	q12–24 h	
	d	50%	
Amikacin	i	q24 h	Yes
	d	20%–30%	
Amlodipine		Unchanged	
Amoxicillin	i	q12–16 h	No
Amphotericin B	i	q24–36 h	No
Amphotericin B cholesteryl sulfate	Unchanged		
Amoxicillin-clavulanic acid	i	q12–24 h	No
Ampicillin	i	q12–24 h	No
Bumetanide		Unchanged	
Caffeine		Unchanged	Yes
Calcitonin		Unchanged	
Captopril	d	50%	
Carbamazepine	d	75%	
Carbenicillin	i	q24–48 h	No
Cefaclor	d	33%	Yes
Cefamandole	i	q8–12 h	No
Cefazolin	i	q24–48 h	No
Cefotaxime	i	q12–24 h	No
Cefoxitin	i	q24–48 h	No
Ceftazidime	i	q24–48 h	No
Ceftriaxone		Unchanged	No
Cefuroxime	i	q48–72 h	Yes
Cephalexin	i	q12–24 h	No
Cephalothin	i	q8–12 h	Yes
Chloral hydrate		Avoid	
Chloramphenicol		Unchanged	No
Cimetidine	d	50%	No
Clavulanic acid	d	50%–75%	No
Clindamycin		Unchanged	No
Dexamethasone		Unchanged	
Diazepam		Unchanged	
Diazoxide		Unchanged	Yes
Dicloxacillin		Unchanged	No
Digitoxin	d	50%–75%	No
Digoxin	i	q48 h	No
	d	10%–25%	No
Diphenhydramine	i	q9–12 h	
Enoxaparin		Not approved	
Erythromycin		Unchanged	No
Ethambutol	i	q48 h	Yes
Fentanyl		30%–50%	
Flucytosine	i	q24–48 h	Yes
	d	20%–30%	
Fluconazole	d	25%	Yes
Furosemide		Unchanged	

TABLE E.1   Drugs Requiring Adjustment in Severe Renal Failure (*Continued*)

Drug	Method	Adjustment	Elimination by PD
Gentamicin	i	q24–48 h	Yes
	d	20%–30%	
Heparin		Unchanged	
Hydrocortisone		Unchanged	
Hydralazine	i	q8–16 h	No
Indomethacin		Unchanged	
Insulin (reg)	d	25%–50%	
Isoniazid		Unchanged	Yes
Kanamycin	i	q24 h	Yes
	d	23%–30%	
Ketoconazole		Unchanged	No
Labetalol		Unchanged	
Lidocaine		Unchanged	
Lorazepam	d	50%	
Meperidine	d	50%	No
Metoprolol		Unchanged	
Metronidazole	i	q12–24 h	No
Morphine		To avoid	
Nafcillin		Unchanged	
Naloxone		Unchanged	No
Nicardipine	d, i	Titrate	?
Oxacillin		Unchanged	
Penicillin G	i	q12–16 h	No
	d	25%–50%	
Pentobarbital		Unchanged	
Phenobarbital	i	q12–16 h	Yes
Phenytoin		Unchanged	
Piperacillin	i	q24 h	No
Prednisone		Unchanged	
Propranolol		Unchanged	
Ranitidine	d	50%	No
Rifampin		Unchanged	No
Secobarbital		Unchanged	No
Sodium nitroprusside		Unchanged	
Theophylline		Unchanged	Yes
Thiazide		Avoid	
Ticarcillin	i	q24–48 h	Yes
Tobramycin	i	q24 h	Yes
	d	20%–30%	
Valproic acid		Unchanged	No
Vancomycin	i	q24 h	No
Verapamil	d	50%–75%	

Renal failure alters the clearance of most drugs to a degree that is inversely proportional to the glomerular filtration rate. Drugs that are entirely cleared by the liver are administered without renal adjustment. Dose is adjusted by either administering a percentage of normal dose (d) or increasing the interval (i) between the doses by hours (18–20). The normal loading dose can be administered for virtually all drugs. Unlike hemodialysis, peritoneal dialysis usually has no significant effect on the clearance of most drugs. However, a supplemental dose is sometimes required. Blood levels of drug, if available, are the best guide. PD, peritoneal dialysis; q, every.

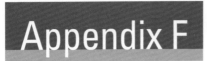

Appendix F

Bedside Checklist for Each Infant while on b-CPAP

To Be Completed by Infant's Nurse Each Shift

Date: _____

Check Points	Time	Time	Time
Blended air/oxygen supply is appropriate			
Flow meter at 5 –7 L/min			
Humidifier water lever is correct			
Excess rainout in the afferent tubing is drained			
Nasal prong size is correct			
Nasal prongs positioned correctly and not touching the septum			
Head cap fits snugly			
Corrugated tubing correctly placed			
Velcro moustache is correctly placed			
Septum is intact			
Neck roll is of correct size and position			
Head position is correct			
Preductal oxygen saturation probe			
Excess rainout in the efferent tube is drained			
Tape at 7 cm at base of bottle			
Sterile water (or acetic acid) level is at 0 cm			
Tubing securely fixed at 5 cm under water			
Gas bubbling in the bottle continuously			
Date circuit is due for a change (7 days max)			
Date CPAP prongs is due for a change (3 days max)			

Nurse Signature

Note: Page numbers followed by "f" refer to figures; page numbers followed by "t" refer to tables.